THE OXFORD HANDBOOK OF

THE HISTORY
OF EUGENICS

THE OXFORD HANDBOOK OF

THE HISTORY
OF EUGENICS

Edited by

ALISON BASHFORD

PHILIPPA LEVINE

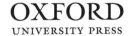

OXFORD

UNIVERSITY PRESS

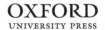

OXFORD
UNIVERSITY PRESS

Oxford University Press is a department of the University of Oxford.
It furthers the University's objective of excellence in research, scholarship,
and education by publishing worldwide.

Oxford   New York
Auckland   Cape Town   Dar es Salaam   Hong Kong   Karachi
Kuala Lumpur   Madrid   Melbourne   Mexico City   Nairobi
New Delhi   Shanghai   Taipei   Toronto

With offices in
Argentina   Austria   Brazil   Chile   Czech Republic   France   Greece
Guatemala   Hungary   Italy   Japan   Poland   Portugal   Singapore
South Korea   Switzerland   Thailand   Turkey   Ukraine   Vietnam

Oxford is a registered trade mark of Oxford University Press
in the UK and certain other countries.

Published in the United States of America by
Oxford University Press
198 Madison Avenue, New York, NY 10016

Library of Congress Cataloging-in-Publication Data
The Oxford handbook of the history of eugenics / edited by
Alison Bashford and Philippa Levine.
p. cm.
Includes index.
ISBN 978-0-19-537314-1 (hardcover); 978-0-19-994505-4 (paperback)
1. Eugenics—History.   I. Bashford, Alison, 1963–   II. Levine, Philippa.
HQ751.O94 2010
363.9'2—dc22   2009051142

Acknowledgments

....

This book has been a pleasurable collaboration across continents and across many years of development. It was initiated during a very early morning coffee in Sydney, Philippa having just flown in from Los Angeles. Crossing academic paths over the next few years, we developed the project in Los Angeles, tightened it in London and Cambridge, and brought it to its production home in New York. We are grateful to our many contributors for their immediate interest and their expertise sought and granted along the way.

There have been three workshops held in the preparation of this volume, and we gratefully acknowledge the University of Southern California and the University of Sydney for funding and facilitating these enjoyable and productive events. With various contributors, we met in Los Angeles in March 2006, in Sydney a year later, and in London in June 2007. It was at one of the fine dinners in Los Angeles that Saul Dubow mentioned how extensive, but also how dispersed, eugenics scholarship was. The project began to reshape at that point into this set of survey chapters that synthesize current knowledge and serve as introductions to further inquiry. The new *Oxford History Handbooks* series emerged as a natural home. Nancy Toff at Oxford has been an exemplary, an efficient, and a wise editor.

We are grateful for the skilled work of our Sydney-based assistants in the preparation of this volume; Annie Briggs and Jeannine Baker have been fine colleagues in this capacity. Thanks also to Matthew Oram, Émilie Paquin, Catie Gilchrist in Sydney, and to the Harvard students in the Fall of 2009, so interested in the comparative history of eugenics. In Los Angeles, we thank Peter Mancall and the USC-Huntington Early Modern Studies Institute staff, as well as Bill Deverell and the Huntington-USC Institute on California and the West for financial, intellectual, and administrative support.

AB
Sydney
PL
Austin, TX

Contents

....

Contributors

SUNIL S. AMRITH is Lecturer in History at Birkbeck College, University of London. He researches the connections between South and Southeast Asia since the late eighteenth century, focusing currently on the history of migration and cultural circulation between south India, Malaya, and Singapore. He has previously written on the international exchange of ideas about health in Asia and is author of *Decolonizing International Health* (2006). He serves as one of the editors of *History Workshop Journal*.

ALISON BASHFORD is Professor of Modern History at the University of Sydney. She has published widely on the modern history of science and medicine, including *Purity and Pollution* (1998) and *Imperial Hygiene* (2004), and has coedited *Contagion* (2001), *Isolation* (2003), and *Medicine at the Border* (2006). She is currently completing a history of geopolitics and the world population problem in the twentieth century. In 2009–2010 she was Visiting Chair of Australian Studies, Harvard University, with the Department of the History of Science.

LUCY BLAND teaches women's studies and history at London Metropolitan University. She has published *Banishing the Beast* (1995) and (with Laura Doan) *Sexology in Culture* and *Sexology Uncensored* (1998). She has written widely on sexuality, feminism, and gender in late-nineteenth- and early-twentieth-century Britain and is on the editorial collective of *Feminist Review*. Her forthcoming book is *Sexual Transgression in the Age of the Flapper: Treacherous Women on Trial*.

MARIA BUCUR's research and teaching interests focus on European history in the modern period, especially social and cultural developments in eastern Europe, with a special interest in Romania (geographically) and gender (thematically). Her publications include *Eugenics and Modernization in Interwar Romania* (2002), *Making Europe* (2007), *Gender and War in Twentieth-Century Eastern Europe* (2006), *Staging the Past* (2001), and *Heroes and Victims: Remembering War in Twentieth-Century Romania* (2009). She is coordinator of the women's and gender history network for the European Social Science History Conference and Director of the Russian and East European Institute at Indiana University.

CHLOE CAMPBELL is author of *Race and Empire: Eugenics in Colonial Kenya* (2007). She is an Honorary Research Fellow at the Psychoanalytic Unit at University College London.

YUEHTSEN JULIETTE CHUNG is Associate Professor of History at the National Tsing Hua University (Taiwan). She has published *Struggle for National Survival: Eugenics in Sino-Japanese Contexts, 1896–1945* (2002). Her forthcoming book is entitled *Science, Biopolitics and Social Nexus: Eugenics in China and its Transnational Context, 1895–2000*.

SAUL DUBOW is Professor of History at the University of Sussex. He has interests in the intellectual, institutional, and political development of segregation and apartheid in modern South Africa, as well as in the history of colonial science, race, and the ideology of empire. He is author of *Racial Segregation and the Origins of Apartheid in South Africa* (1989), *Scientific Racism in Modern South Africa* (1995), and, most recently, *A Commonwealth of Knowledge: Science, Sensibility and White South Africa 1820–2000* (2006).

RAPHAEL FALK studied biology at the Hebrew University and genetics at Stockholms Högskola. He has served on the academic staff at the Hebrew University since 1960. He has been visiting professor at Columbia University (1970–1971) and the University of Oregon (1980–1981); Fellow at the *Wissenschaftskolleg* in Berlin (1983–1984); and Visiting Scientist at the University of Massachusetts (1990–1991) and Harvard University (1994–1995). In addition to historical research, Falk has researched the effects of X-ray induced mutations in *Drosophila melanogaster* and chromosome organization and development in Drosophila. He is author of *Zionism and the Biology of the Jews* (2006) (in Hebrew) and *Genetic Analysis: A History of Genetic Thinking* (2009).

RICHARD S. FOGARTY earned his PhD in history from the University of California, Santa Barbara, in 2002 and specializes in the French colonial empire, the history of race and racism, and World War I. He is currently Associate Professor of History at the University at Albany, State University of New York, and author of *Race and War in France: Colonial Subjects in the French Army, 1914–1918* (2008), winner of the Phi Alpha Theta Best First Book Award.

STEPHEN GARTON is Professor of History and Provost and Deputy Vice Chancellor at the University of Sydney. He is a Fellow of the Australian Academy of the Humanities, the Academy of Social Sciences in Australia, the Royal Australian Historical Society, and the author of four books and over 70 articles and chapters on such areas as the history of psychiatry, social policy, policing, masculinity, and sexuality. Recently he has published on the history of parole in the American South and the emergence of criminal psychiatry in the operation of penitentiaries in New York State.

LESLEY A. HALL is Senior Archivist at the Wellcome Library and Honorary Lecturer in History of Medicine at University College London. She has published extensively on questions of sex, gender, and reproduction in the United Kingdom during the nineteenth and twentieth centuries, including *Sex, Gender and Social Change in*

Britain since 1880 (2000) and *Outspoken Women: Women Writing about Sex, 1870–1969* (2005).

GILBERTO HOCHMAN is Senior Researcher and Professor of History of Science and Health at Oswaldo Cruz Foundation (Rio de Janeiro, Brazil). He has published *A Era do Saneamento—As bases da política de saúde pública no Brasil* (1998) and is coeditor of *Cuidar, Curar* (2004), and *Políticas Públicas no Brasil* (2007). He coedited special issues of *Ciência & Saúde Coletiva* (History of Health Workers, 2008), *Canadian Bulletin of Medical History* (Latin American and International Health, 2007), and *História, Ciências, Saúde-Manguinhos* (History of International Health: Latin American Perspectives, 2006).

SARAH HODGES is Associate Professor of History at the University of Warwick. She has published *Contraception, Colonialism and Commerce: Birth Control in South India, 1920–1940* (2008) and is editor of *Reproductive Health in India: History, Politics, Controversies* (2006).

SUSANNE KLAUSEN is Associate Professor in the Department of History at Carleton University, Ottawa. She writes about reproductive control in twentieth-century South Africa and is author of *Race, Maternity, and the Politics of Birth Control in South Africa, 1910–39* (2004). She is at work on a study of criminalized abortion under apartheid. Klausen has published in numerous journals, including the *Canadian Bulletin of Medical History, Journal of Southern African Studies*, and *South African Historical Journal*.

WENDY KLINE is Associate Professor of History at the University of Cincinnati, where she teaches courses on U.S. women's history, the history of sexuality, women's health, and social movements. She is author of *Building a Better Race: Gender, Sexuality, and Eugenics from the Turn of the Century to the Baby Boom* (2001). Her second monograph is *Bodies of Knowledge: Sexuality, Reproduction, and Women's Health in the Second Wave* (2010). Her article, "'Please Include This in Your Book:' Readers Respond to *Our Bodies, Ourselves*," *Bulletin of the History of Medicine* (Spring 2005), was reprinted in *Major Problems in American Women's History* in 2007. Kline's current research focuses on the recent history of childbirth in the U.S.

NIKOLAI KREMENTSOV is Associate Professor in the Institute for the History and Philosophy of Science and Technology, Toronto University. He is author of *Stalinist Science* (1997), *The Cure: A Story of Cancer and Politics from the Annals of the Cold War* (2002), and *International Science between the World Wars: The Case of Genetics* (2005). His current research interests include the history of biomedical sciences in 1920s Russia and the history of Cold War science.

PHILIPPA LEVINE is the Mary Helen Thompson Centennial Professor in the Humanities and codirector of the Program in British Studies at the University of

Texas at Austin and author of a number of books, including *Prostitution, Race and Politics: Policing Venereal Disease in the British Empire* (2003) and *The British Empire, Sunrise to Sunset* (2007). She is at work on a study of evolution, eugenics, and empire.

NÍSIA TRINDADE LIMA is Senior Researcher and Professor of History of Science and Health at the Oswaldo Cruz Foundation (Rio de Janeiro, Brazil), where she is Scientific Editor of Fundação Oswaldo Cruz Press. She has published *Um sertão chamado Brasil* (1999), is coeditor of *Saúde e Democracia: História e perspectivas do SUS* (2005), *Louis Pasteur & Oswaldo Cruz: Inovação e tradição em saúde* (2005), and *Antropologia Brasiliana: Ciência e educação na obra de Edgard Roquette-Pinto* (2008). She coedited special issues of *História, Ciências, Saúde-Manguinhos* (Pathways, Communications, and the Sciences, 2008), and *Ciência & Saúde Coletiva* (History of Health Workers, 2008).

MARCOS CHOR MAIO is Senior Researcher and Professor of History of Science and Health at Oswaldo Cruz Foundation (Rio de Janeiro, Brazil). He is author of *Nem Rothschild, Nem Trotsky: Pensamento anti-semita de Gustavo Barroso* (1992); coeditor of *Raça, Ciência e Sociedade* (1996); *Ideais de Modernidade e Sociologia no Brasil* (1999); *Divisões Perigosas: Políticas raciais no Brasil Contemporâneo* (2007); and editor of *Ciência, Política e Relações Internacionais: Ensaios sobre Paulo Carneiro* (2004). He coedited special issue of *História, Ciências, Saúde-Manguinhos* (Visions of the Amazon, 2000).

JAMES MOORE is Professor of the History of Science at the Open University (Milton Keynes, UK). His books include *The Post-Darwinian Controversies* (1979), *Religion in Victorian Britain* (1988), *History, Humanity and Evolution* (1989), *The Darwin Legend* (1994), and, with Adrian Desmond, the best-selling biography *Darwin* (1991), which has been widely translated, and *Darwin's Sacred Cause: Race, Slavery and the Quest for Human Origins* (2009).

A. DIRK MOSES is Professor of Global and Colonial History at the European University Institute, Florence, and Associate Professor in History at the University of Sydney. He is author of *German Intellectuals and the Nazi Past* (2007) and editor of *Colonialism and Genocide* (2007, with Dan Stone), *Empire, Colony, Genocide: Conquest, Occupation and Subaltern Resistance in World History* (2008) and *The Oxford Handbook of Genocide Studies* (2010, with Donald Bloxham). He is an editor of the *Journal of Genocide Research*.

VÉRONIQUE MOTTIER is Fellow and Director of Studies in Social and Political Sciences at Jesus College, Cambridge, as well as Professor of Sociology at the University of Lausanne. Her research interests are in the areas of discourse analysis, feminist political theory, eugenics and the state, and the politics of sexuality and gender. Her books include *Sexuality: A Very Short Introduction* (2008), the coedited

Pflege, Stigmatisierung und Eugenik (2007), *Genre et politique* (2000), and *Politics of Sexuality: Identity, Gender, Citizenship* (1999).

MICHAEL A. OSBORNE has published widely on the history of medicine, science, and European imperialism. Formerly Professor of History and Environmental Studies at the University of California, Santa Barbara, where he had the good fortune to begin a series of collaborations with Richard Fogarty, he is currently Professor of History of Science at Oregon State University. His book *Nature, The Exotic, and the Science of French Colonialism* examined how the acquisition of empire transformed sectors of French zoology and botany. His current project analyzes the emergence of tropical medicine in France.

DIANE B. PAUL is Professor Emerita at the University of Massachusetts-Boston, and Research Associate at the Museum of Comparative Zoology, Harvard University. Her publications include *Controlling Human Heredity: 1865 to the Present* (1995) and *The Politics of Heredity: Essays on Eugenics, Biomedicine, and the Nature-Nurture Debate* (1998). Current research interests include historical and policy issues related to newborn screening, the "nature-nurture" debate before Galton, and nineteenth- and twentieth-century attitudes toward first-cousin marriage. She has recently been Visiting Professor at the UCLA Center for Society and Genetics and the Department of Medical History and Bioethics at the University of Wisconsin-Madison.

HANS POLS is Senior Lecturer at the Unit for History and Philosophy of Science at the University of Sydney. He is interested in the history of psychiatry, the medical and social reactions to mental breakdown during war, and the history of medicine in the Dutch East Indies and Indonesia.

MARIA SOPHIA QUINE is author of *Population Politics in the Twentieth Century: Fascist Dictatorships and Liberal Democracies* (1996) and *Italy's Social Revolution: Charity and Welfare from Liberalism to Fascism* (2002). She is formerly Senior Lecturer in Modern European History at Queen Mary, University of London, and is currently Research Fellow in the School of History, University of East Anglia. Her next book is a study of Darwinism and Social Darwinism in Italy, in a transnational perspective.

JENNIFER ROBERTSON is Professor of Anthropology, University of Michigan. Among her books are *Native and Newcomer: Making and Remaking a Japanese City* (1991), *Takarazuka: Sexual Politics and Popular Culture in Modern Japan* (1998), editor, *Same-Sex Cultures and Sexualities: An Anthropological Reader* (2004), and editor, *A Companion to the Anthropology of Japan* (2005). The editor of *Colonialisms,* a book series from the University of California Press, she is presently completing a book on cultures of Japanese colonialism, eugenics, and humanoid robots.

NILS ROLL-HANSEN is Professor Emeritus of History and Philosophy of Science at the University of Oslo. He has published on Pasteur and spontaneous generation, the origins of classical Mendelian genetics, plant breeding, environmental science, and eugenics. *The Lysenko Effect: The Politics of Science* (2005) investigates how certain science policy doctrines undermined the rationality and autonomy of science. *Eugenics and the Welfare State* (1995, 2005), coedited with Gunnar Broberg, investigates eugenics and sterilization policy in Scandinavia. Major present interests include the formation of classical genetics around 1900, and the importance of distinguishing basic and applied research in the politics of science.

CYRUS SCHAYEGH was at the American University of Beirut, 2005–2008, and is now Assistant Professor at Princeton University, where he teaches modern Middle Eastern history. His recent book, *Who Is Knowledgeable Is Strong: Science, Class, and the Formation of Modern Iranian Society, 1900–1950* (2009), explores modern Iranian uses of a variety of bio-medical sciences. His current project reexamines the post-Ottoman, interwar Levant as a region formed by the interplay between new states and cross-border movements of goods and people.

PATIENCE A. SCHELL's work addresses questions of gender, sociability, and the history of science, particularly in Mexico and Chile. She is the author of *Church and State Education in Revolutionary Mexico City* (2003) and coeditor of *The Women's Revolution: Mexico, 1910–1953* (2007). She received her PhD from Oxford University and teaches at the University of Manchester.

JENNIFER A. STEPHEN is Associate Professor of History at York University (Canada). She is author of *"Pick One Intelligent Girl": Employability, Domesticity and the Gendering of Canada's Welfare State, 1939–1947* (2007).

ALEXANDRA MINNA STERN is Zina Pitcher Collegiate Professor in the History of Medicine, Director of the Program in Contemporary History and Health Policy, and Associate Director of the Center for the History of Medicine at the University of Michigan. She is author of many books and articles, including the award-winning *Eugenic Nation: Faults and Frontiers of Better Breeding in Modern America* (2005). Her current research is on the history of genetics and society, and the history of pandemics, particularly the 1918 influenza pandemic.

DAN STONE is Professor of Modern History at Royal Holloway, University of London. His publications include *Breeding Superman: Nietzsche, Race and Eugenics in Edwardian and Interwar Britain* (2002), *Constructing the Holocaust* (2003), *Responses to Nazism in Britain, 1933–1939* (2003), *The Historiography of the Holocaust* (ed., 2004), *History, Memory and Mass Atrocity: Essays on the Holocaust and Genocide* (2006), *Hannah Arendt and the Uses of History: Imperialism, Nation, Empire and Genocide* (ed. with Richard H. King, 2007), *The Historiography of Genocide* (ed., 2008) and *Histories of the Holocaust* (2010). He is editor of the forthcoming *Oxford Handbook of Postwar European History*.

CAROLYN STRANGE has published widely on the history of gender, sexuality, and deviance in nineteenth- and twentieth-century Canada, Australia, and the United States. Her first book, *Toronto's Girl Problem: The Perils and Pleasures of the City, 1880–1930* (1995) examines the implication of law and medicine in the regulation of single wage-earning women. That theme was broadened in *Making Good: Law and Moral Regulation in Canada, 1867–1939* (1996, with Tina Loo), which highlights the management of Canada's marginal populations (in particular, Aboriginal people, non-Anglo-Saxon immigrants, and the poor) in the project of nation building. Her next book touches on nineteenth-century crimino-legal constructions of sanity.

MATHEW THOMSON is Reader in the Department of History at the University of Warwick and is currently Director of Warwick's Centre for the History of Medicine. He is author of *The Problem of Mental Deficiency: Eugenics, Democracy and Social Policy in Britain, 1870–1959* (1998) and *Psychological Subjects: Identity, Health and Culture in Twentieth-Century Britain* (2006). He is currently researching the history of childhood in postwar Britain.

MARIUS TURDA is Reader in Central and Eastern European Biomedicine at Oxford Brookes University and Director of the Cantemir Institute at the University of Oxford. He is author of *Modernism and Eugenics* (2010; French translation 2011), *Eugenism și antropologia rasială în România, 1874–1944* (2008) and editor of *Blood and Homeland: Eugenics and Racial Nationalism in Central and Southeast Europe, 1900–1940* (2007). He is the series editor of *CEU Studies in the History of Medicine*.

MATTIAS TYDÉN has a PhD in history from Stockholm University and is a researcher at the Institute for Futures Studies, Stockholm. He has written extensively on Swedish eugenics and the policies and implementation of sterilization. Other areas of research include the history of individual rights, immigration history, and Sweden during World War II. Among his published works are *Oönskade i folkhemmet: Rashygien och sterilisering i Sverige* [The Excluded: Eugenics and Sterilization in Sweden] (1991, with Gunnar Broberg), *Sverige och Förintelsen: Debatt och dokument om Europas judar 1933–1945* [Sweden and the Holocaust] (1997, with Ingvar Svenberg), and *Sverige och Nazityskland: Skuldfrågor och moraldebatt* [Sweden and Nazi-Germany: On the Question of Guilt] (2007; coedited with Lars M. Andersson).

PAUL WEINDLING is Wellcome Trust Research Professor in the History of Medicine at Oxford Brookes University. He has published *Health, Race and German Politics* (1989), *Epidemics and Genocide in Eastern Europe* (2000), *Nazi Medicine and the Nuremberg Trials* (2004), and *John W. Thompson, Psychiatrist in the Shadow of the Holocaust* (in press). He directs an AHRC-funded project on victims of Nazi human experiments. His research on medical, nursing, and scientific refugees from Nazism in the United Kingdom covers over 5,000 life histories to date.

ABBREVIATIONS

....

AID	artificial insemination by donor
AIWC	All-India Women's Conference
AWARE	Association of Women for Action and Research
BMA	British Medical Association
CGQJ	Commissariat général aux questions juives
CMHA	Canadian Mental Health Association
CNCMH	Canadian National Committee for Mental Hygiene
CS	Conseil Sanitaire
EAC	Economic Advisory Council
EAMJ	East African Medical Journal
EAS	East African Standard
ECT	electroconvulsive treatment
ESC	Eugenics Society of Canada
FPAI	Family Planning Association of India
FPAP	Family Planning Association of Pakistan
FPASL	Family Planning Association of Sri Lanka
IBE	*Izvestiia Biuro po Evgenike*
IEB	Institute of Experimental Biology
IEV	Indo-Europeesch Verbond
IFEO	International Federation of Eugenic Organizations
IMG	Institute of Medical Genetics
INC	Indian National Congress
INED	Institut national d'études démographiques
IUD	intrauterine devices
IUSPP	International Union for the Scientific Investigation of Population Problems
IVF	in vitro fertilization
JSAS	Journal of Southern African Studies
KNA	Kenya National Archives
KSSRI	Kenya Society for the Study of Race Improvement
LNAG	League of Nations Archive, Geneva
MBI	Medical-Biological Institute
MCP	Malayan Communist Party
NGO	nongovernmental organization
NMJC	National Medical Journal of China
NSB	Nationaal-Socialistische Beweging

NSW	New South Wales
OECD	Organisation for Economic Cooperation and Development
OMM	Okhmatmlad
OPR	Office of Population Research
PND	prenatal diagnosis
PZM	*Pod Znamenem Marksizma*
REJ	Russian Eugenics Journal
RES	Russian Eugenics Society
SAJS	South African Journal of Science
SPD	Social Democrat Party
SS	Schutzstaffel
TNA	The National Archives, London
UFA	United Farmers of Alberta
UMNO	United Malays National Organization
UN	United Nations
UNESCO	United Nations Educational, Scientific and Cultural Organization
USPHS	United States Public Health Service
VD	venereal disease
VOC	Vereenigde Oost-Indische Compagnie
WHO	World Health Organization
YMCA	Young Men's Christian Association

THE OXFORD HANDBOOK OF

THE HISTORY OF EUGENICS

INTRODUCTION: EUGENICS AND THE MODERN WORLD

PHILIPPA LEVINE AND
ALISON BASHFORD

"ONE day someone will write a history of the eugenic movement. The historian will have some puzzles to solve."[1] So wrote Alexander Carr-Saunders (1886–1966), author of *Eugenics* (1926) and director of the London School of Economics (1937–1955). Carr-Saunders offered this reflection in his 1935 Galton Lecture for the Eugenics Society in England. It was republished by the *Eugenics Review* in 1968, two years after his death, at a time when eugenics had waned as a serious scientific and policy field but was reemerging as a controversial object of critique. Carr-Saunders would have been surprised by the sudden and sustained historical interest in the field that arose after his lecture was republished.[2] This volume is a result of that large wave of work, a book that summarizes both the history and the historiography of eugenics across the world and that indicates new lines of inquiry that have evolved in recent years.

The aim of most eugenics movements was to affect reproductive practice through the application of theories of heredity. Eugenic practice sometimes aimed to prevent life (sterilization, contraception, segregation, abortion in some instances); it aimed to bring about fitter life (environmental reforms, *puériculture* focused on the training and rearing of children, public health); it aimed to generate more life (pronatalist interventions, treatment of infertility, "eutelegenesis"). And at its most extreme, it ended life (the so-called euthanasia of the disabled, the non-treatment of neonates). Eugenics always had an evaluative logic at its core. Some human life was of more value—to the state, the nation, the race, future generations—than other human life, and thus its advocates sought to implement these practices differentially.

The idea of eugenics grew quickly from the 1880s, reaching its peak in the 1920s. The actual practices and their uptake differed considerably, as the geographically oriented chapters in this volume vividly demonstrate. Yet eugenics rapidly became a shared language and ambition in cultures and locations that were otherwise radically different. Nikolas Rose sees four terms delineating eugenics: "population, quality, territory, and nation."[3] Each of these has a specific modern history, shaped by long-nineteenth-century global changes that accelerated in the dramatic and turbulent history of the early to mid-twentieth century. The emergence of widespread nationalism, important technological changes, and new ways of thinking about populations as a citizenry, as a labor force, and as the generator of future fitness combined to produce an environment sympathetic to claims that preceded Francis Galton, the originator of the term "eugenics," but which he solidified, named, and publicized. Both the broad spread and the timing of the interest in eugenics suggests that it should be interpreted as much with respect to period as to place. Eugenics was, in central ways, about modernity.

WHAT WAS EUGENICS?: HEREDITY, REPRODUCTION, AND FITNESS

From the late eighteenth century, scientists in many countries were intrigued by and actively explored mechanisms and patterns of human, plant, and animal heredity. The term *hérédité* was first used by French physicians in the 1830s, and in both Britain and the U.S. hereditary disease was a subject of study decades before the emergence of Darwinian theory.[4] But while evolutionary thought was popular in the first half of the nineteenth century, it was Darwin's work from the 1850s that foregrounded population-level ideas; his theories of natural and sexual selection put humans *in* nature, and subject *to* natural laws, critically undermining the argument for special creation.

Several authors in this collection (Diane Paul and James Moore; Nils Roll-Hansen; Philippa Levine) demonstrate the ways in which new developments in the biological sciences created the basis for eugenic ideas. Paul and Moore show that Darwin's *Origin of Species* (1859) profoundly influenced his cousin Galton's *Hereditary Genius* (1869), which in turn partly shaped *Descent of Man* (1871). Galton saw eugenics as a means to manipulate natural selection in humankind. Humans could—and should—"replace Natural Selection by other processes that are more merciful and not less effective. This is precisely the aim of Eugenics." By 1908, he understood eugenics as a preferable alternative to natural selection among humans:

Its first object is to check the birth-rate of the Unfit, instead of allowing them to come into being, though doomed in large numbers to perish prematurely. The second object is the improvement of the race by furthering the productivity of the Fit by early marriages and healthful rearing of their children. Natural selection rests upon excessive production and wholesale destruction; Eugenics on bringing no more individuals into the world than can be properly cared for, and those only of the best stock.[5]

As this consideration of "excessive production" shows, Galton and Darwin were heavily reliant on Thomas Malthus's ideas about human population numbers. But if Darwin wrote of "man and nature" as they existed—as they were—then Galton wrote of "man and nature" as they might be, even as they *should* be, through active human intervention on a qualitative basis. The difference between Darwin's description and Galton's prescription was what, in essence, made eugenics political.

Galton understood eugenics to be the rational planning of, and intervention into, human breeding, the application of "selection" to humans based on statistical probability and on an understanding of the mechanisms of heredity. In practice, this materialized both as individuals managing their own reproduction and as state and expert interventions into people's reproductive lives and choices. When in 1904 he wrote that eugenics was a field devoted to "the study of agencies under social control that may improve or impair the racial qualities of future generations, either physically or mentally,"[6] he expressed the twin sides of the eugenic coin: efforts to improve the fertility of some (positive eugenics) while curbing the fertility of others (negative eugenics), depending on which population and which socio-biological problem was being addressed. Many of the essays in this volume show how both "improvement" and "impairment" projects were simultaneously present in most eugenic movements, another reflection of the duality that characterizes both eugenics and its politico-cultural counterpart, modernity.

Not surprisingly, marriage and reproductive activity were invariably central issues. But as John Waller has persuasively argued, the tendency to equate eugenics with Galton is an oversimplification.[7] There is without doubt a longer nineteenth-century history of concern with hereditary disease and of plans to manage marriage for the common good. Statisticians before Galton were motivated to compute the damage done by unfit marriages, suggesting that Galton's timing was ripe. Attempts by the experimental community founded in Oneida, New York, in 1848 to create ideal reproductive unions in a fully controlled way represents an early conflation of social and reproductive utopianism that predates Galtonian eugenics. Not a few regimes over the twentieth century sought similar reproductive control in far more complex and larger societies. Their leaders could only dream of the total submission to the larger good which the Oneida women professed: "We do not belong to *ourselves* in any respect…we have no rights or personal feelings in regard to childbearing…we will, if necessary, become martyrs to science."[8]

Most women, however, needed rather more persuasion, and eugenics frequently interacted with the welfare structures emerging in the modern nation state. Advocates sought the promotion of marriage and the reproduction of individuals and families deemed desirable and fit through state-based financial incentives and endowments. In early-twentieth-century America, the psychologist Leta S. Hollingsworth (1886–1939) explicitly named "adequate compensation" as an "effective social device" that would encourage good child-bearing.[9] Galton envisioned a society in which the state aided the well-born in expanding their families, and in National Socialist Germany, among other states, such state aid materialized rapidly.

In many contexts there was strong support for marriage counseling and the physical and mental screening of intending couples before marriage. In some jurisdictions, legislation prevented the marriage of individuals with certain traits; the 1926 Soviet Civic Code, for example, prohibited marriages between mentally ill parties (see the chapter by Krementsov). Though it failed in more jurisdictions than it succeeded, there were numerous attempts by eugenic associations to make marriage screening compulsory, aiming to restrict the reproduction of those with conditions and diseases considered heritable: syphilis, leprosy, tuberculosis, epilepsy, alcoholism, and less specific conditions such as "criminality" or sexual "tendencies." Galton himself, as Paul and Moore point out in this volume, warned that the day would come when those who reproduced irresponsibly would be considered "enemies to the State."

Eugenics and racism have become almost interchangeable terms, but the association is perhaps too simplistic. Historical work on eugenics shows that much, if not most, eugenic intervention was directed at "degenerates" who already "belonged," racially or ethnically: "internal threats" or "the enemy within," whose continued presence diluted the race. In the Third Reich, the prime target for sterilization and euthanasia was the disabled or "feebleminded" German, rather than the foreigner. For Australian lawmakers, it was the English insane who were to be excluded, through immigration restriction statutes and their eugenic clauses. In twentieth-century South Africa, as Saul Dubow shows, eugenics was often a battle over whiteness. In some American states, sterilization of whites was a critical procedure, a means of stabilizing respectable visions of whiteness in a changing demographic environment. To be sure, these were projects of racial nationalism and indeed racial purity—eugenics was never *not* about race—but the objects of intervention, the subjects understood to be "polluting," were often not racial outsiders, but marginalized insiders whose very existence threatened national and class ideals. This was as much the case in emergent states such as Cuba, as Patience Schell's chapter shows, as in nations with a longer history.

Although eugenics was sometimes applied with rural, peasant, and indigenous populations in mind,[10] more often it concerned the urban "problem populations" of industrialization. In Britain, in particular, eugenics addressed the class issues that had come to dominate domestic British thinking. The urban poor, already regarded as a tenacious problem population, became the focus of a wide range of research.[11] Solutions to the problem of poverty were, in essence, twentieth-century scientific extensions of nineteenth-century social and legislative reform on "pauperism," in which scientific "proofs" of weakness and inferiority bolstered existing moral condemnation. While the massed and urban poor were the main eugenic "problem population" in Britain, the presence of the empire ensured that racial concerns were never wholly muted. Indeed, Dan Stone has argued that race and class were inseparable in the writings of British eugenics advocates. His emphasis on "ethnic exclusivity" is an important corrective to the more common view of British eugenics as driven predominantly by class prejudices.[12]

Wendy Kline shows in this volume that it was poor rural whites, southern European immigrants, and African Americans only a generation or two from slavery who were considered "problem populations" in Progressive Era America. And when eugenicists turned to the postwar global problem of the "Third World," they imagined a globalized pauper class whose advance demanded intervention, action, and expertise. As Susanne Klausen and Alison Bashford's chapter suggests, it was this interest in managing and intervening in the reproductive lives of one particular social group—the poor—that most directly linked neo-Malthusians and eugenicists.

In places as different as the United States, colonized areas of Africa, and Germany, "undesirable" marriage was also understood in racial terms, and anti-miscegenation laws were increasingly driven by eugenic rationales.[13] As Dan Stone and Dirk Moses point out in this volume, anxieties about interracial marriage were frequently linked to colonial rule. Fears over racial mixing reached their nadir in apartheid South Africa, but as Saul Dubow's chapter shows, apartheid was the endpoint of several generations of work, much of it eugenic and scientific, on the perceived problems of race-mixing. Nonetheless, the presence of apartheid politics was not a necessary precondition for hostility to race-mixing. Hans Pols's chapter discusses the race-crossing research undertaken by Ernst Rodenwaldt in the Dutch East Indies, which he took back to Nazi Germany in 1934. And in Australia, scientific policy-makers closely considered the "half-caste problem," implementing a process of biological and cultural assimilation influenced by eugenic ideas. "Half-caste" children were removed from their indigenous families into institutions and then into white communities, with the ultimate aim of "breeding out the colour," as it was often put. Even in non-colonial national contexts with a high degree of social homogeneity, racial "insiders" could become "outsiders" in eugenic initiatives. Véronique Mottier discusses the extensive program of child removal in Switzerland, and Mattias Tydén, the eugenic work of Swedish researchers on the northern Sami minority.[14]

Concerns with population encompassed not only an interest in improving and revitalizing populations to inhabit a modern world, but also the obvious, if sinister, corollary that some populations would be unfit to do so. The prospect of extinction—made so much more viable by new evolutionary theories in the nineteenth century—was applied by eugenically inflected anthropologists to human societies considered too primitive for modern survival (see chapters by Philippa Levine, Mathew Thomson, A. Dirk Moses and Dan Stone). In some contexts, "primitive" societies where weak offspring were not nursed were admired as naturally eugenic, as Saul Dubow points out.

Quantitative and qualitative aspects of population management were almost always entwined, as Schneider showed in his important early study of French eugenics.[15] Susanne Klausen and Alison Bashford discuss here the complicated relationship between the unconditional advocacy of contraception by neo-Malthusians and the cautious ambivalence typical of eugenicists. Eugenic advocates were often concerned with the decline of the middle-class birth rate attributed to contraception, but were simultaneously interested in the provision of contraception to working-class and some non-white populations. In certain colonial and national contexts, eugenics and managed birth control campaigns were virtually indistinguishable, as Sarah Hodges shows for South Asia and Yuehtsen Juliette Chung for Hong Kong. In India, Hodges suggests, organized nationalist feminism articulated some of the strongest advocacy for eugenics in the region, premised on the tight relationship between eugenics and birth control. Sunil Amrith discusses postcolonial renditions of this connection, where the newly independent state of Singapore (like modern China) proceeded strongly with birth control as part of its population policy.

Since eugenics was always concerned with reproductive sex, it was also always about gender, an insight rendered place-specific in chapters by Lucy Bland and Lesley Hall on Britain, Carolyn Strange and Jennifer Stephen on Canada, and Stephen Garton on Australia and New Zealand. Whether arguing for the maintenance of traditional gender roles and thereby increasing the number of fitter families, or for radically new heterosexual formations, eugenics and "the woman question" were inevitably linked. Nor should we be surprised at the sometimes close association between eugenics and the radical politics of sexology in the early twentieth century.[16] In her chapter, Alexandra Stern extends the analysis of eugenics through gender by addressing the question of masculinity and the subjectivity of eugenic advocates.

Eugenics often dovetailed with broad public health and hygiene practices. In eastern Europe, for example, eugenics supporters lobbied for greater spending on public health (see Maria Bucur in this volume), while in early twentieth-century China social hygienists were active in the medical profession, in voluntary organizations such as the YMCA, and in the rapidly expanding nationalist movement (see Chung in this volume). The emphasis on public health was especially, albeit not exclusively, found in national and colonial sites where Lamarckian ideas were dominant, such as France and Latin America. That said, even in the strictest Mendelian versions of eugenics, efforts constantly crossed over into the public health arena and into the management of infectious diseases. The twentieth century saw the adoption in many places of compulsory notification of those with sexually transmissible diseases, leprosy, or tuberculosis, a practice that dovetailed logically with systems for preventing disease carriers from marrying.

Eugenics took the form of mass education that encouraged individual responsibility for sexual and reproductive conduct and for healthy conduct that would benefit a larger collective. Populist campaigns in many settings rewarded eugenic motherhood through "fitter family" competitions. At the same time, eugenics influenced contemporary debates about educability and thus the worth of education. The development of psychometric testing in the early twentieth century (see Thomson and Dubow in particular) was frequently linked to eugenic ideals and concerns. In colonial contexts, as Chloe Campbell's chapter on Kenya demonstrates, entire indigenous populations could be labeled as ineducable and naturally feeble-minded, making their education an expensive irrelevance to the state.

Among the best-known and more radical manifestations of eugenics was the segregation and sterilization of those deemed "defective" to ensure that they did not pass on their defects to the next generation. As Thomson shows, eugenics was closely linked to a much longer history of institutionalization, in particular the proliferation of asylums from the nineteenth century.[17] It was the institutionalized who were most subject to the proliferating practice of sterilization. Conversely, sterilization was commonly understood to be an advantageous and economically efficient alternative to segregation, minimizing the need for, and the longer-term costs of, the latter. Sterilization was fairly widespread by the 1930s, permitted by legislation in many U.S. and Canadian states and provinces, in the Swiss canton of Vaud, in Scandinavian countries, in Germany, Japan, and Veracruz (Mexico), as well as in Czechoslovakia, Yugoslavia, Hungary, Turkey, Latvia, and Cuba. In some places—Russia being a good example—eugenic advocates were nonetheless hostile to the principle of sterilization.

At its most radical, eugenics manifested as both passive withholding of treatment from, and active killing of, disabled people. The German Darwinist Ernst Haeckel had advocated eugenic euthanasia as early as 1868, and in liberal Britain the eugenicist Dr. Robert Rentoul was euthanasia's best-known proponent. Such a practice was undertaken privately by physicians on newborns, probably everywhere, but very publicly in the United States in the early twentieth century when Dr. Harry Haiselden (1870–1919) withheld treatment for deformed newborns in Chicago and actively promoted this eugenic practice as in the interest of the infant, the family, and society.[18] Active "euthanasia" of disabled people on a large scale was authorized by a 1939 Reich Ministry of the Interior decree in Germany, first targeting neonates and children, and subsequently expanding to adult asylum populations.[19]

Eugenics was centrally an evaluative project for the classification of humans. The designations "fit" and "unfit" applied both to populations and to individuals, and eugenic literature is packed with data on human hierarchies, some of it statistical, some of it visual, all of it confident in its ability to evaluate, classify, and fix the characteristics and qualities of humans. Anthropometric photography—much lauded by late nineteenth-century anthropologists and naturalists—measured the particulars of bodies, while the new intelligence testing of the early twentieth century (developed first in France and spreading quickly) determined mental capacity. Where Galton had quantified, in the first instance, the existence and inheritance of "genius," the new testing was often, as in the United States, more concerned with identifying "feeblemindedness," which was regarded as a heritable condition. The Eugenics Record Office, founded in the United States in 1910, compiled a vast database and repository of information on American individuals and families. Records and data were essential to the eugenics project (see Paul Weindling in this volume).

Eugenics experts always had one eye on past generations and one eye on future generations, for what had come before augured what could or would follow. Genealogy—family trees—captured and symbolized this Janus-faced characteristic of eugenics: any individual both received, and potentially passed on, flawed and/or beneficial attributes. One of the commonest images in eugenic publications was the family tree, the "pedigree chart," which tracked the history of talented families, defective families, racially hybrid families, or of leprous, tubercular, epileptic, criminal, and alcoholic families. The pedigree chart was, as Pauline Mazumdar has written, both the research and propaganda methodology of eugenics, especially in its early years.[20] Social and scientific work on genealogy and heredity, on dominant and recessive genes, was eugenics' core business, famously the studies of the Jukes and the Kallikaks, less famously families afflicted with Huntington's disease.[21] Not infrequently, such modern projects were grafted onto preexisting cultural, religious, or folk practice about marriage and family lines. Galton and Darwin were both deeply interested in and concerned about their culture's practice of consanguineous marriage (and Darwin, of course, was himself in such a marriage, having married his first cousin, Emma Wedgwood [1808–1896]), which seemed to bring benefits of familial purity, but problems as well. In his chapter on eugenics and the Jews, Raphael Falk writes about the enthusiasm of some early-twentieth-century rabbis for eugenics, who linked the new science to "breeding problems [that] have always occupied an important role in Jewish life." Many, he writes, claimed a central and long-standing role for eugenics in Jewish tradition.

Galton's work was from the first about genealogy. His earliest eugenic research traced families who possessed what he called "hereditary genius," and with biometrician Karl Pearson (1857–1936), he refined mathematical predictions of the characteristics of later generations, in order to effect change.[22] Pearson—whom historian Judith Walkowitz describes as a man for whom "biology had absolutely determining power"[23]—was the first Galton Chair of Eugenics (later Genetics) in University College London's Department of Applied Statistics; his institutional legacy was enshrined in the journal he founded, *Biometrika*. The actuarial aspect of this work was not lost on life insurance companies, who regularly drew on eugenics research. Conversely, the data held by life insurance companies—about probability of illness and death within families—was of considerable value to eugenic researchers.

If eugenics was about the problems of inheriting the past, it was also about the optimistic possibilities of planning future generations. There was a power in eugenic promise—perfectibility, improvement, the benefits that would accrue from rational planning. Despite the persistence of a degenerationist discourse, eugenics was thus marked by considerable optimism: it was an active creed, an *applied* science. The first pedigrees Galton composed were not of epileptic families, but of the Wedgwood-Darwin-Galton family to which he himself belonged; these studies traced the inheritance of ability. Meliorist terms such as "race betterment" and "race improvement" were titles commonly chosen by and for eugenic associations, especially those with a greater lay and community membership. Eugenics was premised on a belief that science was of necessity reformist in its intentions and aspirations. Thus Cyrus Schayegh notes in his chapter that Reza Shah's modernist plans for a new Iran focused attention on sociocultural reforms effected through bio-medicine. In Soviet Russia, eugenics focused far more on helping and improving the "fit" rather than worrying about the effects of leaving the "unfit" to their own devices. And as Nikolai Krementsov's chapter shows, this unusual emphasis also offered an outlet for an acceptance of some forms of mental illness (what Russian scientists dubbed "pathography"), which linked creativity and mental instability. From family planning to national planning, eugenics often appeared beneficial for future populations.

WHEN WAS EUGENICS?
MODERNITY AND THE NATION STATE

Eugenics as a distinct theory emerged in the 1880s, thrived in the years before and after World War I, came under considerable scientific criticism in the 1930s, and suffered more disabling political criticism after World War II. But as Bashford's epilogue indicates, eugenics continued in various forms as part of the scientific and social development of later-twentieth-century genetics and reproductive technologies.

Writers in the early twentieth century often drew a long genealogy for eugenic ideas and practice, writing about ancient traditions of the withdrawal of aid to weakly children and adults.[24] Eugenics thus gained authority by creating a classical lineage for itself. But modern eugenics was also understood by its advocates to be especially humanitarian compared to the ancients. Galton was insistent that the whole point of eugenics was to substitute "humane" methods for both inhumane practices such as infanticide and for the cruelties, as he saw it, inherent in natural selection. Scholars, too, have located eugenics firmly as an expression and a manifestation of modernity. Frank Dikötter suggests that "Eugenics was not so much a clear set of scientific principles as a 'modern' way of talking about social problems in biologizing terms."[25] What, then, was it in the modern period that was so productive of, and receptive to, eugenic practices and eugenic ideas?

Over the nineteenth century the idea of the state, as well as its practices, underwent massive change. Populations—people and their bodies—increasingly became the business of government, to be improved physically and morally. Statistics— originally the "science of the state"—was brought into the fold of biology in new ways, extending long-standing government interest in "vital statistics." Nineteenth-century governments had become centrally concerned with the size of their populations, and statistics provided them with myriad lifestyle and census-style data.

Though the measures recognizable under the eugenic banner were not always state-initiated, one of the more striking aspects of eugenics is that its presuppositions and premises frequently did feed state policy; the science behind, and the practical applications of, eugenics were taken seriously by states across the globe, especially in the first half of the twentieth century. In many places the state's responsibility for citizens and subjects was freshly assessed, with not a few nations assuming increasing responsibility for health, longevity, and welfare. As nationalism expanded its reach, expectations that states would change and grow catalyzed new notions of the relationship between the individual and the polity.

Eugenics is commonly associated with World War II because of the atrocities committed under Nazi rule. But eugenics historically has at least as much to do with the years around World War I, and the major new political configurations of people and territory it precipitated. Thus, if early historians of eugenics understood the field primarily through the lens of the history of science, a more recent generation takes eugenics to be primarily concerned with the nation and nationalism of the modern period.[26] New kinds of states were emerging everywhere in the modern world. Older empires collapsed and new nations—often ethnically imagined and constituted—were formed and reformed in their place. Maria Bucur's chapter on eastern Europe is a fine example of just how closely eugenics could match and enshrine the aspirations of new nation-states anxious to establish their legitimacy. In a different hemisphere, the Spanish-American War saw the decline of Spanish imperialism and the creation of new domains of U.S. imperial influence, closely attended by health, hygiene, and population questions. In the late nineteenth and early twentieth centuries, a series of states emerged in Central and South America in which population and reproduction were key governance issues, especially in newly proclaimed republics, as the chapters by Patience Schell and by Gilberto Hochman, Nísia Trindade Lima, and Marcos Chor Maio demonstrate. In the same period, Japanese modernization manifested itself as nationalism, again with an attendant concern for population quality and quantity. Jennifer Robertson's chapter shows the extensive Japanese interest in race, nation, and eugenics.[27] Across the British and French Empires, colonial rule continued after World War I, but these empires were increasingly faced with anti-colonial nationalist activity. The latter was as likely to embrace as to reject population and eugenic thinking.

The end of World War II saw another wave of nation-building; population planning—sometimes called "eugenic," sometimes not—was often part of core business. In this vein, eugenics could manifest itself as an aspect of colonial governance, or prove useful for anti-colonial nationalists as they dreamed of, and then implemented, independence. It was population planning, for example, that drove the five-year plans for a new, modernized India. It was "a scientific approach to all our problems and to life itself," as Nehru put it.[28] Sunil Amrith's chapter on eugenics in postcolonial Southeast Asia and Sarah Hodges's chapter on Indian eugenics both demonstrate how population planning could transfer easily from colonial to independent national regimes.

In the early to mid-twentieth century, scientifically authorized projects of race and racial purity were mapped onto this extensive new nation-building. Homogeneity (homo-gene—of the same kind) was characteristically privileged over heterogeneity and became a signature element for the imagining and, in many cases, the establishment of new "racial" nations. Australia is a good example of an early-twentieth-century "racial" nation, where eugenic language took considerable hold, as Garton's chapter demonstrates. In many arenas, blood type determined belonging to territory and nation, as Bucur explains for eastern Europe. Likewise, Robertson's chapter demonstrates how profoundly the idea of blood purity was "an organizing meta-phor" for deciding exactly who was Japanese. Some Zionists, as Raphael Falk's chapter shows, used blood as a claim for a Jewish homeland. Before chromosome-based technologies, blood typing was paramount in technical attempts to classify, include, and exclude groups of people.[29] This new science of blood typing had strong links to older notions of blood as a distinguishing characteristic, whether distinguishing on the basis of class, race, or other sorts of classification. In these ways, eugenics was central to the modern project of racial nationalism and national rejuvenation.

In the turbulent years of the early twentieth century, eugenics offered particular technologies that might be taken up by states, as nations were built and rebuilt, gen-erated and regenerated by scientists, statesmen, and political and economic planners. Véronique Mottier explores the very different *kinds* of states in which eugenics was able to flourish: liberal, totalitarian, social democratic, socialist. Despite the popular link drawn constantly between eugenics and the Nazi regime, there was probably as strong a connection between eugenics and the left, and to progressive and reform politics.[30] The optimism of eugenics, and its aspiration to apply scientific ideas actively, was among the reasons it so frequently attracted progressives and liberals.

Thus, in each of these kinds of modern states—even liberal states—eugenic discourse encouraged hygienic practices for the perceived larger good. As Amir Weiner has succinctly put it: "No longer were self-improvement and perfection the pursuit of the selected few, mainly religious orders…In the modern state, each and every individual counted."[31] Citizens and subjects were to streamline themselves, their families, and their bodies for their new modern state. What Ayça Alemdaroğlu argues of modernizing Turkey is more widely applicable: "Imagining…society as a national organic unity prioritized the duties of citizens over their rights."[32] As we have seen, it was typically the powerless and disenfranchised who were rendered problematic and who were likeliest to experience the effects of eugenic philosophy and practice—rural populations, women, non-white people, the urban underclass. At the same time, these populations were increasingly understood in terms of what Maria Bucur calls "biological capital."

On the one hand, then, eugenics invokes a modern political history in which individuals have been subsumed within collectives and their perceived interests. Eugenic advocates typically had population-level aims firmly in sight, and were concerned less with making individuals happier, healthier, or fitter for their own sake (although for many, this was a perfectly desirable side effect) than with making a significant difference to the physical constitution of future generations. Yet the materialization of the population-level change necessarily entailed intervention into individual lives, mostly though not exclusively managed or promoted by the modern or modernizing state, whether directly or indirectly.

On the other hand, eugenics remains an important part of the history of the modern subject, especially the modern liberal subject whose emerging individual rights—to reproduction, to health, to bodily integrity—were not infrequently asserted and argued in legal cases specifically about eugenic practice, sometimes successfully, sometimes not. The history of eugenic sterilization in particular is a key component of the development of a discourse of "rights" in which reproduction has, in many countries, come to be comprehended.[33] Similar issues arose around the legal concept of consent when Nazi experimentation (including sterilization) was assessed in the postwar Nuremberg trials, as Weindling discusses in this volume.[34]

Eugenics, then, arose out of a constellation of recognizably modern issues, but it soon became a signal for, and almost a symbol of, modernization. States keen to display a commitment to modern planning implemented hygiene and public health measures. Nation-states—China, Japan, and in eastern Europe—and the professionals and experts supporting them, whose reputations depended on their being seen as modernizing, took up eugenics enthusiastically. The modern state's increasing interest and involvement in health practices served as an incentive for doctors to encourage eugenic practices that would increase their status as well as the resources allocated to their work. As many of the chapters that follow reveal, doctors and other medical professionals were often central supporters and advocates of eugenic practices from disease notification to public health campaigns aimed at expanding public understanding of hereditary diseases.

Marius Turda and Paul Weindling have argued that the "modernity" model for understanding eugenics is most appropriate in the case of Britain. In central and southeastern Europe they see other forces at work: "eugenic movements . . . reflected the aspirations of a segment of trained professionals dependent upon the state for funding and legitimacy, and whose main goal was the strengthening of their newly created national states."[35] Maria Bucur and Maria Sophia Quine, too, stress this goal, one that we would argue quite precisely defines eugenics as a moment of modernity. Indeed, as Cyrus Schayegh shows, the aspirations of elite professionals for whom nationalism was an opportunity was manifest not just in European settings but elsewhere in the world—in this case, Iran—suggesting that a global push to modernity helped shape eugenic practice. The formation of nation-states—and in particular the focus on their population's potential at a biological level—*was* an essential element of modernity.

Modernity manifested in—and as—culture, as well as in and as politics and science. Historians of material and mass culture, of literature, and of film have increasingly understood eugenics as a key expression of modernity. Christina Codgell has analyzed the place of eugenics in 1930s design; Martin Pernick links eugenics and the motion picture; Daylanne English has explored the place of eugenics in the Harlem Renaissance; Angelique Richardson looks at eugenics in late-nineteenth-century women's writings.[36] Wendy Kline's chapter shows how, in popular cultural forms, eugenics reached well beyond the constituencies of medicine and politics to become a well-known and popularly supported movement in the United States.

Sociologists of modernity have also found eugenics of interest. As Mottier notes, Zygmunt Bauman writes of the modern state as a "gardening state," weeding and cultivating, selecting out and selecting in the unfit and the fit, the lives deemed not worth reproducing, and even the lives, by expert assessment, deemed not worth living.[37] Bauman argues that the Holocaust, with its emphatic, even obsessive order-making and taxonomizing, was the apogee of modernity. Michel Foucault likewise wrote about a "eugenic ordering of society" fed by "mythical concern with protecting the purity of the blood and ensuring the triumph of the race."[38] "Bio-politics"—the modern optimization of life—has influenced a generation of eugenics scholars and is especially present among recent historians of European eugenics.[39] Bio-politics speaks to the relation between social organization and social power on the one hand, and population and generation of life as the raw material of the social world, on the other. From intervention into the smallest units of life—genes and later molecular biology—to the largest unit of life—species and their interactions—eugenics was always and centrally about life.

For sociologists and political philosophers, then, as well as for historians of science, education, social policy, and culture, eugenics emerged out of, and came to stand for, modernity. It has done so in large part because of the strong popular and scholarly connection drawn even now between eugenics, German National Socialism, and the Holocaust. Our volume shows, however, that the link between modernity and eugenics was about period as much as place; it is less the Nazi version of eugenics than the familiarity of those practices across so many nations and cultures that is the truly astounding element in the history of eugenics.

Where Was Eugenics?
Local and Global Geographies

This book is structured by two aspects of the question of eugenics and place. On the one hand, we recognize the phenomenal transnational uptake of eugenic ideas more or less simultaneously across many parts of the world. Part I analyzes these transnational themes in eugenics. Part II surveys the important question of place-based differences in eugenic aims, methods, policies, and outcome. The geography of eugenics was national in the first instance. But regional and, in some instances, interregional, cultural-scientific alliances were increasingly significant.

Thoughtful historical commentators often understood eugenics as transnational, even global. The cosmopolitan Indian economist Benoy Kumar Sarkar commented in 1936 for example, on the "family likeness" among national "fitness" campaigns: Czech national fitness campaigns, Fascist Italy's "sanitary rejuvenation," and the youth movement of postwar Germany. "India," he wrote, "has thus been touched by the worldwide endeavours of today directed as they are towards race-betterment and conscious 'planning' of physical manhood."[40] His comments highlight the astounding similarity of eugenic ambitions and agendas internationally. In part this stemmed from the modern possibilities of connection: scientific ideas, people, and organizations quickly crossing oceans, exchanging scientific information in journals and papers in any number of new media.

Human movement across the globe on a hitherto unforeseen scale was as much an object of eugenic inquiry and intervention as it was a vehicle for the transmission of eugenic ideas and debate. Forced and free migrations and massive diasporic labor movements prompted ever-tighter restrictions on immigration. Eugenics found another outlet in immigration regulations that attended to heredity and to race in new and distinctly modern modes (see chapters by Cyrus Schayegh; Alison Bashford; Patience Schell; A. Dirk Moses and Dan Stone). Movement of this sort could also feed into eugenic thought in curious ways. Sarah Hodges shows in her chapter how communal unrest in India was sometimes expressed in terms of an originary and an invading race, the latter (in this instance, Indian Muslims) disparaged as essentially foreign and not "naturally" Indian.

The "place" of eugenics, then, was as much a newly international world, as it was the place of new nations. Bashford's chapter explores both the international eugenic associations and the place of eugenics in the League of Nations and, later, the United Nations. In an exemplary instance of the transnationalism of eugenics, Quine analyzes connections between southern Europe and southern and central America. This was formalized as an association of Latin eugenics that explicitly differentiated itself from an Anglophone North American and British eugenics, and to some extent from Scandinavian and German eugenics. A newly imagined "pan-American" region was important, writes Schell of Cuba, Mexico, and Puerto Rico. Not dissimilarly, but less formally, a Francophone eugenics linked experts in France, Quebec, and as Schayegh shows, Iran as well. In such instances, the personal connections between Iranian experts trained in France, or, to take another example, Japanese experts trained in Germany, were critical in the global flow of eugenic ideas.

Eugenic practices were produced by a vast amount of eugenic theory, deriving from any number of nineteenth-century sciences. It was probably the scientific theory that was the most global element of eugenics: a language shared, even if conclusions differed. There were some clear place-bound trends in scientific ideas, however. Historians have traced different national receptions of, and tendencies toward Lamarckian and Mendelian theories of heredity. Nils Roll-Hansen's chapter explains the divergent theories of heredity, and many other chapters analyze the varying implications of derivative social policy. In general, Lamarckian-inclined scientific cultures were more concerned with environmental and public health and hygiene interventions, as Schayegh shows in Iran, Richard Fogarty and Michael Osborne in France, Hochman et al. in Brazil. But chapters here also complicate these long-held views on eugenics as well. Chung's research on China and Hong Kong indicates that these divisions cannot solely be ascribed to national preferences. In China, for instance, differing eugenic camps promoted radically different policies. Social hygienists and nationalists sought—and found—reconciliations between these competing theoretical models. In the early years of the Soviet Union, as Krementsov shows, eugenicists liberally combined disparate elements of eugenic thought to create their own brand of the science. In the Soviet Union, the political role of eugenics was particularly marked in an era in which Lamarckian theories were championed as properly socialist and Russian geneticists increasingly feared for their lives. Indeed, Krementsov's analysis of Russian eugenics makes clear that eugenics could flourish even in environments where few of the major texts of the movement were ever published.

Broad differences between environmental and biological approaches in different contexts are suggested by the terms used for eugenics. Some national cultures used the word "eugenics," derived from *eu* (well or good) and *genus* (born). Other national policy and science groups preferred terms deriving from a root meaning "to cultivate" or "to care for," rather than "to be born": *puériculture* was often used in Francophone contexts, where the term came to mean infant or child health, or methods of rearing and training children.[41] The more generic "homiculture" was also widely used in place of eugenics in Latin America. With a sense of active tilling and tending, homiculture, *puériculture,* and viriculture—broadly consistent with Lamarckian approaches to heredity—held a more social meaning than the biologically oriented "eugenics." Indeed, Galton had early considered "viriculture" as a possible term for his new science.[42] Even earlier, the strange term "stirpiculture" was used to signal the breeding of special stocks, or family lines, with respect to humans. In the late 1840s the leader of the utopian Oneida community in New York, John Humphrey Noyes (1811–1886) used "stirpiculture" to describe his plans and activities for "intelligent, well-ordered procreation," claiming that "scientific combination will be applied to human generation as freely and successfully as it is to that of other animals." This was a plan he and his community put systematically into practice between 1865 and 1878.[43] In this instance, the term "stirp"—broadly meaning a line of descent from a single ancestor, or primary bearer of heredity, and used briefly by Galton—was as significant as the term "culture."

Hygiene was another important term linked to place in the history of eugenics. As Turda's chapter shows, *Rassenhygiene* was deployed first by the German biologist Alfred Ploetz (1860–1940) in 1895, and the term was picked up in Anglophone settings: the Racial Hygiene Association of New South Wales, for example, was an Australian eugenic-feminist organization, which retained its title until 1960. In English-speaking contexts, race was a slippery concept, sometimes meaning "white people," sometimes "English-speaking peoples of the world," but also sometimes "human species." In India, Hodges tells us, "race" and "nation" were terms used largely interchangeably. By the late 1930s, especially during and after World War II, "racial hygiene" came to signal German eugenics specifically, and English eugenicists typically distanced themselves from such associations.

Although eugenic aspirations and ambitions were remarkably common, shared, and agreed across the globe, the methods by which they were realized were often distinct points of difference and comparison. Because eugenics dealt with life and death, the stakes were high and organized religions were involved at both doctrinal and institutional levels, shaping one of the major geographical axes of difference in the history of eugenics. Many of the chapters discuss the significant gap between Protestant- and Catholic-dominated contexts. Catholic opposition was not always directed to eugenics per se, but rather to the specific practices that rendered sex non-reproductive and thus ran up against Catholic doctrine on the sanctity of life and the function of heterosexual marriage: sterilization especially but also contraception. As the chapters by Mottier,

Klausen and Bashford, Schell, and Strange and Stephen discuss, Catholic opposition was organized, strong, and successful in a variety of settings. But it must be remembered that the sterilization procedures so antithetical to Catholic doctrine were highly questionable, even in Protestant and secular states. Moreover, religious unease with eugenics was not limited to Catholics and the Catholic world. In South Africa, pious Afrikaner nationalists feared the implicit challenge to a literal interpretation of the Bible that eugenics, as an evolutionary doctrine, offered, as Dubow explains. In a wholly different vein, in the pre-Stalinist era of the Soviet Union, the geneticist Nikolai Kol'tsov (1872–1940) dreamed of a eugenic religion that would provide meaningful shape to people's lives (see the chapter by Krementsov).

National eugenic cultures were not infrequently defined and compared historically along a voluntary-compulsory continuum, most often with regard to sterilization. After 1933, when a compulsory sterilization law was passed in Germany, proponents of the legalization of voluntary sterilization put considerable effort into distinguishing their ideals from the German model, as Tydén argues of many Scandinavian states. British eugenicists also sought the legalization of sterilization, but voluntary sterilization was always their aim.[44] Australian, New Zealand, and South African jurisdictions were cautious about compulsory laws, influenced by a strong English liberal tradition against state interventions into homes and bodies. Those Canadian provinces that passed sterilization laws were strongly influenced by the United States, which, while always quick to rhetoricize its commitment to the liberty of the subject, initiated the early-twentieth-century wave of compulsory sterilization law, beginning with Indiana's 1907 Act.

Yet the difference between "voluntary" and "coerced" was oftentimes difficult to discern.[45] As Natalia Gerodetti has argued, "the absence or existence of a legislative basis for sterilization is in itself not much of an indicator for its practice…The absence of regulation, furthermore, potentially leaves practices in the hands of gate keepers or institutional policies."[46] Historians know that sterilizations took place in institutions irrespective of legal indications at least until the late twentieth century.[47] Yolanda Eraso, for example, has demonstrated the extent to which biological sterilizations took place in Catholic Argentina for eugenic reasons in the 1930s, despite its clear illegality according to the Penal Code, and despite Catholic opposition.[48] Nonetheless, the question of consent was central for eugenicists, as they developed and argued their cases, and for clinicians who sought to avoid regulation.

CRITICS OF EUGENICS

The successful implementation of actual eugenic practice was sometimes quite limited, or at least not as extensive as the promoters of eugenics hoped. In practice, eugenics was hobbled almost everywhere it emerged, sometimes by outspoken and organized religious opposition, sometimes by skeptical scientists, sometimes by individuals who refused to live the implications of modern dreams of national fitness and efficiency, and perhaps most often by politicians and jurists. Most of these protagonists questioned, either directly or indirectly, the implications of eugenics for relations between the individual and the state in the modern world. Though we tend to think that eugenics became an object of criticism only in the 1970s, it had attracted opponents and critics from the moment of its emergence. The history of eugenics is by no means a linear shift from unqualified support to unqualified resistance. Rather, it is one of simultaneous enthusiasm and disquiet.

Some of the strongest critics of eugenics were scientists, especially geneticists from the 1930s.[49] As Roll-Hansen's chapter demonstrates, the fast-paced development of genetics in the twentieth century threw doubt on the efficacy of eugenic plans to shape future generations by limiting reproduction. Increasing knowledge of dominant and recessive genes suggested that sterilization of ever larger numbers of people with a supposedly inheritable mental or physical condition would have a limited effect. The U.S. geneticist Herbert Jennings (1868–1947) pointed out in the early 1930s that for many problem populations, the defect was not dominant but recessive, and a large group of asymptomatic "carriers" would always continue to pass on the gene to the next generation, no matter what interventions were made to those with the dominant defect. Jennings did signal, however, the as-yet theoretical possibilities of diagnostics: "negative eugenic measures would be made more effective by the discovery of a method of detecting normal carriers of defective genes: but this cannot now be done."[50] Here Jennings anticipated the enormous change that took place after prenatal diagnosis and pre-implantation genetic diagnosis of embryos became possible, developments that Bashford discusses in the epilogue.

Geneticists, then, were particularly critical of the sterilization programs that by the 1920s and 1930s were favored in many countries. But eugenics was also frequently opposed by scientists on political as well as scientific grounds. Having put forward his critique of the efficacy of sterilization, Herbert Jennings pointed out the non-scientific character of much eugenics: "National and racial prejudices have entered largely into eugenic propaganda. One of the commonest objectives has been the maintenance of the purity or the dominance of a certain racial or national group— the group selected for preferences being that to which the selectors belong."[51] While Nazi Germany is always foremost in modern critiques of eugenics, earlier German expressions prompted considerable opposition as well. The British writer G. K. Chesterton (1874–1936) published his scathing *Eugenics and Other Evils* in 1922 in the light of "Prussianism." Chesterton's position on eugenics was, in his words, "a more general critique of a modern craze for scientific officialdom and strict social organization."[52] Critics of eugenics included key geneticists such as William Bateson (1861–1926), Lancelot Hogben (1895–1975), and Raymond Pearl (1879–1940), as well as social scientists like Franz Boas (1858–1942). Sun Benwen (1892–1979) in China, thought the application of animal breeding techniques to humans a dubious science, and he was openly critical of Chinese eugenics (see the chapter by Chung).

Criticism of eugenics sharpened in and over the postwar assessment and trials of Nazi officials. The so-called Doctors' Trials focused attention on the "euthanasia" program, the sterilization experiments, and genetic-oriented twin experiments.[53] As Bashford discusses in the epilogue, the connection between eugenics, sterilization, and Nazi genocidal policies and practices were drawn especially strongly from the 1970s, when disability, feminist, and anti-racist activists and scholars questioned ongoing discriminatory practice in health and reproductive domains, including sterilization. Details of the Tuskegee syphilis experiment begun in the United States in the 1930s, in which treatment was withheld from African American men in the Alabama county of Macon, were widely disseminated from 1972 and crystallized public conversation about race and medical ethics. This was a period of strongly left-oriented intellectual critique of science, the apogee of postwar anti-science, and anti-psychiatry in particular, leading to a generation of individuals who began to seek compensation for past state practices—for eugenic sterilization, for compulsory confinement, for experimental medical practice. This all coincided with and was driven by a wave of new scholarship on the history of eugenics, and by literature on eugenics in almost every genre, from memoir to novel to psychiatrist Peter R. Breggin's piece, "The Psychiatric Holocaust," in a 1979 issue of *Penthouse*.[54]

Conclusion

Mark Adams laid the groundwork for our study two decades ago, in his important comparative collection on Germany, France, Brazil, and Russia.[55] This new collection extends and deepens his important insistence on a comparative approach to the history of eugenics. The chapters that follow survey the global contours of this history, as both a transnational phenomenon of the modern period where particular themes are recognizable in otherwise vastly different locations, and as place-bound histories of colonies, nations, and regions.

The popularity and persistence of what detractors have often called a pseudo-science across such a remarkable variety of political, cultural, and scientific boundaries is itself a phenomenon that demands attention. What made eugenics so attractive, so powerful a pull for policy-makers in the early decades of the twentieth century, and in such different locations? Wherever we look, and whatever other differences marked its emergence, eugenics was always centrally about life—and death—in the new scientific frame of evolution, in new kinds of states, and in a newly globalized world.

NOTES

1. Alexander Carr-Saunders, "Eugenics in the Light of Population Trends," *Eugenics Review* 60 (1968): 46.

2. Important early research in this area includes Daniel Kevles, *In the Name of Eugenics: Genetics and the Uses of Human Heredity* (New York: Knopf, 1985); Mark B.

Adams, ed. *The Wellborn Science: Eugenics in Germany, France, Brazil, and Russia* (New York and Oxford: Oxford University Press, 1990); Nancy Leys Stepan, "*The Hour of Eugenics*": *Race, Gender, and Nation in Latin America* (Ithaca, NY: Cornell University Press, 1991).

3. Nikolas Rose, *The Politics of Life Itself: Biomedicine, Power, and Subjectivity in the Twenty-First Century* (Princeton, NJ: Princeton University Press, 2008), 58.

4. Charles E. Rosenberg, "The Bitter Fruit: Heredity, Disease, and Social Thought," in *No Other Gods: On Science and American Social Thought*, ed. Charles E. Rosenberg, (Baltimore, MD: Johns Hopkins University Press, 1997), 24–53; Carlos Lopez Beltran, "Heredity Old and New," in *A Cultural History of Heredity II* (Berlin: Max Planck Institute for the History of Science, 2003), 10; Roger J. Wood and Vítězslav Orel, *Genetic Prehistory in Selective Breeding: A Prelude to Mendel* (Oxford: Oxford University Press, 2001); Staffan Müller-Wille and Hans-Jörg Rheinberger, eds., *Heredity Produced: At the Crossroads of Biology, Politics, and Culture, 1500–1870* (Cambridge, MA: MIT Press, 2007).

5. Francis Galton, *Memories of My Life* (London: Methuen, 1908), 323.

6. Galton cited in Diane B. Paul, *Controlling Human Heredity: 1865 to the Present* (Atlantic Highlands: Humanities Press, 1995), 3–9.

7. John C. Waller, "Ideas of Heredity, Reproduction and Eugenics in Britain, 1800–1875," *Studies in History and Philosophy of Biological and Biomedical Sciences* 32, no. 3 (2001): 473–475.

8. Hilda Herrick Noyes and George Wallingford Noyes, "The Oneida Community Experiment in Stirpiculture," in *Eugenics, Genetics, and the Family*, eds. Charles Davenport et al. (Baltimore, MD: Williams & Wilkins, 1923), 374–386.

9. Leta S. Hollingsworth, "Social Devices for Impelling Women to Bear and Rear Children," *American Journal of Sociology* 22, no. 1 (1916): 29.

10. For one analysis of eugenics and peasant populations, see Gary Sigley, "Peasants into Chinamen: Population, Reproduction and Eugenics in Contemporary China," *Asian Studies Review* 22, no. 3 (1998): 309–38.

11. Pauline Mazumdar, "The Eugenists and the Residuum: The Problem of the Urban Poor," *Bulletin of the History of Medicine* 54 (1980): 204–215. See also Angelique Richardson, *Love and Eugenics in the Late Nineteenth Century: Rational Reproduction and the New Woman* (Oxford and New York: Oxford University Press, 2003).

12. Dan Stone, *Breeding Superman: Nietzsche, Race and Eugenics in Edwardian and Interwar Britain* (Liverpool: Liverpool University Press, 2002), 102, 95; See also, Lucy Bland, "British Eugenics and 'Race Crossing': A Study of an Interwar Investigation," *New Formations* 60 (2006–2007): 66–78.

13. A considerable feminist literature has examined colonial attitudes to miscegenation. See Persis Charles, "The Name of the Father: Women, Paternity, and British Rule in Nineteenth-Century Jamaica," *International Labor and Working-Class History* 41 (1992): 4–22; Amirah Inglis, *The White Woman's Protection Ordinance: Sexual Anxiety and Politics in Papua* (New York: St. Martin's Press, 1975); Philippa Levine, *Prostitution, Race and Politics: Policing Venereal Disease in the British Empire* (New York and London: Routledge, 2003); Ann Laura Stoler, " 'Mixed-bloods' and the Cultural Politics of European Identity in Colonial Southeast Asia," in *The Decolonization of Imagination. Culture, Knowledge and Power*, eds. Jan Nederveen Pieterse and Bhikhu Parekh (London and New Jersey: Zed Books, 1995), 128–148.

14. For eugenic child-removal in the U.S. context, see, for example, Angela Gonzales, Judy Kertész, and Gabrielle Tayag, "Eugenics as Indian Removal: Sociohistorical Processes and the De(con)struction of American Indians in the Southeast," *The Public Historian* 29, no. 3 (2007): 53–67.

15. William H. Schneider, *Quality and Quantity: The Quest for Biological Regeneration in Twentieth-Century France*, (Cambridge: Cambridge University Press, 1990).

16. See, for example, Kevin Repp, "'More Corporeal, More Concrete:' Liberal Humanism, Eugenics, and German Progressives at the Last Fin de Siècle," *Journal of Modern History* 72, no. 3 (2000): 683–730.

17. See also Pamela Block, "Institutional Utopias, Eugenics, and Intellectual Disability in Brazil," *History and Anthropology* 18, no. 2 (2007): 177–196.

18. Martin S. Pernick, *The Black Stork: Eugenics and the Death of "Defective" Babies in American Medicine and Motion Pictures since 1915* (New York and Oxford: Oxford University Press, 1996), 23.

19. Michael Burleigh, *Death and Deliverance: "Euthanasia" in Germany, 1900–1945* (Cambridge: Cambridge University Press, 1994).

20. Pauline M. H. Mazumdar, *Eugenics, Human Genetics and Human Failings: The Eugenics Society, Its Sources, and Its Critics in Britain* (London and New York: Routledge, 1992), 58–95.

21. Richard L. Dugdale, *The Jukes: A Study in Crime, Pauperism, Disease, and Heredity* (New York and London: G.P. Putnam's, 1877); Nicole Hahn Rafter, *White Trash: The Eugenics Family Studies, 1877–1919* (Boston, MA: Northeastern University Press, 1988); Alice Wexler, *Mapping Fate: A Memoir of Family, Risk, and Genetic Research* (New York: Random House, 1995); Alice Wexler, *The Woman Who Walked into the Sea: Huntington's and the Making of a Genetic Disease* (New Haven, CT: Yale University Press, 2008).

22. Theodore M. Porter, *Karl Pearson: The Scientific Life in a Statistical Age* (Princeton, NJ: Princeton University Press, 2004).

23. Judith R. Walkowitz, "Science, Feminism and Romance: The Men and Women's Club 1885–1889," *History Workshop Journal* 21, no. 1 (1986): 39.

24. Allen G. Roper, *Ancient Eugenics* (Oxford: Blackwell, 1913).

25. Frank Dikötter, "Race Culture: Recent Perspectives on the History of Eugenics," *American Historical Review* 103, no. 2 (1998): 467–478.

26. Marius Turda and Paul J. Weindling, *"Blood and Homeland": Eugenics and Racial Nationalism in Central and Southeast Europe, 1900–1940* (Budapest: Central European University Press, 2007); Alexandra Minna Stern, *Eugenic Nation: Faults and Frontiers of Better Breeding in Modern America* (Berkeley, CA: University of California Press, 2005).

27. See also Tessa Morris-Suzuki, "Debating Racial Science in Wartime Japan," *Osiris* 13 (1998): 354–375.

28. Jawaharlal Nehru to the Indian Science Congress, 1938, cited in Benjamin Zachariah, "The Uses of Scientific Argument," *Economic and Political Weekly* 36, no. 39 (2001): 3693.

29. See, for example, William Schneider, "Hérédité, sang, et opposition à l'immigration dans la France des années trente," *Ethnologie Française* 24 (1994): 104–117.

30. Diane Paul, "Eugenics and the Left," *Journal of the History of Ideas* 45 (1984): 567–590; Kevles, *In the Name of Eugenics*; G.R. Searle, "Eugenics and Politics in Britain in the 1930s," *Annals of Science* 36 (1979): 159–169; Richard Cleminson, "A Century of Civilization under the Influence of Eugenics: Dr. Enrique Diego Madrazo, Socialism, and Scientific Progress," *Dynamis* 26 (2006): 221–251.

31. Amir Weiner, "Introduction: Landscaping the Human Garden," in *Landscaping the Human Garden: Twentieth-Century Population Management in a Comparative Framework*, ed. Amir Weiner (Stanford, CA: Stanford University Press, 2003), 2.

32. Ayça Alemdaroğlu, "Politics of the Body and Eugenic Discourse in Early Republican Turkey," *Body and Society* 11, no. 3 (2005): 63.

33. "The language of rights...has become an integral part of the discussion of reproductive practices [because of] the practice of some states in interfering with the freedom of certain groups of individuals to make choices." Sheila McLean, "The Right to Reproduce," in *Human Rights: From Rhetoric to Reality*, eds. Tom Campbell et al, (Oxford: Basil Blackwell, 1986), 114–115.

34. Paul Weindling, "The Origins of Informed Consent: The International Scientific Commission on Medical War Crimes, and the Nuremberg Code," *Bulletin of the History of Medicine* 75, no. 1 (2001): 37–71.

35. Marius Turda and Paul J. Weindling, "Eugenics, Race and Nation in Central and Southeast Europe, 1900–1940: An Historiographical Overview," in Turda and Weindling, "*Blood and Homeland*," 7.

36. Christina Cogdell, *Eugenic Design: Streamlining America in the 1930s* (Philadelphia, PA: University of Pennsylvania Press, 2004); Pernick, *The Black Stork*; Daylanne K. English, *Unnatural Selections: Eugenics in American Modernism and the Harlem Renaissance* (Chapel Hill, NC: University of North Carolina Press, 2004); Richardson, *Love and Eugenics in the Late Nineteenth Century*. For one analysis of present-day cultural reception of eugenics, see Ralph Brave and Kathryn Sylva, "Exhibiting Eugenics: Response and Resistance to a Hidden History," *The Public Historian* 29, no. 3 (2007): 33–51.

37. Zygmunt Bauman, *Modernity and the Holocaust* (Cambridge: Polity Press, 1989); see also Véronique Mottier and Natalia Gerodetti, "Eugenics and Social Democracy: or, How the European Left Tried to Eliminate the 'Weeds' from its National Gardens," *New Formations* 60 (2006–2007): 35–49.

38. Michel Foucault, *The History of Sexuality: An Introduction* (Harmondsworth: Penguin, 1987), 149. For studies of Foucault, eugenics, and modernity, see C. Hanson, "Biopolitics, Biological Racism and Eugenics," in *Foucault in an Age of Terror: Essays on Biopolitics and the Defence of Society*, eds. Stephen Morton and Stephen Bygrave (Basingstoke: Palgrave, 2008), 106–117; Alan Milchman and Alan Rosenberg, "Michel Foucault, Auschwitz and Modernity," *Philosophy & Social Criticism* 22 (1996): 101–113.

39. For example, Marius Turda, "The Nation as Object: Race, Blood, and Biopolitics in Interwar Romania," *Slavic Review* 66, no. 3 (2007): 413–441; see also, Alison Bashford, *Imperial Hygiene: A Critical History of Colonialism, Nationalism, and Public Health* (Basingstoke: Palgrave, 2004) chap. 7.

40. Benoy Kumar Sarkar, *The Sociology of Population with Special Reference to Optimum, Standard of Living and Progress* (Calcutta: N.M. Ray-Chowdhury, 1936), 18.

41. William Schneider, "Puériculture and the Style of French Eugenics," *History and Philosophy of the Life Sciences* 8 (1986): 265–277.

42. Francis Galton, *Inquiries into Human Faculty and its Development* (London: Macmillan, 1883).

43. John Humphrey Noyes, *First Annual Report of the Oneida Association* (Oneida Reserve: Leonard, 1849), 34; Anita Newcomb McGee, "An Experiment in Human Stirpiculture," *American Anthropologist* 4, no. 4 (1891): 319–326.

44. John Macnicol, "Eugenics and the Campaign for Voluntary Sterilization in Britain Between the Wars," *Social History of Medicine* 2, no. 2 (1989): 147–169.

45. Ian Dowbiggin, *The Sterilization Movement and Global Fertility in the Twentieth Century* (Oxford and New York: Oxford University Press, 2008), 34.

46. Natalia Gerodetti, "From Science to Social Technology: Eugenics and Politics in Twentieth-Century Switzerland," *Social Politics* 13, no. 1 (2006): 69.

47. See, for example, Elena Gutierrez, *Fertile Matters: The Politics of Mexican-Origin Women's Reproduction* (Austin, TX: University of Texas Press, 2008); Alexandra M. Stern,

"Sterilized in the Name of Public Health: Race, Immigration and Reproductive Control in Modern California," *American Journal of Public Health* 95, no. 7 (2005): 1128–1138.

48.   Yolanda Eraso, "Biotypology, Endocrinology, and Sterilization: The Practice of Eugenics in the Treatment of Argentinian Women during the 1930s," *Bulletin of the History of Medicine* 81, no. 4 (2007): 793–822.

49.   Mazumdar, *Eugenics, Human Genetics and Human Failings*, chap. 4; David Barker, "The Biology of Stupidity: Genetics, Eugenics and Mental Deficiency in the Inter-War Years," *British Journal of the History of Science* 22 (1989): 361, 373. For a different argument, see Diane B. Paul, "Did Eugenics Rest on an Elementary Mistake?" in Paul, *The Politics of Heredity: Essays on Eugenics, Biomedicine, and the Nature-Nurture Debate* (Albany, NY: State University of New York Press, 1998), 117–132.

50.   Herbert Jennings, "Eugenics," in *Encyclopedia of the Social Sciences*, eds. Edwin Seligman and Alvin Johnson, vol. 5 (New York: Macmillan, 1931), 619.

51.   Ibid., 620.

52.   G. K. Chesterton, *Eugenics and Other Evils* (London: Cassell, 1922), preface, n.p.

53.   P. J. Weindling, *Nazi Medicine and the Nuremberg Trials: From Medical War Crimes to Informed Consent* (Basingstoke: Palgrave, 2005).

54.   Peter R. Breggin, "The Psychiatric Holocaust," *Penthouse* (January 1979): 81–84.

55.   Adams, *The Wellborn Science*.

PART I

··

TRANSNATIONAL THEMES IN THE HISTORY OF EUGENICS

··

CHAPTER 1

THE DARWINIAN CONTEXT: EVOLUTION AND INHERITANCE

DIANE B. PAUL AND JAMES MOORE

WHETHER efforts to improve the human stock follow logically from Charles Darwin's theory of evolution is a contested and highly sensitive issue. In recent years, defenders of creationism have taken to charging Darwin and his theory with responsibility not just for the rise of eugenics, but for that movement's absolutely worst barbarities. Thus, according to AnswersinGenesis.com, a Web site linked to the recently established Creation Museum in Petersburg, Kentucky:

> Firmly convinced that Darwinian evolution was true, Hitler saw himself as the modern saviour of mankind.... By breeding a superior race, the world would look upon him as the man who pulled humanity up to a higher level of evolutionary development. If Darwinism is true, Hitler was our saviour and we have crucified him. As a result, the human race will grievously suffer. If Darwinism is not true, what Hitler attempted to do must be ranked with the most heinous crimes of history and Darwin as the father of one of the most destructive philosophies of history.[1]

Strong stuff. No wonder feelings run high. But with the "eugenics" label deployed as a weapon of war against evolution, sometimes crudely, sometimes cleverly, the temptation to take no prisoners besets both sides. Those anxious to defend Darwin acknowledge that eugenicists often invoked his theory but condemn them for perverting its intent and substance. In their counter-framing of history, Darwin himself would have been appalled to find others drawing social implications from his strictly scientific work.

As often occurs when the past is used by partisans, historical nuance is lost. These dueling accounts caricature both Darwin (1809–1882) and the theory of evolution by natural selection as he and his peers conceived it. Darwin was not a proponent of eugenics, much less a proto-Nazi. Yet his theories and his own writings on social evolution, especially the 1871 *Descent of Man,* played a vital role in shaping scientific and popular attitudes on questions related to human breeding. In this chapter, we aim to show how this came about.

IMPLICATIONS OF THE *ORIGIN OF SPECIES:* FRANCIS GALTON

Anxieties about Darwin's theory of evolution by natural selection explain why it was not until the late nineteenth century that a concept endorsed by Plato and Aristotle helped underwrite a social movement. Although Darwin avoided discussing "man" in the *Origin of Species,* there was widespread unease about the book's human implications. Controversy immediately centered on the "monkey question": Were humans descended from apes and, if so, what were the implications for morality and society? If humans had reached their current high estate through a process in which the weak in mind and body were constantly eliminated through natural selection, weren't public charities, vaccinations, sanitary measures and the like counterproductive? Didn't they allow the less adequate members of society to survive and reproduce? Wouldn't these people eventually swamp the more capable and thus reverse the direction of evolution? And if progress were threatened, what could and should be done to maintain it? Withdraw aid to the mentally and physically weak? Continue to salvage the sickly but discourage or prevent them from reproducing? Encourage the capable to marry early and produce many children?

Such questions vexed Darwin and many of his contemporaries, such as the retired mill owner William Rathbone Greg (1809–1881), who argued that natural selection was failing in the case of humans and that in a sensible world, only those who passed a competitive examination would be allowed to breed.[2] But the first to publicize unease about the relaxation of selection in "civilized societies" was Darwin's half first cousin, Francis Galton (1822–1911).[3] His intervention was also the most influential, not least because of its impact on Darwin.

In his memoirs, Galton recalled that the *Origin* had extinguished his Christian beliefs like a nightmare exposed to the light of day and had aroused in him "a spirit of rebellion against all ancient authorities whose positive and unauthenticated statements were contradicted by modern science." Darwin inspired Galton to pursue a long-standing interest in the topics of heredity "and the possible improvement of the Human Race."[4] The first fruits of his research were two articles entitled

"Hereditary Talent and Character."[5] Published in 1865 in a highly respectable monthly aimed at an upper-middle-class audience, the article argued that the laws of inheritance applied to humans just as much as they did to other animals, and that mental and temperamental as well as physical traits were inherited from both parents. Galton also proposed that human mentality and character could be improved through institutionalized good breeding. Four years later, Galton expanded the argument into a book, *Hereditary Genius.*[6]

The ideas Galton advanced in the 1860s hardly arose *de novo* with him. As John Waller has argued, the common view of Galton as the founder of eugenics has led to a neglect of an earlier discourse on the transmission of hereditary disease and its reproductive implications.[7] The science of phrenology, which related the shape of the skull to specific human propensities such as friendship, compassion, and envy, was also an element in this context. Phrenology's founder, Franz Joseph Gall (1758–1828), argued that intellectual and moral faculties were innate; the work of Gall and his successors was held in high respect by some quite eminent Victorians.[8]

The practical implications of these doctrines had also been much debated. In the 1840s, the relative importance of "innate character" and "institutional arrangements" in explaining human differences was central to bitter disputes over the "Irish problem" and the status of black labor in Jamaica. The philosopher and economist John Stuart Mill (1806–1873) took the lead in arguing that human behavior and social relationships were the product of history and culture and so were malleable, while his nemesis Thomas Carlyle (1795–1881) insisted that they were fixed by nature.[9] Mill's famous assertion, "Of all the vulgar modes of escaping from the consideration of the social and moral influences on the human mind, the most vulgar is that of attributing the diversities of conduct and character to inherent natural differences," appeared in the first edition of his *Principles of Political Economy*, published in 1848 long before Galton's article and Darwin's *Origin.*[10]

That a debate had already begun does not reduce the importance of Galton. His intervention was the first framing of the issue to be inspired by the *Origin:* the first to make an *evolutionary* argument about human nature and to link questions of human breeding to the anxieties about biological decline that Darwin had provoked. Galton also advanced for the first time a "hard" concept of heredity, repudiating the conventional "soft" or Lamarckian belief in the inheritance of acquired characters. And he embarked on the first systematic empirical inquiry into inheritance, with statistical studies that proved convincing to some prominent contemporaries, not all of whom shared his political inclinations. A favorable review of *Hereditary Genius* by Alfred Russel Wallace (1823–1913), an Owenite socialist, was only the beginning of his support for Galton's project. Although Wallace could be a severe critic of eugenics, he always showed the greatest respect for Galton's empirical work, which convinced him that both individual and national differences are in large part hereditary and that in respect to innate quality, modern Britons compared poorly with ancient Athenians.[11] Of Galton's project, Ruth Schwartz Cowan has noted that "rarely in the history of science has such an important generalization been made on the basis of so little concrete evidence, so badly put, and so naively conceived."[12] But several prominent scientists among his contemporaries thought Galton entirely plausible.

What was Galton's case? He began by acknowledging that little was known of the laws of inheritance. However, he argued, we need not understand exactly *how* traits are inherited to recognize that in humans, as in other animals, offspring tend to resemble their parents both mentally and physically. To establish this, Galton used biographical reference works to show that scientists, statesmen, artists, and others "eminent" enough to be listed were more likely than the general population to have close male relatives also eminent enough to be listed. From this apparent fact that high achievement runs in families, Galton concluded that the traits making for success were transmitted from parent to child in the hereditary material: all human qualities and faculties, physical, moral, mental, and religious, were essentially fixed at birth and that when people succeeded in life it was because they had inherited the necessary traits, and that when they failed, it was because they had not.

Making eminence a fair test of natural ability was controversial, as Galton well knew. Thus he sought to minimize other causes of professional success, such as education and family connections. Against the presumed skeptics, he asserted that, in general, the truly gifted would succeed in life however impoverished their environment, while those who lacked ability (a combination of intelligence, energy, and perseverance) would fail, however favorable their education and training or influential their social connections. Or at least these results would hold in the fields Galton considered meritocracies, such as science and the law.

Having made his case for the inheritance of ability, Galton went on to argue that the least capable members of society were reproducing too rapidly. Darwin had shown that progress depended on a struggle in which the fittest survived and reproduced. It now seemed as though this process was being halted. Civilized societies restrained the natural culling process, allowing those to survive and reproduce who in earlier ages would have succumbed to starvation, cold, or disease. Meanwhile, the most gifted individuals were producing fewer offspring. Unless these trends were reversed, the quality of civilized populations would continue to decline. Galton told Darwin that he feared natural selection was spoiling rather than improving the human race because "it is the classes of coarser organisation who seem on the whole most favoured...and who survive to become the parents of the next [generation]."[13]

Hereditary Genius included a chapter analyzing the comparative worth of different races. By estimating the proportion of eminent men in each race, Galton calculated that black Africans ranked on average two grades below whites in natural ability, and Australian Aborigines three. The ablest race in history was the ancient Greeks, especially the Athenians. But the high "Athenian breed" declined and eventually disappeared because emigration and immigration weakened the race and the most gifted Athenian women failed to marry and reproduce.[14]

Galton did not consider the "savage" races to be a threat.[15] He assumed that the stronger would eventually extirpate the weaker in a process that was already well advanced. The fate of Anglo-Saxons was another matter: Galton believed his own race was following the Athenians by failing to breed from the best; degeneration would render the English unfit to cope with the demands of an increasingly complex world.

What to do about it? Galton proposed that humans should deliberately take charge of their own evolution, doing for themselves what breeders did for domestic plants and animals. This was what Galton would later call "positive" eugenics—increasing the proportion of individuals with desirable traits. ("Negative" eugenics decreased the proportion of those with undesirable traits.) The most pressing task for Galton was to enrich society with outstanding individuals. And he thought the best way to achieve this was to induce the sort of men celebrated in *Hereditary Genius* to marry similarly gifted women. Eventually, their intermarried dynasties, isolated from the main population, would constitute a new human breed. "[B]y selecting men and women of rare and similar talent, and mating them together, generation after generation, an extraordinarily gifted race might be developed," he predicted.[16] The superiority of this race would become evident as natural selection culled its competitors. As proof, Galton pointed to the United States, where the most extraordinary Europeans had been selectively isolated for generations and were now breeding at the expense of the inferior indigenous races.

In his 1865 article, Galton imagined a Utopia where marriages among those receiving the highest marks in state-administered competitive exams were celebrated at Westminster Abbey and rewarded with wedding presents generous enough to allow them to start a family immediately. If only 5 percent of what was spent to improve breeds of horses and cattle were expended on measures to enhance the human race, he mused, "what a galaxy of genius might we not create!"[17] It was less clear what might be done in the here-and-now. In the 1860s, Galton made his breeding schemes conditional on inheritance in humans being as well understood as it was in domestic animals.

Later, Galton floated other ideas for inducing "fit" people to have more children: competitions for state "dowries" to encourage early marriage; subsidized housing "settlements" where gifted couples could raise large families; and even eugenic farms. Rich landowners on "liberally-managed" estates could take in promising young people, gathering "fine specimens of humanity" around them in the same way they "procure and maintain fine breeds of cattle." The youths would then naturally "marry early and suitably" among themselves, and secure "favour for their subsequent offspring"—the first-fruit of human husbandry.[18] In 1890, Galton proposed to Henry Sidgwick (1838–1900), the cofounder of Newnham College, that Cambridge University women of superior health and intellect should receive £50 if they married before age 26 and £25 on the birth of each child: "It is a monstrous shame to use any of these gifted girls for hack work, such as bread winning…as bad as using up the winners of the Oaks in harness work."[19]

FROM *HEREDITARY GENIUS* TO *THE DESCENT OF MAN*

While reading *Hereditary Genius,* Darwin wrote to congratulate his cousin: "I must exhale myself, else something will go wrong in my inside. I do not think I ever in all my life read anything more interesting and original."[20] He agreed with "every word" in Wallace's favorable review and, for all their differences, told him so.[21] Darwin's high opinion of the book and preceding articles is perhaps most evident from his frequent citations in *The Descent of Man.*

What did he so admire in Galton's work and how did he deploy its arguments? Darwin would surely have felt flattered by Galton's chapter on scientific men, in which the Darwin family loomed large, and there were more substantive reasons why Galton's claims about the inheritance of talent and character must have appealed to him. Darwin's theory rested on the assumption of heritable variations for morphological, physiological, and behavioral traits. Those heritable differences constituted "the raw material from which natural selection would choose its winners and losers."[22] Galton's work rested on the same assumption.

Despite Darwin's claim that his cousin partly converted him to natural ability rather than "zeal and hard work" as the root of genius, he may have already been convinced of that.[23] In any case, the *Descent* maintains that most human traits are innate. Mental characters are inherited in domestic animals and in families alike; and "we now know through the admirable labours of Mr. Galton that genius…tends to be inherited; and on the other hand, it is too certain that insanity and deteriorated mental powers likewise run in the same families."[24] In his autobiography Darwin was "inclined to agree with Francis Galton…that education and environment produce only a small effect on the mind of any one, and that most of our qualities are innate."[25] Thus he criticized John Stuart Mill for believing that education and environment powerfully shape human nature. He may have admired Mill's intellect and at least sometimes his politics, but he took issue in the *Descent* with Mill's environmentalism, and in the second edition even added a note: "The ignoring of all transmitted mental qualities will, as it seems to me, be hereafter judged as a most serious blemish in the works of Mr. Mill."[26]

If human qualities are innate, they must be both the product of natural selection and subject to its continuing action: "Man, like every other animal, has no doubt advanced to his present high condition through a struggle for existence consequent on his rapid multiplication; and if he is to advance still higher, it is to be feared that he must remain subject to a severe struggle."[27] Given that selection follows from the struggle for existence, what are the likely consequences of mitigating that struggle? In his chapter on "civilized nations," Darwin tried to account for the social world of his day, its character, development, and future progress, in the light of natural selection. What he saw was the individually and racially fittest being swamped by the less fit. The phrases he used to refer to the former include: "the able in body and mind," "the finest young men," "the intellectually superior," "civilised races," "the frugal, foreseeing, self-respecting, ambitious Scot," "the English," "Canadians of English...extraction," and "Anglo-Saxon people." The less fit are characterized as the "shorter and feebler men, with poor constitutions," "melancholic and insane persons," "violent and quarrelsome men," "profligate women," "parents who are short-lived," "the reckless and improvident," "the vicious and otherwise inferior members of society," "the poorest classes," "Celts," "Canadians of...French extraction," and "the careless, squalid, unaspiring Irishman."

It seemed to Darwin that the less fit were reproductively more successful than the rest. The prudent waited to marry until they could afford to raise children; the improvident married young and had many children born during their mothers' prime of life to inherit strong constitutions. The less fit also survived because civilized societies actively checked the struggle for existence, building asylums for the sick, imbecile, and insane, vaccinating against smallpox, and in other ways preserving the weak. Darwin attributed success in domestic-animal breeding to the "elimination of those individuals...which are in any marked manner inferior." Blackness in sheep was as undesirable as "black sheep" in a family, "men" whose bad dispositions "may perhaps be reversions to a savage state." "Hardly anyone is so ignorant as to allow his worst animals to breed," yet civilized people permit the "weak members" of their societies to "propagate their kind." This "must be highly injurious to the race." Except, no (Darwin balked), to do otherwise would have a worse effect, eroding "the noblest part of our nature," the moral sentiments, which have themselves evolved.[28]

Here Darwin vacillated and hesitated. He sometimes wrote as though the need for social intervention was urgent. Thus he remarked that if various checks "do not prevent the reckless, the vicious, and the otherwise inferior members of society from increasing at a quicker rate than the better class of men, the nation will retrograde, as has occurred too often in the history of the world."[29] Yet he also thought selection continued to work in a positive direction. Mortality was high among the feckless poor and among irresponsible women who married very young. Criminals and the insane died disproportionately often by their own or others' hands; imbeciles and others in institutions were kept from reproducing. Profligate men and women frequently became infertile from disease, while the incurably restless tended to emigrate. Even among the very poor, the more intelligent and thrifty had some edge over their "stupid" and "restless" fellows and so tended to leave more offspring.

In the *Descent's* concluding pages, Darwin comes as close as he ever would to stating how humans could improve themselves by selective breeding. Selection, he wrote, might enhance man's body, intellect, and morals, and the sort he recommended was purely voluntary and individualistic: abstinence from marriage. Beyond this, all hopes for bettering humanity were "Utopian and will never be even partially realised until the laws of inheritance are thoroughly known." The crucial word here is "until." Darwin did *not*—nor did he ever—rule out a society (Utopian or otherwise) in which the artificial selection of humans would be *other* than voluntary and individualistic. This is evident from his slap at Parliament for rejecting a proposal—his own in fact—to shed light on at least one law of inheritance: "whether or not consanguineous marriages are injurious to man."[30] Had such a law been discovered, Darwin would surely have wished legislation to be guided by it: his own sick children were the offspring of a first-cousin marriage.

LAWS OF INHERITANCE

Both Darwin and Galton realized that efforts to improve human populations through breeding were limited by ignorance of the laws of inheritance. But as each worked intently to understand those laws, their perspectives increasingly diverged.

Darwin knew a great deal about the mechanics of reproduction. It could even be said that he was obsessed with the subject. But the *results* of sex baffled him. Why do offspring differ from their parents? Why do they resemble one parent more than the other, or resemble grandparents or more distant relatives, or occasionally resemble no one in the family? Why do defects and monstrosities occur? To all such questions, each edition of the *Origin of Species* solemnly replied: "No one can say."[31]

He did have certain fundamental beliefs about inheritance. After all, he had studied the subject all of his life and probably knew as much about its *phenomena*—what the unknown "laws of inheritance" had to explain—as any living person. He read the great treatises on heredity, tapped breeders' lore, solicited facts from around the world, and undertook his own observations and experiments. In the course of these investigations, he developed ideas about how the baffling phenomena were produced. One premise of everything Darwin believed about inheritance was that characters acquired during an organism's lifetime could be transmitted to their offspring. These included the effects of habit and "use and disuse" of organs, and to some extent the direct effects of the environment. In this sense, Darwin was a life-long Lamarckian, though he still believed that natural selection was, on the whole, the most potent cause of evolution.

But Lamarckian inheritance lacked a mechanism. In *The Variation of Animals and Plants under Domestication* (1868) and again in *The Descent of Man*, Darwin sought to supply one in his "provisional hypothesis of pangenesis," a plausible speculation to account for the appearance of individual variations, the phenomena of atavism (the reappearance of characters of distant relatives), the intermediate nature of hybrids, and the non-inheritance of characters in offspring.

According to the hypothesis, cells in the body throw off minute copies of themselves. These "gemmules" circulate throughout the body, collect in the reproductive organs, and mix with the gemmules of another organism during fertilization. Darwin compared the gemmules to seeds in a "bed of mould," noting that some will germinate quickly, others not at all, and that some will lie dormant for a period, appearing later in life or in a future generation. "When we hear it said that a man carries in his constitution the seeds of an inherited disease, there is much literal truth in the expression."[32] Only some mechanism such as pangenesis could explain how changed conditions of life or the long-continued use and disuse of bodily organs produced inherited modifications.

It is crucial, from this perspective, that parents were able to increase the biological as well as the social endowment they bequeathed to their children. Whatever their social assets, a family could, to an extent, enhance their biological fortunes through education, exercise, good nourishment, and the pursuit of "higher" pleasures such as music and art. Good gemmules, like precious gems, could be amassed and bequeathed to posterity by parents who led prudent lives. The same principle applied to society. Improved social conditions could, at least in some cir-cumstances, benefit future generations by improving people's bodies and thus the gemmules they pass on. So in Darwin and Galton's day, a "hereditarian" position was not necessarily pessimistic. Even if pauperism, criminality, and other undesir-able behaviors were attributable to bad heredity, they could in principle be amelio-rated through environmental improvements. In this way, Lamarckian heredity seemed to bolster the case for correcting unhealthy habits and conditions. Although some Lamarckians argued that deterioration continued for several generations would become, for all practical purposes, irreversible, their "soft" view of heredity was generally associated with an optimistic and socially reformist spirit.

But what if acquired characters were *not* inherited? What if one's best efforts to live well did not benefit one's offspring? What if their biological endowment had little or nothing to do with parental investment? What if improvements in social condi-tions had no direct effect on the hereditary quality of a population? This was the prospect raised by Galton. The consequences he foresaw were radically far-reaching.

In his article "Hereditary Talent and Character" Galton grasped the nettle firmly: "Can we hand anything down to our children, that we have fairly won by our own independent exertions?...Or are we no more than passive transmitters of a nature we have received, and which we have no power to modify?" In short, are acquired charac-ters inherited? Galton thought not; or at least the inherited effect was minimal. Individual variations arose "we know not how"; "moral monstrosities" were born, not made. Social influences altered inborn dispositions only through selection. Thus gen-erations of European misfits were selected, or selected themselves, to emigrate to America, and from their "exceedingly varied, and usually extreme" inborn disposi-tions, a nation of roughnecks had been born, "restless...enterprising, defiant, and touchy...very tolerant of fraud and violence...strongly addicted to cant."[33]

While studying Darwin's *Variation of Animals and Plants,* Galton saw how the pangenesis hypothesis could be tested. He took Darwin's statement that the gem-mules "circulate freely throughout the system" to mean they were carried in the bloodstream to the sex organs. If this was right, Galton reasoned, it should be pos-sible to transfuse blood between animals and give the recipients' progeny the qual-ities of the donors. In consultation with Darwin, Galton embarked on a series of experiments with rabbits, transfusing silver-greys with blood from other strains. The male and female silver-greys were then mated. Two years and many litters later,

Galton had found no evidence of transmitted characters in the transfused blood, and in March 1871, he reported his negative results to the Royal Society.[34]

Galton believed he had refuted the pangenesis hypothesis. The distinction *between* inheritance *and* acquired characters hardened in his mind, and he began to tackle the social implications. With artificial selection now the sole remaining means of heritable human improvement, society had to aim to "breed out feeble constitutions, and petty and ignoble instincts, and to breed in those which are vigorous and noble and social." Individuals should submit themselves "like bees or ants" to this collective task. "I do not for a moment contemplate coercion," Galton added, anticipating political flak, but he did let slip that it was "easy to believe the time may come" when those who persistently "procreate children, inferior in moral, intellectual and physical qualities...would be considered as enemies to the State, and to have forfeited all claims to kindness." Meanwhile, to promote good breeding, science would have to be mobilized. "Some society" was needed to advise the state, a body that would study breeding in a "purely scientific" way.[35]

What was the proposed society's field of work to be called? "We greatly want a brief word to express the science of improving stock," Galton wrote in 1883. "The word *eugenics* would sufficiently express the idea." Eugenics, he explained, from Greek, meaning "good in stock, hereditarily endowed with noble qualities," was "equally applicable to men, brutes, and plants," though he regretted that breeding in all these branches was as yet unequally understood. "Investigation of human eugenics...is at present extremely hampered by the want of full family histories, both medical and general, extending over three or four generations. There was no such difficulty in investigating animal eugenics," which benefited from stud books and the like. But once human breeding was as well understood as that of animals—once the human equivalent of a national stud book had been established—the state could begin to act. Of all eugenic policies, "the most merciful...would consist in watching for the indications of superior strains or races, and in favouring them that their progeny shall outnumber and gradually replace that of the old one." To cooperate thus for Great—and a greater—Britain's sake, or indeed to submit one's family tree to pruning, would be a new form of religious obligation. Eugenics to Galton was the ethical heart and soul of a Church Scientific, with cousin Charles as its patron saint. Man's duty henceforth would be to "further evolution" through good breeding.[36]

TROUBLED TIMES

Hereditary Genius had a tepid reception.[37] Although it impressed Darwin, Wallace, and a few other men of science, reviewers in political, literary, and theological journals were unenthusiastic and the book sold poorly. Given the number of conventional beliefs it challenged, that was not surprising. Galton, anti-clerical and openly skeptical of religious doctrines, explained religious sentiment by natural selection, denied the soul's existence, and belittled the doctrine of Original Sin. Flawed human nature was not the result of Adam's Fall but a biological inheritance from animal ancestors, the product of an unfinished evolution. Man's immediate ancestors were barbarians, fitted by natural selection to their conditions of life; and selection had not caught up with the requirements of a civilized state. Accordingly, moral struggle was futile. Galton had little patience with "tales written to teach children to be good—that babies are born pretty much alike and that the sole agencies in creating differences between boy and boy, and man and man, are steady application and moral effort."[38] Virtue and vice were fixed in men by nature and ultimately beyond individual control. Moral responsibility was not to be inculcated but in-bred.

Galton's audacity was breathtaking. He stood all but alone, lacking a scientific consensus to support his biological premises. Natural selection had few adherents, and many converts to evolution, still accepting Lamarckian inheritance, doubted selection's sufficiency. Worse, Galton had little basis for applying selection to humans. He lacked data on the inheritance of mental and moral traits for *any* population, and his pedigree research was restricted to eminent families. Given the prevailing assumption of "soft" heredity, social reform was viewed as a plausible solution even to admitted hereditary problems. Galton's claim that the mentally and morally worst were swamping the best was based on theoretical considerations, not thorough research. Thus his work was initially greeted with skepticism.

But thirty years later the new science caught on. Galton bankrolled the Eugenics Record Office at University College in 1904 and transformed it under his disciple Karl Pearson (1857–1936) in 1907 into the Francis Galton Laboratory for the Study of National Eugenics. For decades, Galton had sought to capture the nation's interest in breeding by publishing articles about "trotting horses," "pedigree moths," and "three generations of lunatic cats." He had even perfected fingerprinting as a method of identifying criminals (his most famous legacy), and now in his eighties, he finally realized his pet project, a society for promoting eugenics.[39]

By the first decade of the twentieth century, Galton's "hard" view of heredity had been reinforced by the German cytologist August Weismann's research on the cell nucleus. In 1883, Weismann (1834–1914) identified two distinct cell types: germ cells, present in the gonads, which give rise to sperm and eggs; and somatic cells, present in all other bodily tissues. He went further: germ cells were completely isolated from somatic cells. Although the latter could be affected by the environment, the hereditary units in the former were inviolate and transmitted unaltered down the generations. Hard though parents might strive to improve their minds or bodies, their children would reap no benefit; and no environmental tinkering would improve the hereditary endowment of populations. Weismann himself concluded that the only route to race improvement lay in selective breeding. His doctrines did not immediately sweep the field, but they found many more immediate adherents than Galton's had at first.

While Weismann and Galton laid the theoretical groundwork for eugenics, a raft of statistical studies seemed to demonstrate national decline in Britain.[40] Galton (like Darwin) had expressed dismay at the fecundity of the poor, but he had data for only a select and narrow slice of society. By the turn of the century, alarmist fears about degeneration seemed amply confirmed. The end of the Boer War (1899–1902) was followed by shocking reports of the number of recruits deemed unfit for military service, which raised the question of whether hereditary weakness would not fatally undermine Britain's capacity for exercising imperial power.[41] Meanwhile, demographic studies demonstrated an inverse correlation between fertility and socioeconomic status, with the birthrate apparently falling much more sharply among the middle and upper-middle classes than among workers and agricultural laborers.[42] Now the old problem of the "differential birthrate" became shockingly real. If the wretched poor were wretched by nature, a nature that was fixed, their apparent high fertility seemed to justify the gloomiest of Darwin's predictions and demand urgent action.

Galton used the new evidence to dramatic effect in his 1901 Huxley Lecture to the Anthropological Institute in London, "The Possible Improvement of the Human Breed, under the Existing Conditions of Law and Sentiment." The tone and content contrasted sharply with Galton's 1865 articles. By 1901, Galton had available some of Charles Booth's 17-volume survey, *Life and Labour of the People in London* (1889–1903), with its statistical evidence for the class divisions of London society.[43] Galton manipulated the data, quietly generalizing it to the whole country *and* subdividing the nation's classes into the "same proportions" found in "East London," stating that though "certainly not accurate," the results were "probably not far wrong."[44] As the East End's social structure was then even less typical of Britain's than it is today, we may surmise that Galton viewed the nation through a badly distorting lens, the population appearing to him more like Jack London's outcast *People of the Abyss* (1903) than a fair use of the evidence would warrant.[45] But the point is: there *was* evidence now, however questionable, which—on the basis of increasingly shared assumptions about evolution and heredity—pointed to a troubled future.

Galton in 1865 had tabled an uplifting spiritual agenda, the epitome of high Victorian optimism. How different he sounded in 1901! The Huxley lecture ended in a bright haze—"we plant our stock all over the world"—but in general the tone was dark. Galton played up the threat from Booth's lowest class, the hereditary "barbarians," whom he says it would be "an economy and a great benefit to the country" to segregate "under merciful surveillance," and deny "opportunities for producing offspring." Eugenics was no longer just about breeding *from* the right people, though this remained his chief concern; it was also about identifying those who ought *not* to breed. Both sort of eugenics—positive and negative—Galton believed "raise the average, the latter by reducing the undesirables, the former by increasing those who will become the lights of the nation."[46]

One who agreed wholeheartedly, and more, was Karl Pearson. Appointed the first Galton Professor of Eugenics at University College London, thanks to a £45,000 bequest in Galton's will, he shared his mentor's belief in hard heredity and fascination with statistics. Pearson may have been a social and political radical, but his militaristic and imperialist eugenics was much harsher than Galton's, and even more strongly inflected by racism.

In his well-known 1901 lecture "National Life from the Standpoint of Science," Pearson argued that it was not the individual but "the herd, the tribe, or the nation which forms the fundamental unit in the evolution of man." Evolution is driven by a global struggle among such units for living space and raw materials. Superior and inferior races cannot coexist; if the former are to make effective use of global resources, the latter must be extirpated. To keep the nation to "a high pitch of internal efficiency," its members should be replenished from the best stock; to maintain external efficiency, the nation must beat inferiors and fight equals for trade routes and resources. Pearson ended the lecture on a bleak note indeed: "Mankind...advances through pain and suffering only. The path of progress is strewn with the wreck of nations; traces are everywhere to be seen of the hecatombs of inferior races, and of victims who found not the narrow way to the greater perfection."[47] As the twentieth century wore on, these dark motifs became increasingly prominent among eugenicists worldwide.

NOTES

1. J. Bergman, "Darwinism and the Nazi Race Holocaust," *Technical Journal* 13 (1999): 101–111, www.answersingenesis.org/tj/v13/i2/nazi.asp (accessed 15 April 2008).

2. William Greg, "On the Failure of 'Natural Selection' in the Case of Man," *Fraser's Magazine* 68 (1868): 353–362.

3. Galton's mother was a Darwin, the first daughter of Charles Darwin's grandfather's second marriage, which made Francis and Charles half first-cousins.

4. Francis Galton, *Memories of My Life* (London: Methuen, 1908), 298.

5. Francis Galton, "Hereditary Talent and Character," *Macmillan's Magazine* 12 (1865): 157–166, 318–327.

6. Francis Galton, *Hereditary Genius: An Inquiry into Its Laws and Consequences* (London: Macmillan, 1869).

7. John C. Waller, "Ideas of Heredity, Reproduction and Eugenics in Britain, 1800–1875," *Studies in History and Philosophy of Biological and Biomedical Sciences* 32, no. 3 (2001): 458, 463.

8. Franz Joseph Gall, *On the Function of the Brain and of Each of Its Parts: With Observations on the Possibility of Determining the Instincts, Propensities, and Talents, or the Moral and Intellectual Dispositions of Men and Animals, by the Configuration of the Brain and Head* (Boston, MA: Marsh, Capen & Lyon, 1835); Franz Joseph Gall and Johann Gaspar Spurzheim, *Anatomie et physiologie du système nerveux en général et du cerveau en particulier; avec des observations sur la possibilité de reconnaître plusieurs dispositions intellectuelles et morales de l'homme et des animaux par la configuration de leur têtes,* 4 vols. and atlas (Paris: F. Schoell, 1810–1819). [Spurzheim coauthored the first two volumes; Gall was sole author of the remaining two]; George Combe, *The Constitution of Man Considered in Relation to External Objects,* 8th ed. (Edinburgh: Maclachlan, 1847).

9. Diane B. Paul and Ben Day, "John Stuart Mill, Innate Differences, and the Regulation of Reproduction," *Studies in History and Philosophy of Biological and Biomedical Sciences* 39, no. 2 (2008): 222–231.

10. John Stuart Mill, "Principles of Political Economy, with Some of Their Applications to Social Philosophy," in *Collected Works of John Stuart Mill*, vols. 2–3, ed. J. M. Robson (London: John W. Parker, 1848; Toronto: University of Toronto Press, 1965).

11. Diane B. Paul, "Wallace, Women, and Eugenics," in *Natural Selection and Beyond: The Intellectual Legacy of Alfred Russel Wallace*, eds. Charles Smith and George Beccaloni (Oxford: Oxford University Press, 2008), 264–268.

12. Ruth Schwartz Cowan, "Nature and Nurture: The Interplay of Biology and Politics in the Work of Francis Galton," *Studies in the History of Biology* 1 (1977): 135.

13. Greta Jones, "Theoretical Foundations of Eugenics," in *Essays in the History of Eugenics*, ed. Robert A. Peel (London: The Galton Institute, 1998), 9.

14. Galton, *Hereditary Genius*, 331.

15. Nancy Stepan, *The Idea of Race in Science: Great Britain 1800–1960* (Hamden, CT: Archon Books, 1982).

16. Galton, "Hereditary Talent and Character," 79.

17. Ibid., 165.

18. Francis Galton, "The Possible Improvement of the Human Breed, under the Existing Conditions of Law and Sentiment," *Essays in Eugenics* (London: Eugenics Education Society, 1909), 31–32.

19. R. Tullberg McWilliams, *Women at Cambridge*, rev. ed (Cambridge: Cambridge University Press, 1998).

20. Francis Darwin and A. C. Seward, eds., *More Letters of Charles Darwin* (London: John Murray, 1903), 41.

21. James Marchant, *Alfred Russel Wallace: Letters and Reminiscences* (New York: Harper & Brothers, 1916), 206.

22. Martin Brookes, *Extreme Measures: The Dark Vision and Bright Ideas of Francis Galton* (New York and London: Bloomsbury Publishing, 2004), 171.

23. Galton, *Memories*, 290.

24. Charles R. Darwin, *The Descent of Man, and Selection in Relation to Sex*, eds. James Moore and Adrian Desmond (London: John Murray, 1871; 2nd ed., final printing 1879; London: Penguin, 2004), 46.

25. Charles R. Darwin, *The Autobiography of Charles Darwin, 1809–1882: With Original Omissions Restored*, ed. Nora Barlow (New York: Harcourt Brace, 1958), 43.

26. Darwin, *Descent*, 121, n. 5.

27. Ibid., 688.

28. Ibid., 158–169.

29. Ibid., 166. Wallace noted that in one of their last conversations, Darwin expressed gloomy views about the future: "in our modern civilisation natural selection had no play, and the fittest did not survive." Alfred Russel Wallace, *My Life: A Record of Events and Opinions*, 2 vols. (London: Chapman and Hall, 1905), 2: 509.

30. Darwin, *Descent*, 688. The comment refers to Darwin's failed efforts to have a question on cousin-marriage included in the 1871 census.

31. Morse Peckham, ed., *The Origin of Species by Charles Darwin: A Variorum Text* (Philadelphia, PA: University of Pennsylvania Press, 1959).

32. Charles Darwin, *The Variation of Animals and Plants under Domestication*, 2 vols. (London: John Murray, 1868; rev. ed. 1875; facsmile with a new foreword by Harriet Ritvo, Baltimore, MD: Johns Hopkins University Press, 1998), 397.

33. Galton, "Hereditary Talent and Character," 75–76, 77, 79.

34. On Galton and pangenesis, see Brookes, *Extreme Measures*, 174–177; Michael Bulmer, *Francis Galton: Pioneer of Heredity and Biometry* (Baltimore, MD: Johns Hopkins

University Press, 2003), 116–118; Nicholas Wright Gilham, *A Life of Sir Francis Galton: From African Exploration to the Birth of Eugenics* (Oxford: Oxford University Press, 2001). The historian of psychology Raymond Fancher is also preparing a new Galton biography.

35. Francis Galton, "Hereditary Improvement," *Fraser's Magazine,* new series, 7 (1873): 116, 120, 124, 129.

36. Francis Galton, *Inquiries into Human Faculty and Its Development* (London: Macmillan, 1883), 24 n5, 44, 307, 337.

37. Emel Aileen Gökyigit, "The Reception of Francis Galton's 'Hereditary Genius' in the Victorian Periodical Press," *Journal of the History of Biology* 27 (1994): 215–240.

38. Galton, *Hereditary Genius,* 291.

39. Karl Pearson, *The Life, Letters and Labours of Francis Galton,* 3 vols. in 4 (Cambridge: Cambridge University Press, 1914–1930), 3a: 391.

40. Richard Soloway's factors include: *fin de siècle* soul-searching; a long agricultural and industrial depression; economic challenges from the United States and Germany; imperial rivalries in Africa and elsewhere; political ferment, including the rise of socialism; humiliating defeats in the Boer War; the declining birthrate both absolutely and relative to that of competitor nations; the differential fertility of social classes, raising fears of physical and mental deterioration and the degeneration of the "race." Richard A. Soloway, *Demography and Degeneration: Eugenics and the Declining Birth-rate in Twentieth-Century Britain* (Chapel Hill, NC: University of North Carolina Press, 1990). Daniel Kevles mentions some of Soloway's factors in generalizing about industrialization and urbanization, the growth of big business, and mass migrations to the cities both from the countryside and abroad, which provoked racism and anti-Semitism. He adds the advent of Mendelian genetics, a spate of "social-Darwinist writings" backed up by Charles Booth's social survey, and taxpayers' resentment at the growing burden of poor relief. Daniel J. Kevles, *In the Name of Eugenics: Genetics and the Uses of Human Heredity* (Cambridge, MA: Harvard University Press, 1995), chap. 5.

41. Isaac Kramnick and Barry Sheerman, *Harold Laski: A Life on the Left* (New York: Penguin, 1993), 38–39.

42. Soloway, *Demography and Degeneration,* 10–17.

43. Charles Booth, *Life and Labour of the People in London,* 17 vols. (London: Macmillan, 1889–1903).

44. Galton, "Possible Improvement," 8. Although not published until 1909, the lecture was given October 29, 1901.

45. Jack London, *The People of the Abyss* (New York: Macmillan, 1903).

46. Galton, "Possible Improvement," 20–24.

47. Karl Pearson, *National Life from the Standpoint of Science* (London: Adam and Charles Black, 1901), 21, 43–44, 53, 61–62.

FURTHER READING

Browne, Janet. *Charles Darwin: The Power of Place* (Princeton, NJ: Princeton University Press, 2003).

Darwin, Charles. *The Descent of Man, and Selection in Relation to Sex,* eds. James Moore and Adrian Desmond (London: John Murray. first published 1871; 2nd ed., final printing 1879; London, Penguin, 2004).

Desmond, Adrian, and James Moore. *Darwin* (New York: W. W. Norton, 1994).

Gayon, Jean. *Darwinism's Struggle for Survival: Heredity and the Hypothesis of Natural Selection* (Cambridge: Cambridge University Press, 2007).

Gilham, Nicholas Wright. *A Life of Sir Francis Galton: From African Exploration to the Birth of Eugenics* (Oxford: Oxford University Press, 2001).

Kevles, Daniel J. *In the Name of Eugenics: Genetics and the Uses of Human Heredity* (Cambridge, MA: Harvard University Press, 1995).

Paul, Diane B., and Ben Day. "John Stuart Mill, Innate Differences, and the Regulation of Reproduction," *Studies in History and Philosophy of Biological and Biomedical Sciences* 39, no. 2 (2008): 222–231.

Porter, Theodore M. *Karl Pearson: The Scientific Life in a Statistical Age* (Princeton, NJ: Princeton University Press, 2005).

Searle, G. R. *The Quest for National Efficiency: A Study in British Politics and Political Thought, 1899–1914,* 2nd ed. (Amherst, NY: Humanity Books, 1990).

Waller, John C. "Ideas of Heredity, Reproduction and Eugenics in Britain, 1800–1875," *Studies in History and Philosophy of Biological and Biomedical Sciences* 32, no. 3 (2001): 457–489.

CHAPTER 2

....

ANTHROPOLOGY, COLONIALISM, AND EUGENICS

....

PHILIPPA LEVINE

IT was in the 1910s and 1920s that eugenic policies designed to limit reproduction among the "unfit" and encourage it among the favored first received political and governmental imprimatur, but the principles governing such policies had already been the subject of some few decades of research and discussion. This chapter traces what catalyzed such ideas, what gave them weight in an increasingly precise scientific environment. While it would certainly be folly to try to identify an origin for eugenic principles or to imply a Whiggish inevitability through a "pre-history," we may nonetheless find, in the potent mid-nineteenth-century combination of anthropology and colonialism, ideas that prefigured and helped generate the subsequent acceptance of eugenics as a serious scientific and increasingly social endeavor. That both anthropology and colonialism were expanding heartily at the "Darwinian moment" is also of some importance, not only (and obviously) because eugenics engaged directly with questions of heredity, but because the emerging terms of the evolutionary debate also shaped anthropological ideas, and gave new and often controversial meaning to old ethnological debates.[1] New ideas about heredity and evolution, coupled with a growing interest in colonial populations and mostly celebratory attitudes toward European imperial expansion, set the stage for the acceptance of eugenics in the twentieth century. In particular, these strands coalesced in ideas about "savage" populations and their relationship to the modernity felt to be enshrined in colonialism. The nineteenth century saw what Patrick Brantlinger terms a "crescendo" of interest in what became known as the dying or doomed races, and indeed, he draws an explicit link between this interest and the development of eugenics. Henrika Kuklick posits an equally compelling association between the emergence of anthropology and a growing interest in dying race theory.[2] Discussions of the "savage" in the nineteenth century deployed a range of ideas and terms around heredity, extinction, degeneration, and regression that were central both to scientific and imperial culture. In this coalescence we may see ideas by no means unfamiliar to later generations of eugenicists, and marked by debates circulating in anthropology and around colonial practice.

Anthropology and Imperialism

Anthropology famously derived its raison d'être, it earliest subject matter, and its justification from the colonial practices increasingly important for European nations. Over the course of the nineteenth century, anthropology became ever more closely associated with the practice and methods of science. Science lent authority and weight with its growing claims to neutrality and objectivity, its measurement and scaling of materials. Thomas Huxley (1825–1895) claimed in 1873 that anthropology was "a section of ZOOLOGY, which again is the animal half of BIOLOGY—the science of life and living things."[3] Nicholas Thomas describes anthropology as subsuming "humanity to the grand narratives and analogies of natural history," in which populations were read as species with distinctive systems and characteristics.[4] That this change coincided with the waning of liberal humanitarianism in any number of colonial contexts suggests strong links to colonialism.[5] With the abolition of slavery, critiques of colonial practice as detrimental to "natives" (which argued that colonialism's mission was to uplift ignorant populations, not to oppress or exterminate them) were drowned out by the growing imperial model of ruling indigenous populations with a small field staff. This new form of colonialism fundamentally altered both labor practices and modes of governance, as well as solidifying already negative attitudes toward colonial peoples.

From an early date anthropology—or more properly, its predecessor, ethnology—had distinct camps. The critical divide concerned whether humans derived from a single origin, a controversy George Stocking describes as the "primary focal point of anthropological thought well into the nineteenth century."[6] This was a widespread debate among anthropologists in Germany, France, Britain, South Africa, and the United States. Over time this debate blended to some extent with the growing camps of progressionist and degenerationist anthropologists, a divide palpably shaped by the new Darwinian version of evolutionary theory. Both these flashpoints of conflict played a key role in the discussion of the modern "savage." Primitive manners and practices, argued anthropologists, needed to be captured and recorded before they were either transformed or destroyed by colonial contact.[7]

Colonialism and anthropology shared a roster of concerns. In his 1903 presidential address to the Anthropological Institute of Great Britain and Ireland,

Alfred Cort Haddon (1855–1940), perhaps the most influential field anthropologist of his generation, praised "all that is being done for Anthropology by the various Governments that constitute the British Empire."[8] His tactic was designed to stimulate further investment in the discipline, and in truth the state's generosity was not bountiful. By allying anthropology, however, to colonial governance, Haddon hoped to secure its institutional footing on a firmer basis. And while government, as ever, preferred to receive its expertise on the cheap, the link Haddon drew was not an imaginary one. Patrick Harries asserts that "the conquest that accompanied the spread of Empire also required a thorough knowledge of aboriginal cultures."[9] And Donna Haraway, deliberately echoing one of the most influential scientific phrases of the high Victorian period, has pointedly called imperialism, "the silent, if deeply constitutive, axis in Victorian debates on 'man's place in nature.'"[10]

One of the main tasks of anthropology was to define and measure civilization—and its absence—as a justification for and of imperial expansion. The close association that was mooted between civilization and the modern European colonial impulse was critical to the spread of anthropology throughout Europe and America, as well as in white settler colonies such as Australia and Canada, struggling with the plight of aboriginal populations massively displaced by generations of settlers. In the Netherlands, colonial officials received anthropological and ethnological training before they took up their posts, the better to understand their charges. Civilization and imperialism were both upward, progressive, and beneficent movements, wholly unlike the world of the savage, whose primitive lack of progress marked her as unfit and unmodern. And anthropology at this juncture was vitally and essentially concerned with the prospect of human extinction, for without progress there could only be decline. Even those critical of imperialism for its tendency to usher in indigenous depopulation saw the issue at stake in oppositional terms: primitivism versus civilization. James Cowles Prichard (1786–1848), sometimes labeled the founder of British anthropology and a persistent critic of colonial practice, noted in 1839 that "wherever Europeans have settled, their arrival has been the harbinger of extermination to the native tribes. Whenever the simple pastoral tribes come into relations with the more civilised agricultural nations, the allotted time of their destruction is at hand."[11] Savage and primitive peoples were under threat, and the most urgent threat they faced was from colonial contact. Olive Dickason goes so far as to claim that the very distinction between a "savage," and a "civilized" human itself "paved the way" for the European colonization of North America.[12]

SAVAGES

But who or what was this savage, so markedly different from the civilized peoples of the Western world? The term "savage" seems to have become widespread toward the end of the sixteenth century, but was palpably burdened with a variety of meanings.[13] Réal Ouellet and Mylene Tremblay find vast and competing descriptions of the savage in European accounts of Amerindian peoples in the early modern period. The savage could be beautiful, diabolical and cruel, intelligent, degenerate and even helpful, suggesting remarkable variety in the meaning and use of the term.[14] At different moments, certainly, particular images prevailed, but however contradictory these depictions might be, there was generally a strong sense of what Ian Duncan has usefully termed the recognition of "radical strangeness."[15] Such strangeness could reside in clothing or its lack, skin color, hair texture, the shape of the skull and of the nose. As Matthew Day has noted, erasing evidence of religious sentiment among savages was a clever way to drive home radical difference in an age suffused with Christianity.[16] For the more politically inclined, it was forms of governance or attitudes toward land ownership that marked the critical difference.

Such representations downplayed humanity and individuality (the province of reason and civilization). Writing in the *Journal of the Anthropological Society of London,* Richard Lee claimed that "the man who now wanders free through the unknown wilds of Australia represents nothing."[17] Novelist and evolutionist Grant Allen (1848–1899) was confident that in

> a race of hunting savages, in the earliest, lowest, and most undifferentiated stage, we shall get really next to no personal peculiarities or idiosyncrasies of any sort amongst them. Every one of them would be a good hunter, a good fisherman, a good scalper, and a good manufacturer of bows and arrows...but of spontaneity, originality, initiative, variability, not a single spark. Know one savage of the tribe, and you know them all.[18]

The savage, the condition of savagery, was a cipher, allowing comparison and justification, and establishing a set of criteria for modernity and civilization. The savage, unburdened by property and unschooled in the higher arts, unkempt and unclean, by turns cruel and sensitive, rational and violent, compliant and unruly, was an imaginary but nonetheless palpable entity whose purpose was to bear the weight of discussion about those fundamentally eugenic topics: fitness and capacity for civilization. Sir Alexander Grant (1826–1884), principal of Edinburgh University in the mid-nineteenth century, called savages "the swamps and backwaters of the stream of noble humanity."[19] And even Darwin, although warning in *The Descent of Man* that "savages...are not nearly so uniform in character, as has often been asserted," nonetheless tended to blur their individuality.[20]

These mostly unflattering pictures of what appeared to be immutable difference fueled the ongoing debate between monogenists and polygenists, a debate with theological as well as scientific significance. The idea of the savage fed assumptions that would be picked up by eugenics on such topics as reproductive capacity, the idea of generational "throwbacks," and crucially what role the environment played in promoting or preventing development. In one form or another, this was a long-standing, complex, and often bitterly waged battle, in which both physical and mental differences were scrutinized.

By the mid-nineteenth century the debate was firmly racialized, with racial difference frequently mapped onto notions of primitive and civilized. Nicholas Hudson helpfully reminds us that Europeans considered themselves superior to other peoples long before race acquired its modern definition, and that superiority was earlier measured by degrees of civilization.[21] Even in the nineteenth century, race was frequently measured by variables other than skin color. Head shape—the cephalic index—was a typical measure of racial difference. Likewise, hair texture, body proportion, nose shape, and a host of other visual and measurable traits were described as racial. Both the monogenist and polygenist camps ranked different populations in racial hierarchies that read whites as more advanced, and as the possessors and founders of modernity. While polygenists saw this as the outcome of species difference for the most part, monogenists mostly stressed environment as the major explanatory factor determining inequality. As a number of commentators have also noted, while such prominent scientists as Huxley and Darwin remained committed in fundamental ways to a monogenist position, their work still allows for a truce with polygenesis by acknowledging the lengthy history of difference.[22] More often than not, the primitive was racially distinct from the civilized white, mirroring later eugenic distinctions (also often racialized) between fit and unfit populations.

THE PRIMITIVE AND THE MODERN: DYING RACES AND HUMAN EXTINCTION

This racialized ranking took a number of forms, all of them marking difference and often expressing the inevitability of the extinction of primitives facing the modern. Alfred Haddon, for example, approvingly duplicated another observer's description of the South Sea Islands as a "museum of living specimens," conjuring up the idea of people whose progress had halted, whose lives and lands had become a laboratory and spectacle, frozen in a pre-modern moment.[23] As late as 1947, A. O. Neville (1875–1954), Chief Protector of Aborigines in Western Australia from 1915 to 1936, recognized that many (he did not include himself) saw "the native as a 'static' being incapable of advancement."[24] A vast literature over a considerable time span echoed his contention. James Hunt (1833–1869), the polygenist president of the Anthropological Society in the 1860s, claimed that in the 1866 uprising in Jamaica, "the Negro found himself overmatched" by Europeans, while the New Zealand writer Alfred Grace (1867–1942), in a collection of colorful if patronizing tales of Maori life, insisted that it was simply impossible for indigenous New Zealanders to stop fighting: "nothing could assuage the Maori's thirst for fighting."[25] And if such pronouncements insinuate the possibility of eradication, they also celebrate a narrative of progress, "a dynamic scheme of evolutionary destiny" in which there was little room for the savage.[26]

The forward march of civilization, always meliorative, could nonetheless leave in its wake destruction. The modern savage, out of time, was civilization's likeliest victim. In a distinctly Spencerian turn of phrase, Canon Tristram (1822–1906) claimed in 1871 that "the weaker must perish in the struggle for existence."[27] Though Darwin stopped short of such pronouncements, he nonetheless accepted differences in human evolutionary development, as we have seen.[28] In this broad view there were, then, humans unfit to acquire, understand, or inherit modern civilization: they were, simply put, in the wrong place at the wrong time, and their demise was inevitable. The notion of the dying race ranged across a host of disciplines and positions. Common among settlers and humanitarians alike, it was developed in the nineteenth century through anthropology; Charles Hursthouse, a New Zealand settler, spoke of the "ethnological law that the black savage shall disappear before the white settler."[29] By the early twentieth century, explanations of such unfitness had entered the realm of psychology. The ethnologist C. G. Seligman (1873–1940) saw Britain's mental deficients and "primitive" peoples sharing brain structures in which the poor development of the "supragranular" layer inhibited their adaptation to higher civilization.[30]

Francis Galton (1822–1911) had earlier applied these ideas to what he called the "dregs" of civilized society, arguing that inheritance was the key to understanding and solving the social problems savagery provoked even in modern times. Addressing the British Association for the Advancement of Science in 1877, Galton referred approvingly to Richard Dugdale's recently published American study of the criminal genealogy of the Jukes family, one of the early classics of eugenic literature. Describing the progenitor of the clan as a "somewhat good specimen of a half-savage," Galton argued that subsequent generations could not adapt to civilization because of the "gipsy-like character of the race." As a result, "hereditary moral weaknesses" surfaced generation after generation.[31] This fear that primitivity continued to lurk even within the confines of civilization spurred both eugenic policy and anthropological research closer to home. To have civilization held back by the undesirable was unacceptable. And while later generations of eugenicists would in some cases successfully press for radical measures to stem such a possibility in Western arenas, the savage in colonial and tropical environments was a different matter. There were fears that some non-Western populations might, far from disappearing, out-reproduce the West, but the more widespread assumption was that some peoples would, over time, weaken and die out, a phenomenon usually dubbed "doomed race" or "dying race" theory.[32]

Fiona Stafford sees this "last-of-the-race" myth fully fledged by the end of the eighteenth century.[33] The clamor of voices pronouncing the ineluctable, certain disappearance of those unable to adapt to the modern world reached its apogee, however, in the mid- and late nineteenth century, strengthened by the new evolutionary theories. In the *Popular Magazine of Anthropology* in 1866, one writer was adamant that "savage races...are formed for the wilderness and die when *it* is reclaimed."[34] Robert Chambers (1802–1871), author of *Vestiges of Creation* (1844), regarded both imperialism and the extinction of primitive species as part of the pattern of human biological progress.[35] In *Descent of Man*, Darwin more than once reiterated extinction as a sad fact. In Chapter 5, he noted that "At the present day civilised nations are everywhere supplanting barbarous nations," and in Chapter 7, he devoted an entire section to human extinction, declaring that when the civilized and the primitive meet, "the struggle is short."[36] For Darwin such destruction, as Ian Duncan notes, was less catastrophic than a "steady seepage" over time, lending it a poignant inevitability.[37] Opinions such as these, expressed in popular and in specialized publications, legitimized annihilation as an unfortunate but necessary effect of modernity.

Common in the arsenal of inevitability arguments was the theme of self-immolation, that extinction was self-inflicted and could not be blamed on contact. We see this at work in Alfred Grace's claim that the Maori were incapable of peaceful coexistence with one another. Colonists were welcomed, he argued, for the weaponry they could provide Maori "to exterminate each other. This they almost accomplished, and now the assimilation of a civilisation they do not understand is finishing the work."[38] Grace's views were published early in the twentieth century, but his sentiments had a far longer history. Almost a century previously, a writer in the *Quarterly Review* had made exactly the same argument with respect to Native Americans. "The natives have nearly completed their own extermination with weapons put into their hands."[39] In 1845 William Porter (1805–1880), attorney general at the Cape Colony, wondered if blaming settlers for "the extinction of the coloured races," was fair. Might not "their defective form of civilisation" instead be the engine of their destruction?[40] Such opinions both naturalized the prospect of extinction and underlined the relationship between modernity and fitness in an uncanny echo of the eugenic principles that would soon follow.

The contradictions that emerged in explaining extinction were themselves revealing of broader instabilities in defining savagery. Many, like Alfred Grace, saw in the savage an unchecked aggression and bloodthirstiness, a literal savageness that was responsible for ending life. John Calder, defending the record of white settlers in nineteenth-century Tasmania, dwelled on Aboriginal belligerence and on the impossibility of "a fair and open fight" against such "acute and crafty" assailants. Yet he simultaneously displayed his Aboriginal foe as far likelier to succumb to respiratory infections than hardier and more sensible settlers.[41] One of the commonest adjectives used to describe the savage throughout the nineteenth century was "feeble." Such palpable contradictions—between warrior status and constitutional frailty, between aggression and weakness—could be, at least in part, smoothed over by an argument derived from evolutionary fitness and adaptation.

Russell McGregor points out that the Spencerian maxim of the "survival of the fittest" replaced "Divine Providence as the cornerstone of the doomed race idea."[42] Couched in what Tony Barta dubs the "language of inevitable demise," the new science could be used to legitimize the extinction-as-inevitable position.[43] In Peter Bowler's words, savages were thus "relics of the past doomed to be swept away."[44] They had no role to play in advancing "the inescapable, progressive logic of European history."[45] In his handbook to the British empire, W. H. Mercer distinguished two types of colonies, employing the French terminology of *colonies d'exploitation* and *colonies de peuplement.* It is the latter that he dubbed "the true colonies" and it was in them, he predicted, that "the natives are to a great extent, in face of the struggle for predominance, expelled or exterminated."[46] In short, the native is unfit, not up to the tasks associated with white settlement, making her demise unfortunate but irresistible. True colonialism, for Mercer, led to native extinction.

"How many whole races have become extinct," asked James Cowles Prichard, "during the few centuries which have elapsed since the modern system of colonisation commenced?"[47] Canon Tristram said much the same some thirty years later, while working to distinguish "natural" and therefore unavoidable extinction from that precipitated by human neglect, greed, or malice. Too many people, he thought, tacitly accepted that "the decay and extinction of every aboriginal race before the presence of the white man is a necessity, mournful, perhaps, but not the less inevitable."[48] Brantlinger's labeling of extinction discourse as "a specific branch of the dual ideologies of imperialism and racism" makes sense of such utterances.[49] Their biologization, achieved through making progress a factor of heredity, sealed for the Victorians the fate of modern primitives, doomed to die out as progress—the cornerstone of the eugenic ideal—continued on its steady march. Watching European plantings overrun native flora in the colonies, many analogized from plants to humans, the "stronger" stock "weeding out" the weaker. Gardening metaphors would figure strongly in twentieth-century eugenic language; in nineteenth-century extinction discourse, we might recognize their forerunners.

DECADENCE AND DEGENERATION

Yet there was a disturbing possibility that progress might itself prove unstable. While it is certainly the case that nineteenth-century anthropologists operated out of a "salvage motive," hoping to conserve fragments of dying cultures, languages, and societies, conservation also operated in more complex ways.[50] Donna Haraway has argued that "decadence was the threat against which exhibition, conservation, and eugenics were all directed as prophylaxis for an endangered body politic."[51] But what was or ought to be conserved could be a divisive question, and itself raised the prospect of white European degeneration. Was degradation the inability to maintain progress, or was it an inexorable sliding from a higher place? Might the civilized nations praised for their modernity one day slip from the pinnacle? These are questions that haunted eugenicists as much as anthropologists, historians (all of whom were familiar with the fate of the Roman Empire) as much as social theorists. Writing in 1861 in *Blackwood's Edinburgh Magazine,* one commentator admitted that "Many of the things noticeable as characteristics of the savages are found lingering amongst ourselves, either in remote provinces, in uncultivated classes, or in children."[52]

By the close of the nineteenth century, fears of degeneration were widespread in Europe and settler colonies as well as in America, manifested in race-based immigration controls. But such ideas were by no means new. There was, of course, a long-standing biblical version of degeneration theory: the fall from grace. This reading of degeneration was concerned with moral behaviors rather than physical and cultural decline, but it was by no means wholly buried in the new degeneration-ist clamor of the *fin de siècle,* so central to eugenics. Settler colonialism in the eighteenth century had also provoked debate over what changes among settlers—for good or for ill—were attributable to colonization.[53] One of the most potent fears in degeneration theory was of a moral slide, although it was often allied to physical signs of decadence. In a controversial critique of the work of anthropologists Edward Tylor (1832–1917) and John Lubbock (1834–1913), the renegade Catholic scientist St. George Jackson Mivart (1827–1900) declared that post-colonial Spain had undergone "partial regression" and that "no one will probably contest the inferiority, in many respects, of the Greece of our day to that which listened to the voices of Aristotle or Plato."[54] The Italian criminologist Cesare Lombroso (1835–1909) and his followers drew direct links between criminal behavior and physical appearance, in which racial marking was prominent. The modern European criminal was, for this school, a primitive throwback whose appearance, language, and acts indicated a lesser evolution akin to that found in the dying races.[55] Francis Galton, concerned primarily with the problems he thought beset Britain, regarded the welfare aspects of civilization as having disrupted the process of natural selection, producing degeneration. This routing of biology by the social helped him see the possibilities as well as the drawbacks of engineering human as well as animal breeding.

There was no great distance to travel from these assumptions to the fear that Europeans in tropical colonial environments might risk reversion, shedding the refinements and civilities that marked them as modern. This concern, of course, reflected an older anxiety about environment rather than heredity, thus destabilizing not only the twin powers of civilization and colonialism, but the new hereditarian orthodoxy out of which eugenics was born. It harked back to old arguments about whether extinction (a cousin to degeneration) was a consequence of contact or a biological absolute. Was European degeneration the product of bad genes or bad environments? Often, of course, the answer depended on class. Well-born Europeans isolated in hostile tropical environments were victims of a difficult geography, while the poor, on the other hand, came from lesser stock, which they blithely and all too promiscuously passed on.

CLASS, POVERTY, AND FECUNDITY

Implicit in this class distinction was another issue linking eugenics and colonialism. The Malthusian undergirding to these arguments saw the poor as irresponsible breeders, fecund beyond their limited resources and unconcerned at bringing weak or poor stock into the world. A parallel debate feared that settlers and other

Europeans in the colonies would be "swamped" by rapid growth among Asian populations. In 1891 the American suffragist Victoria Woodhull Martin (1838–1927) warned that the "vast hordes" of China and India "may yet overrun and wipe out western civilization."[56] Commentators conjured up visions of a world in which white Europeans were heavily outnumbered, a constant theme in twentieth-century discussions of population control. Books such as Étienne Dennery's (1903–1979) 1931 treatise (quickly translated into English), *Asia's Teeming Millions: And Its Problems for the West,* fed fears of the impact of Asian population growth on Western prowess and prosperity. Madison Grant's (1865–1937) *The Passing of The Great Race* (1916), with its prediction that new and inferior immigrants would breed faster than America's elite, was typical of this fare. In a 1907 book on the *Asiatic Danger in the Colonies,* South African L. E. Neame was clear that:

> An influx of Asiatics inevitably means first a lowering of the standard of living for the white worker, and then his gradual elimination; it means that the country becomes of no value to the empire as a home for the surplus population of the United Kingdom, and in the end it means that it becomes a diminished commercial asset, and a greater strain upon the defensive forces of England.[57]

His ideas followed those of James Bryce (1838–1922), the liberal explorer, historian, and foe of slavery, who noted in his *Impressions of South Africa,* first published in 1897, that "Kaffirs were fast increasing and would swamp the whites," even while the dying races (in this case Bushmen and Hottentots) were rapidly waning in number.[58] In white settler colonies these concerns precipitated immigration restrictions: laws in New Zealand between 1899 and 1908, in Australia (1901), and in Canada (1910) were designed to exclude populations regarded as overly fecund, as was America's 1924 Immigration Restriction Act. In these enactments the hand of eugenics is not hard to discern. It was a common Malthusian-derived eugenic belief that "inferior" races bred at a higher rate than their betters.[59] The assimilationist policies of mid-twentieth-century Australia were prompted in part by fears that in remote parts of the country, children of mixed Aboriginal and European parentage, known as half-castes, would outnumber white settlers.[60] The removal of part-aboriginal children from their natal families ensured, among other things, that this threat could be countered.

MISCEGENATION

The Australian approach of "breeding out" Aboriginality—often known as breeding out the color—was a radical one, to be sure. Far more common was a fear of mixed-race coupling focused on a belief that offspring would inherit only the worst parental traits, a view picked up by eugenicists concerned with bad stock being passed on. The Societé d'Anthropologie de Paris created a commission "for the Study of Métis" in 1907, which sent questionnaires to colonists inviting their observation of mixed-race progeny.[61] This was an arena where the conflict between hereditary and environmental theory was clear. Brazilian scientists argued that miscegenation was vital to white survival in the tropics, whites acquiring through such liaisons resistance to harsh climatic conditions.[62] Australian politician J. Mildred Creed (1842–1930) thought it "natural" that Aboriginal Australians would mingle most with the "lowest whites," but strenuously insisted that in more cultivated environments, they could "rise" above such influences.[63] A. O. Neville, architect of the child-removal programs in Western Australia, agreed, arguing that "the more they mix with us the more like us they become, the less the likelihood of reversion to the aboriginal type."[64] Neville was unusual in prescribing intermarriage as a solution, since the suspicion that miscegenation would either result in weaker, more vicious offspring, or in sterility was more common. Nineteenth-century polygenists, in particular, wedded to the notion that there were different species of humans, assumed "hybrids" would be weaker and less fertile, even becoming infertile in a third generation. Interracial (or as the polygenists would have it, inter-species) breeding could thus be deployed either to predict over-population on the part of the undesirable, or its effective opposite, a waning of fertility. Neither scenario was reassuring for those who hewed to a degenerationist framework in which the key question centered inevitably on whether all populations were ultimately vulnerable to decline. The newly repopularized notion of cyclical history invoked by scholars such as Arnold Toynbee implied that decay would occur—and naturally—in time. The growing use of birth control among more affluent Britons toward the end of the nineteenth century, like the dip in the French birthrate in the same period, fueled both eugenic policy and the related belief that the declining middle-class birthrate signaled the beginning of the end for Western civilization. Arthur de Gobineau (1816–1882) had made similar arguments in France in the 1850s, fearing that debased bloodlines caused by "blending" would sap racial vitality.[65] Gobineau linked degeneration to extinction. The *dégénéré* "whose value has been gradually modified by successive blending...shall definitely perish, and his civilisation with him."[66] Such fatalism lay at the root of the appointment in Britain of the 1904 Committee on Physical Deterioration, prompted by fears that receding working-class vitality would leave Britain without a military bulwark for the defense of empire.

A parallel anxiety questioned whether whites could survive or prosper in tropical environments. This latter concern encompassed both alarm that neurasthenia would engulf those posted to the tropics, and a concern that white laborers might not be able to withstand tropical conditions.[67] The enthusiasm for healthy climates that would stimulate human as well as agricultural productivity was, by the late nineteenth century, matched by widespread skepticism that tropical lassitude could be overcome. Closely related to fears of degeneration "at home," these misgivings left no clear division between environment and heredity, but they palpably led to a pessimistic assessment of the future of both civilization and of colonialism. If tropical climates catalyzed degeneration, or even more alarmingly, if some peoples could degenerate or fail to progress, did that signal a potentially similar fate for all humans? The experimental genetics of the 1890s and early 1900s made the possibility of reversion to an earlier type plausible, even likely, and while much of this work (as was so for Weismann and Mendel) was focused on plant inheritance, there were always social theorists eager to translate modestly conceived and experimental findings into a broader and human application. Progress and regression or degeneration, then, were cut from the same conceptual cloth, at least in the popular imagination.

SEXUAL DIFFERENCE

In this haunting fear of regression we can also discern the centrality of sexual difference. It was a widespread scientific maxim of the nineteenth century that differences between men and women were a mark of progress and that their greater differentiation separated the primitive from the civilized. Darwin suspected that gender equality might itself give rise to regression, and that evolution necessarily produced male superiority.[68] The influential American palaeontologist Alpheus Hyatt (1838–1902) warned that sexual equality, which he represented as the feminization of men and the emasculation of women, would indicate that humans had "entered upon the retrogressive period of their evolution."[69] Luke Owen Pike (1835–1915), known primarily as a legal historian, warned that encouraging intellectualism in women spelled humanity's extinction: it represented "neither more nor less than the abolition of motherhood."[70] It was Herbert Spencer's (1820–1903) conviction that the conservation of her energies for reproduction necessarily arrested a woman's development in other areas.[71] Inequality, in these terms, was a law of nature, as biologist George Romanes (1848–1894) asserted in 1887.[72] The argument was similar to that claimed for the allegedly biological differences between the savage and the civilized, and another element tying these together (as much for some eugenic constituencies as for nineteenth-century biologists and anthropologists) was the association of women *with* primitivity. McGrigor Allan saw menstruation as proof that women were closer to the "lower" animals and primitive men, while the craniometrists found as much significance in women's smaller cranial capacity as they had in the skulls of non-white men.[73] In the third of his *Lectures on Man,* published in English in 1864, Swiss scientist Carl Vogt (1817–1895) asserted that the "female skull approaches, in many respects, that of the infant, and in a still greater degree that of the lower races."[74] Women's brains were likened to those of children as well as of "primitive" peoples, tempting Thomas Huxley into declaring that the majority of women, "will stop in the doll stage of evolution to be…the drag on the civilisation."[75] Women were not merely, by these lights, possessed of lesser cranial capacity and therefore a less deep intelligence, but like savages, they were also by nature less attuned to and appreciative of the benefits of progress. It was a suspicion that science often bolstered. For Lombroso, women demonstrated an atavism seen also in savages.[76] Vogt thought women insusceptible to radical change.[77] Here was the "angel in the house" garbed in the cloak of neutral science.

DIFFERENCE AND EUGENICS

This insistence that difference was both a biological fact and vital to humanity's future looked back to the simultaneous attention to the differences said to define the primitive and the civilized. "Lower races represented the 'female' type of the human species, and females the 'lower races' of gender."[78] It was a perfect recipe, too, for imperial justification: "male genius was synonymous with British civilization, which depended heavily on the establishment of the empire of science, if not of empire itself."[79] And this was surely the same set of principles that would motivate eugenics as the nineteenth century came to a close. The perpetuation of an imperially fit nation of British men preoccupied Galton, his best-known follower Karl Pearson (1857–1936), and most of the prominent eugenicists of the first decades of the twentieth century. Galton's early work on hereditary genius and Pearson's meticulous statistical studies of the Jewish child set out to reveal which populations should be encouraged to breed and thrive.[80] While the new biometrics of the twentieth century brought statistical rigor to these ideas, they still owed much to an earlier tradition of anthropometrics and anthropology born both of the new scientific practices of the nineteenth century and of the colonial endeavor. In the early twentieth century, the potent brew that brought together evolution, eugenics, and empire prescribed lessons in maternalism for the faulty working-class mother and improved medical services for her sons—the potential foot-soldiers of empire—and encouraged the eugenically fit of the motherland to breed, and to breed carefully and well.

CONCLUSION

We can see, then, much the same vocabulary as well as thinking animating the anthropological concerns of the nineteenth century, and still at work in the practice and policies of eugenics in the early years of the twentieth century. Whether one looks at the biometric or the Mendelian eugenicists, the stress on hereditary fitness was crucial. It was fitness and betterment—especially racial betterment—that lay at the heart of eugenic thinking, a philosophy and practice that combined an earlier optimism in science as progress with a later nineteenth-century pessimism around degeneration. The existence of the latter helped push the prospect of the former into the limelight, most especially in an era of high and even hysterical imperialism. And the years between the Berlin Congress in the 1880s and World War I were

among the most tense and aggressive eras of colonial rivalry and tension. The culmination of scientific growth and imperial expansion certainly created a receptive
climate for culturing eugenic ideas. Martin Fichman argues that science in Britain
enjoyed considerable "cultural and institutional security" in the later years of the
nineteenth century, at a point when the British empire seemed unassailable in its
preeminence.[81] Making the case for eugenics late in his life, Galton saw eugenic
practice as enabling the "race" to "be better fitted to fulfil our vast imperial
opportunities."[82] It was a clear statement of intent, of destiny, and of desire, and
only five years later it was echoed in the words of the ardent eugenicist Caleb Saleeby
(1878–1940), who proclaimed that eugenics was the path to rebuilding "the living
foundations of empire."[83]

Nancy Stepan has argued that Galton "linked race and eugenics from the first,"
but his ability to do so was fostered in a climate suffused with notions of European
imperial superiority bolstered by a growingly confident scientific establishment, at
the core of which was a wide-ranging biology of humanity in which the measurement
and scaling of difference played a devastating central role.[84] Colonialism twinned
with the new methods and presumptions of anthropology and evolutionary biology
provided a vigorous environment for the growth of eugenic principles.

NOTES

1. For a discussion of the distinction between anthropology and ethnology, see
Michael T. Bravo, "Ethnological Encounters," in *Cultures of Natural History*, eds. Nicholas
Jardine, James A. Secord, and E. C. Spary (Cambridge: Cambridge University Press, 1996),
338–357.

2. Patrick Brantlinger, *Dark Vanishings. Discourse on the Extinction of Primitive Races,
1800–1930* (Ithaca, NY: Cornell University Press, 2003), 5; Henrika Kuklick, "Introduction,"
in *A New History of Anthropology*, ed. Henrika Kuklick (Malden and Oxford: Blackwell,
2008), 5.

3. Thomas Henry Huxley, *Critiques and Addresses* (London: Macmillan, 1873), 134
[original emphasis]. See also George W. Stocking, "What's in a Name? The Origins of the
Royal Anthropological Institute," *Man* 6, no. 3 (1971): 374.

4. Nicholas Thomas, *Colonialism's Culture: Anthropology, Travel and Government*
(Princeton, NJ: Princeton University Press, 1994), 6.

5. Andrew Bank, "Losing Faith in the Civilizing Mission: The Premature Decline of
Humanitarian Liberalism at the Cape, 1840–1860," in *Empire and Others: British Encounters
with Indigenous Peoples, 1600–1850*, ed. Martin Daunton and Rick Halpern (Philadelphia,
PA: University of Pennsylvania Press, 1999), 365.

6. George Stocking, *Race, Culture and Evolution: Essays in the History of Anthropology*
(New York and London: The Free Press, 1968), 44–45. While in Britain monogenists
remained largely dominant, many German scientists favored polygenist theories. See
Henretta Trent Band, "Nineteenth Century Arguments on Mankind and Polygenesis and
Definition of Species in Darwin's 1859 *Origin of Species*," *Michigan Academician* 31, no. 3
(1999): 351–353. Blair G. Nelson argues that it was in America that polygenesis was most

favorably received: "'Men before Adam!': American Debates over the Unity and Antiquity of Humanity," in *When Science and Christianity Meet,* eds. David C. Lindberg and Ronald L. Numbers (Chicago, IL: University of Chicago Press, 2003), 166.

7. Patrick Harries, "Anthropology," in *Missions and Empire,* ed. Norman Etherington (Oxford: Oxford University Press, 2005), 246; James R. Ryan, *Picturing Empire: Photography and the Visualization of the British Empire* (Chicago, IL: University of Chicago Press, 1997), 151.

8. A. C. Haddon, "President's Address. Anthropology, Its Position and Needs," *Journal of the Anthropological Institute of Great Britain and Ireland* 33 (Jan–Jun 1903): 20.

9. Harries, "Anthropology," 245.

10. Donna Haraway, *The Haraway Reader* (London and New York: Routledge, 2004), 144. See also Stocking, *Race, Culture and Evolution,* 234.

11. James Cowles Prichard, *On the Extinction of Human Races* (London: Aborigines Protection Society, 1839), 3.

12. Olive P. Dickason, "The Concept of *L'Homme Sauvage* and Early French Colonialism in the Americas," *Revue Francaise d'Histoire d'outre-mer* 64, no. 234 (1977): 30.

13. Ibid., 8.

14. Réal Ouellet and Mylene Tremblay, "From the Good Savage to the Degenerate Indian: The Amerindian in the Accounts of Travel to America," in *Decentring the Renaissance. Canada and Europe in Multidisciplinary Perspective, 1500–1700,* eds. Germaine Warkentin and Carolyn Podruchny (Toronto: University of Toronto Press, 2001), 159–170. In *The Spirit of the Law* (1748; Cambridge: Cambridge University Press, 1989), Montesquieu distinguished between the "savage" and the "barbarian," the former being hunters and the latter pastoral peoples. See too Bruce Buchan, "The Empire of Political Thought: Civilization, Savagery and Perceptions of Indigenous Government," *History of the Human Sciences* 18, no. 2 (2005): 8–10.

15. Ian Duncan, "Darwin and the Savages," *Yale Journal of Criticism* 4, no. 2 (1991): 14. See too Mathias Georg Guenther, "From 'Brutal Savages' to 'Harmless People:' Notes on the Changing Western Image of the Bushmen," *Paideuma* 26 (1980): 125–127.

16. Matthew Day, "Godless Savages and Superstitious Dogs: Charles Darwin, Imperial Ethnography, and the Problem of Human Uniqueness," *Journal of the History of Ideas* 69, no. 1 (2008): 49–70.

17. Richard Lee, "The Extinction of Races," *Journal of the Anthropological Society of London* 2 (1864), xcviii.

18. Grant Allen, "The Recipe for Genius," *Cornhill Magazine* 5, new series (October 1885): 408, 410–411.

19. Alexander Grant, "Philosophy and Mr. Darwin," *Contemporary Review* 17 (1871): 281.

20. Charles Darwin, *The Descent of Man and Selection in Relation to Sex,* 2nd ed. (1879; London: Penguin Books, 2004), 203.

21. Nicholas Hudson, "From 'Nation' to 'Race': The Origin of Racial Classification in Eighteenth-Century Thought," *Eighteenth-Century Studies* 29, no. 3 (1996): 249.

22. For example, Stephen G. Alter, "Race, Language, and Mental Evolution in Darwin's *Descent of Man,*" *Journal of the History of the Behavioral Sciences* 43, no. 3. (2007): 239–255; Duncan, "Darwin and the Savages," Cannon Schmitt, "Darwin's Savage Mnemonics," *Representations* 88 (2004): 55–80. See also Huxley, *Critiques and Addresses,* 163; Peter J. Bowler, "From 'Savage' to 'Primitive:' Victorian Evolutionism and the Interpretation of Marginalized Peoples," *Antiquity* 66 (1992): 721–729; Stocking, *Race, Culture and Evolution,* 46; Nancy Leys Stepan, *The Idea of Race in Science: Great Britain, 1800–1960* (Hamden, CT:

Archon Books, 1982), 85. As Thomas Glick has noted, Darwin rejected polygenesis but embraced recapitulation, a theory that easily allowed for critical distinctions between primitives and moderns, even if they lived at the same time. Thomas F. Glick, "The Anthropology of Race across the Darwinian Revolution," in Kuklick, *A New History of Anthropology,* 240.

23. Haddon, "President's Address," 22.

24. A. O. Neville, *Australia's Coloured Minority: Its Place in the Community* (Sydney: Currawong Publishing, 1947), 26.

25. James Hunt, "Address Delivered at the Third Anniversary Meeting of the Anthropological Society of London," *Journal of the Anthropological Society of London* 4 (1866), lxxviii; Alfred A. Grace, *Tales of a Dying Race* (London: Chatto & Windus, 1901), v–vi.

26. Matt Matsuda, "In the Revolutionary Garden: Memories of Savages and Civilization," *Historical Journal* 22, no. 2 (1996): 317.

27. Canon Tristram, "Mr. Wallace on the Conservation of Native Races," *Contemporary Review* 16 (1871): 546.

28. Bowler, "From 'Savage' to 'Primitive,'" 724–725. See also Adrian Desmond and James Moore, *Darwin's Sacred Cause: Race, Slavery and the Quest for Human Origins* (London: Allen Lane, 2009).

29. Charles Hursthouse, *New Zealand, or Zealandia, the Britain of the South,* 2 vols. (London: Edward Stanford, 1857), 1: 159–160. Quoted in Toeolesulusulu Damon Salesa, "'The Power of the Physician:' Doctors and the 'Dying Maori' in Early Colonial New Zealand," *Health and History* 3 (2001): 20.

30. Mathew Thomson, "'Savage Civilisation': Race, Culture and Mind in Britain, 1898–1939," in *Race, Science and Medicine, 1700–1960,* eds. Waltraud Ernst and Bernard Harris (London: Routledge, 1999), 241–242. It is perhaps not insignificant that Seligman had been a member of the team who had traveled in 1898 to the Torres Straits to conduct some of the earliest major field work in British anthropology.

31. Francis Galton, *Address to the Anthropological Department of the British Association, Plymouth, 1877* (London: William Clowes and Son), 13.

32. See especially Brantlinger, *Dark Vanishings*; and Russell McGregor, *Imagined Destinies: Aboriginal Australians and the Doomed Race Theory, 1880–1939* (Carlton: Melbourne University Press, 1997)for modern interpretations.

33. Fiona J. Stafford, *The Last of the Race: The Growth of a Myth from Milton to Darwin* (Oxford: Clarendon Press, 1994), 134.

34. Anon, "On Aboriginal Savage Races of Men," *Popular Magazine of Anthropology* 1, no. 2 (April 1866): 50. Ellipsis in original.

35. Brantlinger, *Dark Vanishings*, 22.

36. Darwin, *Descent of Man*, 153, 212.

37. Duncan, "Darwin and the Savages," 35.

38. Grace, *Tales of a Dying Race*, vii.

39. "Gass's Voyages and Travels," *Quarterly Review* 1 (1809): 293.

40. Quoted in Bank, "Losing Faith in the Civilizing Mission," 370.

41. J. E. Calder, "Some Account of the Wars of Extirpation and Habits of the Native Tribes of Tasmania," n.p., n.d., bound into Volume 14 (Tract no. 9) of the *Tracts Relating to the Science of Man*, formerly the collection of A. H. L. F. Pitt-Rivers, now held at the Haddon Library, University of Cambridge, 7; 14.

42. McGregor, *Imagined Destinies*, 48.

43. Tony Barta, "Mr. Darwin's Shooters: On Natural Selection and the Naturalizing of Genocide," *Patterns of Prejudice* 39, no. 2 (2005): 127; Roy MacLeod and Philip F. Rehbock,

"Introduction," in *Darwin's Laboratory: Evolutionary Theory and Natural History in the Pacific*, eds. Roy MacLeod and Philip F. Rehbock (Honolulu, HI: University of Hawaii Press, 1994), 12–13.

44. Bowler, "From 'Savage' to 'Primitive,'" 726.

45. Matsuda, "In the Revolutionary Garden," 316.

46. W. H. Mercer, *A Handbook of the British Colonial Empire* (London: Waterlow & Sons, 1906), 2.

47. Bowler, *On the Extinction of Races*, 3.

48. Tristram, "Mr. Wallace," 536.

49. Brantlinger, *Dark Vanishings*, 1.

50. Ryan, *Picturing Empire*, 149–150; Kuklick, *A New History of Anthropology*, 5

51. Donna Haraway, "Teddy Bear Patriarchy: Taxidermy in the Garden of Eden, New York City, 1908–1936," in Haraway, *The Haraway Reader*, 187.

52. "Uncivilised Man," *Blackwood's Edinburgh Magazine* 89 (1861): 39.

53. Jonathan Lamb, "Metamorphosis and Settlement: The Enlightened Anthropology of Colonial Societies," in *The Anthropology of the Enlightenment*, eds. Larry Wolff and Marco Cipolloni (Stanford, CA: Stanford University Press, 2007), 281–282.

54. St. George Mivart, "The Descent of Man," *Quarterly Review* 131 (1871): 65.

55. For a useful discussion of this, see David G. Horn, "The Norm Which Is Not One: Reading the Female Body in Lombroso's Anthropology," in *Deviant Bodies: Critical Perspectives on Difference in Science and Popular Culture*, eds. Jennifer Terry and Jacqueline Urla (Bloomington, IN: Indiana University Press, 1995), 109–128 and Daniel Pick, *Faces of Degeneration: A European Disorder, c. 1848–1918* (Cambridge: Cambridge University Press, 1989).

56. Victoria C. Woodhull Martin, *The Rapid Multiplication of the Unfit* (New York: The Women's Anthropological Society of America, 1891), 19.

57. L. E. Neame, *The Asiatic Danger in the Colonies* (London: George Routledge and Sons, 1907), 107.

58. James Bryce, *Impressions of South Africa* (London: Macmillan, 1897), 71.

59. David M. Levy and Sandra J. Peart, "Statistical Prejudice: From Eugenics to Immigrants," *European Journal of Political Economy* 20, no. 1 (2004): 18.

60. Heidi Zogbaum, "Herbert Basedow and the Removal of Aboriginal Children of Mixed Descent from their Families," *Australian Historical Studies* 34, no. 121 (2003): 127.

61. Claude Blanckaert, "Of Monstrous Métis? Hybridity, Fear of Miscegenation, and Patriotism from Buffon to Paul Broca," in *The Color of Liberty: Histories of Race in France*, eds. Sue Peabody and Tyler Stovall (Durham, NC: Duke University Press, 2003), 42.

62. Glick, "The Anthropology of Race," 240.

63. J. Mildred Creed, "The Position of the Australian Aborigines in the Scale of Human Intelligence," *The Nineteenth Century and After* 57, no. 325 (1905): 89.

64. Neville, *Australia's Coloured Minority*, 63, 57.

65. Matsuda, "Revolutionary Garden," 314.

66. Arthur de Gobineau, *Essai sur l'inégalité des races humaines* (Paris, 1853–1855), quoted in Sean Quinlan, "The Racial Imagery of Degeneration and Depopulation: Georges Vacher de Lapouge and 'Anthroposociology' in Fin-de-Siècle France," *History of European Ideas* 24, no. 6 (1998): 58–59.

67. Warwick H. Anderson, *The Cultivation of Whiteness: Science, Health and Racial Destiny in Australia* (Carlton: Melbourne University Press, 2002), part 2; Alison Bashford, *Imperial Hygiene: A Critical History of Colonialism, Nationalism and Public Health* (Basingstoke: Palgrave, 2004), chap. 6.

68. Darwin, *Descent of Man*, esp. 630.

69. Alpheus Hyatt, "The Influence of Woman in the Evolution of the Human Race," *Natural Science* 11 (August 1897): 91.

70. Luke Owen Pike, "On the Claims of Women to Political Power," *Journal of the Anthropological Society of London* 7 (1869): liv.

71. Herbert Spencer, *The Study of Sociology*, quoted in Susan Sleeth Mosedale, "Science Corrupted: Victorian Biologists Consider 'The Woman Question,'" *Journal of the History of Biology* 11, no. 1 (1978): 10.

72. George J. Romanes, "Mental Differences between Men and Women," *The Nineteenth Century* 21 (1887): 664.

73. Allan, "On the Real Difference in the Minds of Men and Women," cxcvii; Evelleen Richards, "Huxley and Woman's Place in Science: The 'Woman Question' and the Control of Victorian Anthropology," in *History, Humanity and Evolution: Essays for John C. Greene*, ed. James R. Moore (Cambridge: Cambridge University Press, 1989), 264–265; Nancy Leys Stepan, "Race and Gender: The Role of Analogy in Science," *Isis* 77 (1976): 269.

74. Carl Vogt, *Lectures on Man: His Place in Creation, and in the History of the Earth*, ed. James Hunt (London: Longman, Green, Longman and Roberts, 1864), 81.

75. Leonard Huxley, *Life and Letters of Thomas Henry Huxley*, 2 vols. (London: Macmillan, 1900), 1: 212.

76. Horn, "The Norm Which Is Not One," 115–117.

77. Vogt, *Lectures on Man*, 82; and see Richards, "Huxley," 266.

78. Stepan, "Race and Gender," 264.

79. Flavia Alaya, "Victorian Science and the 'Genius' of Women," *Journal of the History of Ideas* 38, no. 2 (1977): 268.

80. Francis Galton, *Hereditary Genius: An Inquiry into Its Laws and Consequences* (London: Macmillan, 1869); Karl Pearson and Margaret Moul, "The Problem of Alien Immigration into Great Britain, Illustrated by an Examination of Russian and Polish Jewish Children," *Annals of Eugenics* 1 (1925): 5–55, 56–127.

81. Martin Fichman, "Biology and Politics: Defining the Boundaries," in *Victorian Science in Context*, ed. Bernard Lightman (Chicago, IL: University of Chicago Press, 1997), 100.

82. Francis Galton, "Eugenics: Its Definition, Scope, and Aims," *American Journal of Sociology* 10, no. 1 (July 1904): 3.

83. Caleb Williams Saleeby, *Parenthood and Race Culture: An Outline of Eugenics* (London: Cassell, 1909), 34.

84. Stepan, *The Idea of Race in Science*, 126.

FURTHER READING

Bowler, Peter J. "From 'Savage' to 'Primitive': Victorian Evolutionism and the Interpretation of Marginalized Peoples," *Antiquity* 66, no. 252 (1992): 721–729.

Brantlinger, Patrick. *Dark Vanishings: Discourse on the Extinction of Primitive Races, 1800–1930* (Ithaca, NY: Cornell University Press, 2003).

McGregor, Russell. *Imagined Destinies: Aboriginal Australians and the Doomed Race Theory, 1880–1939* (Carlton: Melbourne University Press, 1997).

Pick, Daniel. *Faces of Degeneration. A European Disorder, c. 1848–1918* (Cambridge: Cambridge University Press, 1989).

Prichard, James Cowles. *On the Extinction of Human Races* (London: Aborigines Protection Society, 1839).

Stafford, Fiona J. *The Last of the Race: The Growth of a Myth from Milton to Darwin* (Oxford: Clarendon Press, 1994).

Stepan, Nancy Leys. *The Idea of Race in Science: Great Britain, 1800–1960* (Hamden, CT: Archon Books, 1982).

Stocking, George. *Race, Culture and Evolution: Essays in the History of Anthropology* (New York and London: The Free Press, 1968).

CHAPTER 3

RACE, SCIENCE, AND EUGENICS IN THE TWENTIETH CENTURY

MARIUS TURDA

To say that race is central to eugenics is no exaggeration. Even a cursory review of the most important scholarly analyses of eugenics makes this abundantly clear.[1] Race, along with class and gender,[2] is considered by many scholars to be an essential component of the ever-changing matrix of eugenic thinking and its associated politics. Already in 1963, in one of the first sustained scholarly efforts to introduce the history of eugenics to the general public, Mark Haller devoted an entire chapter to the relationship between eugenics and race. Haller believed that "a mutual attraction brought on the marriage of racism with eugenics,"[3] basing his interpretation on the involvement of eugenicists in debates on immigration and miscegenation in the United States, and by highlighting the work of authors like Madison Grant and Harry Hamilton Laughlin in particular. More nuanced interpretations of American eugenics have since been proposed,[4] yet the view persists that American eugenicists were, by and large, racist. This association of race and eugenics is by no means confined to the American case. Discussing eugenics in South Africa, Saul Dubow remarked that, at least partially, "eugenics reflected a triumphant confidence in the superiority of the Anglo-Saxon race."[5] Chloe Campbell, writing about colonial Kenya, similarly argued that "eugenics emerged at a time when racist thinking was becoming increasingly dominant: the language of race abounded in eugenic discourse."[6] While acknowledging that British eugenicists "may not have been especially preoccupied with race," Campbell nevertheless insists that eugenics "supplied the basis for a scientific justification of racist thought."[7] Another scholar, Stefan Kühl, in his discussion of German and American eugenic movements, proposed the term "eugenic racism" to refer to those eugenicists who accepted "a genetic under-standing of race. Race, in this view is regarded as unity of procreation, preservation, and development. It is an attempt to define group cohesion biologically, but without referring to a fixed typology of qualitative differences."[8]

These interpretations, relevant as they are in many respects, are too broad to reflect accurately the many nuances and complex relationships that connected race and eugenics. Undoubtedly, although numerous eugenicists were racists, eugenics as such was not necessarily a racist movement: indeed, arguing that eugenics was "racist" tells us very little.[9] In this chapter, I chart some of the coordinates of that ever-changing matrix of eugenic thinking and its associated racial component.

The idea of race played a seminal and decisive role in the ideological growth of eugenics during the late nineteenth and the first half of the twentieth centuries. To use Stephen Jay Gould's expression, eugenics was in many ways a form of "biological determinism" presupposing that "shared behavioral norms, and the social and economic differences between human groups—primarily races, classes, and sexes—arise from inherited, inborn distinctions and that society, in this sense, is an accurate reflection of biology."[10] To understand the affinities between traditions and practices of race and eugenics one hence needs to concentrate on the myriad interfaces between scientific and political forces across national borders, as well as to explore the histor-ical usage of the term "race" by the eugenicists, hermeneutically and conceptually. In this way a careful investigation of the relationship between race and eugenics and, above all, the scientific privileges ascribed to them, suggest the need for a more subtle and comparative understanding of eugenic and racial terminology.

Paul Weindling, in his thoughtful and provocative history of German eugenics, advised against a simplified understanding of eugenics, urging scholars to "tran-scend the limitations of the conventional history of German racism."[11] Without dis-cussing primary eugenic texts one cannot fully grasp the host of conflicts that existed between local and international eugenic traditions and technologies of race. In this chapter, therefore, I aim to go beyond the existing scholarship on eugenics and to point out the complex intertwining of visions of racial improvement with eugenic hybrids during the twentieth century. By considering how prominent European and American eugenicists expressed ideas about race and science from the late nineteenth century onward, this epistemologically oriented approach engages critically with those lines of reasoning that, after 1945, depicted eugenics as "pseudo-science,"[12] as a form of "reactionary bourgeois irrationalism,"[13] unworthy of the same critical hermeneutics applied to other disciplines in the social sciences and the humanities. As Lene Koch perceptively argued, "eugenics as such should not be dismissed as an unscientific, amateurish activity."[14] This recent scholarship appropriately evaluates the degree and nature of conceptual transfers of eugenic knowledge and ideas and addresses eugenics' key components as they were formu-lated on the basis of a comparative analysis of various authors. Such an approach also necessitates testing the value of eugenic interpretative models linked to notions such as race. Ultimately, by offering an insight into the convoluted relationship bet-ween race and eugenics, I not only hope to shed light on how eugenics functioned in and as part of other scientific disciplines,[15] but also to contribute to the increasingly polarized current discussion about what Jean Gayon and Daniel Jacobi have inspiringly termed the "eternal return of eugenics."[16]

EUGENICS AND RACIAL HYGIENE

In his 1883 *Inquiries into Human Faculty and Its Development,* Francis Galton (1822–1911) engaged with "various topics more or less connected with that of the cultivation of the race, or, as we may call it, with 'eugenic' questions."[17] He defined eugenics as "the science of improving the stock, which is by no means confined to questions of judicious mating, but which especially in the case of man, takes cognisance of all influences that tend in however remote a degree to give to the more suitable races or strains of blood a better chance of prevailing speedily over the less suitable than they otherwise would have had."[18] Although he would use the term "race" in abundance, Galton did not define it explicitly, but it was understood biologically, as a community of people sharing similar physiological and psychological characteristics transmitted from generation to generation. "Race" was used to refer to a complex amalgam of biological factors determined by heredity and determining the close bond between the individual and the society at large.

Other eugenicists in Europe and the United States followed a similar hereditarian and biological understanding of race. In his 1895 *Grundlinien einer Rassen-Hygiene* (The Foundations of Racial Hygiene) Alfred Ploetz (1860–1940), the founder of the German eugenic movement, shifted the focus of eugenics from a preoccupation with the individual's inherited qualities to those of the broader national community.[19] If for Galton the improvement of the race was a prerequisite for the success of eugenics, for Ploetz it was the most important goal of eugenics: "Race hygiene treats the sum of the most favourable conditions for the preservation and development of our race."[20] Yet the divergence between his understanding of eugenics and that of Galton's were not as significant as one may assume.[21] Writing in 1924, the German geneticist Fritz Lenz (1887–1976) claimed that Ploetz, although conversant with the work of Darwin, Wallace, and Haeckel, was not familiar with "Galton's pioneering work."[22] Lenz claimed that, as "the word 'eugenics' was unknown" to Ploetz when he wrote his 1895 book, "he gave the name of 'Rassenhygiene' to the study of the best conditions for the maintenance and development of the race. The word means exactly the same as the word 'eugenics' which Galton introduced." As a consequence, Lenz argued, 'Rassenhygiene' "is therefore best translated into English not [as] 'race hygiene,' as seems to be customary, but simply 'eugenics.' "[23]

It was after launching the *Journal of Social and Racial Biology* in 1904 that Ploetz became interested in Galton's work. One of Galton's articles on eugenics was translated and published in the *Journal* in 1905, and Ploetz expressed his hope that Galton—described in one letter as "the senior of the practical application of the principles of evolution on man"—would find the time, "in an hour of leisure" to read his work and write him his "cool judgment." Referring to his 1895 book, Ploetz remarked candidly that it was "written mostly in a small town, where I practiced as a physician, absent from a good library and therefore without much knowledge of current literature" on eugenics. More importantly, Ploetz described his choice of terminology to Galton: "I started from an English use of the word 'race' and tried to investigate the conditions of preserving and developing a race-hygiene ('Rassen-hygiene'). Afterwards, in the first introducing [sic] article of our *Archiv,* I tried to sharpen the meaning of the word 'race,' so as to make it suitable for the theoretical and practical needs of a man, who will seize the real *long* (beyond the individuals) lasting unities of life, their conditions of preservations [sic] and development."[24] The Hungarian eugenicist István Apáthy (1863–1922) put forward a similar perspective: "Racial hygiene (*fajegészségtana*) is practically what Galton means by *Eugenics.*"[25]

Race, according to these authors, broadened the social and national sphere considered worthy of eugenic intervention.[26] Going beyond the stylized idea of a "racial-soul" (*Rassenseele*), which was fashionable in Germany at that time due to the popularity of the works of Houston Stewart Chamberlain,[27] and its neo-classicized version popularized by Ludwig Woltmann, Ploetz and Apáthy conceptualized race as both something singular—an ethnic group displaying similar physical and mental traits—and universal—humanity. Contrary to Apáthy's view, Ploetz's idea of eugenics, however, was fittingly ornamented with cultural representations of the "Aryan" race long popular in German thinking: "The hygiene of the entire human race converges with that of the Aryan race, which apart from a few small races, like the Jewish race—itself quite probably overwhelmingly Aryan in composition—is the cultural race *par excellence.* To advance it is tantamount to the advancement of all humanity."[28]

Ploetz endeavored to establish racial hygiene as a discipline in its own right, rather than being a mere subdiscipline of social hygiene, as the influential social hygienist Alfred Grotjahn (1869–1931) had maintained.[29] Racial hygiene, according to Ploetz, was exclusively concerned with the hereditary qualities of the population, and its aims were twofold: to both increase and further those hereditarily "superior" individuals, and to decrease—if elimination was not possible—those considered racially undesirable. Contrary to social hygiene, which focused on the protection of *existing* hereditary qualities, eugenics was *future* oriented as its driving force was toward building a new racial community.[30]

Ploetz and other German racial hygienists' approach to eugenics was rarely very different than that adopted by British, American, or Scandinavian authors: there was a general theoretical consensus within the international eugenic community. An exception was Wilhelm Schallmayer (1857–1919) and his revolt against the usage of race in the definition of eugenics.[31] In 1931, the German Society for Racial Hygiene even added "Eugenik" (Eugenics) to its official name, indicating—in the words of the Catholic eugenicist and head of the Kaiser Wilhelm Institute for Anthropology, Human Heredity, and Eugenics during the 1930s, Hermann Muckermann (1877–1962)—the return to "the historical line" of the movement, namely the "non-Aryan-supremacist eugenics movement."[32] Sheila

Weiss interprets this change of terminology as crucial to the international acceptance of German racial hygiene during the last years of the Weimar republic. "Had the Nazis not forced a drastic change in course in 1933," she argued, "there is every reason to believe that [the German eugenic] movement would have become even more similar to its counterpart in Britain."[33] In 1934, illustrating these political changes, Fritz Lenz eliminated *Eugenik* from the society's official name and reverted to the old name, *German Society for Racial Hygiene.*

THE EUGENIC LANGUAGE OF RACE

Notwithstanding these debates over terminology, the fundamental reality was that eugenics was born into a period when European and American societies thought in terms of racial categories, and believed in the existence of "superior" and "inferior" races.[34] After World War I, eugenics intensified its racial content, accentuating its ambition to reconfigure the national community according to hereditarian programs based on the biological selection of valuable racial elements.

Most eugenic and anthropological texts written between 1900 and 1945 understand race as both a physical entity—described by one anthropologist as being the "sum-total of somatological characteristics"[35]—and a cultural artifact, the result of specific historical conditions.[36] The German eugenicist Hermann W. Siemens (1891–1969), for example, offered a two-pronged definition of race. There was a "system race: a subdivision of a species in a natural-science system" and a "vital race: the super-individual unit of continuing life, which is represented by a circle of similar individuals who live in sexual commerce with one another; the body of the people continuously living on."[37] There was no consensus on what actually constituted a "race," nor did anthropologists agree on how many races populated Europe. Attempts to work through this problem are detectable in the effort to standardize racial cartography. Here, three models competed for prominence. The first was proposed by the French naturalist and anthropologist Joseph Deniker (1852–1918), who identified six primary races: Northern; Eastern; Ibero-Insular; Western or Cenevole; Littoral or Atlanto-Mediterranean; and Adriatic or Dinaric; along with four sub-races: sub-Northern; Vistulian; North-Western; and sub-Adriatic.[38] Another model was outlined by the American racial cartographer William Z. Ripley (1867–1941), who insisted that there were only three European races: Teutonic; Alpine (Celtic); and Mediterranean.[39] In turn, the German racial anthropologist Hans F. K. Günther (1891–1968) suggested that there were five European races: Nordic; Western; Dinaric; Eastern; and Baltic.[40] Eugenicists, although often skeptical of these racial classifications, proposed eugenic theories of social and biological improvement that characterized, classified, and utilized national identities in a climate where cultural and racial definitions of the nation competed for legitimacy.

Stefan Kühl, one of the scholars to analyze most closely how racism shaped American and German eugenics, has suggested that one "useful way to distinguish between strands in the eugenics movement is to emphasize their differing conceptions of race improvement." Kühl further noted that "all eugenicists held the idea that it was possible to distinguish between inferior and superior elements of society, but all traced inferiority directly to an ethnic basis."[41] As a cluster of social, biological, and cultural ideas centered on the redefinition of the individual and the national community according to the laws of natural selection and heredity, eugenics promoted a regenerative racial program. Two directions were generally followed: discouraging those individuals categorized as "inferior" to reproduce; and encouraging those deemed "superior" to value their hereditary importance for the general health of the nation. Eugenics, therefore, defined a dominant ethnic group as the repository of the nation's racial qualities and pursued biological, social, and political means to assess and eliminate the factors seen as contributing to its degeneration. During the interwar period, especially, eugenic ideas of racial superiority were revived and replicated in political discourses, whether it was about miscegenation in the United States, the British Empire, or Germany. And although the scientific challenges prompted by the development of genetics did not eliminate the overt usage of racial determinism by the eugenicists, the eroding of the conventional, "natural" hierarchy of races inevitably furthered the growth of alternate ways of eugenic thinking, notably in France and Britain. Even in Germany, where the concept of race was intensely cultivated by National Socialist ideology, eugenicists often specifically rejected racism. In their widely disseminated book on *Human Heredity* (1931), Erwin Baur (1875–1933), Eugen Fischer (1874–1967), and Fritz Lenz hoped to dispel the accusations of racial supremacy associated with German racial hygiene. It is, therefore, worth reproducing Lenz's argument at length:

> The recognition that race is the substratum of all civilization must not, however, lead anyone to feel that membership to a superior race is a sort of comfortable couch on which he can go to sleep. For that reason, I must not conclude my account of the mental peculiarities of the races without expressingly insisting that the biological heritage of the mind is no more imperishable than the biological heritage of the body. If we continue to squander that biological mental heritage as we have been squandering it during the last few decades, it will not be many generations before we cease to be the superiors of the Mongols. Our ethnological studies must lead us not to arrogance but to action—to eugenics.[42]

According to Sheila Weiss, although Lenz "fully recognized physical differences between the world's races, he found these uninteresting in themselves and sometimes unreliable when it came to assessing an individual's racial type. Lenz concentrated almost exclusively on what he called the *seelische* (spiritual) differences, by which he meant the sum total of all non-physical qualities of the major races."[43] By the late 1930s, however, most German eugenicists were too deeply involved with the biopolitical National Socialist regime not to be affected by its insistence on race, as understood by Günther and other racists. Even when they were breaking new ground in genetics, psychiatry, or general biology, most German eugenicists situated their eugenic ideas within the generalized racial discursive field choreographed by Nazi politics. Their example, one should remember, unequivocally demonstrates not only that the realm of eugenics was as much scientific as social and political, but also that eugenicists saw themselves as both scientists and modern-day nation builders. Indeed, for many of them, protecting the race took on the qualities of a new and more direct and interfering strategy for improving society and the individual within it.

NATURE AND NURTURE

Race was a central component in the eugenic imagination, and what this centrality provides is, in fact, an insight into a larger debate, one which came to be known from the middle of the nineteenth century as the nature-nurture debate.[44] Eugenicists in Europe and North America, although aware of the importance of environment and education in shaping individual life and human behavior,[45] were generally hereditarian in their interpretation of social and national improvement. Francis Galton phrased the debate in terms of "race" and "nurture." In his 1873 study "Hereditary Improvement," Galton accepted that nurture was essential to eugenic betterment. "An improvement in the nurture of the race," he noted, "will eradicate inherited diseases; consequently, it is beyond dispute that if our future population were reared under more favourable conditions than at present, both their health and that of their descendants would be greatly improved." In his commending of nurture, Galton dwelt on the need to create an effective correlation between social environment, education, and sanitary welfare, warning that the race's quality would be damaged if these conditions were not strengthened. Yet, nurture was only secondary in importance. "I look upon race," Galton emphasized, "as far more important than nurture. Race has a double effect, it creates better and more intelligent individuals, and these become more competent than their predecessors to make laws and customs, whose effects shall favourably react on their own health and on the nurture of their children."[46] Envisioning a shared role for racial and cultural development, Galton nevertheless imparted the contributions unevenly: although nurture could serve social improvement, it was, for him, nature that served as the foundation for eugenics.

Galton returned to the importance of race in shaping eugenic and demographic policies in his 1892 presidential address to the Seventh International Congress of Hygiene and Demography. "The importance to be attached to the race," he emphasized, "is a question that deserves a far larger measure of exact investigations than it receives. We are exceedingly ignorant of the respective ranges of the natural and acquired faculties in different races, and there is far too great a tendency among writers to dogmatise wildly about them, some grossly magnifying, others as greatly minimising their several provinces."[47] This criticism illustrates that a great deal of misunderstanding and conceptual confusion about race persisted among eugenicists and other social theorists. But it also indicates the tendency toward finding a way to integrate race successfully within eugenics, rather than to distance race from it. Drawing on the same set of arguments, the British eugenicist Caleb Saleeby (1878–1940) even ventured to propose the division between "Natural Eugenics," based on "all the aspects of heredity," and a "Nurtural Eugenics, which has regard to all the aspects of environment."[48] The same inclination toward a synthesis between heredity and society appealed to later eugenicists— Karl Pearson (1857–1936), Charles Davenport (1866–1944), Leonard Darwin (1850–1943), and the like—who were directly associated with Galton's theories.

New developments in the burgeoning field of genetics after 1900 were, to the development of eugenics, what the seminal theory of natural selection was to the development of biology in the nineteenth century. Darwin believed that improvements to the social environment and education would prove beneficial to the transmission of acquired characteristics to offspring. But the new mechanisms of heredity proposed by August Weismann (1834–1914), who stressed the non-heritability of acquired characteristics (the continuity of the germ plasm), and the hereditary model proposed by the Moravian monk Gregor Mendel (1822–1884), later known as the system of Mendelian inheritance, challenged not only the theory of blending inheritance but also revolutionized evolutionary biology. It likewise changed the history of eugenics. Seeking scientific dogma to enforce their biological agendas, eugenicists immediately seized upon the possibility of transferring genetic theories from experimental laboratories to human society. It was a convoluted process of adaptation and appropriation, with implications for the usage of race in eugenic narratives of human improvement.

When the British geneticist William Bateson (1861–1926) popularized Mendelian genetics in Britain, he experienced constant opposition from the biometric school of heredity led by Karl Pearson and W. F. R. Weldon (1860–1906).[49] In 1901, Pearson, Weldon, and Francis Galton founded the journal *Biometrika*, in which they endeavored to apply modern statistical and biometrical methods to biological development and hereditarian social policies. In their approach, the supporters of the biometrical school followed Charles Darwin's theory of gradual evolution, and it was this mechanism of natural selection that was severely criticized by Mendelians. Having worked on morphology and environmental influences on the inheritance of characteristics, Bateson believed in discontinuous evolution, one that occurred through saltations. It was this model that perfectly matched Mendel's discontinuous model of heredity, which ultimately Bateson integrated into his own theories.[50]

In Germany, the geneticist and president of the Stuttgart Society for Racial Hygiene, Wilhelm Weinberg (1862–1937) proposed mathematical models of Mendelian inheritance, which he then applied to eugenics.[51] Following Weinberg's method, the psychiatrist Ernst Rüdin (1874–1952), another important member of the German eugenic movement, applied the theory of recessive Mendelian inheritance to psychiatry. It was an important moment for eugenics, as is illustrated by the reception of Rüdin's 1916 book on *Dementia praecox* in *The Journal of Racial and Social Biology*. "Up till the present," the reviewer remarked, "medical research on heredity has been rather dilettantish: this work now puts it on a methodologically impeccable basis. It must finally be recognised that it is not enough to throw together a few pedigrees to solve the problem of inheritance."[52]

The case of the American eugenicist Charles Davenport is equally illustrative.[53] In his 1911 *Heredity in Relation to Eugenics*, Davenport fused Mendelian genetics with quantitative approaches to biology to promote his eugenic program. "Eugenics," Davenport believed, was "the science of the improvement of the human race by better breeding." To convey his ideas, Davenport employed analogies from both animal and plant breeding: "The eugenical standpoint is that of the agriculturalist who, while recognizing the value of culture, believes that permanent advance is to be made only by securing the best 'blood.' "[54] Based on this argument, "the experience of animal and plant breeders who have been able by appropriate crosses to increase the vigor and productivity of their stock and crops should lead us to see that proper matings are the greatest means of permanently improving the human race—of saving it from imbecility, poverty, disease and immorality." According to Davenport, eugenics could ultimately offer "the salvation of the race through heredity."[55] It was this form of racial eugenics and the rejection of environmentalism that Davenport would later employ in his studies of racial crossing in Jamaica.[56]

If developments in the agricultural sciences and animal breeding provided an important source of inspiration to those interested in eugenic theories of racial improvement, discoveries made in microbiology and serology provided another. Following Karl Landsteiner's (1868–1943) discovery of the blood groups (A, B, O) around 1900, the Polish microbiologist Ludwik Hirszfeld (1884–1954) confirmed that the percentage of blood groups in a population varied according to their respective racial origins. These authors not only helped sustain the emergence of serology as a discipline preoccupied with deciphering the chemical properties of blood groups for the benefit of improving medical care (such as blood transfusions), and the discovery of new vaccines, but also brought the fascination with blood into the mainstream of the racial imagination. The idea of "biochemical races," as Hirszfeld called them, echoed particularly widely and provided eugenics with a new method for classifying human groups by more accurate, biochemical means rather than the highly contested anthropometric characteristics advocated by anthropology.[57]

Equally important, serology also demonstrated that blood groups were inherited according to Mendelian laws of heredity, thus impregnating the individual with one distinguishing attribute, one impervious to internal or external influences. As racial measurements had proven incapable of providing definitive answers to historical questions about racial identity, eugenicists hoped that heredity and serology could offer the scientific certainty needed to legitimize theories of biological uniqueness. The eugenic narrative that emerged thus had broader implications for the understanding of theories of the nation and race when cast in terms of the dichotomy between the perennial nature of blood and the ephemeral, atavistic impact of culture and history. As Pauline Mazumdar has explained: "Blood-group serology offered a model system for human genetics, and for its practical arms, eugenics and racial hygiene. The blood groups themselves provided a race-maker that attracted the attention of

German *völkisch* anthropologists. Blood promised to be a new and scientific way to define populations, to distinguish races from each other, and to trace their origins, migrations routes, and boundaries."[58] Illustrating this new trend in racial biology, anthropology, and eugenics, a German Society for Blood Group Research was established by the eugenicist and anthropologist Otto Reche (1879–1966) in 1926.[59] All the while, however, diverse interpretations of race continued to fluctuate widely among eugenicists.

Karl Pearson attempted to clarify the meaning of race in his 1911 *The Academic Aspect of the Science of National Eugenics,* where he spoke of "racial character, one which is the product of many centuries of selection, one which passes from generation to generation, and one which is not fundamentally modified if a child be born to the race in India, Canada, or Australia." Pearson portrayed race as a living organism, functioning according to hereditary laws, and contended that this was what Galton intended in his definition of eugenics: "There is not the least doubt in my mind that the author of our definition was convinced that the physical and mental qualities he was speaking of were essentially *hereditary.*"[60] Yet, such a strong emphasis on the hereditarian nature of race allowed for an equally strong interest in cultural and environmental factors. "Hence," Pearson continued, "in using the term *racial,* which signifies ultimately hereditary qualities, we are not *a priori* refusing to consider how far nature and environment affect physical or mental characters. On the contrary, we assert that the relative intensity of nature and nurture with regard to both physical and mental qualities is directly prescribed in our definition as part of the study of eugenics."[61] This outlook, in its broadest outlines, was congruent with the "biological imperative" articulated by the American sociologist Lester F. Ward (1841–1913).[62]

A similar explanation was offered by Hermann Muckermann (1877–1962), who suggested that "the words 'race' and 'racial' seem to have been used by Galton to mean the genetic heritage ('the inborn qualities or stock of some one human population') without specifying whether he meant any particular race—say, the English race, or the human race."[63] It was the process of biological determinism, the trend to ascribe certain racial qualities to certain nations, that Pearson and Muckermann broadly rejected. Within this climate, one must mention another critique of the eugenic idea of race vividly embodied in the anthropological theories of Franz Boas (1858–1942). As one of the most powerful authorities in twentieth-century anthropology, Boas is described as the founder of cultural relativism and one of the first detractors of the scientific racism that dominated American and European anthropology at the beginning of the twentieth century.[64]

Boas argued that eugenics' strong hereditarian basis precluded the generalized application of biology to the development of human society. "It would seem, therefore, that the first duty of the eugenicist should be to determine empirically and without bias what features are hereditary and what not. Unfortunately, Boas continued, "this has not been the method pursued; but the battle-cry of the eugenicists, 'Nature not nurture,' has been raised to the rank of a dogma, and the environmental conditions that make and unmake man, physically and mentally, have been relegated to the background." In contrast to the eugenicist who assumes that "higher civilization is due to a higher type; that better health depends upon a better hereditary stock; and so on," the anthropologist "believes that different types of man may reach the same civilization, that better health may be produced by better bringing up of any existing types of man."[65] Eugenicists saw their efforts within the broad context of a battle against biological and social degeneration, the ultimate aim being the creation of a healthy racial community.

To further elaborate on the claim that eugenics was "a panacea for human ills," Boas sought not only to separate biology from nature, but, in the process, to introduce a new anthropological interpretation of human development. He thus rejected eugenic rational programs to control a population's racial improvement first on moral grounds. Eugenics, Boas maintained, should, therefore, "not be allowed to deceive us into the belief that we should try to raise a race of supermen, nor that it should be our aim to eliminate all suffering and pain." To follow a strict selectionist agenda based on scientifically sound hereditarian principles was what eugenicists should do: "The attempt to suppress those defective classes whose deficiencies can be proved by rigid methods to be due to hereditary causes, and to prevent unions that will unavoidably lead to the birth of disease-stricken progeny, is the proper field of eugenics. How much can be and should be attempted in this field depends upon the results of careful studies of the law of heredity." Ultimately, Boas warned, "Eugenics is not a panacea that will cure human ills; it is rather a dangerous sword that may turn its edge against those who rely on its strength."[66]

In the decades that followed, biologists and geneticists took up the critique of eugenics' racial overtones. In 1935, the evolutionary biologist Julian S. Huxley (1887–1975) and anthropologist Alfred C. Haddon (1855–1940) published *We Europeans*, a devastating critique of ideas of racial superiority.[67] In a 1936 article, Huxley echoed many of the ideas voiced by Boas but phrased them in the light of new developments in biology and genetics.[68] "Once the full implications of evolutionary biology are grasped," Huxley maintained, "eugenics will inevitably become part of the religion of the future, or of whatever complex of sentiments may in the future take the place of organized religion."[69] When it came to race, Huxley reiterated that the term "only has meaning in the description of somewhat hypothetical entities or as a goal for even more hypothetical future ideals"; racial characteristics were without any "genetic or eugenic significance."[70]

Huxley's avowed purpose was to transcend the reigning racial ideas of his time regarding eugenics and society. It is thus quite fitting that his ideas of scientific objectivity should tend toward a new eugenic synthesis: "Science is simultaneously both theory and practice, both knowledge and control. For the applied science of eugenics to neglect the environment is a source both of confusion and of practical weakness."[71] If Boas invited eugenicists to embrace anthropology's cultural relativism, Huxley urged them to "familiarize [themselves] with the outlook and the concepts of sociology, with the technique and practice of social reform; for they are an indispensable part of the machinery we need to realise our aims."[72] Other eugenicists thought along the same lines. The American eugenicist Frederick Osborn

(1889–1981) correspondingly spoke of a new and less dogmatic "eugenic philosophy," which acknowledged "the present scientific knowledge [of] human inheritance and its relations to our social system."[73] But there was more than just skepticism in Osborn's argument. Like Huxley, Osborn chided those eugenicists who yielded to racial views, inviting them to adopt a more reconciliatory stance toward the social sciences and their methodologies.

CONCLUSION

"Eugenics," the British eugenicist Caleb W. Saleeby noted in 1909, "is at once a science, and a religion, based upon the laws of life, and recognising in them the foundation of society."[74] It was this portrayal of eugenics that Michael Burleigh elicited when he defined eugenics as a "collectivist, materialist, technocratic creed which promised to conquer in a Promethean way, nature's final frontier and which, like socialism itself, had evolved from primitive utopianism into a secular religion with scientific pretensions."[75] What Burleigh emphasized was the fusion between scientific language and forms of religious and political rituals. Galton considered eugenics to be "the science which deals with those social agencies that influence, mentally or physically, the racial qualities of future generations."[76] Any attempt, therefore, to recapture how twentieth-century eugenicists formulated their ideas of race and science must inevitably contain an understanding of how ideas of evolution and heredity have battled traditional forces, like religion, for supremacy over the human body. At the heart of all these conflicts there was, in fact, a characteristically scientistic attitude, one that Galton described as "the religious significance of the doctrine of evolution."[77] When Galton spoke of eugenics as the "new religion of the future," he not only hoped to convert coming generations to the new scientistic faith, but also that these new converts would establish eugenics as a universally recognized science for the improvement of the human race.

What Michelle Brattain has said about the evolution of race after World War II can appropriately be applied to eugenics as well: "What race *was* is not what race *is*, but understanding how it has been constructed in the past is essential to understanding and contributing to debate about its current construction."[78] One can nevertheless suggest, in George Fredrickson's words, that the post-1945 period established "patterns of thought and action concerning race and racism that would endure for the rest of the century."[79] Yet, what eugenics was during the interwar period is certainly not what the new genetics of today is, although I share Merryn Ekberg's reflection that "it would be naïve to assume the old eugenics differs from the new genetics because the old eugenics was faulty and the new genetics is faultless, or that the old eugenics was based on science fiction and the new genetics is based on science fact."[80]

The examples of eugenic thinking on race provided in this chapter, it should be said, are among the more salient and more readily traceable ones in the history of eugenics and race; but they were also key sources for the numerous post-1945 works that denied the concept of race any scientific validity, culminating in the 1952 UNESCO declaration on race. The scientific community had, by then, reached a general consensus about the usage of race as a valid biological concept.[81] The same cannot be said about eugenics.[82] Recently, moreover, eugenics has come to offer a conceptual background for debates on cloning and *in vitro* fertilization among many more. Aware of the general sensitivity surrounding these topics, specialists and lay observers alike have attempted to disassociate themselves from the interwar history of eugenics. But there is little heuristic value in conceptualizing between "bad" eugenics (namely racist) and "good" eugenics (critical of Nazi racism).[83] Perhaps more helpful is a counternarrative that highlights the cultural memory of eugenics in recent debates on genetic engineering.[84]

As this volume powerfully illustrates, the study of twentieth-century eugenics is currently undergoing a remarkable transformation, one framed by society's need to engage with scientific advances and the ethical dilemmas they raise on the one hand, and the inclusion of hitherto neglected case studies on the other. The historiography on eugenics is now re-adapting its epistemological foundation to reflect developments in the history of biology and medicine as well as the history of ideas and political ideologies. The latter field, especially, has contributed in new and refreshing ways to our understanding of eugenics and race. Attempts have been made, most prominently by Zygmunt Bauman, Tzvetan Todorov, Edward Ross Dickinson, Roger Griffin, and Aristotle Kallis, to integrate eugenics into the general discussion of the links between fascism and modernity. These authors suggest that eugenics should not be treated as an extraordinary episode removed from sociopolitical life, as a deviation from the norm that found its culmination in Nazi policies of genocide, but as an integral part of European modernity in which the state and the individual embarked on an unprecedented quest for the renewal of an idealized racial community.[85] The new scholarship on eugenics, therefore, must take these new developments in the history of science, medicine, and political ideologies into account. Only then we will be able to convincingly and precisely reconstruct how the relationship between race, science, and eugenics became possible in the first place, so that we can move forward and contextualize those instances where this relationship was obstructed, and ultimately rejected.

NOTES

1. Classics include Richard Hofstadter, *Social Darwinism in American Thought, 1860–1915* (Philadelphia, PA: University of Pennsylvania Press, 1944); Mark H. Haller, *Eugenics: Hereditarian Attitudes in American Thought* (New Brunswick, NJ: Rutgers University Press, 1963); Allan Chase, *The Legacy of Malthus: The Social Costs of the New Scientific Racism* (New York: Alfred A. Knopf, 1977); and Daniel J. Kevles, *In the Name of Eugenics: Genetics and the Uses of Human Heredity* (New York: Alfred A. Knopf, 1985).

2. For class see G. R. Searle, *Eugenics and Politics in Britain, 1900–1914* (Leyden: Noordhoff International Publishing, 1976); for gender, see Angelique Richardson, *Love and Eugenics in the Late Nineteenth Century: Rational Reproduction and the New Woman* (Oxford: Oxford University Press, 2003).

3. Haller, *Eugenics,* 144.

4. See, for example, Garland E. Allen, "The Misuse of Biological Hierarchies: The American Eugenics Movement, 1900–1940," *History and Philosophy of the Life Sciences* 5, no. 2 (1983): 105–128; Edwin Black, *War against the Weak: Eugenics and America's Campaign to Create a Master Race* (New York: Thunder's Mouth Press, 2003); Alexandra Minna Stern, *Eugenic Nation: Faults and Frontiers of Better Breeding in Modern America* (Berkeley, CA: University of California Press, 2005).

5. Saul Dubow, *Scientific Racism in Modern South Africa* (Cambridge: Cambridge University Press, 1995), 121.

6. Chloe Campbell, *Race and Empire: Eugenics in Colonial Kenya* (Manchester: Manchester University Press, 2007), 19.

7. Ibid., 20.

8. Stefan Kühl, *The Nazi Connection: Eugenics, American Racism, and German National Socialism* (Oxford and New York: Oxford University Press, 1994), 70–71.

9. For an early discussion of this aspect in the Anglo-American context see Lyndsay A. Farrall, "The History of Eugenics: A Bibliographical Review," *Annals of Science* 36, no. 2 (1979): 111–123; in the case of German eugenics, see Sheila Faith Weiss, "The Race Hygiene Movement in Germany," *Osiris* 3, 2nd series (1987): 193–236.

10. Stephen Jay Gould, *The Mismeasure of Man* (New York: W. W. Norton, 1981), 20.

11. Paul Weindling, *Health, Race and German Politics between National Unification and Nazism, 1870–1945* (Cambridge: Cambridge University Press, 1989), 6.

12. See Joseph L. Graves, Jr., *The Emperor's New Clothes: Biological Theories of Race at the Millennium* (New Brunswick, NJ: Rutgers University Press, 2001).

13. See Georg Lukács, *The Destruction of Reason*, trans. Peter Palmer (London: Merlin Press, 1980) [original German edition, 1952].

14. Lene Koch, "The Meaning of Eugenics: Reflections on the Government of Genetic Knowledge in the Past and Present," *Science in Context* 17, no. 3 (2004): 323. See also Robert A. Nye, "The Rise and Fall of the Eugenics Empire: Recent Perspectives on the Impact of Biomedical Thought in Modern Society," *The Historical Journal* 36, no. 3 (1993): 687–700.

15. See chapters in this volume by Philippa Levine (chap. 2), Nils Roll-Hansen (chap. 4), and Mathew Thomson (chap. 6).

16. Jean Gayon and Daniel Jacobi, eds., *L'éternal retour de l'eugénisme* (Paris: Presses Universitaires de France, 2006).

17. Francis Galton, *Inquiries into Human Faculty and Its Development* (London: Macmillan, 1883), 17.

18. Ibid.

19. Alfred Ploetz, *Grundlinien einer Rassen-Hygiene* (Berlin: S. Fischer, 1895).

20. Alfred Ploetz, "Neo-Malthusianism and Race Hygiene," in *Problems in Eugenics. Report of Proceedings of the First International Eugenics Congress*, 2 vols. (London: The Eugenics Education Society, 1913), 2: 183.

21. Sheila Faith Weiss, for example, considers that "the German term *Rassenhygiene* (race hygiene) had a broader scope than the English word *eugenics*. It included not only attempts aimed at 'improving' the hereditary quality of a population but also measures directed toward an absolute increase in population." Weiss, "The Race Hygiene Movement in Germany," 193. This view echoes that of many early twentieth-century eugenicists. Géza

von Hoffmann, the Hungarian eugenicist, defined the two terms thus: "The motto of eugenics we may define as 'Quality, not quantity.' Race hygiene says 'Quality *and* quantity.'" In "Eugenics in the Central Empires since 1914," *Social Hygiene* 7, no. 3 (1921): 286.

22. Fritz Lenz, "Eugenics in Germany," *The Journal of Heredity* 15, no. 5 (1924): 223.

23. Ibid.

24. Ploetz's letter to Galton, 17 August 1905, in *The Life, Letters and Labours of Francis Galton*, ed. Karl Pearson, vol. IIIB (Cambridge: University Press, 1930), 546.

25. István Apáthy, "A faj egészségtana," *Magyar Társadalomtudományi Szemle* 4 (1911): 265. See also Marius Turda, "'A New Religion:' Eugenics and Racial Scientism in Pre-World War I Hungary," *Totalitarian Movements and Political Religions* 7, no. 3 (2006): 303–325.

26. For some authors, like Robert Reid Rentoul, the eugenic protection of the race meant complete eradication of degeneracy through sterilization, as developed in *Race Culture, or Race Suicide? (A Plea for the Unborn)* (London: Walter Scott, 1906), while for others, like Susanna Way Dodds, it meant the popularization of modern ideas of motherhood, as illustrated in *Race Culture: Mother and Child* (London: L. N. Fowler, 1910).

27. See Marius Turda, *The Idea of National Superiority in Central Europe, 1880–1918* (New York: Edwin Mellen Press, 2005).

28. Ploetz, *Grundlinien einer Rassen-Hygiene*, 5.

29. Alfred Grotjahn proposed the term *Fortpflanzungshygiene* (reproductive hygiene) instead. See his *Die Hygiene der menschlichen Fortpflanzung. Versuch einer praktischen Eugenik* (Berlin: Urban & Schwarzenberg, 1926).

30. I have discussed this aspect elsewhere. See Marius Turda, *Modernism and Eugenics* (Basingstoke: Palgrave, 2010).

31. Wilhelm Schallmayer, the other towering figure of German eugenics, suggested the terms *Rassenhygiene* (the hygiene of the race) and *Vererbungshygiene* (hereditary hygiene). See his *Vererbung und Auslese im Lebenslauf der Völker: Eine staatswissenschaftliche Studie auf Grund der neueren Biologie* (Jena: Gustav Fischer, 1903).

32. See Weiss, "Race Hygiene in Germany," 222.

33. Ibid.

34. From an immense literature, see Nancy Stepan, *The Idea of Race in Science: Great Britain, 1800–1960* (London: Macmillan, 1982); Emmanuel Chukwudi Eze, *Race and the Enlightenment: A Reader* (Oxford: Blackwell, 1997); Lee D. Baker, *From Savage to Negro: Anthropology and the Construction of Race, 1896–1954* (Berkeley, CA: University of California Press, 1998); and George M. Fredrickson, *Racism: A Short History* (Princeton, NJ: Princeton University Press, 2003).

35. J. Deniker, *The Races of Man: An Outline of Anthropology and Ethnography* (London: Walter Scott, 1900), 8.

36. Paul Topinard, "De la notion de race en anthropologie," *Revue d'anthropologie* 8, no. 2 (1879): 589–660.

37. Hermann W. Siemens, *Race Hygiene and Heredity* (New York: D. Appleton, 1924), 175.

38. Deniker, *The Races of Man*, 325–335.

39. William Z. Ripley, *The Races of Europe: A Sociological Study* (New York: D. Appleton, 1899).

40. Hans F. K. Günther, *Rassenkunde Europas*, 2nd ed. (Munich: J. F. Lehmann, 1925; Munich: J. F. Lehmann, 1926). See also Amos Morris-Reich, "Race, Ideas, and Ideals: A Comparison of Franz Boas and Hans F. K. Günther," *History of European Ideas* 32, no. 3 (2006): 313–332. For a description see Carlos C. Closson, "The Hierarchy of European Races," *The American Journal of Sociology* 3, no. 3 (1897): 314–327. For how ideas of racial classification were used in different institutional contexts, see Frederik Barth, Andre

Gingrich, Robert Parkin, and Sydel Silverman, *One Discipline, Four Ways: British, German, French, and American Anthropology* (Chicago, IL: University of Chicago Press, 2005).

41. Kühl, *The Nazi Connection*, 70.

42. Fritz Lenz, "The Inheritance of Intellectual Gifts," in Erwin Baur, Eugen Fischer, and Fritz Lenz, *Human Heredity*, trans. Eden and Cedar Paul (London: George Allen & Unwin, 1931), 699.

43. Weiss, "Race Hygiene in Germany," 215.

44. For a recent treatment, see Aaron Gillette, *Eugenics and the Nature-Nurture Debate in the Twentieth Century* (New York: Palgrave, 2007).

45. To be sure, neo-Lamarckian interpretations of social and biological degeneration found supporters among many Latin American, French, Italian, and Romanian health reformers and eugenicists. See chapters in this volume by Maria Sophia Quine (chap. 22) and Patience A. Schell (chap. 28). See also Yolanda Eraso, "Biotypology, Endocrinology, and Sterilization: The Practice of Eugenics in the Treatment of Argentinian Women during the 1930s," *Bulletin of the History of Medicine* 81, no. 4 (2007): 793–822.

46. Francis Galton, "Hereditary Improvement," *Fraser's Magazine* 7, no. 37 (1873): 116.

47. Francis Galton, "Presidential Address," in *Transactions of the Seventh International Congress of Hygiene and Demography, London, August 10th–17th, 1891*, ed. C. E. Shelly, vol. 10, *Demography* (London: Eyre and Spottiswoode, 1892–1893), 11.

48. C. W. Saleeby, *The Methods of Race Regeneration* (London: Cassell, 1911), 9.

49. The bibliography on this subject is voluminous. See, for example, William B. Provine, *The Origins of Theoretical Population Genetics* (Chicago, IL: Chicago University Press, 1971); Donald Mackenzie, "Sociobiologies in Competition: The Biometrician-Mendelian Debate," in *Biology, Medicine and Society 1840–1940*, ed. Charles Webster (Cambridge: Cambridge University Press, 1981), 243–288; Peter J. Bowler, *The Mendelian Revolution: The Emergence of Hereditarian Concepts in Modern Science and Society* (London: The Athlone Press, 1989); Pauline M. H. Mazumdar, *Eugenics, Human Genetics and Human Failings: The Eugenics Society, Its Sources and Its Critics* (London and New York: Routledge, 2002); and Margaret Morrison, "Modelling Populations: Pearson and Fischer on Mendelism and Biometry," *British Society for the Philosophy of Science* 53, no. 1 (2002): 39–68.

50. William Bateson, *Mendel's Principles of Heredity* (Cambridge: University Press, 1902).

51. P. M. H. Mazumdar, "Two Models for Human Genetics: Blood Grouping and Psychiatry in Germany between the World Wars," *Bulletin of the History of Medicine* 70, no. 4 (1996): 609–657.

52. Quoted in ibid., 614.

53. See Jan A. Witkowski and John R. Inglis, eds., *Davenport's Dream: 21ˢᵗ Century Reflections on Heredity and Eugenics* (New York: Cold Spring Harbor Laboratory, 2005).

54. Charles Benedict Davenport, *Heredity in Relation to Eugenics* (New York: Henry Holt, 1911), 1.

55. Ibid., 260.

56. See Charles Benedict Davenport and Morris Steggerda, *Race Crossing in Jamaica* (Washington, D.C.: Carnegie Institute, 1929). For a discussion of Davenport's racial studies, see Elazar Barkan, *The Retreat of Scientific Racism: Changing Concepts of Race in Britain and the United States between the World Wars* (Cambridge: Cambridge University Press, 1992).

57. L. Hirschfeld and H. Hirschfeld, "Serological Differences between the Blood of Different Races," *The Lancet* 197, no. 2 (18 October 1919): 675–679. See also Ludwik

Hirszfeld, *Konstitutionsserologie und Blutgruppenforschung* (Berlin: Julius Springer, 1928); Laurence H. Snyder, *Blood Grouping in Relation to Clinical and Legal Medicine* (Baltimore: Williams and Wilkins, 1929); and Fritz Schiff, *Die Blutgruppen und ihre Anwendungsgebiete* (Berlin: Julius Springer, 1933). Secondary literature includes W. H. Schneider, "Chance and Social Setting in the Application of the Discovery of Blood Groups," *Bulletin of the History of Medicine* 57, no. 4 (1983): 545–562; and P. M. Mazumdar, "Blood and Soil: The Serology of the Aryan Racial State," *Bulletin of the History of Medicine* 64, no. 2 (1990): 187–219.

58. Mazumdar, "Two Models for Human Genetics," 620.

59. Michael Hesch and Günther Spannaus, eds., *Kultur unde Rasse: Otto Reche zum 60. Geburtstag gewidmet von Schülern und Freuden* (Munich: J. F. Lehmann, 1939).

60. Karl Pearson, *The Academic Aspect of the Science of National Eugenics* (London: Dulau, 1911), 5.

61. Ibid., 6.

62. Lester F. Ward, "Eugenics, Euthenics, and Eudemics," *The American Journal of Sociology* 18, no. 6 (1913): 737–754.

63. Hermann Muckermann, "Eugenics and Catholicism," in *The Eugenics Movement: An International Perspective*, ed. Pauline M. H. Mazumdar, 6 vols. (London and New York: Routledge, 2007), 4: 25.

64. See Franz Boas, *Race, Language, and Culture* (Chicago, IL: University of Chicago Press, 1940); George W. Stocking, Jr., ed., *The Franz Boas Reader: The Shaping of American Anthropology, 1883–1911* (Chicago, IL: University of Chicago Press, 1989); and Vernon J. Williams, Jr., *Rethinking Race: Franz Boas and His Contemporaries* (Lexington, KY: The University Press of Kentucky, 1996).

65. Franz Boas, "Eugenics," *The Scientific Monthly* 3, no. 5 (1916): 472.

66. Ibid., 478.

67. Julian S. Huxley and A. C. Haddon, *We Europeans: A Survey of "Racial Problems"* (London: Jonathan Cape, 1935). See also Michelle Brattain, "Race, Racism, and Anti-Racism: UNESCO and the Politics of Presenting Science to the Postwar Public," *American Historical Review* 112, no. 5 (2007): 1386–1413.

68. Julian S. Huxley, "Eugenics and Society," *The Eugenics Review* 28, no. 1 (1936): 11–31.

69. Ibid., 11.

70. Ibid., 17.

71. Ibid., 25.

72. Ibid., 31.

73. Frederick Osborn, "Development of a Eugenic Philosophy," *American Sociological Review* 2, no. 3 (1937): 389.

74. Caleb Williams Saleeby, *Parenthood and Race Culture: An Outline of Eugenics* (London: Cassell, 1909), ix.

75. Michael Burleigh, "Eugenic Utopias and the Genetic Present," *Totalitarian Movements and Political Religions* 1, no. 1 (2000): 64.

76. Francis Galton, "Studies in Eugenics," *The American Journal of Sociology* 11, no. 1 (1905): 11.

77. Francis Galton, *Inquiries into Human Faculty and Its Development*, 220.

78. Brattain, "Race, Racism, and Anti-Racism," 1413.

79. Fredrickson, *Racism*, 127.

80. Merryn Ekberg, "The Old Eugenics and the New Genetics Compared," *Social History of Medicine* 20, no. 3 (2007): 591.

81. See Snait B. Gissis, "When Is 'Race' a 'Race'? 1946–2003," *Studies in History and Philosophy of Biological and Medical Sciences* 39, no. 4 (2008): 437–450.

82. To give just a few examples: *The Hellenic Eugenics Society* was established in 1953, while the journals *The Eugenics Review* (UK) and *Eugenics Quarterly* (U.S.) continued their

publication until 1968, when the first was discontinued and the second renamed *Social Biology*.

83. For example John Glad, *Future Human Evolution: Eugenics in the Twenty-first Century* (Schuylkill Haven, PA: Hermitage Publishers, 2006). Glad does not declare race to be the crux of twenty-first century eugenics, but the concern for future generations.

84. Jürgen Habermas, *The Future of Human Nature* (London: Polity Press, 2003); and Nicholas Agar, *Liberal Eugenics: In Defence Of Human Enhancement* (Oxford: Blackwell, 2004). For a discussion of these trends, see Marius Turda, "Recent Scholarship on Race and Eugenics," *The Historical Journal* 51, no. 4 (2008): 1115–1124. See also Bashford's epilogue in this volume.

85. Zygmunt Bauman, *Modernity and Ambivalence* (London: Polity Press, 1991); Edward Ross Dickinson, "Biopolitics, Fascism, Democracy: Some Reflections on Our Discourse about 'Modernity,'" *Central European History* 37, no. 1 (2004): 1–48; Tzvetan Todorov, *Hope and Memory: Lessons from the Twentieth Century* (Princeton, NJ: Princeton University Press, 2004); Roger Griffin, *Modernism and Fascism: The Sense of a New Beginning under Mussolini and Hitler* (Basingstoke: Palgrave, 2007); and Aristotle Kallis, *Genocide and Fascism: The Eliminationist Drive in Fascist Europe* (London and New York: Routledge, 2009).

FURTHER READING

Adams, Mark B., ed. *The Wellborn Science: Eugenics in Germany, France, Brazil, and Russia* (New York: Oxford University Press, 1990).

Engs, Ruth C. *The Eugenics Movement: An Encyclopaedia* (Westport, CT: Greenwood Press, 2005).

Jones, Greta. *Social Hygiene in Twentieth Century Britain* (London: Croom Helm, 1986).

Koch, Lene. "Past Futures: On the Conceptual History of Eugenics—A Social Technology of the Past," *Technology Analysis & Strategic Management* 18, no. 3–4 (2006): 329–344.

Mazumdar, Pauline M. H., ed. *The Eugenics Movement: An International Perspective*, 6 vols. (New York: Routledge, 2007).

Paul, Diane B. *Controlling Human Heredity: 1865 to the Present* (New York: Humanity Books, 1998).

Peel, Robert A., ed. *Essays in the History of Eugenics* (London: The Galton Institute, 1998).

Schmuhl, Hans-Walter. *The Kaiser Wilhelm Institute for Anthropology, Human Heredity, and Eugenics, 1927–1945* (Dordrecht: Springer, 2008).

Schneider, William H. *Quality and Quantity: The Quest for Biological Regeneration in Twentieth-Century France* (Cambridge: Cambridge University Press, 1990).

Stepan, Nancy Leys. *"The Hour of Eugenics:" Race, Gender, and Nation in Latin America* (Ithaca, NY: Cornell University Press, 1991).

Stone, Dan. *Breeding Superman: Nietzsche, Race and Eugenics in Edwardian and Interwar Britain* (Liverpool: Liverpool University Press, 2002).

Turda, Marius. *Modernism and Eugenics* (Basingstoke: Palgrave, 2010).

Turda, Marius. *Eugenism şi antropologie rasială în România, 1874–1944* (Bucharest: Cuvântul, 2008).

Turda, Marius, and Paul J. Weindling, eds. *Blood and Homeland: Eugenics and Racial Nationalism in Central and Southeast Europe, 1900–1940* (Budapest and New York: Central European University Press, 2007).

CHAPTER 4

....

EUGENICS AND THE SCIENCE OF GENETICS

....

NILS ROLL-HANSEN

EUGENICS as an ideology and a social movement emerged in the late nineteenth century inspired by worries about human degeneration under the impact of industrialization and modern urban living. The movement drew its scientific concepts and its scientific authority from the newly established Darwinian theory of evolution, which supported a naturalistic view of humankind. Human beings were seen as an integral part of living nature, descended from the same ancestors as other animals, and subject to the same causal laws. In particular, the same mechanism of evolution by natural selection applied to humans as to other living organisms, with the important caveat that "natural" be interpreted in a broad sense, including not only physical and biological but also social factors, like sexual selection. The effects of human breeding on plants and animals played a central role in Darwin's argument in *On the Origin of Species*. This naturalism implied that helping weak and disadvantaged individuals to live and reproduce would promote degeneration, suppressing the elimination of dysfunctional properties via natural selection. However, the real impact of such degeneration, which many understood to be created by the new institutions of social and medical assistance, was highly dependent on mechanisms of biological heredity, still mostly unknown at the turn of the century. Whether such degeneration would appear in a couple of generations or take hundreds of years to become a serious problem was unknowable without a more precise understanding of heredity itself.

The last decades of the nineteenth and the first decade of the twentieth century saw revolutionary new discoveries about the structure and function of the cells that make up all living organisms. In particular, the behavior of the intracellular bodies called chromosomes attracted much attention because they seemed so closely linked to reproduction and heredity. At the same time, studies of variation and experience in breeding, especially plant breeding, suggested that Darwin's ideas about heredity were radically inadequate. From the new understanding of life processes on the microscopic level, along with the practical experiences of a vigorously expanding modern agriculture, grew the new science of genetics—classical genetics, as it is usually called. Its basic principles were fully formed by around 1915.[1] But it took another couple of decades before the ideas of biological heredity were generally accepted by the broader community of biological scientists. The pre-genetic orthodox Darwinian conceptions of heredity thus continued to play an important role in popular thinking as well as political decision-making well into the middle of the twentieth century.

Eugenics started as a science-based movement to combat threatening degeneration. It was initiated by idealistic scientists and was inspired by a humanistic Enlightenment ideal of science as the servant of human welfare, in which the general goal was to improve the biological heredity of human populations. In the abstract this appeared as a good and unobjectionable aim—provided the means were acceptable. Before the 1930s and the traumatic experiences of Nazi population policies, the word "eugenics" had mostly positive connotations. Even the Catholic Church accepted eugenic policies, as long as there was no unacceptable interference with natural biological processes through abortion, sterilization, prohibition of marriage, or contraceptive techniques.[2] There was broad acceptance that the knowledge of genetics and other biological science should inform social policy.

EVOLUTION AND THE PROBLEM OF HEREDITY

The emergence of classical genetics in the early twentieth century radically changed the theory of evolution by natural selection. According to Darwin's theory the advantages that certain kinds of variation offer in the struggle to survive and procreate is the driving force in the evolution of species. Individuals with the most advantageous properties are "selected" as parents for the next generation. But to have an effect on the following generations the properties had to be inherited, and Darwin lacked an adequate theory of variation and heredity. He held on to a traditional theory of pangenesis formulated by Hippocrates and others. As Paul and Moore elaborate in their chapter in this volume, the hereditary material transmitted to the progeny consisted of particles ("gemmules") from all parts of the parent organism. This collection of particles provided the starting point for developing similar parts and properties in the new individual.

Heredity on the individual level was an obvious phenomenon, but it also appeared as capricious and unpredictable. Sometimes characteristic traits of a parent would reemerge in its child, at other times not. And sometimes it would be the characteristic of a more or less distant forebear that showed up. How was this apparent arbitrariness to be explained? Was there a basis in some kind of causal regularity?

The nature and source of variation between individuals, in particular between parents and offspring, was another pressing question. Not all characteristic variation was inherited. Was there an underlying difference between hereditary and non-hereditary variation? Some variations appeared as adaptations to environmental influence or demand. The same kind of plant would look very different when grown in humid and in dry climates, or at sea level and in the high mountains. To what extent, if at all, were such differences inherited? And what would the underlying mechanism be? The French biologist Jean Baptiste Lamarck (1744–1829) thought that the adaptations of the individual organism to meet the challenges of its environment were in part hereditary, and a main source of evolutionary change. Darwin introduced natural selection as a crucial mechanism in the evolution of species.[3] Yet he retained Lamarck's idea that individual adaptation was a major source of hereditary variation. Indeed this idea of inheritance of acquired characters—Lamarckism, as it is still called—took on increasing importance in consecutive editions of *Origin of Species*.

The inadequacy of traditional theories of pangenesis became more and more obvious as microscopic biology developed through the second half of the nineteenth century. The new knowledge about cells, their interaction, and their internal structure led to a revolution in the understanding of biological heredity. The Dutch botanist Hugo de Vries (1848–1935) believed in hereditary particles, but not that they moved between cells. He called his theory "intracellular pangenesis." Francis Galton advanced the idea of a "stirp," or rootstock, of underlying hereditary material running through the generations. Each individual developed directly from the stirp and varied according to prevailing local conditions, while the stirp remained unaffected by these variations.

The germ-line theory of August Weismann (1834–1914) was another alternative to pangenesis and to Lamarckian inheritance of acquired characters. He observed that sex organs in animals grew directly from the zygote (the fertilized egg-cell), in contrast to the other specialized cells of the organism. This germ-line runs through the generations without being influenced by the other cell of the organism, the soma. Weismann tested this conclusion by simple experiments, for example, cutting off the tails of mice through many generations, to no effect. He also developed an elaborate theory of embryological development built on discoveries of the 1880s and 1890s about the behavior of the chromosomes. He saw differentiation as a result of cells receiving different kinds of hereditary particles. This fit well with the germ-lines observed in animals, but not with the well-known botanical phenomenon that whole new individuals could be reproduced asexually from many different parts of a plant, so-called cloning.

THE NEW SCIENCE OF GENETICS

It was the discovery that phenomena of inheritance could best be explained by underlying stable factors that laid the foundation of genetics, what Ernst Mayr (1904–2005) called "hard" heredity.[4] Already in the 1860s, Gregor Mendel (1822–1884) had proposed that law-like inheritance in plants of such properties as color and form of seed or flowers were determined by factors transmitted unchanged through the generations. But his discovery was little known and generally disregarded until it was rediscovered in 1900. Mendel's idea was contrary to Darwin's theory of evolution by natural selection, which assumed that heredity changed continuously, both through time and in each character of the organism. This meant that hereditary variation in all directions was always available for the force of natural selection to sculpt biological form, adapting it to the demands of environment. By the end of the nineteenth century, this belief in evolution based on continuous variation in heredity was sharply challenged.

The pugnacious British biologist William Bateson (1861–1926) criticized the so-called biometricians, in particular the physicist and mathematician Karl Pearson (1857–1936) and the zoologist Frank Raphael Weldon (1860–1906), for their belief in continuous variation of heredity. In 1894 Bateson published a collection of *Materials for the Study of Variation* to show that variation had to be discontinuous. And in 1900 he quickly picked up the rediscovery of Mendel's laws and soon became the most influential propagandist for the new science of heredity.[5] He was the first to use the term "genetics" publicly (in 1906). Likewise, de Vries experimented with selection of specific botanical characters, like the number of petals in a flower or rows of seed on a corncob, and found that hereditary variation was not continuous. He concluded that in well-defined and homogeneous varieties, also called "elementary species," heredity was generally fixed. New elementary species arose occasionally through sudden change, claimed de Vries. His term for this phenomenon, "mutation," became the hallmark of hereditary discontinuity in the new science of genetics, though de Vries's own explanation was soon abandoned.[6] In support of the mutation theory he pointed to recent experience in plant breeding: the method of mass selection, substituting human demands for environmental pressure, often failed when specific goals were sought, for instance increased winter-hardiness of wheat, or stiffer straw in barley. New and more successful methods of pedigree breeding were developed, recognizing the presence of multiple stable types within an apparently homogeneous population.[7]

Classical genetics was established by extending explanation in terms of hard heredity throughout the plant and animal world, to quantitative as well as qualitative characters. A full-fledged genetic theory was achieved when a group of fruit fly geneticists led by American embryologist Thomas Hunt Morgan (1866–1945) succeeded in mapping specific factors responsible for determining characters onto the chromosomes. They produced a theoretical synthesis in their modest, lucid, and epoch-making monograph, *The Mechanism of Mendelian Heredity*, in 1915.[8]

A clear and experimentally operational distinction between genotype and phenotype was essential to this achievement, that is, between the underlying biological type and the concrete shape of individuals under varying environmental conditions. Danish botanist Wilhelm Johannsen (1857–1927) introduced and defined the terms "genotype" and "phenotype" in 1909, building on an experiment selecting for weight and shape of bean seed.[9] His clever move was to use pure lines, that is, populations descending from a single individual. In self-fertilizing organisms like beans, such in-breeding populations are genetically highly uniform. Latching onto the controversy between de Vries and the biometricians, he wanted to test how much of the pheno-typic variation is inherited. In contradiction to the biometricians, he found no inher-itance in the case of self-fertilizing pure lines. Galton's contrary result with sweet peas, a plant with a similarly sexually reproductive biology to that of beans, was simply a result of using genetically non-homogeneous material. Galton had selected from a population that contained many lines with different heredity, Johannsen explained.[10] In this elegant way, Johannsen was able precisely to separate hereditary variation, with evolutionary and breeding relevance, from mere phenotypic variation. His theory of a stable genotype was soon extended to selection experiments in cross-breeding and genetically non-homogeneous lines of organisms like corn and chicken.[11]

The experimental demonstration of hard heredity, the stability of genotype, had two important implications: there was neither continuous change in heredity nor inheritance of individually acquired character. According to Johannsen's inter-pretation, strictly continuous variation was only found on the phenotypic level, where an incalculable number of environmental factors contributed to the formation of the individual organism. Nevertheless, continuous versus discontinuous heredi-tary variation continued for a long time to be a key question in the theoretical debates among geneticists. As late as 1916, William Castle (1867–1962), one of the founding fathers of genetics in America, argued that elementary hereditary factors were subject to continuous change.

However, in other areas of biology—embryology, systematics, ecology, paleon-tology—the inheritance of acquired characters was still widely considered to be an important basic alternative to the principles of classical genetics as late as the 1930s and 1940s. And the *possibility* that there existed such mechanisms with significance for evolution as well as practical breeding was recognized throughout the twentieth century. Reports that such inheritance had been observed continued to attract much interest. The great political scandal of twentieth-century science—the suppression of classical genetics in the Soviet Union from the 1930s to the 1960s—was inspired by reports of this kind, which turned out to be largely illusory.[12] Indeed, to date, a number of molecular mechanisms have been discovered that can support inheri-tance of acquired characters for one or a few generations and thus play a significant role in evolution. Contrary to "the central dogma" of early molecular genetics, information can to some extent flow from phenotype to genome (genotype).[13]

RISING GENETIC CRITICISM OF EUGENICS

The main scientific input to the birth of eugenics was the Darwinian theory of evo-lution. But originally this had a thin, even nonexistent explanation of the actual mechanism of heredity. There was plenty of room for popular, common-sensical, and even mythical ideas about human inheritance, to be linked to evolutionary ideas generally, and eugenics specifically. Only with the development of a coherent and substantial theory of classical genetics in the second decade of the twentieth century did a reliable scientific basis for criticism of popular eugenic ideas start to develop. Historian Daniel Kevles introduced the terms "mainline" and "reform" eugenics to distinguish the early racist, anti-feminist, and authoritarian trend from the liberal and democratic social and population policies that were developed through the 1920s and 1930s, consciously based on the new science of genetics, that came to be supported by liberal and left-wing geneticists toward the end of that period.[14] Yet "mainline" and "reform" eugenics continued to exist side by side for decades. There was no rapid transition from one to the other, but rather a gradual shift.[15]

In the early twentieth century many pioneers of classical genetics joined eugenic organizations.[16] The American Breeders Association was for some time both the main scientific society for genetic science and a primary promoter of eugenic ideas in the United States. T. H. Morgan, for instance, was a member of the association's Committee on Animal Breeding, but by 1915 reacted strongly against what he regarded as loose and outdated genetic speculation. He criticized "the reckless statements and the unreliability of a good deal that is said" in the association's *Journal of Heredity*, arguing that such claims could be used to support tempting goals with untenable arguments and inefficient means.[17]

By the beginning of World War I, there was widespread and growing concern among professors of biology and medicine in the United States that "hasty and ill-advised legislation" could result from "eugenic zeal without sufficient eugenic knowledge."[18] The same worries were developing among liberal and left-wing scientists in Europe. Their criticism came to have a strong restraining impact on eugenic legislative proposals concerning marriage and sterilization in the 1920s and 1930s.[19]

An example of a geneticist and medical doctor who picked up the genetic criticism of mainline eugenics at an early stage and pursued it into the complex international struggles over science and politics during the period around World War II was Otto Lous Mohr (1886–1967). In 1915 he sharply attacked Jon Alfred Mjøen (1860–1939), pharmacist and leader of the popular eugenics movement in Norway, a man active in international eugenic organizations. Mohr claimed that Mjøen was a dilettante in genetics, and that his proposal for eugenic policies lacked a factual scientific basis and would likely produce more harm than good. His attack effectively marginalized Mjøen and mainline eugenics in Norway. Mohr's combination of advanced scientific knowledge and liberal social engagement made him an influential actor in local eugenic and sterilization politics.[20] Studies of cytology in Belgium and genetics with the Morgan group introduced him to the international network of geneticists. As chair of the Permanent International Committee of Genetics, he later played a crucial role in relocating the Seventh International Congress of Genetics from Moscow to Edinburgh, when he and his colleagues found the tightening of political control of science accompanying the start of Stalinist purges in 1936 incompatible with traditional scientific autonomy and freedom. They were fighting scientific obscurantism on two fronts: communist Lamarckism on one, and Nazi mainline eugenics on the other.[21]

The distinction between positive and negative eugenics was central to eugenic policy discussions. Judgments about good and desirable as well as bad and undesirable inheritance differed greatly and it was hard to agree on general criteria, except in one area: genetically derived illness and severe disability. The simple idea of negative eugenics was that if people with such ailments did not have children, the occurrence of these ailments would decrease in coming generations. However, the appealing idea of combating hereditary illness through negative eugenics soon started to fade in the face of growing genetic knowledge. If the cause of an ailment was recessive rather than dominant, it would take generations to achieve a significant effect. It was a simple calculation of elementary Mendelian theory that if 1 percent of the population suffered from a condition caused by one recessive gene, around 10 percent would have a single gene of the same kind and only about 20 percent of the unwanted genes would be eliminated if those suffering from the ailment produced no offspring. As most kinds of hereditary illness and disability have a frequency much less than 1 percent, and as it gradually became clear that these are mainly recessive, negative eugenics lost its attraction. Proponents nevertheless continued to argue that a reduction on the order of 10 percent per generation was important. They pointed to what was then called feeblemindedness (mental retardation), which was assumed to affect about 1 percent of the population and likely to be due to one recessive gene.[22]

Old fears of hereditary degeneration were also dispelled by the new concepts and theories of genetics. The stability of the genes and the understanding of their fundamental difference from individually developed characters—only the former were transmitted to offspring—gradually dispelled ideas about the causes and mechanisms of degeneration. The lack of demographic data to demonstrate progressive racial degeneration confirmed that the fear had been exaggerated.[23]

The fundamental distinction between genotype and phenotype implied that environment was as indispensable and fundamental to the development of an individual as heredity. It also soon became clear that there is no one-to-one relationship between hereditary factors and the characters of the organism. The relation is complex, with each gene affecting many characters and each character being affected by many genes. This had been clearly stated in *The Mechanism of Mendelian Heredity*, which Morgan and his students published in 1915. Empirical population studies, like those of Russian-American geneticist Theodosius Dobzhansky (1900–1975), demonstrated the great genetic diversity and variability of natural populations.[24] Theoretical population genetics developed formal tools to analyze complex interactions between genes and environment in evolution. Nevertheless, the ideas of a "unit character" and "gene for" continued to flourish, especially in popular discourse on genetics. The persistence of such terminology suggests that simple determinism may still be widespread in the early twenty-first century.

It took time for the new picture of human heredity to become clearly developed in genetic science and even longer to make an impact on popular and political thinking. The mid-twentieth century saw two major reactionary movements in which traditional popular conceptions of heredity inspired political suppression and perversion of genetic science: Nazi population policies in Germany, and Lysenkoist "genetics" in the Soviet Union.

GENETICS VERSUS RACISM

The racism of mainline eugenics referred to pre-genetic physical anthropology and evolutionary theory. The validity of such scientific support had been contested already before the turn of the century, for instance by the German-American anthropologist Franz Boas (1858–1942).[25] Criticism of racism from the new science of genetics developed gradually during the 1910s and 1920s, and was radically sharpened in response to Nazi ideology and population policies in the 1930s.

After World War I, the idea that some races have a general genetical superiority to others had lost plausibility in scientific debates. But the possibility was raised that race crossings could produce genetically unbalanced and thus inferior hybrids. This became a central topic in the dispute between eugenics and genetics. At the 1921 International Congress of Eugenics in New York, Jon Alfred Mjøen attracted considerable public attention when he argued that race interbreeding might lead to offspring with physical and mental qualities that were not well balanced. He pointed to his own experiments with rabbits, where offspring had a mixture of upright and hanging ears, as well as to the "deplorable" social conditions of mixed Nordic and Sami families. This fed into an existing American debate spearheaded by Charles Davenport (1866–1944).[26] But not all American geneticists concurred with Davenport. William Castle criticized Mjøen for neglecting social inheritance. "Much that is the best in human existence is a matter of social inheritance, not biological," argued Castle, concluding, "so far as biological considerations are concerned, there is no race problem in the United States."[27]

Davenport, in a study on *Race Crossing in Jamaica* (1929), had found only scant evidence of disharmony in physical characters, but still claimed that mental ones could be important. His study was severely criticized by Karl Pearson (1857–1936) for its statistical methods. Davenport gave no convincing reasons for assuming a specific genetic basis for mental imbalances, and other genetic and anthropological studies of the period found no significant physical disharmonies.[28]

Sharp public criticism of mainline eugenic policies and proposals emerged in the 1930s, spearheaded by leading experts on genetics and evolution, including Americans like Herbert Jennings (1868–1947) and Nobel Prize winner Hermann J. Muller (1890–1967), Britons like J. B. S. Haldane (1892–1964), Julian Huxley (1887–1975), and Lancelot Hogben (1895–1975), as well as Scandinavians such as Gunnar

Dahlberg (1893–1956) and Otto Lous Mohr. Less well-known outside scientific circles, but very important in the long run, was the work of Lionel Penrose (1898–1972) on the biological basis of mental retardation. He displayed a detailed picture of how different kinds of mental retardation depended on different environmental and hereditary factors. For these progressive scientists, the racist politics emerging in Nazi Germany was a major political threat, and it became a duty for politically conscious liberal and left-wing scientists to reveal its lack of scientific validity.[29]

A Liberal Consensus

The intensity of geneticists' campaigns against the ideas of mainline eugenics grew with the increasing political tensions in 1930s Europe. They sharply rejected the idea that some human races are genetically superior to others, as well as the simple genetic determinism that characterized mainline eugenics. They insisted that radical social reforms, improvement of living conditions for the poor, and emancipation of women were necessary to create a just society, but they were not opposed to eugenics in principle. They believed in the possibility of important genetic improvement within populations in the long run.

Such a view was expressed in the so-called "Geneticists' Manifesto" formulated by H. J. Muller and signed by a representative group of leading American and European geneticists in August 1939, as the Seventh International Congress of Genetics hurriedly disbanded on the eve of World War II. The signatories included such leading critics of older eugenics as Huxley, Haldane, Hogben, and Dahlberg. This document, entitled "Social Biology and Population Improvement," was a response to a survey by the Science Service of Washington, D.C., which asked the explicitly eugenic question: "How could the world's population be improved most effectively genetically?"[30]

The message of the geneticists was that radical reforms of social equality and justice were needed before any kind of eugenic policy could become effective and truly beneficial. The first step had to be a good physical and social environment for all. It was not possible to "estimate and compare the intrinsic worth of different individuals...without equal opportunities for all members of society." And the elimination of hereditarian prejudices against races or groups would not be possible until "the conditions which make for war and economic exploitation have been eliminated." The manifesto also called for protection and support for women to ensure that a woman's "reproductive duties do not interfere too greatly with her opportunities to participate in the life and work of the community at large."[31] The geneticists' manifesto illustrates how liberal left-wing geneticists in 1939 gave first priority to a just social system. Only on this basis could human genetics contribute to sound social policy. Social reform in the spirit of social democratic movements across northern Europe was the primary need.

This critical attitude to contemporary eugenics was manifested in the nature of the sterilization laws in the Scandinavian countries in the 1930s, characterized by strong concern for the principle of voluntariness and the priority of social reforms.[32] This was in accordance with the views of geneticists such as Mohr and Dahlberg, who acted as influential advisors to their respective governments in Norway and Sweden. They were highly critical of the radical eugenic policies of the German Nazi regime, which enforced sterilization on hereditarian criteria.

The 1934 Norwegian sterilization law is an example of the different place of genetic criteria for sterilization in Nazi Germany and in Scandinavian social democracies. This law permitted biological heredity as an acceptable reason for sterilization only when there was danger of an affliction being directly transmitted to offspring. This was not a eugenic justification in the strict sense, because it was not pursued with an entire population in mind. It was an individual medical approach similar to that of medical genetic counselling in the postwar period. The primary criterion of the Norwegian law was social and not biological: lacking the ability to take care of children. This applied to those with full legal right who applied for sterilization on their own behalf as well as to those who were under guardianship of others due to mental retardation or insanity. Thus the Norwegian law was directly contrary to the German law of 1933, which only allowed sterilization on grounds of biological heredity: social grounds were illegal.[33]

Geneticists and the UNESCO Declaration on Race

A strong and politically motivated anti-racism accompanied the formation of the United Nations at the end of World War II. There was broad agreement among social as well as natural scientists that the theories about hereditary differences between human races on which Nazi ideology was based were untenable, and that preventing new racist catastrophes meant making this clear, worldwide. The United Nations itself was established in the hope of preventing future wars, while UNESCO's particular aim was to harness and utilize educational and scientific means to achieve this end. This was the context within which the two UNESCO declarations on race, in 1950 and 1951, were forged. Inevitably, scientists' ideas differed on how best to achieve these ends. While the first declaration expressed a view widespread among social scientists, the second was written and supported primarily by geneticists, and it offered a markedly different approach to issues of race.[34]

The view of human heredity behind the first declaration is exemplified in physical anthropologist Ashley Montague's *Man's Most Dangerous Myth: The Fallacy of Race,* which built on the critique of racism articulated by Franz Boas half a century earlier. The purpose of Montague's book was to clarify "thinking upon an important subject about which clear thinking is generally avoided."[35] He proposed to exchange the tainted word "race" with "ethnic group," defined in terms of what contemporary biologists knew about races. Montague pronounced the old concept of race to be "meaningless."[36] Most geneticists, however, took a different approach, arguing that popularizing existing knowledge of genetics and its limited implications for human population policy was the most effective protection against dangerous racist doctrines.

The 1947 book *Heredity, Race and Society* by geneticists Leslie Dunn and Theodosius Dobzhansky was representative of the views behind the second UNESCO declaration on race. Its opening claim was: "One of the most important facts about human beings is that they are not all alike." The geneticists claimed that it was essential to understand that two fundamentally different factors caused human difference: the inherited and the environmental. Dunn and Dobzhansky took for granted the existence of genetically different human groups, traditionally called races, but stressed that there were no pure races. They wholly rejected theories of biologically superior races, but argued that abolishing the term "race" could as easily aggravate the political problem as solve it: "Some have used 'ethnic group' in place of race; but unfortunately 'ethnic group prejudice' is easily exchangeable for 'race prejudice'; and one can hate 'ethnic groups' just as venomously as real or imaginary races."[37]

An introductory note to the second UNESCO declaration explains that in the first declaration "it was chiefly sociologists who gave their opinion...That statement had good effect but it did not carry the authority of just those groups within whose special province fall the biological problems of race." In discussing the social and political implications of genetics and evolution, this second statement used the word "race" without hesitation and was open to the possibility of significant hereditary differences between human races. Nevertheless, the second statement ended in political harmony with the first. There was, it concluded, good support for "the view that genetic differences are of little significance in determining the social and cultural differences between different groups of men." And there was "no evidence that race mixture produces disadvantageous results from a biological point of view."[38]

The difference between geneticists and social anthropologists persisted in UNESCO's anti-racist activities. Dahlberg's UNESCO-sponsored educational pamphlet *Raser och Folk* (Races and People) describes the different human races and their origin according to genetic and evolutionary theory, denies the existence of a "higher" race, and ends with current sociopolitical problems connected to increased immigration.[39] Social scientists, on the other hand, showed little interest in popularizing modern scientific knowledge about human heredity, instead challenging racism by arguing that current concepts of race were scientifically unsound and politically obnoxious, and calling for rejection of the word "race" altogether. For many social scientists, Boas's *The Mind of Primitive Man* offered the key argument against eugenics. However, successive editions of this classic work relied more on the "ancestral heredity" of nine-

teenth-century biometric theory than on the classical genetics of the early twentieth century. Boas's essay lacked the deeper scientific understanding of the
nature/nurture question that the new concepts of genotype, phenotype, and
gene provided. In his foreword to a 1963 reprint, the anthropologist Melville J.
Herskovits (1895–1963), a central actor in UNESCO debates, makes no mention
that the essay was biologically outdated.[40]

EUGENICS AND GENETICS
IN THE 1950S AND 1960S

The experience with Nazism radically reduced the attractiveness of eugenic policies.
Nonetheless, there was no sudden abandonment of eugenics after World War II.
Moderate non-racist versions continued in some contexts. It had been clear by the
1930s that simple hereditary models, such as identifying one recessive gene as the
cause of a wide range of mental retardation, were untenable. But some moderate
eugenicists like the Swedish zoologist Nils von Hofsten (1881–1967), an influential
government advisor on eugenics, and the Danish human geneticist Tage Kemp
(1896–1964), organizer of the first international conference of human genetics in
Copenhagen in 1956, still argued that sterilization of the mentally retarded could
have significant eugenic effect. These two together with the Norwegian director of
health services, Karl Evang (1902–1981), continued to promote eugenic sterilization
of the mentally retarded as late as the 1950s. Within the medical profession, psychiatrists in particular held on to a strong genetic determinism.[41] But around 1960 the
rapid development of human genetics, in particular cytogenetics, made this view
scientifically obsolete.[42]

By the 1960s the word "eugenics" had practically disappeared from public
discourse. But many scientists were still interested in the long-term steering of
human evolution in a spirit similar to that of the Geneticists' Manifesto of 1939. An
example is the collection of articles *Control of Human Heredity and Evolution* (1965)
dedicated to the memory of Herbert Jennings, "father of the genetics of unicellular
organisms and leading educator of the general public of his generation in the
bearing of biological, and chiefly genetic, knowledge on human affairs."[43] Among
the contributors were Nobel Prize geneticists S. E. Luria (1912–1991), Edward Tatum
(1909–1975), and Muller. A comment on Muller's talk on the future possibility of
"genetic surgery," or what we today call gene technology, stressed how much more
knowledge was needed before such technology would be possible. Such detailed
knowledge of the structure and function of "man's genetic equipment" would
"hardly be available in the twenty-first century, if ever."[44] A decade after the discovery of the structure of DNA, geneticists were careful in not promising much
advance in genetic engineering for the near future.

CONCLUSION

The willingness of most German scientists, including geneticists, to cooperate in the extreme eugenic and racist population policies of the Nazi regime is one of the most sinister phenomena of twentieth-century science. Only very few of the leaders of German eugenics avoided the embrace of the Nazis.[45] The voluntary partnership of science with a totalitarian regime raises deep and troubling questions concerning the traditional Enlightenment view of science. Can the idea of mutual support and alliance between science and social progress in any way be saved? Around World War II, the scientific tradition was widely perceived as the anchor of intellectual freedom and of a lasting liberal democratic society. In recent years this view has been criticized as invalid, a "naive and self-serving" idea by which scientists have promoted their own interest.[46] In a generally pessimistic survey of German anthropological and genetic science during the Nazi period, Hans-Walter Schmuhl nevertheless ends on a cautiously optimistic note, quoting Dostojewski on the difference between "true" and "untrue" scholarship.[47]

Strong claims about political influence on scientific views have been made in recent decades. For instance, William Provine argued that between 1930 and 1950 geneticists "did revise their biology to fit their feelings of revulsion" against Nazism. Earlier in the century many scientists regarded wide race crosses as biologically harmful, and later argued that they were "at worst biologically harmless."[48] This argument is not sufficiently careful in distinguishing the strictly scientific claims from the political statements geneticists made on the basis of this science. Indeed, this chapter points to strong criticism of claims about harmfulness in the 1920s. Agnosticism appears to have been the more common position among leading geneticists. Progress in genetic theory from the 1920s through the 1940s strengthened the criticism and supported claims to harmlessness. The history of the UNESCO declarations of the early 1950s shows how many geneticists held agnostic views on genetic differences between human races, and reacted against political pressure to revise their scientific claims to suit an anti-racist agenda. This resistance was at the core of their disagreement with social scientists. Geneticists recognized that racism was a major political problem and that it was often supported by "facts" without sound scientific foundation. But at the same time, most scientists were not willing to make political compromises on what they agreed was sound scientific knowledge.[49]

The discovery of the chemical structure of DNA in 1953 was the starting point of a revolution in knowledge about heredity and development on the chemical level. Nevertheless, classical genetics, with its methods of hybridization and selection supported by cytological study of chromosomes, was the main basis of the most important practical applications of genetics through the remainder of the twentieth century. The greatest practical success was probably the green revolution in agriculture, which culminated around the 1980s. Medical genetics, with prenatal diagnostics as a central technology, has grown steadily in practical power and breadth of applications since the 1970s, including increasingly sophisticated molecular methods.

The molecular "genetic surgery" that Muller speculated on in the mid-1960s has been introduced in the chemical industry, for instance in the production of pharmaceuticals by manipulated microorganisms. It is now making its way into the breeding of pest-resistant plants, although it is still far from an effective chemical technology of human heredity.

The completion of the Human Genome Project in 2003 provided a general map of the DNA sequences of the human genome. Popularizations of this great scientific achievement sometimes give the impression that a map of an individual's DNA sequences also maps the "genes" that determine her or his behavior, a situation that would open a completely new situation not only for medical genetics but also for eugenics. In fact, the map of the human genome has reinforced scientific awareness of the complexity of the genome and its interaction with the rest of the organism, as well as with its external environment. The idea of the gene as a DNA sequence is dissolving in the complexity of the architecture and dynamics of the chemical machinery of the cell. This complexity does not necessarily mean that utopias of genetic engineering, producing human designer babies at will, can never be reached. It simply means that we still do not know how far it is possible to develop practical methods in this direction.[50]

By the 1990s it was once more politically acceptable to argue that eugenics is not necessarily a bad thing.[51] It might even be an inevitable consequence of molecular genetic knowledge that was growing much faster than the geneticists of the 1960s believed. And we had better make the best out of it by establishing effective democratic political control of its practical applications. Philosophers have emphasized how our modern society appears to be faced with "Inescapable Eugenics."[52] They have argued that the new genetic technologies force us to face truly eugenic problems, even if they are not applied with eugenic purpose. The individual choices made by parents can produce significant genetic changes at the population level. The social consequences of these choices have to be addressed by this generation, as their predecessors tackled the eugenic and genetic debates of the early to mid-twentieth century.[53]

NOTES

1. For a general overview of genetics in its social context up to the twenty-first century, see Staffan Müller-Wille and Hans-Jörg Rheinberger, *Vererbung: Geschichte und Kultur eines biologischen Konzepts* [Heredity: History and Culture of a Biological Concept] (Frankfurt: Fischer Taschenbuch Verlag, 2009; English translation under preparation).

2. Papal Encyclical, *Casti connubii*, 1930. See, for example, Daniel Kevles, *In the Name of Eugenics: Genetics and the Uses of Human Heredity* (New York: Alfred A. Knopf, 1985), 119.

3. Darwin and Lamarck differed fundamentally over descent. According to Darwin, present existing species had common forebears. Ultimately they had one or a few ancestors in the form of simple, probably unicellular, organisms. According to Lamarck, there was no branching "tree of evolution." Each presently existing species represented one line of

evolution leading to more and more complex organisms. Simple organisms continued to come into existence spontaneously from inorganic matter. Thus to Lamarck the most complex species were the oldest, and the simplest were the youngest. See, for example, Wolfgang Lefèvre, "Jean Baptiste Lamarck," in *Lexikon der bedeutenden Naturwissenschaftler*, eds. Dieter Hoffmann, Hubert Laitko, and Staffan Müller-Wille, 3 vols. (Heidelberg: Spektrum Akademischer Verlag, 2003–2004), 2: 358–363.

4. See Ernst Mayr, "Prologue: Some Thoughts on the History of the Evolutionary Synthesis," in *The Evolutionary Synthesis: Perspectives on the Unification of Biology*, eds. Ernst Mayr and William B. Provine (Cambridge, MA: Harvard University Press, 1980), 1–48.

5. W. Bateson, *Mendel's Principles of Heredity: A Defence* (Cambridge: University Press, 1902).

6. H. de Vries, *Die Mutationstheorie* [The theory of mutation], vol. 1 (Leipzig: Verlag von Weit, 1901).

7. See, for instance, Nils Roll-Hansen, "Svalöf and the Origins of Classical Genetics," in *Svalöf 1886–1986: Research and Results in Plant Breeding*, ed. Gösta Olsson (Stockholm: LTS Förlag, 1986), 35–43.

8. T. H. Morgan, A. H. Sturtevant, H. J. Muller, and C. B. Bridges, *The Mechanism of Mendelian Heredity* (New York: Henry Holt, 1915).

9. Wilhelm Johannsen, *Elemente der Exakten Erblichkeitslehre* (Jena: Gustav Fischer, 1909).

10. Nils Roll-Hansen, "Sources of Wilhelm Johannsen's Genotype Theory," *Journal of the History of Biology* 42, no. 3 (2009): 457–493.

11. A milestone event was the presentation of Johannsen's genotype theory to the American society of naturalists in December 1910. Wilhelm Johannsen, "The Genotype Conception of Heredity," *American Naturalist* 45, no. 531 (1911): 129–159.

12. See, for instance, Zhorez Medvedev, *The Rise and Fall of T. D. Lysenko* (New York: Columbia University Press, 1969); David Joravsky, *The Lysenko Affair* (Cambridge, MA: Harvard University Press, 1970); Valery Soyfer, *Lysenko and the Tragedy of Soviet Science* (New Brunswick, NJ: Rutgers University Press, 1994); Nils Roll-Hansen, *The Lysenko Effect: The Politics of Science* (Amherst, MA: Humanity Books, 2005).

13. Eva Jablonka and Marion J. Lamb, *Evolution in Four Dimensions: Genetic, Epigenetic, Behavioral, and Symbolic Variation in the History of Life* (Cambridge, MA and London: MIT Press, 2005).

14. Kevles, *In the Name of Eugenics*, 172–175.

15. A politically important difference was the attitude toward racism. The genetic superiority of Europeans was often taken for granted before World War I. But the experience of war created a new social and political climate. Revolutionary demands for a more just and egalitarian society forced a conscious reconsideration of the meaning and implications of race differences.

16. Kenneth M. Ludmerer, *Genetics and American Society: A Historical Appraisal* (Baltimore, MD: Johns Hopkins University Press, 1972), 34–43.

17. Quoted in Garland Allen, *Thomas Hunt Morgan* (Princeton, NJ: Princeton University Press, 1972), 229.

18. Lewellys F. Barker, "Foreword," in *Eugenics: Twelve University Lectures* (New York: Dodd, Mead, 1914), xi.

19. Øyvind Giæver, "Marriage and Madness: Expert Advice and the Eugenic Issue in Twentieth Century Norwegian Marriage Legislation," *Science Studies* 16, no. 1 (2003): 3–21; Nils Roll-Hansen, "Norwegian Eugenics: Sterilization as Social Reform," and "Conclusion:

Scandinavian Eugenics in the International Context," in *Eugenics and the Welfare State: Sterilization Policy in Denmark, Sweden, Norway, and Finland*, eds. Gunnar Broberg and Nils Roll-Hansen, 2nd ed. (East Lansing, MI: Michigan State University Press, 2005), 151–194, 259–271.

20. Roll-Hansen, "Norwegian Eugenics," 158–160, 169–175.

21. Roll-Hansen, *The Lysenko Effect*, 230–243.

22. For a broad presentation of debates about eugenics and recessive heredity through the first decades of the twentieth century, see Diane B. Paul, "Did Eugenics Rest on an Elementary Mistake?" in Diane B. Paul, *The Politics of Heredity: Essays on Eugenics, Biomedicine, and the Nature-Nurture Debate* (Albany, NY: State University of New York Press, 1998), 117–132.

23. See, for example, Roll-Hansen, "Norwegian Eugenics," 156–158.

24. Mark B. Adams, ed., *The Evolution of Theodosius Dobzhansky* (Princeton, NJ: Princeton University Press, 1994).

25. Franz Boas, "Human Faculty as Determined by Race," *Proceedings of the American Association for the Advancement of Science, 43rd Annual Meeting 1894*, (Salem: Fredric W. Putnam, 1895), 301–327; Boas, "The Mind of Primitive Man," *Science* 13, no. 321 (22 February 1901): 281–289.

26. William B. Provine, "Geneticists and the Biology of Race Crossing," *Science* 182, no. 4114 (23 November 1973): 790–796.

27. W. E. Castle, "Biological and Social Consequences of Race-Crossing," *Journal of Heredity* 15, no. 9 (1924): 365–366.

28. Provine, "Geneticists and the Biology of Race Crossing," 793–794.

29. For a general account and analysis of this development see Barkan, *Retreat of Scientific Racism*, and Kevles, *In the Name of Eugenics*. For a contemporary testimony, see Gunnar Dahlberg, *Race, Reason and Rubbish* (London: Allen & Unwin, 1942). The book was first published in Swedish in 1940 and translated into English by Lancelot Hogben when he was forced by the German invasion of Norway in April 1940 to flee to Sweden and had to wait for passage through Russia back to England.

30. "Social Biology and Population Improvement," *Nature* 144, no. 3646 (16 September 1939): 521–522.

31. Ibid.

32. These laws were passed by overwhelming parliamentary majorities. In Norway there was one vote against, in Sweden and Denmark a very small minority. This meant that the laws included some amount of compromise to appease eugenics enthusiasts.

33. The situation was similar in Sweden. Thus Peter Weingart's "Science and Political Culture: Eugenics in Comparative Perspective," *Scandinavian Journal of History* 24, no. 2 (1999): 163–177, presents a distorted picture of the situation in Sweden in the 1930s and 1940s when he writes (173) that there was "a virtual identity of the eugenic and race-hygiene discourse in Sweden and Germany as well as a striking similarity in the steriliza-tion practice." A similarly misleading picture has been widespread in recent historiography of eugenics. See Broberg and Roll-Hansen, *Eugenics and the Welfare State*, preface.

34. For analysis of the role of genetic science, see Stefan Kühl, *Die Internationale der Rassisten. Aufstieg und Niedergang der internationalen Bewegung für Eugenik und Rassenhygiene im 20. Jahrhundert* (Frankfurt/Main: Campus Verlag, 1997); Jean Gayon, "Do Biologists Need the Expression 'Human Races?' UNESCO 1950–51," in *Bioethical and Ethical Issues Surrounding the Trials and Code of Nuremberg*, ed. Jacques J. Rozenberg (Lewiston, NY: Edwin Mellen Press, 2003); Staffan Müller-Wille, "Race et appartenance ethnique: La diversité humaine et l'UNESCO. Les Déclarations sur la race 1950 et 1951,"

in *UNESCO, 60 ans d'histoire de l'UNESCO. Actes du colloque international, Paris, 16–18 novembre 2005 Maison de l'UNESCO, Paris* (Paris: UNESCO 2007), 211–220. Jean Gayon, "Commentaire," ibid., 223–227.

35. M. F. A. Montague, *Man's Most Dangerous Myth: The Fallacy of Race*, 2nd ed. (New York: Columbia University Press, 1945), ix.

36. Montague's argument was based on a radically empiricist philosophy of science insisting that theoretical concepts be directly derived from observed facts.

37. L. C. Dunn and Theodosius Dobzhansky, *Heredity, Race, and Society* (New York: Penguin Books, 1947), 94.

38. See "Race," in *Encyclopedia of Human Rights*, ed. Edward Lawson, 2nd ed. (Washington, DC: Taylor & Francis, 1996), 1217.

39. Gunnar Dhalberg, *Raser och Folk* [Races and People] (Stockholm: Ehlins, 1955).

40. Melville J. Herskovits, "Foreword," in Franz Boas, *The Mind of Primitive Man* (Westport, CT: Greenwood Press, 1963), 5–12. Boas's essay was first published in 1911 and reprinted a number of times. A German version, *Kultur und Rasse*, was published in 1914, and a thoroughly revised English version in 1938.

41. Nils Roll-Hansen, "Eugenic Sterilization and the Role of Science: The Scandinavian Case," in *Legacies of Modernism: Art and Politics in Northern Europe, 1890–1950*, eds. Patrizia C. McBride, Richard W. McCormick, and Monika Zagar (New York: Palgrave, 2007), 72–74.

42. L. C. Dunn, "Cross Currents in the History of Human Genetics," *American Journal of Human Genetics* 14, no. 1 (1962): 1–13.

43. T. M. Sonneborn, ed., *The Control of Human Heredity and Evolution* (New York: Macmillan, 1965).

44. Ibid., 125.

45. Hermann Muckermann was one exception. He was a practicing Catholic who had been forced out of eugenic research and teaching by the Nazis; he continued to pursue a scientific humanism after the end of World War II. See Hans Ebert, "Hermann Muckermann, Profil eines Theologen, Widerstandskämpfers und Hochschullehrers der Technischen Universität Berlin," *Humanismus und Technik* 20, no. 1 (1976): 29–40.

46. Carola Sachse and Mark Walker, "Introduction: A Comparative Perspective," in *Osiris* 20, 2nd series, Politics and Science in Wartime: Comparative International Perspectives on the Kaiser Wilhelm Institute (2005): 1–20. They wrote: "Our collective analysis also reinforces the recent rejection of the naive and self-serving, or alternatively arrogant and conceited, belief that science flourishes best, or even can only really flourish, in a Western-style liberal democracy" (17). The rejected view is exemplified by quotations from the sociologist of science Robert Merton.

47. Hans-Walter Schmuhl, *Grenzüberschreitungen: Das Kaiser-Wilhelm-Institut für Anthropologie, menschliche Erblehre und Eugenik 1927–1945* (Göttingen: Wallstein Verlag, 2005), 541.

48. Provine, "Geneticists and the Biology of Race Crossing," 796.

49. This was essential, for instance, in the "ethics of knowledge" that the French molecular geneticist Jacques Monod formulated as his response to Marxist theories about science in the 1960s. Jacques Monod, *Le hasard et la necessité, essai sur la philosophie naturelle de la biologie moderne* (Paris: Editions du Seuil, 1970), 52.

50. Michel Morange, *The Misunderstood Gene* (Cambridge, MA: Harvard University Press, 2001). Müller-Wille and Rheinberger, *Vererbung*, chap. 8.

51. See for instance, Arthur Caplan, Glenn McGee, and David Magnus, "What Is Immoral about Eugenics?" *British Medical Journal* 319, no. 7220 (13 November 1999): 1284.

52. Philip Kitcher, *The Lives to Come: The Genetic Revolution and Human Possibilities* (New York: Simon and Schuster, 1997), chap. 8.

53. Diane B. Paul, *Controlling Human Heredity: 1865 to the Present* (Atlantic Highlands, NJ: Humanities Press, 1995), 132–135; Allen Buchanan, Dan W. Brock, Norman Daniels, and Daniel Wikler, *From Chance to Choice: Genetics and Justice* (Cambridge: Cambridge University Press, 2000).

FURTHER READING

Barkan, Elazar. *The Retreat of Scientific Racism: Changing Concepts of Race in Britain and the United States between the World Wars* (Cambridge and New York: Cambridge University Press, 1992).

Broberg, Gunnar, and Nils Roll-Hansen, eds. *Eugenics and the Welfare State: Sterilization Policy in Denmark, Sweden, Norway and Finland* (East Lansing, MI: Michigan State University Press, 1996).

Buchanan, Allen, Dan W. Brock, Norman Daniels, and Daniel Wikler. *From Chance to Choice: Genetics and Justice* (Cambridge: Cambridge University Press, 2000).

Jablonka, Eva, and Marion J. Lamb. *Evolution in Four Dimensions: Genetic, Epigenetic, Behavioral, and Symbolic Variation in the History of Life* (Cambridge, MA and London: MIT Press, 2005).

Kevles, Daniel. *In the Name of Eugenics: Genetics and the Uses of Human Heredity* (New York: Alfred A. Knopf, 1985).

Ludmerer, Kenneth M. *Genetics and American Society: A Historical Appraisal* (Baltimore, MD: Johns Hopkins University Press, 1972).

Müller-Wille, Staffan, and Hans-Jörg Rheinberger. *Vererbung: Geschichte und Kultur eines biologischen Konzepts* [Heredity: History and Culture of a Biological Concept] (Frankfurt: Fischer Taschenbuch Verlag, 2009).

Paul, Diane B. *The Politics of Heredity: Essays on Eugenics, Biomedicine, and the Nature-Nurture Debate* (Albany, NY: State University of New York Press, 1998).

Weindling, Paul. *Health, Race and German Politics between National Unification and Nazism, 1870–1945* (Cambridge and New York: Cambridge University Press, 1989).

CHAPTER 5

FERTILITY CONTROL: EUGENICS, NEO-MALTHUSIANISM, AND FEMINISM

SUSANNE KLAUSEN AND
ALISON BASHFORD

BY the turn of the twentieth century, colonial as well as national states were greatly alarmed by new knowledge that uncontrolled demographic changes were underway. The massive European population increases of the eighteenth and early nineteenth centuries suddenly slowed from the 1880s, a shift that by the early twentieth century was widely construed as a key component of "degeneration."[1] Consequently, the rational planning of future populations—their quality and quantity—was increasingly perceived as core political business. Similarly, eugenicists believed that demographic change should be managed by the state, acting on their advice. Anxiety about the implications of uncoordinated population changes for race, nation, and/or empire was the lifeblood of eugenics movements everywhere, and it fueled a long-standing, though uneasy, preoccupation with reproductive regulation. Eugenicists' relationship to the issue of fertility regulation was intellectually and politically complicated but, given their focus on selective breeding, one they could not avoid. For historians, too, the connections are simultaneously critical and difficult to disentangle. But one thing is certain: the fundamental aspiration of eugenicists the world over was to entrench the systematic regulation of human reproduction in order to bring about desired demographic change—at once a means and an end.

This chapter analyzes the preoccupation of eugenics with fertility control—a broad term denoting all methods by which humans seek to induce, prevent, or terminate pregnancy.[2] Eugenicists' approaches were inevitably complex and contingent. But it is possible to trace a shift over several generations from a position of great wariness, if not outright antagonism to measures aimed at reducing fertility, to a point at which eugenics was defined by faith in them. As the twentieth century progressed, eugenicists increasingly aligned themselves with advocates of contraception (commonly called birth control), out of recognition that they needed to be part of the birth control "revolution" that was taking place, or risk being left behind. Looking forward to a new policy for his Eugenics Society, English social scientist Alexander Carr-Saunders (1886–1966) summed up this realization when he observed: "whether we take long or short views, voluntary parenthood occupies the centre of the field."[3] In some contexts, it was eugenicists who were among the first to establish birth control clinics, and to advocate for more controversial technologies of reproductive control such as sterilization and sometimes abortion.

Birth Control

Today, campaigns for birth control are typically remembered for their prominent role in feminism's ongoing struggle for women's reproductive freedom. But it is important to recall that in the nineteenth and early twentieth centuries the advocates of contraceptive technologies were often men, occasionally as feminist sympathizers but more frequently as neo-Malthusians. Early neo-Malthusians established the Malthusian League in England in 1877, to promote greater public awareness of Thomas Malthus's law of population (first published in 1798).[4] Malthus (1766–1834) had argued that over-population created and exacerbated poverty, and that restricting births was one of the means by which to achieve economic security.[5] A clergyman, he approved the use of "moral" forms of birth control only, namely abstinence and delayed marriage. Neo-Malthusians embraced Malthus's economic ideas but combined them with advocacy of contraceptive technologies. What is important to highlight is that Malthusianism—old and new—was first and foremost an economic theory. Malthus's intellectual descendants aimed to reduce poverty, first at familial and national levels, and eventually internationally, through curbing population growth.

Early eugenicists typically disagreed with neo-Malthusianism on the question of fertility restriction. Indeed, the first generation of English eugenicists advocated positive eugenics, meaning population *growth* among select groups. Francis Galton (1822–1911) himself was predisposed toward positive eugenics, believing that moral persuasion, public education, and appropriate social policy could convince "fitter" members of society to have more children. He proposed the adoption of a policy of "befriendment" of growing families to encourage reproduction of the fit. Similarly, the likeminded W. C. D. Whetham proposed that old age pensions be based on the number of children raised, that scholarships be set aside for the children of the middle class, and that posts in the empire be guaranteed to the sons of the gentry.[6] By contrast, Charles Vickery Drysdale (1874–1961), long-serving president of the Malthusian League (and son of its founder, Charles Robert Drysdale, 1829–1907), declared in 1909 that neo-Malthusians did not agree with positive eugenics, since their objective was an overall decline of population growth rates, irrespective of class.[7]

Galton, Whetham, and others were wary of birth control because they feared it would contribute to "race suicide," meaning the disappearance of putatively better quality middle- and upper-class members of society. "I protest," said Galton, "against the abler races being encouraged to withdraw in this way from the struggle for existence."[8] The marked demographic change toward the small family system was celebrated by neo-Malthusians, but worried early eugenicists anxious about differential fertility on both class and race grounds.

Despite Galton's enthusiasm for positive eugenics, subsequent eugenicists in Anglo-America—and many other modernizing countries in the non-Catholic world—began in pragmatic fashion to incorporate negative eugenics (and therefore fertility control) into theory and practice. Relying on the "fit" to boost their numbers was unlikely to succeed, they increasingly realized, not least because many members of the "fitter" classes were the most diligent practitioners of birth control; curbing the population growth of dysgenic groups was soon understood to be the better approach. In the United States in the early twentieth century, eugenicists fearful of the declining birth rate of native-born Americans and steeped in the proliferating social sciences were initially wary of promoting birth control in a general way, but suggested that aiming it at the "unfit" could be useful. Paul Popenoe (1888–1979) captured this view in 1917 when he asked in *Birth Control Review,* "Is the practice of birth control eugenic?" He thought not, because it was generally practiced by the "superior classes." But universal knowledge of birth control "can not now be stopped," so rather than being opposed ought to be extended to "the inefficient part of the population."[9]

Similarly, C. V. Drysdale in Britain began subscribing to eugenic ideas and to view neo-Malthusianism and eugenics as mutually compatible. By 1912 he considered a general reduction in the birth rate a necessary pre-condition for successful eugenics: "at the very outset of the neo-Malthusian propaganda it was predicted that a movement in favour of rational selection would arise as soon as the birth-rate was sufficiently reduced, and the Eugenics movement has justified this prophecy."[10] In his mind, far from being oppositional, the "quality" and "quantity" problems plaguing populations, as well as their solutions, were complementary.

The rapprochement between eugenics and the birth-control movement began to be forged at a series of meetings organized by neo-Malthusians. From the outset, British neo-Malthusians engaged likeminded thinkers and activists elsewhere—in France, Belgium, the United States, India—and starting in the early twentieth century they arranged a series of International Neo-Malthusian Conferences that brought together activists who advocated fertility control. Although small, these meetings are significant because they evolved into the much larger birth control conferences of the 1920s and 1930s, key meetings where the relationship between fertility control and eugenics was renegotiated. Neo-Malthusians also established organizations that in some contexts were the earliest sites of development and dissemination of eugenic ideas. William Schneider has noted that in France *Le Malthusien* was one of the only journals to use the word "eugenics" before the International Congress in London in 1912. Indeed, after that meeting the journal changed its title to *Le Malthusien: Revue eugéniste.*[11] In Australia—like France a low-fertility nation—neo-Malthusian men were among the earliest and most vocal eugenicists. Statistician Sir George Knibbs (1858–1929), for example, was a regular participant in international neo-Malthusian as well as international eugenic conferences, and a key demographer who sounded the alarm about world overpopulation as early as 1916.[12]

In India as well, it was neo-Malthusian organizations and personnel who first discussed eugenics, blending together and often blurring the line between economic and biological arguments for reducing population growth. Knibbs's neo-Malthusian publications on global overpopulation were read carefully by a core group of Indian scholars, extending the long colonial and local traditions of economic and scientific research on population issues. In Madras, a Hindu Neo-Malthusian organization was established as early as 1882, remerging in 1928 as the Madras Neo-Malthusian League, run by elites, publishing in English, and as Sarah Hodges shows in this volume, explicitly incorporating eugenics. Aiming for "human welfare through birth control," its objectives included giving medical instruction on contraceptive methods "to all married people who desire to limit their families or who are in any way unfit for parenthood."[13] The *Madras Birth Control Bulletin* regularly discussed the core eugenic question of differential fertility, of "the relative proportion of different classes in the population."[14] Eugenics and neo-Malthusianism were increasingly interchangeable ideas, practices, and movements. Biology professor Gopaljee Ahluwalia created the Indian Eugenics Society in Lahore in 1921 and the Indian Birth Control Society in Delhi the following year.[15] These Indian neo-Malthusians published widely in English eugenic and birth control presses, and they engaged key figures such as American birth-control activist Margaret Sanger (1879–1966) in their efforts.[16]

Sanger herself was instrumental in linking neo-Malthusianism and eugenics. With her long-standing interest in social issues like poverty and pacifism, in addition to her fundamental concern for women's health, Sanger was early influenced by the arguments of British Malthusians, and consistently constructed her own political genealogy in these terms. Historical interpretations of her career have tended to minimize the neo-Malthusian connection, however. Hodgson and Watkins argue that her links with prominent neo-Malthusians Edward Alsworth Ross (1866–1951) and Clarence Little (1888–1971) were strategic rather than genuine.[17] Angus McLaren similarly distances Sanger from a neo-Malthusian position, arguing that in coining the term "birth control," she replaced "the old, gloomy economic label, 'neo-Malthusianism' and began to separate the issue of fertility restriction from its nineteenth-century political and economic associations."[18] But the themes of reproduction, poverty, and population growth remained intimately intertwined in Sanger's political economy (as they did for most other advocates of birth control), even as she and other feminist birth controllers such as Edith How-Martyn (1875–1954) emphasized gendered power relations in reproduction.

Starting in the 1920s, Sanger, rebuffed by the American medical establishment and vociferously opposed by the Catholic Church, sought an alliance with the eugenics movement. She organized the 1927 World Population Congress in Geneva, a watershed event billed initially as the Seventh International Neo-Malthusian Conference. Despite the title, the meeting was as much about "quality" as "quantity" issues: speakers from Italy, Germany, Sweden, and Britain spoke on differential fertility, a core eugenic concern. Her co-organizer was Clarence Little (1888–1971), sometime president of the American Eugenics Society and member of the American Birth Control League.[19] Like so many of his counterparts, especially in the Anglophone world, Little fully subscribed to neo-Malthusianism alongside and as part of his eugenics.

In Catholic France advocacy of any method of restricting births was increasingly politically difficult. Anxiety about fertility decline produced a strident and official pro-natalism, backed up by the criminalization of contraception from 1920. This did not affect population trends but did render politically marginal movements and individuals who sought to validate, or argue for the extension of, birth-control services. It also shaped the nature of eugenics toward Lamarckian *puériculture*—a hygiene-based model of preventive and environmental health—that would become influential in the Middle East and in Latin America, as chapters in this volume show.

In contexts outside the Catholic world, however, eugenicists began to shift their stance toward a more pragmatic accommodation of birth control, realizing that positive eugenics had failed. Sterilization no longer held much scientific validity on genetic and statistical grounds, and many states would continue steadfastly to refuse to implement coercive measures. By 1933, the American Eugenics Society formally endorsed Margaret Sanger's birth-control campaign, and Henry Pratt Fairchild (1880–1956) announced in 1940 that "these two great movements [eugenics and birth control] have now come to such a thorough understanding and have drawn so close together as to be almost indistinguishable."[20] In Britain, too, under the leadership of birth-control advocate C. P. Blacker (1895–1975), the Eugenics Society shared premises, resources, personnel, and objectives with various birth-control organizations.

Eugenicists' support for birth control went beyond mere advocacy. They were often involved in establishing birth-control clinics and other schemes for the distribution of information among the poor, in both working-class districts in industrializing nations and rural centers in some agricultural-based economies. It was this interest in managing and intervening in the reproductive lives of one particular social group—the poor—that most directly linked neo-Malthusians and eugenicists. Clinics engaged variously in advising and distributing contraceptive information and technologies, including the cap, diaphragm, condom, intra-uterine device, sponge, and spermicides.

In settler colonial contexts particularly, eugenics and birth control often dovetailed neatly. Racial dynamics commonly focused expert attention on the qualities of white settler populations. In Australia, eugenic organizations were centrally concerned with improving the mental and physical health of the white population. Measures they promoted included mental and physical health screening of migrants from Britain, marriage certificates, birth control for married women, and sterilization for some.[21] In South Africa, the small but determined eugenics movement that emerged during the Great Depression was a pioneering and leading force in favor of institutionalizing birth control. This was a radical proposition in a society where, as almost everywhere, "unnatural devices" of contraception were perceived by settlers to hasten rather than prevent race suicide. Indeed, the Race Welfare Society in Johannesburg, which comprised highly respected eugenicists, opened the first birth-control clinic in the colony in 1932. Its opening is explained by the racial/ethnic context within which eugenics took root: in South Africa, eugenicists were afraid that the minority white population (about 20 percent of the total population) would be "swamped" by the subjugated black majority. Their fear led them to conclude that the best way to preserve white supremacy was to strengthen the white race by making birth control available to "unfit" "poor whites," who were prolific relative to middle-class whites, and whose poverty was intensified and made even more visible in urban centers during the Great Depression. Along with maternal feminists, the eugenics movement in South Africa succeeded in convincing the state to subsidize birth-control clinics for women in 1937, decades ahead of other British colonies and Britain itself.[22]

Early birth-control clinics were often an amalgam of neo-Malthusian, eugenic, and feminist impulses, and it is important to understand that for activists and experts at the time, these discourses were not necessarily contradictory. The Racial Hygiene Association of New South Wales, for example, which became the Family Planning Association of Australia in 1960, began as an initiative of the Feminist Club in the 1920s and was strongly supported by the state's leading eugenicist, Member of Parliament and sometime Minister of Health, Dr. Richard Arthur (1865–1932). Fully understanding that women sought birth control for varied reasons, the Association categorized attendances at its clinic along "health," "economic," or "eugenic" criteria.[23] Similarly, data collected over seven years from 55 clinics in Germany, the United States, and Britain, presented at the 1930 International Birth Control Conference in Zurich, gave indications for women's attendance: "Health Only," "Economic," or "Eugenic."[24] In India, to take another example, the Sholapur Eugenics Education Society ran a "Wives' Clinic," headed by A. P. Pillay (1890–1956). A handbill of the day catches perfectly the frequently linked feminist, eugenic, and neo-Malthusian discourses. It began with the classic definition of eugenics and then indicated that contraceptive information would be offered to married women who were too young, ill, or weak for pregnancy, or who experienced pregnancy too frequently. Women whose husbands had venereal disease or conditions that might be transmitted to offspring (insanity, idiocy, epilepsy, criminality) were also to be offered information. Finally—revealing the original Malthusian (economic) logic—information was available to women whose husbands "have too small an income to rear up a large family."[25] In some instances, eugenics and birth control came to be more or less interchangeable terms, one selected over the other according to locally expedient politics. In 1937 the new Hong Kong birth-control group (discussed in Chung's chapter in this volume) called themselves the Hong Kong Eugenics League, explaining: "The name 'Eugenics' is selected because it is thought that it will appeal more to the Chinese mind than birth control. However the object and functions of the League are purely those of birth control."[26] Such ambiguity in motives and terminology has often been overlooked by both scholars and partisans, who have oversimplified the eugenic agenda on the part of birth-control activists. Yet, we should properly *expect* many advocates of accessible contraceptives to have linked neo-Malthusianism, feminism, and eugenics in this period.[27] All three had in common the belief in the social efficacy of fertility control under particular circumstances, and the political lines dividing each ideology were not necessarily clear to their advocates. The eugenic component of birth control campaigns needs to be appreciated as historically commonplace.

STERILIZATION

The degree to which users should have control over contraceptive technologies was often a key point of difference between groups with an investment in fertility control. Eugenicists, who were usually members of the social elite, generally advocated methods that could be closely managed by authorities, from state policies designed to prevent or delay marriage through various forms of health certificates and legal regulation, segregation of the "unfit," sterilization of social undesirables, and withholding public health services from social "incapables."[28] As Karl Pearson (1857–1936) ominously declared as early as 1897, "Society will have in some fashion to interfere with and to restrict the anti-social in the matter of child-bearing."[29] This was quite a different stance from that taken by neo-Malthusians and feminists, who advocated methods such as condoms and diaphragms that could be controlled in private by individuals and couples.

Sterilization was a technology that lent itself particularly well to control by experts. It was usually achieved through surgical methods for both women and men, although biological methods (the injection of sheep spermatozoid, for example) and X-ray methods were also used.[30] While there were some eugenic endeavors in the 1920s and 1930s that ventured into sterilization as a form of birth control available through clinics (A. R. Kaufman's clinics in Canada are a notable example),[31] typically sterilization was envisioned as part of the management of institutionalized "problem populations," namely those housed in asylums, prisons, and hospitals; these were groups comprised disproportionately of poor, non-white, or otherwise socially marginal people. In fascist Germany, targeting specific groups for sterilization became official policy.[32] Nazi eugenics included policies and practices that aimed simultaneously to increase the fertility rate of members of the German stock deemed "racially pure" and decrease the number of those labeled racial degenerates. As Wilhelm Frick, the Reich minister for the interior, explained in 1933, the new population and race policy would have regard for the "insights of genetics, selection of life, and racial hygiene...In order to raise the number of hereditarily healthy progeny we have, above all, the duty to diminish the expenses for the asocial, inferior and hopelessly hereditarily ill and to prevent the procreation of hereditarily tainted persons."[33] In practice this led to the forced sterilization of mentally and physically disabled people, including proletarian women whose supposed promiscuity was perceived as a symptom of mental deficiency.[34]

One of the great national differences in the world history of eugenics is found in the comparative success and failure of sterilization laws. In Catholic contexts, as Mottier and Quine detail in this volume, sterilization was rarely promoted by eugenicists and was intricately connected to public debate on birth control in general. In France, Quebec, and many Latin American contexts, Catholic opposition was solidified in the light of the Papal Encyclical *Casti Connubii* of 1930.[35] As Schneider notes, this represented the first organized opposition to eugenic intervention in reproductive bodies.[36] Combined with the *puériculture* environmentalist and non-Mendelian cast of Francophone eugenics, then, there were major parts of the world where sterilization was simply not on the agenda.

Overall, as Mottier shows, the less Catholic and the more Protestant the context, the more likely were eugenicists to promote, and sometimes achieve, the legalization of eugenic sterilization: the Scandinavian countries, the western Canadian provinces, various states within the United States, Germany, and the Swiss canton of Vaud.[37] And in contexts where Christian doctrine was not particularly relevant—such as India and Japan, for example—sterilization was readily discussed and eventually endorsed in law. As a subcommittee of the Indian National Congress resolved in 1938:

> The state should follow a eugenic programme to make the race physically and mentally healthy. This would discourage marriages of unfit persons and provide for the sterilization of persons suffering from transmissible diseases of a serious nature such as insanity or epilepsy.[38]

After independence, Jawaharlal Nehru chaired the National Planning Commission, and its 1951 report called for free sterilization and contraception on medical, social, and economic grounds, as well as birth-control research.[39]

Yet even in Protestant-dominated contexts, Catholic opposition was often vocal and sometimes successful in blocking the translation of eugenic campaigns into law. Combined Catholic and Labour Party opposition, for example, blocked the British Eugenic Society's intense efforts to legalize voluntary sterilization during the interwar period.[40] In some colonial contexts—such as Hong Kong—officials who happened to be Catholic were effective in limiting the extent and nature of birth-control clinics, including discussion of sterilization.[41] Similarly, Catholic chaplains in the U.S. occupying force in postwar Japan were vocal in their opposition to any form of birth control, then being promoted implicitly by the United States and explicitly by the Japanese government: "'Any use of the Marriage Act that robs the act of its natural power to generate life is an abuse of nature; and those who so use the act are guilty of a serious sin against God.' Such is the doctrine laid down by Pius XI."[42]

In jurisdictions governed by British common law and closely linked to British political developments, sterilization laws were also stymied by arguments in favor of the liberty of the subject. Moreover, sterilization was extremely controversial in part because of previous, negative experiences with the state attempting to compel medical procedures. In England and Wales in 1853, vaccination was made mandatory for all infants, swiftly sparking an intense public backlash, and in the 1860s the British Parliament, concerned about the high rate of venereal disease in the armed forces, passed a series of laws making the medical treatment of infected prostitutes compulsory, provoking major opposition. In many "British world" contexts, then, including some (but not all) Canadian provinces, Australia, South Africa, and New Zealand, early bids for even "voluntary" sterilization requiring the consent of the (usually) institutionalized patient were unsuccessful. Moreover, by the 1930s eugenicists everywhere were being confronted with a new challenge to their campaigns for eugenic sterilization, namely growing scientific criticism of its efficacy. Geneticists and statisticians argued that there was no evidence that most genetic defects would be diminished at a population level through a program of sterilization (see Roll-Hansen, chapter 4 of this volume).

Finally, when discussing the controversial issue of sterilization it is important to take heed of historian Johanna Schoen's recent reminder that reproductive technologies are neither inherently liberating nor oppressive.[43] Depending on context, she notes, they can hold myriad meanings. In fact, women in many contexts have pursued sterilization as a reliable and permanent means of preventing pregnancy. In Schoen's words, in North Carolina and elsewhere, sterilization "that violated a young girl in the name of eugenics brought relief to her overburdened mother."[44] Sterilization took place in multiple social spaces and types of clinical encounters— it was both forced upon the incarcerated and institutionalized in the name of eugenics, and actively sought by women in private consultation in doctors' rooms and in the growing number of birth-control clinics.

ABORTION

Abortion was widely considered sinful in both Protestant and Catholic contexts and was illegal in many jurisdictions by the early twentieth century. Eugenicists rarely supported abortion.[45] Weimar Germany was one exception; feminists from the 1910s utilized eugenic thinking to agitate for accessible abortion and birth control.[46] More commonly, though, feminist neo-Malthusians and some eugenicists advocated greater access to mechanical, and later biological, contraceptives, as well as sterilization, as means by which the number of illegal, dangerous (and for many, unethical) abortions would be reduced.

One national context where abortion was promoted in eugenic terms was post-World War II Japan where in 1948 the Eugenic Protection Law legalized abortion to "prevent the birth of eugenically inferior offspring, and to protect maternal health and life." Sterilization had already been legalized with the National Eugenics Law, passed in 1940, for the same reason.[47] The laws reflected the U.S. occupation force's and Japanese experts' anxiety about population growth, as well as the concerns of socialists, feminists, and eugenic birth-control activists.[48] In the 1948 law in particular, the conflation of eugenic, neo-Malthusian, and feminist rationales for fertility control is clear. It permitted abortion if the woman or spouse had "a mental illness, mental deficiency, psychopathic disorder, hereditary physical ailment or hereditary deformity." Abortion was also permitted if the woman had leprosy (understood to transfer to offspring), if the pregnancy resulted from rape, or "if the continuation of pregnancy or childbirth is likely to seriously harm the mother's health for physical or economic reasons."[49] The inclusion of this economic indication meant that abortion and sterilization services became both available and widely used. According to one report, in 1951 alone there were around one million abortions and 23,000 sterilizations in Japan. Only 717 of these sterilizations were notified for the eugenic criteria above; the rest were sought and granted on the "economic" criterion, that is, as a form of birth control.[50] The eugenic laws in postwar Japan were in effect delivering radical reproductive choice to many women in the absence of effective contraception.

Considered within a narrow history of eugenics, this law might be considered anachronistic: a strange postwar deployment of eugenic ideology which had recently been "discredited by Nazi abuses."[51] Yet once neo-Malthusian, feminist, and eugenic strands are tied together as part of a linked, if complicated, twentieth-century story of fertility control, this law can also be understood as a precursor of the widespread liberalization of abortion laws that would follow in the 1960s and 1970s. That is, the health and economic terms on which both sterilization and abortion became legal in Japan are recognizably the same terms by which termination of pregnancy later became legal in many other jurisdictions. The "eugenic" criterion also continued in the legalization of abortion of a fetus considered "handicapped" or "abnormal." For example, in the United Kingdom, the 1967 Abortion Act permitted the procedure on a similar criterion, "that there is a substantial risk that if the child were born it would suffer from such physical or mental abnormalities as to be seriously handicapped."[52] Similarly, in South Africa the Abortion and Sterilization Act (1975) permitted medical abortion when there was a "serious risk that the child to be born will suffer from a physical or mental defect of such a nature that he will be irreparably seriously handicapped."[53] In this sense, far from fading away, eugenic-derived practices became increasingly normalized.

EUGENICS, FERTILITY CONTROL, AND FEMINISM

Intervening in populations' rate of growth has vastly different implications for men and women. Historians have shown how the rise of nationalism and visions of patriotic motherhood commonly went together in the early twentieth century: examples include modernizing Turkey, British Edwardian imperialism, Puerto Rican nationalism, and German expansionism.[54] Eugenics, too, with its focus on selective breeding, typically placed women at the center of its project. As Argentinean doctor José Beruti explained in 1934, "maternity…encompasses most of the eugenic problems requiring urgent solution."[55] Inevitably, therefore, eugenics' concern with manipulating fertility led to close encounters with another movement preoccupied with the social implications of women's reproductive capacity: feminism.

First-wave feminism comprised many strands, each with its own particular goal—moral reform, political emancipation, economic independence.[56] Unsurprisingly, class, nationalism, imperialism and anti-colonialism shaped feminist agendas differently. Yet despite ideological and political differences, feminists were linked by a belief in the principle of voluntary motherhood: women should be able to avoid unwanted pregnancy. But they disagreed over what constituted the best means by which to do so. Some called for temporary or complete abstinence, others for the rhythm method, while a small minority advocated contraceptive technologies. At best, feminism was initially highly ambivalent about contraception out of concern that the separation of sex and reproduction would erode women's already limited power within marriage, and public endorsement was rare until the 1920s. This is also unsurprising, given pressures of respectability, the often illegal status of circulation of information about contraception, strident Catholic opposition, grudging Protestant toleration, and many feminists' conviction that advocacy of birth control would harm the "cause."

However, some early feminists—typically those connected to Malthusian political and economic theory—did advocate the use of contraceptives, both for the sake of women's health and as a means to address chronic familial and national poverty. Women like Annie Besant (1847–1933) and Alice Vickery Drysdale (1844–1929) (partner of Charles Robert Drysdale and mother of C. V. Drysdale) introduced an important feminist dimension to the debate, one which subsequent activists like Sanger, How-Martyn, and Lady Rama Rao in India made remarkably successful: they promoted contraceptives on the basis of women's health (by arguing their use would diminish dangerous abortion and give women time to rest between pregnancies) and economic stability for women and their smaller families. Very occasionally—and most radically in the first two decades of the twentieth century—feminists such as Emma Goldman (1869–1940) and Marie Stopes (1880–1958) advocated the use of contraceptives to separate sex from reproduction for the sake of women's sexual pleasure.[57]

Today it is widely understood that feminism played a major role in the social acceptance of technologies of reproductive control; some may even assume that feminists alone achieved this. However, the history is far more complex. As we have seen, eugenics, too, was significant. Eugenics and feminism have often been interpreted as inherently antagonistic on the matter of reproductive control, and for good reason: just as feminism was starting to promote voluntary motherhood, eugenics was arguing that women's reproductive capacity was too important to the race/nation to be left in women's charge. Put simply, eugenicists saw women's social role as determined by their reproductive function; as Karl Pearson wrote, "women's child-bearing activity is essentially part of her contribution to social needs."[58] Not infrequently, eugenicists were intensely anti-feminist, opposed to the individualism that shaped a major strand of late-nineteenth and twentieth-century Western feminism (more precisely, a "new woman" culture), and were acutely unhappy that "fit" women, who often supported the women's movement, were avoiding pregnancy. Eugenic scientists invested in the biology of sexual difference sometimes claimed that women's new social and political aspirations "unsexed" them.[59] And so when English sexologist Havelock Ellis (1859–1939) claimed that "the question of Eugenics is to a great extent one with the woman question," this had both feminist and anti-feminist implications.[60] Nonetheless, at times the two social movements actually had a more amenable relationship than is commonly supposed. Indeed, eugenics, with its emphasis on the heritability of health, made it possible for some feminists to rethink their position on contraception. It provided a respectable justification for using and making available contraceptives, especially for poor women.

Historians disagree, however, over the nature of the relationship between feminism and eugenics. Some have downplayed the genuine interest many feminists had in eugenic ideas and policies aimed at improving the race through selective breeding. They have tended to interpret feminists' relationship to eugenics as strategic only, perceiving them as deploying eugenic arguments about the health of the race as a tactic in a larger fight for women's emancipation. Angus McLaren, for example, writes that social purity campaigners drew upon eugenic arguments to strengthen their criticism of men who infected their wives with venereal disease contracted through sex with prostitutes.[61] Linda Gordon argues, similarly, that in the nineteenth century feminists, like many other social reformers, drew on the legitimacy of science in the form of evolutionary theory to buttress their radical claims.[62] Dorothy Porter claims that in Britain and Sweden some feminists "separated the rights of women to control their own fertility and eugenic concerns about racial improvement," but without noting the corollary: that some feminists combined them.[63] Porter sees Italian feminists utilizing arguments about women's crucial role as "bearers and nurturers of future citizens" as a rhetorical device in their bid for political equality and full citizenship.[64] And according to Susan Pedersen, feminists adopted eugenic arguments as a means of deflecting anti-feminist accusations that they were shirking motherhood. Thus feminists fighting for family allowances in the 1920s and 1930s "accepted" the eugenic claim that social success was evidence of biological fitness as a means of winning sufficient political support.[65] To these scholars, feminists harnessed eugenic rhetoric to their aspirations solely for pragmatic political reasons.

Other historians perceive a less utilitarian relationship between the two movements, suggesting that eugenic ideas were an integral dimension of feminist theory and action. Lucy Bland, for example, argues that some feminists believed women, as reproducers of "fit" offspring and moral saviors, could "purify" the race and employed a biologized discourse of class as well as of the superiority of the white Anglo-Saxon race over its colonial subjects.[66] Lesley Hall observes that feminists believed that improving the conditions and status of motherhood was key to revitalizing the nation.[67] Nancy Ordover agrees with Linda Gordon and Angela Davis that Margaret Sanger was a genuine and consistent advocate of fertility limitation for the biologically "unfit."[68] And the most famous British feminist advocate of birth control, Marie Stopes, promoted the sterilization of the "hopelessly rotten and racially diseased," as she once put it.[69] Historian Ann Taylor Allen declares that "eugenic theory was a basic and formative, not an incidental, part of feminist positions on the vitally important themes of motherhood, reproduction, and the state," and critiques historians' reluctance to acknowledge the genuine interest many feminists had in eugenic ideas and policies aimed at improving the race through selective breeding.[70] All over the world, as many chapters in this volume show, feminist movements did more than use eugenic ideas as instruments in their efforts to combat representations of women as mere breeders with the new ideal of "responsible" motherhood; they enthusiastically produced and incorporated eugenics in their campaigns.[71]

Despite a sometimes uneasy relationship between eugenicists and feminists, the issue of birth control ultimately proved to be a key point of connection between them. Feminists drew upon eugenic arguments about the importance of rational, responsible parenthood in their growing demands for accessible birth control. And eugenicists increasingly took up the feminist-Malthusian argument that poor women's ability to space or limit pregnancies would benefit the race, nation, and latterly, the "Third World."

CONCLUSION

In many countries, eugenics succeeded in entrenching the idea that selective breeding is a social good. Starting in the late nineteenth century, eugenicists engaged in a long-running campaign to instill in their societies the sense that a good pregnancy is a planned pregnancy, and one that will lead to the birth of a "healthy" child. Their success was in large part due to the organizational and discursive overlap with neo-Malthusians and feminists. And although fertility control is most readily associated with the history of feminism, as we have seen, the activists that secured philanthropic and, later, state sponsorship of accessible methods of fertility control were as likely to be motivated by neo-Malthusian and eugenic ideas as by feminist ideas. Men like Clarence Little in the United States, A. R. Kaufman in Canada, Clarence Gamble in Puerto Rico, H. B. Fantham in South Africa, C. P. Blacker in Britain, Richard Arthur in Australia, and A. P. Pillay in India—all were instrumental in promoting fertility control and linking it to eugenics. In the same way that not all feminists were "birth controllers," not all "birth controllers" were feminists.

The assumption that people should plan their families "responsibly" and avoid having "abnormal" offspring is now somewhere near normative in many national contexts, although the *method* of this avoidance remains as controversial as it was in the early twentieth century, if not more so. The widely shared belief in the value of selective breeding (for individuals, if not for populations) is a major legacy of eugenics: the men cited above would be pleased to know how commonplace both the notion and the practice have become. But this norm was not produced by eugenics alone. As we have seen, feminists, too, played a vital role, working hand in glove with eugenicists to popularize the notion of rational family planning. Feminist eugenicists and eugenic feminists—often connected by neo-Malthusian ideas— have been "strange bedfellows" who together played a leading role in developing new reproductive technologies, as well as making commonplace the contemporary belief that individuals have the right, and should have the means, to take steps to prevent giving birth to "unfit" children.

NOTES

1. Simon Szreter, *Fertility, Class, and Gender in Britain, 1860–1940* (Cambridge: Cambridge University Press, 1996); Hera Cook, *The Long Sexual Revolution: English Women, Sex, and Contraception, 1800–1975* (Oxford: Oxford University Press, 2004).

2. Kate Fisher, *Birth Control, Sex, and Marriage in Britain, 1918–1960* (Oxford: Oxford University Press, 2006), 2.

3. A. M. Carr-Saunders, "Eugenics in the Light of Population Trends," *Eugenics Review* 60 (1968): 55. This was a republication of Carr-Saunders's 1935 Galton lecture.

4. Thomas Malthus, *An Essay on the Principle of Population* (London: J. Johnson, 1798).

5. Rosanna Ledbetter, *A History of the Malthusian League, 1877–1927* (Columbus, OH: Ohio State University Press, 1976), 66; Richard Soloway, *Birth Control and the Population Question in England, 1877–1930* (Chapel Hill, NC: University of North Carolina Press, 1982).

6. Angus McLaren, *Birth Control in Nineteenth-Century England* (London: Croom Helm, 1978), 148–149.

7. Charles Vickery Drysdale, "The Eugenics Review and the Malthusian," *The Malthusian* 33, no. 12 (1909).

8. Cited in McLaren, *Birth Control*, 144.

9. Paul Popenoe, "Birth Control and Eugenics," *Birth Control Review* 1, no. 3 (1917): 6.

10. C. V. Drysdale, *Neo-Malthusianism and Eugenics* (London: William Bele, 1912).

11. William H. Schneider, *Quality and Quantity: The Quest for Biological Regeneration in Twentieth-Century France* (Cambridge: Cambridge University Press, 1990), 37.

12. Sir George Handley Knibbs, *Shadow of the World's Future* (London: Ernest Benn, 1928), 19–20.

13. *Madras Birth Control Bulletin* 6, no. 1 (Jan–Feb 1936), in Eileen Palmer Papers, British Library of Political and Economic Science, London (hereafter Eileen Palmer Papers), COLL MS 639/1/25.

14. Ibid. The Bombay Birth Control League was established in 1923, and in 1930 Dr. Sailendranath Singh established the Neo-Malthusian Society of Bengal. See Mausumi Manna, "Approach Towards Birth Control: Indian Women in the Early Twentieth Century," *Indian Economic and Social History Review* 35, no. 1 (1998): 38.

15. See Sanjam Ahluwalia, *Reproductive Restraints: Birth Control in India, 1877–1947* (Urbana, IL: University of Illinois Press, 2008), 30–32.

16. For example, Narayam Sitaram Phadke, *Sex Problems in India* (Bombay: Taraporevala Sons, 1927); see Barbara Ramusack, "Embattled Advocates: The Debate over Birth Control in India, 1920–40," *Journal of Women's History* 1, no. 2 (1989): 34–64.

17. Dennis Hodgson and Susan Cotts Watkins, "Feminists and Neo-Malthusians: Past and Present Alliances," *Population and Development Review* 23, no. 3 (1997): 475–476.

18. Angus McLaren, *Twentieth Century Sexuality: A History* (Oxford and Malden: Blackwell, 1999), 65.

19. Alison Bashford, "Nation, Empire, Globe: The Spaces of Population Debate in the Interwar Years," *Comparative Studies in Society and History* 49, no. 1 (2007): 170–201.

20. Fairchild cited in Hodgson and Watkins, "Feminists and Neo-Malthusians," 478.

21. Alison Bashford, *Imperial Hygiene: A Critical History of Colonialism, Nationalism, and Public Health* (Basingstoke: Palgrave, 2004), chap. 7.

22. Susanne Klausen, *Race, Maternity and the Politics of Birth Control in South Africa, 1910–39* (Basingstoke: Palgrave, 2004).

23. Émilie Paquin, *Social Hygiene in New South Wales, Ontario and Quebec: A Comparative History of Two Organisations, 1919–1939* (MPhil diss., University of Sydney, 2008).

24. Birth Control Clinics, Conference File, Margaret Sanger Papers, Library of Congress, Washington DC, MS 38,919, Box 193.

25. Brochure, Sholapur Eugenics Education Society, n.d. Eugenics Society Papers, Wellcome Library, London, SA/EUG/E/10.

26. K. C. Yeo to How-Martyn, 11 Feburary 1937, Eileen Palmer Papers, COLL MISC 639/1/9.

27. "The Truth about Margaret Sanger," *Citizen*, 20 January 1992, www.blackgenocide.org/sanger.html (accessed 15 October 2008). For an excellent discussion of 1970s interpretations of sterilization as genocide, see Laura Briggs, *Reproducing Empire: Race, Sex, Science, and US Imperialism in Puerto Rico* (Berkeley, CA: University of California Press, 2002), 142–152.

28. McLaren, *Birth Control*, 149–50.

29. Karl Pearson, *Chances of Death* (London: E. Arnold, 1897), 129.

30. See for example, Yolanda Eraso, "Biotypology, Endocrinology, and Sterilization: The Practice of Eugenics in the Treatment of Argentinian Women during the 1930s," *Bulletin of the History of Medicine* 81, no. 4 (2007): 817.

31. Linda Revie, "'More than Just Boots!' The Eugenic and Commercial Concerns behind A. R. Kaufman's Birth Controlling Activities," *Canadian Bulletin of Medical History / Bulletin canadien d'histoire de la médecine* 23, no. 1 (2006): 119–143.

32. Gisela Bock, "Antinatalism, Maternity and Paternity in National Socialist Racism," in *Maternity and Gender Policies: Women and the Rise of the European Welfare States, 1880s–1950s*, eds. Gisela Bock and Pat Thane (London and New York: Routledge, 1991),

233–255. As Bock shows, Nazi sterilization policy represented a continuity with the overall consensus among Weimar eugenicists that sterilization of those deemed "unfit" was desirable.

33. Cited in Gisela Bock, "Nazi Sterilization and Reproductive Politics," in *Deadly Medicine: Creating the Master Race,* ed. Sara Bloomfield (Washington, DC: United States Holocaust Museum, 2004), 62.

34. Dagmar Herzog, *Sex after Fascism: Memory and Morality in Twentieth-Century Germany* (Princeton, NJ: Princeton University Press, 2005), 4.

35. See John Macnicol, "Eugenics and the Campaign for Voluntary Sterilization in Britain Between the Wars," *Social History of Medicine* 2, no. 2 (1989): 161–162. See also Matthew Connelly, *Fatal Misconception: The Struggle to Control World Population* (Cambridge, MA: Harvard University Press, 2008), 85–86; Nancy Leys Stepan, *"The Hour of Eugenics:" Race, Gender, and Nation in Latin America* (Ithaca, NY: Cornell University Press, 1991).

36. Schneider, *Quality and Quantity,* 285.

37. See Mottier, chap. 7; Natalia Gerodetti, "From Science to Social Technology: Eugenics and Politics in Twentieth-Century Switzerland," *Social Politics* 13, no. 1 (2006): 59–88. An exception is Mexico, which passed a 1932 eugenic sterilization law as an expression of anti-clericalism and secularism. Stepan, *"The Hour of Eugenics,"* 130–133.

38. National Planning Committee Report, 1938, quoted in Benjamin Zachariah, "The Uses of Scientific Argument: The Case of 'Development' in India, c. 1930–1950," *Economic and Political Weekly* 36, no. 39 (2001): 3695.

39. Connelly, *Fatal Misconception,* 141–146. See also Hodges, chap. 12 of this volume.

40. Macnicol, "Eugenics and the Campaign for Voluntary Sterilization."

41. K. C. Yeo to How-Martyn, 11 Feburary 1937, Eileen Palmer Papers, COLL MISC 639/1/9.

42. "Birth Control Opposed," *Nippon Times,* 30 April 1949.

43. Johanna Schoen, *Choice and Coercion: Birth Control, Sterilization, and Abortion in Public Health and Welfare* (Chapel Hill, NC: University of North Carolina Press, 2005).

44. Ibid., 3.

45. For connections between abortion and sterilization debates, see Marius Turda, "'To End the Degeneration of a Nation': Debates on Eugenic Sterilization in Inter-war Romania," *Medical History* 53, no. 1 (2009): 77–104; Henry P. David, Jochen Fleischhacker, and Charlotte Hohn, "Abortion and Eugenics in Nazi Germany," *Population and Development Review* 14, no. 1 (1988): 81–112; Øyvind Giæver, "Abortion and Eugenics: The Role of Eugenic Arguments in Norwegian Abortion Debates and Legislation," *Scandinavian Journal of History* 30, no. 1 (2005): 21–44; Jean Elisabeth Pedersen, "Regulating Abortion and Birth Control: Gender, Medicine, and Republican Politics in France 1870–1920," *French Historical Studies* 19, no. 3 (1996): 673–98. If eugenicists rarely supported abortion, the same can be said for feminists. Stella Browne was exceptional among feminists in her advocacy of legal abortion. See Stella Browne, "The Right to Abortion," in *World League for Sexual Reform: Proceedings of the Third Congress, London, 1929,* ed. Norman Haire (London: Kegan Paul, Trench, Trubner, 1930), 178–181.

46. Atina Grossmann, *Reforming Sex: The German Movement for Birth Control and Abortion Reform, 1920–1950* (Oxford and New York: Oxford University Press, 1995).

47. "Eugenic Protection Law (1948)," in Tiana Norgren, *Abortion before Birth Control: The Politics of Reproduction in Postwar Japan* (Princeton, NJ: Princeton University Press, 2001), Appendix 1, 149. See also Robertson, chap. 25 of this volume.

48. Norgren, *Abortion before Birth Control,* 36–44.

49. Ibid., 149.

50. Yoshio Koya, "The Program for Family Planning in Japan: In Reference to the Results of the Study on the Three Test Villages in Japan," n.d, in Rockefeller Family Papers, Rockefeller Archives Centre, Tarrytown NY, Record Group 5, Series 1, Box 80, Folder 671.

51. Norgren, *Abortion before Birth Control,* 4.

52. For the original legislation in full see British Abortion Act (1967), www.statutelaw.gov.uk.

53. Susanne Klausen, "'Reclaiming the White Daughter's Purity': Afrikaner Nationalism, Racialized Sexuality, and the 1975 Abortion and Sterilization Act in Apartheid South Africa," *Journal of Women's History* 22, no. 3 (2010).

54. Anna Davin, "Imperialism and Motherhood," *History Workshop* 5 (1978): 9–65; Briggs, *Reproducing Empire*; Cornelie Usborne, *The Politics of the Body in Weimar Germany* (Ann Arbor, MI: University of Michigan Press, 1992); Ayça Alemdaroğlu, "Politics of the Body and Eugenic Discourse in Early Republican Turkey," *Body and Society* 11, no. 3 (2005): 61–76.

55. José Beruti (1934) cited in Eraso, "Biotypology, Endocrinology, and Sterilization," 793.

56. Marlene LeGates, *In Their Time: A History of Feminism in Western Society* (London and New York: Routledge, 2001).

57. Linda Gordon, *The Moral Property of Women: A History of Birth Control Politics in America* (Urbana, IL: University of Illinois Press, 2002), 141–148. Marie Stopes, it should be noted, was contemptuous of the Malthusian League and entirely dismissive of economic arguments for birth control.

58. Pearson, *The Chances of Death,* 251, cited in McLaren, *Birth Control,* 146.

59. Cynthia Russett, *Sexual Science: The Victorian Construction of Womanhood* (Cambridge, MA: Harvard University Press, 1989).

60. Havelock Ellis, *The Task of Social Hygiene* (London: Constable, 1912), 46–47. See also Daniel Kevles, *In the Name of Eugenics: Genetics and the Uses of Human Heredity* (New York: Alfred A. Knopf, 1985), 87.

61. McLaren, *Birth Control,* 199–200.

62. Gordon, *Moral Property of Women,* 68.

63. Dorothy Porter, *Health, Civilization, and the State: A History of Public Health from Ancient to Modern Times* (London and New York: Routledge, 1999), 189.

64. Ibid., 183.

65. Susan Pedersen, *Family, Dependence, and the Origins of the Welfare State: Britain and France, 1914–1945* (Cambridge and New York: Cambridge University Press, 1993), 42, 318.

66. Lucy Bland, *Banishing the Beast, English Feminism and Sexual Morality, 1885–1914* (London: Penguin, 1995), 222, 231.

67. Lesley A. Hall, "Women, Feminism and Eugenics," in *Essays in the History of Eugenics,* ed. Robert A. Peel (London: The Galton Institute, 1998), 36.

68. Nancy Ordover, *American Eugenics: Race, Queer Anatomy, and the Science of Nationalism* (Minneapolis, MN: University of Minnesota Press, 2003).

69. Hall, "Women, Feminism and Eugenics," 40.

70. Ann Taylor Allen, "Feminism and Eugenics in Germany and Britain, 1900–1940: A Comparative Perspective," *German Studies Review* 23 no. 3 (2000): 477–505.

71. See also Angelique Richardson, *Love and Eugenics in the Late Nineteenth Century: Rational Reproduction and the New Woman* (Oxford and New York: Oxford University Press, 2003); Greta Jones, "Women and Eugenics in Britain: The Case of Mary Scharlieb, Elizabeth Sloan Chesser, and Stella Browne," *Annals of Science* 52, no. 5 (1995): 481–502;

George Robb, "The Way of All Flesh: Degeneration, Eugenics, and the Gospel of Free Love," *Journal of the History of Sexuality* 6, no. 4 (1996): 589–603; Grossman, *Reforming Sex*, 70–75; Usborne, *The Politics of the Body in Weimar Germany,* 102–136.

FURTHER READING

Connelly, Matthew. *Fatal Misconception: The Struggle to Control World Population* (Cambridge, MA: Harvard University Press, 2008).

Dowbiggin, Ian. *The Sterilization Movement and Global Fertility in the Twentieth Century* (Oxford and New York: Oxford University Press, 2008).

Hodges, Sarah, ed. *Reproductive Health In India: History, Politics, Controversies* (New Delhi: Orient Longman, 2006).

Hodgson, Dennis, and Susan Cotts Watkins. "Feminists and Neo-Malthusians: Past and Present Alliances," *Population and Development Review* 23, no. 3 (1997): 469–523.

Klausen, Susanne. *Race, Maternity and the Politics of Birth Control in South Africa, 1910–39* (Basingstoke: Palgrave, 2004).

Giæver, Øyvind. "Abortion and Eugenics: The Role of Eugenic Arguments in Norwegian Abortion Debates and Legislation," *Scandinavian Journal of History* 30, no. 1 (2005): 21–44.

McLaren, Angus. *Twentieth Century Sexuality* (Oxford: Blackwell, 1999).

Quine, Maria Sophia. *Population Politics in Twentieth-Century Europe* (London and New York: Routledge, 1996).

Richardson, Angelique. *Love and Eugenics in the Late Nineteenth Century: Rational Reproduction and the New Woman* (Oxford and New York: Oxford University Press, 2003).

CHAPTER 6

DISABILITY, PSYCHIATRY, AND EUGENICS

MATHEW THOMSON

PSYCHIATRY and mental disability appear central in the story of eugenics at its most influential, in the period from the eve of World War I to the end of World War II. This chapter reviews assumptions about this centrality, explaining why the mentally disabled, more than the mentally ill or the physically disabled, became the focus of eugenic anxiety as well as policy. It also examines why such policies were taken further in some countries than others, and whether the focus on mental disability applies equally to eugenics within a colonial setting. It argues that the primacy of the mentally disabled does not necessarily equate with the primacy of psychiatry: the development of eugenic policies toward the mentally disabled in this period was more crucially a consequence of political and economic context than of the influence of psychiatry itself. Finally, it concludes with an exploration of the history of disability, psychiatry, and eugenics since World War II.

MENTAL DISABILITY AND THE EUGENICS OF SEGREGATION

To understand this story, we need to begin by looking at why mental illness, and more particularly mental disability, emerged as a major subject of concern in relation to the health of the broader population at the end of the nineteenth century. This entails first looking back to the rise of the mental asylum. The idea that this was part of a "great confinement" of the unruly, driven by concerns about discipline, and backed by the state, has little support now from historians of the subject.[1] Pioneering efforts in fact depended on philanthropy and drew on Enlightenment ideals of reform through moral therapy for the mentally ill (as at the York Retreat in England) and reeducation for the mentally disabled (as inspired by Edouard Séguin, first in France and then in the United States).[2] Nevertheless, the nineteenth century saw an inexorable demand for such specialized institutional care, from families unable to cope, and from work-houses, reformatories, and prisons, which identified recidivism as a sign of inherent mental incapacity. By the end of the century, public funds in North America, Europe, and Britain and its settler societies of the Empire had invariably been drawn upon to support what, in the context of the time, were among the most impressive achieve-ments of state welfare in a generally laissez-faire age. Without the therapeutic weapons of the pharmaceutical revolution that followed World War II, and often shackled by a legalism among cultures suspicious of placing control of liberty in medical hands, it proved hard for inmates once incarcerated to escape the public asylum. Asylums expanded accordingly, becoming overcrowded and increasingly swamped by a long-term population of the chronically sick, incapable, and aging.[3] It is generally agreed that this was a crucial factor in a mounting therapeutic nihilism and an association between the problem of mental illness and theories of degeneration. The latter, of course, was a broad cultural movement, its anxieties reaching far beyond the problem of the asylum; its advocates were more likely to be writers and intellectuals than psychiatrists.[4] Nevertheless, the doctors who worked in or with the population of the asylums—who came, gradually, to identify themselves as psychiatrists, through specialist organizations and journals—did occasionally take a prominent role. In France, psychiatrist Bénédict Augustin Morel (1809–1873) popularized the term "degeneration" to describe the individual descent into mental illness.[5] And in Britain, Henry Maudsley (1835–1918) has attracted interest for his increasingly pessimistic view of medicine's power to cure insanity.[6] These ideas came in an era before the emer-gence of a popular eugenics movement, and they played a part in providing an envi-ronment for the success of this movement when it did emerge.

Nineteenth-century asylum records make it clear that well before the age of eugenics or genetics it was common to attribute mental illness to heredity. Yet his-torians of the process of admission to asylums have offered little indication that hereditary concerns were a major factor in the decision for confinement before the late nineteenth century. Doctors, in any case, were less often the crucial voices that historians have assumed them to be. Lay magistrates, lawyers, and families were more influential, and here issues of manageability and violent or dangerous behavior were the important factors in the decision to confine.[7]

In the early decades of the twentieth century, this situation changed. Concern about heredity of mental disorder, in particularly of mental disability—in the language of the time the "mental defective" or the "feebleminded"—emerged as an important factor in debate about the need for an expansion and specialization of institutional care.[8] In Britain, the birthplace of eugenics, an idea turned into a movement in part through bringing together a broad coalition of parties around this issue and through the success of a new system of institutions for the "feebleminded" under the Mental

Deficiency Act of 1913.[9] The clamor for action drew on ideas about potential inheritance (even if there was little agreement as to the exact mechanism) and thus a fear that feeblemindedness would spread unless this population was confined. But political success depended on the conjuncture of this hereditarianism with the existence of powerful social and moral justifications for ensuring that the danger of the feebleminded was contained.[10] In fact, the fragility of the scientific basis for an argument about heredity, as well as a general suspicion about placing too much power in the hands of medical experts, meant that the political campaign had to be cautious about its use of a language of "eugenics."[11] Nevertheless, the Mental Deficiency Act was the most substantial achievement of the British eugenics lobby. The Eugenics Education Society, founded in 1907 and coming to maturity in Britain in the midst of the campaign, was eager to support this view.[12] And the idea that legislation on mental deficiency was a first and fundamental step in any modern approach to eugenics was a model that would be exported well beyond Britain itself. However, more broadly, it might be characterized as less innovative, indicative of a general modernization of systems of care for the mentally disordered. Even in Britain itself, specialization had already been developing since the 1870s, in part through the recognition of the feebleminded within the poor law system, in part through the recognition of ineducable children within the universal elementary education system first introduced in 1870. In Europe and particularly in North America, a new type of institution—the colony—had already emerged, less focused on cure and containment than the asylum, and more concerned with providing sheltered work in self-supporting communities safely set apart from the broader community. As belief in the eugenic danger of the mentally defective became widespread in the first decades of the century, the colony-style institution seemed to offer an ideal solution: safely segregated, economical, expandable, and modern. This helped make segregation the first and foremost eugenic policy of the day.

Why were the feebleminded, rather than the mentally ill or the physically disabled, the key target of this early-twentieth-century eugenics? There was certainly a belief that some forms of blindness or deafness were hereditary, and there were intersections between movements for care in these areas and the eugenicists. In the United States, for instance, Alexander Graham Bell (1847–1922), inventor of the telephone, was a founding figure of the Eugenics Society and an advocate of sterilization and the outlawing of marriage for the deaf. But eugenic concern about these disabilities remained on the periphery. When it came to mental illness, psychiatrists throughout the nineteenth century had tended rather casually to record heredity as a likely cause. Some psychiatrists, particularly in Germany, the leader in this period in a scientific approach to researching mental illness, began to explore inheritance in more detail.[13] However, mental illness invariably manifested itself as temporary or at least as something that emerged at a certain point in the life cycle. Because of this, the efforts of psychiatric reform and public sympathy increasingly looked to forms of temporary and voluntary admission to catch cases in the early, treatable stages and toward the use of psychotherapy for the mass of mental health problems within the community in order to prevent decline into certifiable mental illness.[14] The mental defective was different because the condition was congenital and thus seemed incurable. More fundamentally still, the highest grade of mental defective—the feebleminded—could readily pass as normal (unlike the physically disabled), and thus there was widespread belief that the scale of the problem had been underreported and that many of the major social problems of the day might be accounted for in this way. The idea of the mental defective provided a viable target for the theories and anxieties about degeneration that preceded and now found further ammunition in the science of eugenics. The defective introduced into the population a degenerate, hereditable strain, which could manifest itself in crime, pauperism, and immorality. Worse still, such social and moral failings led to profligate breeding (just as the fertility of the responsible classes appeared to be falling) and thus a future generation that would replicate such biological, social, and moral decline on an ever larger scale, over time dragging down the overall fitness of the population.[15]

Crucial to the eugenic fear surrounding the feebleminded was the mapping of individual mental (and thus social) inadequacy onto thinking about the population as a whole. This appealed, politically and culturally, in the early twentieth century because it paralleled an international climate of concern about national efficiency in an era of escalating international competition in the years before World War I.[16] And it was made possible because increasingly interventionist states provided new resources and techniques for viewing individual ability in relation to that of the population.[17] Feeblemindedness could emerge not just as an individual but also as a eugenic and social problem of huge scale because the expansion of systems of state and voluntary welfare and surveillance, crucially assisted by the public-spiritedness and social investigation of women social workers, made not just the scale but also the genealogical nature of the condition visible. Represented through compelling stories of families like the Jukes and the Kallikaks in the United States and through the visual logic of family tree diagrams, this new representation of defective heredity had the potential to reach far beyond a medical audience, helping to turn eugenics into a popular movement, gaining the attention of the political classes and the state. Perhaps most crucially, the new intelligence test, which emerged in large part through the concern about mental deficiency in the first decade of the century, provided an apparently scientific and efficient way to identify and grade mental defect, thus turning eugenic policy into a practical possibility.[18] Moreover, in setting the mentally defective on a bell curve of intelligence for the population as a whole, testing presented not just the feebleminded, but even their dull and backward offspring and relatives, as a eugenic disaster for the state of the nation.[19]

BEYOND SEGREGATION

Given the way that this conjuncture of factors acted to escalate fears about the scale of the problem of low intelligence early in the century, not only eugenicists but also governments concerned with national efficiency began to think beyond institutional segregation. In the United States, Canada, and Australasia, immigration became a focus for eugenic concern. Here, psychiatrists took a lead role in warning of the potentially dysgenic effect of unrestricted immigration, pushing for a greater role in this area and often favoring the deportation of the mentally disordered. Yet immigration policy tended to be shaped more by the politics of ethnicity (with attempts to restrict the proportion of southern and eastern Europeans in favor of the Nordic).[20] There were also experiments with laws prohibiting marriage among defectives. In the United States, the first state to introduce such a law was Connecticut in 1895; by the mid-1930s over 40 states had laws relating to the marriage of the feebleminded and insane. However, eugenicists questioned the success of these policies, viewing them as difficult to enforce, often inconsistent with genetic understanding, and as potentially dysgenic in discouraging the fit from breeding.[21]

The policies of sexual sterilization widely discussed in this volume had roots in the 1890s in the United States, where castration was used in some penal institutions, partly to control masturbation and sexual appetites. It is important to recognize, however, that the expansion of this policy depended on it being directed at the problem of mental deficiency, and as a result it was often closely associated with psychiatry. Initially, doctors were wary of an operation that was of no obvious medical benefit to the patient, but when in 1899 Dr. Harry Sharp of the Indiana State Reformatory developed the new operation of vasectomy, which was simple to perform and relatively safe, the situation changed. The new eugenic climate was also crucial to this medical change of heart. In 1907, Indiana was the pioneer in legalizing compulsory sterilization, still directed mostly at criminals and rapists, though now also targeting the insane, epileptics, and idiots on purely eugenic grounds. Wherever sterilization was legalized in the interwar period, its main focus was the mental defective: in the United States, Canada, Scandinavia, and Switzerland. And in Germany, which saw by far the most substantial program (375,00 operations), this was again by some distance the leading category of operations (52.9 percent); though other disabled groups were also covered, including schizophrenics (25.4 percent) and hereditary epileptics (14 percent), as well as smaller numbers of cases of hereditary physical deformity (6.3 percent), manic depression (3.2 percent), severe alcoholism (2.4 percent), hereditary deafness (1 percent), hereditary blindness (0.6 percent), and Huntington's Chorea (0.2 percent).[22]

Though the scale and breadth of the Nazi policy overshadows the history of eugenic sterilization, there has been a tendency in recent work on the subject to downplay exceptionality. It is now recognized that the United States was the pioneer in the area of sterilization (and thus an influence and inspiration for Germany) and also that within Germany itself the emergence of a law on sterilization as well as the rise of eugenics predated the Nazi assumption of power.[23] Research on Scandinavia, meanwhile, has highlighted the way that sterilization could be attractive to governments on the Left as well as the Right.[24] On the other hand, the disproportionate scale of the Nazi policy clearly does demand special explanation, and historians have looked toward a complex interplay of professional, political, and economic contexts.

By the 1930s, German psychiatry was at the forefront of research into the biological basis of mental illness, building on a tradition introduced by Emil Kraepelin (1856–1926) at the start of the century. It moved forward as a properly funded and dedicated research field with specialized research centers able to take advantage of the latest developments in medical science, rather than leaving research to isolated asylum doctors weighed down by the pressures of daily management of huge institutions, as was the case, for instance, in Britain. By the 1930s, the genetic (and racial) basis of mental disorder was at the cutting edge of such research. Indeed, the Rockefeller Foundation in the United States saw it as so important to its broader program of research in "psychobiology" that it continued to offer financial support until 1939.[25] The Nazi assumption of power did not redirect this research toward heredity, but it did provide a crucial political and ideological context as well as a system of patronage that encouraged and radicalized such a focus, and this in turn helped legitimize the implementation of policy.[26] Psychiatrists benefited economically and in terms of status from their involvement in the apparatus for prosecuting a policy of sterilization in Germany, assuming new roles in relation to training, administration, and adjudication of the law.[27] Nevertheless, comparative research would suggest that the political and legal context, not science, was most crucial to the scale of sterilization in Germany.

In Britain, one of the stumbling blocks for proposals on sterilization was concern about liberty of the subject; and there was a fundamental contradiction in arguing that mental defectives—by definition incapable—could be sterilized on a "voluntary" basis. In the United States, the Supreme Court in the 1927 case of *Buck v. Bell* (centering on Carrie Buck, a "feebleminded" girl from Virginia) upheld the legality of compulsory sterilization, but the federal system meant that law depended on individual state initiatives. Thus a state like Virginia, where the issue had gained popular local support, introduced a law in 1930 giving the superintendents of five state institutions the power to request sterilization of inmates.[28] But with persistent debate about legality as well as discontinuity of political control at the state level, there was never the political framework for the type of mass national program seen in Germany. The willingness of psychiatrists to cooperate in such schemes was never enough on its own to ensure effective implementation.

Ongoing scientific dispute about the hereditary basis of feeblemindedness was also an obstacle, with a move during the 1920s and 1930s toward recognizing that some of the early crude models, that like-begets-like, or that one form of degeneration could manifest itself in another in the next generation, were no longer sustainable. Increasingly, inheritance was recast as a complex multifactorial model. Generally, this was debated, not by psychiatrists, but by geneticists. Within this context, a genetically orientated psychiatrist, such as Lionel Penrose (1898–1972) in Britain, could emerge as an opponent rather than a supporter of eugenics.[29]

Psychiatrists were important, however, for a different reason. They looked at the issues of mental deficiency and illness from their perspective as custodians of institutions that already housed this population. Nations that had been pioneers in providing special institutional care for the mentally ill and the mentally handicapped in the nineteenth and early twentieth century now found themselves stretched economically by the challenge of extending systems of welfare and medicine to workers, pensioners, mothers, and children. Spending more on institutions for the mentally ill and defective was a decreasing political priority in an era of expanding democracy and the need for state welfare to satisfy the new political constituencies of the working class, women, and the increasingly influential parties of the Left. The result for asylum patients was overcrowding and terrible conditions. In World War I, huge numbers of patients in German hospitals died as food shortages exacerbated already poor conditions; arguably this established a significant precedent that may have affected the acceptability of later treatment in mental hospitals during the economic crises of the next war.[30] The economic challenge never went away, but it returned with a vengeance in the Depression, with unemployment and welfare cuts in the 1930s. This was a crucial context for sterilization not just in Germany (where numbers in fact declined from 1937 in part because pressure on the institutions had by then been alleviated) but also in the United States.[31] In California, for instance, which developed one of the most substantial programs of involuntary sterilization in the country, the policy emerged as a way to alleviate pressure on mental hospitals, enabling the parole of mentally ill and feebleminded patients who were there in large part because of the eugenic argument. Here, sterilization—with over 11,000 operations between 1930 and 1944—became a handmaiden for aftercare in the community, appealing to psychiatrists struggling to overcome the image of the mental hospital as a dumping ground, and eager to be associated with new medical therapeutics.[32] In Britain, on the other hand, psychiatrists were wary of any further stigma that might arise from association with sterilization.[33] Whatever the case, in policy terms, the economic rationale for sterilization depended less on the support of the psychiatrists than on those who paid for institutions.

Interwar psychiatry also looked to advance its status by escaping the asylum altogether, allying with a broader public and political interest in preventive medicine in the closely related mental hygiene, race hygiene, and eugenics movements of the era. This involved dialogue at both a national and an international level, and with pressure groups as well as the state, and was thus potentially hugely attractive in advancing the individual status of the psychiatrist as well as the collective status of the profession. Psychiatrists were not the foot soldiers of the eugenics movements of the era, which drew very broadly on the professional and middle classes, but in most countries they were important and sympathetic allies. In a few instances, they did assume a leadership role. The secretary and driving force behind the Eugenics Society in London was psychiatrist C. P. Blacker (1895–1975); in Germany, the psychiatrist Ernst Rüdin (1874–1952), who went on to be a key figure in the Nazi eugenics program, had previously represented Germany at international congresses of eugenics and mental hygiene. We also find psychiatrists seeking status, which was unavailable to them as mere managers of mental institutions, through offering expert advice to states increasingly concerned with eugenic fitness. In Canada, psychiatrists advised on immigration control; psychology, with its mental tests, was also crucial in this regard, notably in the United States.[34] Even in Britain, there were opportunities for advancement in undertaking surveys of the mental fitness of the population, and here psychiatrists were important in guiding the government on the need to address eugenics, first in the Mental Deficiency Act of 1913, and then again in the revival of concerns and linkage to the "social problem group" in the 1930s.[35]

This was not just the case in countries with a comparatively well-developed system of psychiatric care; the appeal of the modernity of eugenics as a preventive route in mental hygiene and as a way to gain support from pressure groups and the state was just as likely where the psychiatric profession was less secure.[36] The comparative study of the involvement of psychiatrists in eugenics in Latin America in the first half of the twentieth century is particularly suggestive in this respect.[37] In Brazil, the links between psychiatry and eugenics appear particularly strong, with the founding of the Liga Brasileira de Higiene Mental in 1923 to support a program of mental prophylaxis focused on the mentally deficient.[38]

There were the same opportunities for psychiatrists to gain a public platform through eugenics in the former white colonies of Britain's Empire, such as Canada, Australia, and South Africa, where eugenics had a similar attraction as part of a nation-building project. These countries tended to follow and share the anxieties of the British (and in the Canadian case, also those of the United States) in the potential threat of the feebleminded to the overall quality of the population, and they too began to establish specialized institutions and new systems for testing and surveying borderline individuals. They also had particular concerns about ensuring that immigrants were not feebleminded. Such eugenic policies focused on the mental qualities of the white settler populations. Thus the Australians considered new legislation on mental deficiency because of the British Royal Commission on the Feeble-Minded of 1908, and though it was deemed unnecessary immediately to follow Britain's 1913 legislation in establishing a system for segregation of mental defectives, legislation followed in Tasmania (1920), Victoria (1922), Queensland (1938), and New South Wales (1939).[39]

Psychiatry also studied the mind of indigenous populations, and tended to conclude that there was a fundamental biological difference in the brain, perhaps akin to that of the mental defective, that helped to account for intellectual inferiority.[40] If it had been needed, such research might have been deployed to provide supposedly scientific justification for the absence of equal rights and for policies of racial segregation.[41] Perhaps most importantly, in an era in which there was such a strong current of belief that it was best that these defectives should never be born, such views contributed to an acceptance that race suicide was a natural and even a progressive event: the primitive mind was simply unable to cope with the complex demands of a civilizing culture. Ultimately, however, mental disorder of native populations in these nation-building settler colonies was of little eugenic concern to the white populations; rather, building a fitter nation meant policing the fertility of, and weeding out the feebleminded among, the white population. In Australasia and South Africa, given the virtual absence of the Aboriginal populations from mental hospitals (partly a result of segregation but more fundamentally because of a lack of concern about extending mental welfare beyond the white population), they never became the focus of a potential conjuncture of eugenic, racial, and economic concern that they might have been in the 1930s. Canada appears an exception to this rule.[42] Thus, psychiatry and its theories of the primitive mind and brain provided further legitimacy for racial segregation and discrimination, but did not generally encounter the Aboriginal populations as a eugenic problem. Even in the southern states of the United States, the almost exclusive focus of psychiatric eugenics in this period was white feeblemindedness. The black population was too low a priority to merit the cost of specialized care (they were more likely to be placed in general asylums or to be dealt with in the penal system). Assertions about their intellectual inferiority tended to be accepted as a given. And the degree to which they represented a eugenic threat was lessened by racial segregation.[43] In the history of psychiatry under European colonialism in an area like Africa, we again see psychiatry operating to account for racial difference—via the idea of a primitive "African mind"—and thus as a tool of Empire, but we do not see it operating as a tool of eugenics.[44] Mental hospitals for the native population tended to be a last resort to control the dangerous and violent. There was no attempt to use them as a tool to improve the eugenic quality of either the native populations or the relatively small number of white colonists within these settings.

PSYCHIATRY, DISABILITY, AND EUGENICS AFTER WORLD WAR II

The conjuncture of eugenics and psychiatry can be seen therefore as a particular feature of modernizing nation-states in the early twentieth century, a manifestation of nationalist anxieties about the qualities of the dominant racial group itself, and thus less characteristic of policy toward colonized and subordinate races. What happened to the anxieties that were so acute, and so characteristic of modernity, particularly in Europe and North America, in the first four decades of the century? This is a central question for a history of psychiatry, disability, and eugenics. It is often assumed that the stigma of association with Nazism was fundamentally important in turning professional, popular, and political support away from eugenics in the second half of the century. Undoubtedly, in the short term, and perhaps just as importantly in the long term, this has been very important in undermining any legitimacy for eugenics. This was partly because the war provided conditions to radicalize eugenics in Germany and to foster its links to the broader racial ambitions of the Nazi regime. Eugenics was largely released from limits arising from free opposition. And it was provided with an economic crisis that magnified the burden of the mental institution. Psychiatrists, competing for professional influence and resources, and often ideologically committed to the regime's ambitions of placing the eugenic fitness of the society above concern for individual well-being and even the life of their patients, were deeply involved and culpable in this process. Under such circumstances, as Weindling discusses, between 70,000 and 95,000 people in mental institutions (including 6,000 handicapped children) were killed under the guise of "euthanasia," and thus with the assistance of medical and other workers, including psychiatrists, within these institutions. Psychiatrists, through such involvement, were able to strengthen their control over institutions for the seriously handicapped, which had earlier been run by the church.[45] Due to public pressure, this euthanasia policy was ended in 1941, though in fact historians have now traced clear continuities to the expansion of the ideology and techniques of psychiatric "euthanasia" as part of the killing on a much greater scale within concentration camps.[46]

The short-term impact of the war on the international reputation and practice of eugenics can nevertheless be overstated. In Britain and the United States, a scientific critique of eugenics was mounting well before the war; even psychiatrists were less sympathetic or confident about support in the 1930s than they had been a decade earlier.[47] Elements of postwar continuity also need to be recognized. Sterilization, for instance, was not necessarily regarded—before, during, or after the war—as a Nazi policy. Hence, people who had undergone compulsory sterilization were excluded from receipt of compensation by the Federal German government in 1960–1961; not until 1981 was the illegitimacy of the policy officially acknowledged.[48] In Japan, a Eugenic Protection Law was passed in 1948. It was particularly directed at postwar anxieties about unwanted pregnancies and illicit abortion, but it would also cover persons with hereditary diseases, including feeblemindedness.[49] In Canada, sterilization in Alberta and British Columbia continued until repeal of the law in 1972.[50] In Denmark, occupied by the Nazis in the war, sterilization in fact increased after the departure of the Germans.[51] In Sweden, sterilization peaked around 1950 and the practice continued right up to the abolition of the law in 1975.[52] In Norway, which had introduced its sterilization law in 1934, it was also after the end of Nazi occupation that levels rose, with a total of 40,891 up to 1976. And in Finland there were 56,080 operations between 1951 and 1970.[53] It does need to be recognized that sterilization in such contexts was increasingly operating as a form of birth control, but such policies were still often targeted at those deemed to be in most need of radical intervention: the mentally dull, backward, and defective.

Even in a country like Britain that had never introduced sterilization, there is plenty of evidence that a significant body of psychiatrists continued to believe that sterilization of mental defectives, if it had not been for political sensitivities, would have been a good thing for the mental health and social well-being of the community. Psychiatrists recognized that the language and policies of "eugenics" had to be rejected as "quite impracticable in a democracy," but they remained frustrated advocates of limiting the fertility of those they regarded as mentally unfit.[54] Even if conditions were not directly hereditable—and there was a general recognition that the psychiatry of the interwar period had been far too incautious and crude in its attitude here—ongoing study of "problem families" showed that the interplay of environmental deprivation and genetics—and thus individuals of allegedly low intelligence and social incompetence—remained a key problem and one that potentially undermined the strength of a welfare state.[55] The Scandinavian postwar sterilization programs were largely justified on such social grounds, with the proportion of operations justified alone on eugenic (or medical) grounds an increasingly small proportion of the whole. The coupling of the social and the biological in fact offered a more effective tool for controlling the fertility of the section of society—involved in crime, poverty, ill-health, poorly educated, and with a high birthrate—that had always been the ultimate target for eugenicists before the war via the focus on mental deficiency (even if sterilization itself had tended to focus on assisting the release of mental defectives in institutions).[56]

A potentially powerful new eugenic tool in addressing disability was the coupling of prenatal testing and selective abortion. By 1961, prenatal screening for likelihood of Down's Syndrome was readily available in Britain.[57] This introduced a new era in which the patients were increasingly given choices of whether to go ahead with pregnancies likely to result in physically or mentally handicapped offspring. Though this may not have been the determining factor in individual choice, over time such policy has had outcomes that could be deemed to be eugenic. One influential account of the process has described this as opening a "backdoor to eugenics."[58]

If advance in human genetics has led to a return of eugenics, it is important to emphasize that it is eugenics of a very different brand than that which characterized the first half of the century; and arguably, the important differences make the analogy unhelpful and at times a hindrance to our understanding of the nature of recent developments. The eugenics of the first half of the century was driven by the eugenic aims of encouraging the fit to breed and preventing the unfit; in contrast, the human genetics of recent decades is cautious on eugenic aims (seeing choice and rights as equally important), though it may ultimately have eugenic ends. And while the eugenics of the first half of the century was willing to go down the route of compulsion, the new human genetics centers on the provision of individual and parental choice (even if we recognize that free choice, without the sway of social pressure and professional guidance, is difficult to achieve in practice).

These are crucial differences. In assessing the relationship between psychiatry, disability, and eugenics, there are three features that suggest a rupture between the history of the first half of the century and the present. First, the new focus on the genetics of disability takes place within a context in which anxiety about being overrun by a population of mental defectives, or even simply of the social and economic "burden" of this population, is now almost wholly silenced within public debate, if not absent altogether. In this respect, it is important to recognize that the final decades of the twentieth century were a period in which the most important and least controversial eugenic policy for restricting the fertility of the mentally disabled—the development of systems of lifetime segregation—was now being dismantled, with no eugenic outcry. Second, the genetic causes of disability, not the carriers of this disability, were now at the center of attention. And this has meant that psychiatry, as the expertise for managing the behavior of the key carrier group, has also been decentered. Third, the changes brought about by the disability rights movement, calling for respect for difference and recasting disability as a social construction, has radically circumscribed the possibilities for any new eugenics, particularly in those countries where a rights agenda is most fully developed. In fact, it was partly the influence of this group that lay behind the return of a discourse of "eugenics," now as a mode of critique (and particularly associated with Nazism) rather than as a program for support. Critics emerging out of this context condemned the offering of choice over termination of a disabled fetus as being in conflict with an ideology of respect for all, and as a new form of fascist "euthanasia."[59] They also drew an analogy with the Nazis in their attacks on proposals for physician-assisted suicide that they feared might introduce a new "euthanasia" of the disabled.[60] And they warned that the long-term result of individual choices based on human genetics could be to exacerbate ongoing prejudice toward disability: reducing numbers of the disabled and making disability an issue of parental responsibility and fault.[61] Undoubtedly, such a voice from below, and crucially from the disabled and their advocates, has ensured that there is now a serious ethical and political barrier to a eugenics that ignored the rights and individual interests of the disabled patient; something that had been almost exclusively absent in the first half of the century.[62]

By the end of the century, the prospects of a new eugenic assault on disability were arguably greater in parts of the world relatively untouched by the first phase of eugenics—places now driven by concerns around national efficiency and modernization and not yet overly concerned with respect for the rights of the disabled. Indeed, looking not just to China but to other emerging populous powers such as India and Russia, one commentator to the *British Medical Journal* suggested that "people who condemn eugenics may be in a minority now."[63] China is the most obvious example of the possibility for thinking about such a new eugenics. Here, the emergence of a new eugenics has been closely linked to the introduction of a one-child policy since 1979, which focused attention on the quality of births and the prevention of somatic and genetic defects. In fact, Chinese eugenics also had much longer-term roots. Modernizing elites had looked to eugenics from the first decades of the century, and there was a long tradition of accepting considerable control over the female population as well as prioritizing the good of the collective over the individual.[64] These factors were significant in the blossoming of eugenic policy in the 1990s. In the mid-1980s, an experiment in Gansu province, known for its high population of people with learning difficulties, introduced new guidelines on premarital checkups, which prohibited marriage between close relatives and involving retarded and mentally ill people, and required intellectually impaired people to undergo sterilization if they married. In 1995, a Eugenics Law covering all of China was introduced, though following criticism the title was changed to the Maternal and Infant Health Care Law.[65] The new law made prenatal testing and the termination of pregnancies involving a genetic or somatic disorder compulsory.[66] The situation in China posed a dilemma for psychiatry in countries that had been through the political rejection of eugenics but which recognized the science of the new genetics. This was ultimately an ethical issue. Given its own eugenic past, the potential for accusations of further Western moral and psychiatric imperialism, and its own sympathies for the new genetics, Western psychiatry was poorly placed to condemn outright a modernizing China that regarded its policies as having a scientific basis.[67]

CONCLUSION

This chapter has argued that mental disability was at the very forefront of eugenic anxieties and actions in the first decades of the twentieth century. There were two main reasons for this. First, this was a problem that eugenics itself had inherited. The nineteenth century had seen the rapid expansion of systems of asylums for the mentally ill and disabled, and eugenics movements emerged in part in response to the question of what to do about this situation, and how to prevent its further expansion. Second, the existence of the feebleminded at large within the community provided a hereditary explanation not just for apparently rising levels of mental disability but also for individual failure, manifest in crime, unemployment, poverty and immorality, and rooted in mental and thus social inefficiency. The link between mental, social, and national failure was readily made at the turn of the century, and this provided a political mandate for eugenic action in countries that could afford a more expansive policy of segregating not just the insane but now also the mentally deficient or feebleminded. Psychiatry could benefit from, play an active role in administering, and to a degree provide legitimacy for such a development, but its ambitions were never enough to dictate development where the political will and economic means were lacking. Thus, in colonial settings, psychiatry may have viewed native populations as racially inferior, but this did not translate into using the asylum as a tool of eugenics. The eugenic segregation of the mentally disabled was characteristic of the wealthier and more modern nation-states of the period.

Democracy and concern about rights provided only a partial obstacle to the advance of eugenics when it came to the target of the mentally disabled in the interwar period. Thus, the lack of such restraints was a factor in the scale of sterilization in Nazi Germany, but sterilization was also widespread in the democracies of North America and Scandinavia. The attraction of the policy was often associated with the problems of sustaining systems of institutional care in the midst of economic crisis, and this affected countries with more advanced welfare systems in the 1930s. Psychiatry was attracted by any policy that could bring therapeutic optimism, though it also had some concerns that association with such an operation risked further stigmatizing the field. Once again, it is hard to see psychiatry itself as the driving force for eugenic policy on mental disability. World War II changed the political acceptability of eugenics. Whether it resulted in a fundamental shift in attitudes toward eugenics within psychiatry is more questionable. In the aftermath of the war, the feeling that the mentally less fit were a eugenic and social problem lingered, and in some settings the policy of sterilization continued; increasingly as a form of birth control, but often still targeted at those deemed mentally less able.

However, the language of eugenics had virtually disappeared. And the eugenic and economic concerns about the mentally disabled now appeared marginal, set alongside the vast demands of increasingly ambitious welfare states.

The debate about eugenics and disability resurfaced in the final decades of the century for two reasons. First, advances in human genetics were leading to a much greater potential than ever before for eugenic engineering. Second, the climate surrounding the rights of the disabled had fundamentally changed, and eugenics returned in part as a language of critique that connected the apparent genetic choices of the present with the discredited eugenics of the past. In fact, a closer analogy to the policies of the first half of the century was the type of state eugenics emerging in a country like China, where the concerns about the rights of the disabled were far less developed. In the countries that had seen mental disability playing such a key part in the emergence of eugenics at the start of the century, the disabled now played a key role in demanding that the specter of eugenics act as a check on the new genetics. A similar critical role for psychiatry, close companion to eugenics in the first half of the century, and now witness to increasing evidence of the genetic basis of mental disorders, is harder to discern.

ACKNOWLEDGMENTS

I would like to thank the Wellcome Trust for funding support and Dr. Katherine Angel for assistance with the research for this chapter.

NOTES

1. Michel Foucault, *Madness and Civilisation: A History of Insanity in the Age of Reason* (New York: Vintage, 1972).

2. On Séguin, see Carolyn Steedman, "Bodies, Figures and Physiology: Margaret McMillan and the Late Nineteenth-Century Remaking of Working-Class Childhood," in *In the Name of the Child: Health and Welfare, 1880–1940*, ed. Roger Cooter (London and New York: Routledge, 1992), 19–44; James Trent Jr., *Inventing the Feeble Mind: A History of Mental Retardation in the United States* (Berkeley, CA: University of California Press, 1994), 40–59. On the York Retreat and moral therapy, see Anne Digby, *Madness, Morality and Medicine: A Study of the York Retreat* (Cambridge: Cambridge University Press, 1985).

3. For instance, see Andrew Scull, *The Most Solitary of Afflictions: Madness and Society in Britain, 1700–1900* (New Haven, CT and London: Yale University Press, 1993).

4. Daniel Pick, *Faces of Degeneration: A European Disorder, c. 1848–1918* (Cambridge: Cambridge University Press, 1989); Mark H. Haller, *Eugenics: Hereditarian Attitudes in American Thought* (New Brunswick, NJ: Rutgers University Press, 1963).

5. Ian Dowbiggin, *Inheriting Madness: Professionalization and Psychiatric Knowledge in Nineteenth-Century France* (Berkeley, CA: University of California Press, 1991); Robert Nye,

Crime, Madness, and Politics in Modern France: The Medical Concept of National Decline (Princeton, NJ: Princeton University Press, 1984).

6. Trevor Turner, "Henry Maudsley—Psychiatrist, Philosopher and Entrepreneur," *Psychological Medicine*, 18, no. 3 (1988): 551–574; Pick, *Faces of Degeneration*, 203–216.

7. David Wright, "Getting out of the Asylum: Understanding the Confinement of the Insane in the Nineteenth Century," *Social History of Medicine* 10, no. 1 (1997): 137–155.

8. The term "mental deficiency" was prevalent in Britain and within its imperial sphere of influence, with three grades of intelligence from low to high: idiots, imbeciles, and the feebleminded. In North American, the dominant term for all categories was the feebleminded.

9. Mathew Thomson, *The Problem of Mental Deficiency: Eugenics, Social Policy and Democracy in Britain, 1870–1959* (Oxford: Oxford University Press, 1998); Mark Jackson, *The Borderland of Imbecility: Medicine, Society and the Fabrication of the Feeble Mind in Late-Victorian and Edwardian England* (Manchester: Manchester University Press, 2000).

10. Harvey G. Simmons, "Explaining Social Policy: The English Mental Deficiency Act of 1913," *Journal of Social History* 11, no. 2 (1978): 387–403.

11. Edward J. Larson, "The Rhetoric of Eugenics: Expert Authority and the Mental Deficiency Bill," *The British Journal for the History of Science* 24, no. 1 (1991): 45–60.

12. On the Eugenics Society, see Pauline M.H. Mazumdar, *Eugenics, Human Genetics and Human Failings: The Eugenics Society, Its Sources, and Its Critics in Britain* (New York and London: Routledge, 1991).

13. For a picture of Germany's preeminence in a scientific approach to psychiatry, see Katherine Angel, Edgar Jones, and Michael Neve, eds., "European Psychiatry on the Eve of War: Aubrey Lewis, the Maudsley Hospital and the Rockefeller Foundation in the 1930s," *Medical History*, supplement no. 22 (London: Wellcome Trust Centre for the History of Medicine at UCL, 2003).

14. This is nicely summarized for Britain in Roy Porter, "Two Cheers for Psychiatry! The Social History of Mental Disorder in Twentieth Century Britain," in *150 Years of British Psychiatry*, vol. 2, *The Aftermath*, eds. German Berrios and Hugh Freeman (London: Athlone, 1996), 383–406; also Mathew Thomson, *Psychological Subjects: Identity, Culture and Health in Twentieth-Century Britain* (Oxford: Oxford University Press, 2006), 173–206.

15. For the relationship between demography, the differences in fertility across classes, and eugenics, see Richard A. Soloway, *Demography and Degeneration: Eugenics and the Declining Birthrate in Twentieth-Century Britain* (Chapel Hill, NC: University of North Carolina Press, 1990).

16. Geoffrey Searle, *The Quest for National Efficiency* (Oxford: Oxford University Press, 1971).

17. Nikolas Rose, *The Psychological Complex: Psychology, Politics and Society in England, 1869–1939* (London and New York: Routledge, 1985).

18. Leila Zenderland, *Measuring Minds: Henry Herbert Goddard and the Origins of American Intelligence Testing* (Cambridge: Cambridge University Press, 1998).

19. Rose, *Psychological Complex*, 112–145.

20. Ian Dowbiggin, *Keeping American Sane: Psychiatry and Eugenics in the United States and Canada, 1880–1940* (Ithaca, NY and London: Cornell University Press, 1997), 134–158, 191–231.

21. Ibid., 75–76.

22. Anne Kerr and Tom Shakespeare, *Genetic Politics: From Eugenics to Genome* (Cheltenham: New Clarion, 2002), 27–28. Kerr and Shakespeare provide a figure of 375,000, which is cited elsewhere. A figure of 360,000 is included in Paul Weindling's definitive

study of eugenics in Germany, *Health, Race and German Politics between National Unification and Nazism, 1870–1945* (Cambridge: Cambridge University Press, 1989), 533.

23. On the influence of American eugenics on Germany, see Stefan Kühl, *The Nazi Connection: Eugenics, American Racism, and German National Socialism* (New York: Oxford University Press, 1994). On the Weimar roots of the law on sterilization, see Paul Weindling, "Compulsory Sterilization in National Socialist Germany," *German History* 5, no. 1 (1987): 10–24.

24. See Mattias Tydén, chapter 21, this volume.

25. Mathew Thomson, "Mental Hygiene as an International Movement," in *International Health Organisations and Movements 1918–1939*, ed. Paul Weindling (Cambridge: Cambridge University Press, 1995), 290–296.

26. Weindling, *Health, Race and German Politics.*

27. Ibid., 525.

28. Troy Duster, *Backdoor to Eugenics* (New York: Routledge, 2003), 141.

29. Mazumdar, *Eugenics, Human Genetics and Human Failings*, 198–255.

30. Weindling, *Health, Race and German Politics*, 289.

31. Ibid., 533.

32. Joel Braslow, *Mental Ills and Bodily Cures: Psychiatric Treatment in the First Half of the Twentieth Century* (Berkeley, CA: University of California Press, 1997), 54–70.

33. Thomson, *Problem of Mental Deficiency*, 110–148.

34. Ian Dowbiggin's study of Canada and the United States, *Keeping America Sane*, is the most searching account to date of the complex interplay between the professional interests of psychiatry and eugenic policy.

35. Thomson, *Problem of Mental Deficiency.*

36. On links between eugenics and mental hygiene in interwar Australia, see Stephen Garton, "Sound Minds and Healthy Bodies: Re-Considering Eugenics in Australia, 1914–1940," *Australian Historical Studies* 26, no. 103 (1994): 163–181.

37. Nancy Leys Stepan, *"The Hour of Eugenics": Race, Gender and Nation in Latin America* (Ithaca, NY and London: Cornell University Press, 1991).

38. Ibid., 51; Nancy Leys Stepan, "Eugenics in Brazil, 1917–1940," in *The Wellborn Science: Eugenics in Germany, France, Brazil, and Russia*, ed. Mark Adams (New York and Oxford: Oxford University Press, 1990), 111–144.

39. Garton, "Sound Minds and Healthy Bodies," 163–164; C. L. Bacchi, "The Nature-Nurture Debate in Australia, 1900–1914," *Historical Studies* 19, no. 75 (1980): 199–212; Stephen Garton, "Sir Charles Mackellar: Psychiatry, Eugenics, and Child Welfare in New South Wales, 1900–1914," *Historical Studies* 22, no. 86 (1986): 21–34.

40. Mathew Thomson, "'Savage Civilisation': Race, Culture, and Mind in Britain, 1898–1939," in *Race, Science and Medicine, 1700–1960*, eds. Waltraud Ernst and Bernard Harris (London and New York: Routledge, 1999), 235–258.

41. On South Africa, see Saul Dubow, *Scientific Racism in Modern South Africa* (Cambridge: Cambridge University Press, 1995).

42. See Carolyn Strange and Jennifer A. Stephen, chap. 31, this volume.

43. Steven Noll, *The Feeble-Minded in Our Midst: Institutions for the Mentally Retarded in the South, 1900–1940*, (Chapel Hill, NC: University of North Carolina Press, 1995), 89–103; Edward Larson, *Sex, Race and Science: Eugenics in the Deep South* (Baltimore, MD: Johns Hopkins University Press, 1995), 9, 93–94.

44. Jock McCulloch, *Colonial Psychiatry and the "African Mind"* (Cambridge: Cambridge University Press, 1995); Jonathan Sadowsky, *Imperial Bedlam: Institutions of Madness in Colonial Southwest Nigeria* (Berkeley, CA: University of California Press, 1999).

45. Weindling, *Health, Race and German Politics*, 544.

46. Ibid., 550–551; Gotz Aly, Peter Chroust and Christian Pross, *Cleansing the Fatherland: Nazi Medicine and Racial Hygiene* (Baltimore, MD: Johns Hopkins University Press, 1994); Michael Burleigh, *Death and Deliverance: "Euthanasia" in Germany 1900–1945* (Cambridge: Cambridge University Press, 1994).

47. On Britain, see Thomson, *Problem of Mental Deficiency*, 199–201. On the critique within science, see Elazar Barkan, *The Decline of Scientific Racism: Changing Conceptions of Race in Britain and the United States between the World Wars* (Cambridge: Cambridge University Press, 1992).

48. Burleigh, *Death and Deliverance*, 287–288.

49. Sandra Buckley, "Body Politics: Abortion Law Reform," in *The Japanese Trajectory: Modernization and Beyond*, eds. Gavan McCormack and Yoshio Sugimoto (Cambridge: Cambridge University Press, 1988), 205–217.

50. Dowbiggin, *Keeping America Sane*, 188; Angus McLaren, *Our Own Master Race: Eugenics in Canada, 1885–1945* (Toronto: McClelland & Stewart, 1990).

51. Gunnar Broberg and Nils Roll-Hansen eds, *Eugenics and the Welfare State: Sterilization Policy in Denmark, Sweden, Norway and Finland* (East Lansing, MI: Michigan State University Press, 1996), 60–61.

52. Ibid., 109–113.

53. Ibid., 234–240.

54. See, for instance, A. A. W. Petrie, "Presidential Address," *Journal of Mental Science* 91 (July 1945), 270.

55. For the evolution of eugenics via the "problem family" and the social, see Gillian Swanson, "Serenity, Self-Regard and the Genetic Sequence: Social Psychiatry and Preventive Eugenics in Britain, 1930s to 1950s," *New Formations*, 60 (2007): 50–65. On the move to "sitting on the fence" in regard to genetics, see J. E. Cawte, "A Note on the Future of Phenylketonuria," *Journal of Mental Science* 102 (October 1956): 805–11. For criticism of the predictions of the genetic effect of segregation and sterilization, see Ørnulv Ødegård, "The Future of Psychiatry: Predictions Past and Present," *British Journal of Psychiatry* 121 (1972): 579–589.

56. Stephen Trombley, *The Right to Reproduce: A History of Coercive Sterilisation* (London: Weidenfeld and Nicolson, 1988), 159–174, 210–213.

57. Kerr and Shakespeare, *Genetic Politics*, 70.

58. Duster, *Backdoor to Eugenics*.

59. Patricia J. Rock, "Eugenics and Euthanasia: A Cause for Concern for Disabled People, Particularly Disabled Women," *Disability and Society* 11, no. 1 (1996): 121–127.

60. Doris James Fleischer and Freida Zames, *The Disability Rights Movement: From Charity to Confrontation* (Philadelphia, PA: Temple University Press, 2001).

61. Adele Clarke, "Is Non-Directive Genetic Counselling Possible?," *Lancet* 338, no. 8773 (1991): 998–1000.

62. Within the disability movement there is also some recognition that not all forms of genetic counseling merit opposition: Tom Shakespeare, "Losing the Plot? Discourses on Genetics and Disability," *Sociology of Health and Illness* 21, no. 5 (1999), 669–688; Tom Shakespeare, *Disability Rights and Wrongs* (London and New York: Routledge, 2006).

63. Riccardo Baschetti, "People Who Condemn Eugenics May Be in Minority Now [letter to the editor]," *British Medical Journal* 319 (30 October 1999): 1196.

64. Frank Dikötter, *Imperfect Conceptions: Medical Knowledge, Birth Defects and Eugenics in China* (New York: Columbia University Press, 1998).

65. Veronica Pearson, "Population Policy and Eugenics in China," *British Journal of Psychiatry* 167, no. 1 (1995): 1–4.

66. "Western Eyes on China's Eugenic Law," *The Lancet* 346, no. 8968 (15 July 1995): 131.

67. Pearson, "Population Policy and Eugenics in China." For the suggestion that the role of psychiatrists in Nazi eugenics presented a dilemma in regard to psychiatric genetics: Anne Farmer and Michael Owen, "Genomics: The Next Psychiatric Revolution?," *British Journal of Psychiatry* 169, no. 2 (1996): 135–138.

FURTHER READING

Broberg, Gunnar, and Nils Roll-Hansen, eds. *Eugenics and the Welfare State: Sterilization Policy in Denmark, Sweden, Norway and Finland* (East Lansing, MI: Michigan State University Press, 1996).

Dikötter, Frank. *Imperfect Conceptions: Medical Knowledge, Birth Defects and Eugenics in China* (New York: Columbia University Press, 1998).

Dowbiggin, Ian. *Keeping American Sane: Psychiatry and Eugenics in the United States and Canada, 1880–1940* (Ithaca, NY: Cornell University Press, 1997).

Duster, Troy. *Backdoor to Eugenics* (London and New York: Routledge, 2003).

Kerr, Anne, and Tom Shakespeare. *Genetic Politics: From Eugenics to Genome* (Cheltenham: New Clarion Press, 2002).

Thomson, Mathew. *The Problem of Mental Deficiency: Eugenics, Democracy, and Social Policy in Britain, 1870–1959* (Oxford: Oxford University Press, 1998).

Trent, James, Jr. *Inventing the Feeble Mind: A History of Mental Retardation in the United States* (Berkeley, CA: University of California Press, 1994).

Weindling, Paul. *Health, Race, and German Politics between National Unification and Nazism, 1870–1945* (Cambridge: Cambridge University Press, 1989).

CHAPTER 7

....

EUGENICS AND THE STATE: POLICY-MAKING IN COMPARATIVE PERSPECTIVE

....

VÉRONIQUE MOTTIER

EMERGING in the late nineteenth century, the new science of eugenics aimed to assist states in implementing social policies that would improve the quality of the national "breed." In opposition to the laissez-faire principles of political liberalism, eugenicists advocated active social engineering and state intervention in the most private areas of citizens' lives, including their reproductive sexuality. The individual had a patriotic duty to contribute to the improvement of the nation through what Sir Francis Galton's (1822–1911) student Karl Pearson (1857–1936) termed a "conscious race-culture."[1] Eugenics was thus from its origins deeply intertwined with social and political aims, emerging as both a science and a social movement. The term caught on rapidly, and numerous eugenics societies were established in Great Britain and other countries, followed by the creation of International and World Leagues.[2] Through such social reform societies, as well as scientific disciplines such as anthropology, psychiatry, sexology, and biology, eugenic science acquired institutional support and legitimacy. A closer look at the history of eugenics shows the pitfalls of assuming a simple "diffusion" model of eugenic science, however. There have been important variations in the ways in which eugenic science developed in different national settings, as well as significant differences in the practical implementation of eugenic ideas. Consequently, we have much to gain from comparative analysis.

Against this backdrop, this chapter proposes to shift the focus from eugenic science to its translation into concrete policy practices, adopting a comparative perspective. I will draw on examples of eugenic policy-making in the United States, the United Kingdom, Switzerland, Sweden, and Germany to explore the relation between eugenic science and the state, examining the impact of different state formations on cross-national variations in the political trajectories of eugenics.

COLONIAL STATES AND EUGENIC NATIONS

States that adopted eugenic policies provide historical examples of "gardening states," to borrow a term from the social theorist Zygmunt Bauman,[3] states that were concerned with eliminating the "bad weeds" from the national garden and thereby constructed sharply exclusionary boundaries around the nation. Frequently drawing on such horticultural metaphors, eugenic science served to legitimize practices such as coerced sterilization or castration, which aimed to exclude "unfit" categories of the population from the (future) nation.

Research on the development of eugenics worldwide has highlighted the centrality of nineteenth-century biological understandings of "race" for the early development of eugenic science, as well as the impact of colonization and empire. The eugenic concern with the improvement of the national "race" via the surveillance of citizens' reproductive sexuality by the state emerged in the political context of colonial rule. As Philippa Levine points out in chapter 2 in this volume, fears about degeneracy of the national "race" were intertwined with anxieties about miscegenation or "blending" with colonial "others" in colonizing states such as the United Kingdom, France, and Germany. Former white settler colonies such as the United States, Australia, Canada, and New Zealand introduced immigration restrictions in the first decades of the twentieth century that were at least partly driven by eugenic concerns about differential birth rates, as has been illustrated by Alexandra Stern and Nancy Leys Stepan.[4]

And yet, in countries such as Switzerland, Sweden, Norway, Denmark, and Finland, eugenic science and practices developed within an entirely different political landscape. Switzerland was never a colonizing state, and the Scandinavian countries no longer had colonies (with the partial exception of Denmark) by the time eugenics emerged. Moreover, their respective populations were racially homogeneous[5] in the early decades of the twentieth century (preceding, in the case of Switzerland, later waves of immigration that would fundamentally transform its demographic composition). A collective preoccupation with the "racial hygiene" of the nation nevertheless strongly developed in these non-colonial states. While the eugenic project in some national and colonial contexts was concerned with both "external" and "internal" others, in Switzerland and Scandinavia, the focus was almost exclusively on populations already within a national border. Eugenic gardening efforts thus turned primarily to "internal others" within the nation such as the mentally ill, the physically disabled, and those members of the underclass whose behavior was considered socially unacceptable, such as unmarried mothers. It is one of the great paradoxes of the history of eugenics that the category of "race"—notoriously fuzzy anyway—was no less important to the eugenic ideas and practices developing within states that experienced little actual racial diversity.

In the Swedish context, racial biology and anthropology thus exercised considerable influence, especially in the first decades of the twentieth century, when eugenicists promoted the idea of a distinct Nordic race, as Broberg and Tydén have established.[6] The first state Institute for Race Biology in the world was founded in Uppsala in 1922, having been voted by the Swedish parliament and ratified by the king. Directed by Herman Lundborg (1868–1943), Sweden's most prominent eugenic scientist at the time, one of its first tasks was mapping the racial features of the Swedish nation.[7] On the basis of measuring the physical attributes of 100,000 Swedes—two-thirds of whom were army recruits and a significant part of the remainder, prison inmates—*The Racial Character of the Swedish Nation* appeared in 1926 to international acclaim. Concerns with racial purity and the dangers of miscegenation to the Swedish nation were further exemplified with Lundborg's attempts in the 1930s to produce a full inventory of the Sami people in Lapland, and in collaborative plans with the American eugenicists Samuel Holmes (1868–1964) and Charles Davenport (1866–1944) to establish institutes in Central America and Africa for eugenic research and promotion.[8] The influence of racial biology waned in Sweden as a result of the rise in genetic understandings of heredity and the promotion of non-racial versions of eugenics by prominent social-democrat ideologues such as Alva Myrdal (1902–1986) and Gunnar Myrdal (1898–1987), founders of the modern Swedish welfare state, leading to what Daniel Kevles describes as a shift from "mainline" to "reform" eugenics in the 1930s and 1940s. However, as Broberg and Tydén point out, that was "largely an academic affair" since Swedish state agencies often continued to engage in the racialization of social problems. A stark illustration is provided by the fact that the "Tattare" (a term used at the time to designate Romani travelers living in Sweden and Norway) were considered a "burden to Swedish society," "both from a biological and a social point of view," as the Swedish National Board on Social Welfare put it in 1940.[9] In reality, the Tattare did not constitute a specific ethnic group. Rather, they formed a catch-all category in which state authorities lumped together individuals accused of having disorderly, unproductive lives, vagrants, as well as traditional "travelers;" the association between racialization and actual racial diversity within non-colonial states was thus often tenuous.

Swiss eugenics was similarly intertwined with racial concerns and marked by the specific processes of nation-building and unifying efforts that followed the 1848 foundation of the Swiss federal state in response to a one-month civil war between Catholic and Protestant cantons. The terms "racial hygiene" and "eugenics" were used interchangeably in Switzerland from the end of the nineteenth century onward, though the former seems to have been used more widely. The physical anthropologist

Otto Schlaginhaufen (1879–1973) was one of the key proponents of racial hygiene in Switzerland, and the first president of the Julius Klaus Foundation for Heredity Research, Social Anthropology and Racial Hygiene, founded in Zürich in 1922 to promote "all scientifically based efforts, whose ultimate goal is the preparation and realisation of practical reforms to improve the white race," including special efforts "for the benefit of the physically and mentally inferior."[10] Schlaginhaufen engaged for several decades in an obsessive but ultimately fruitless search for the "pure Swiss race," which was to be called *Homo Alpinus Helveticus.* The mapping of the racial structure of the Swiss nation was, for Schlaginhaufen as for others, an "important scientific, and patriotic task."[11] Echoing the Swedish efforts, his team of researchers measured the bodily characteristics of over 35,000 male army recruits from 1927 to 1932, creating complex racial categories and crafting extensive series of maps representing the racial variations found within the Swiss nation. Its results were published in 1946 in *Die Anthropologie der Eidgenossenschaft* (The Anthropology of the Confederation). *Homo Alpinus* proved elusive, however: following Schlaginhaufen's own criteria, only 8.661 percent of the Swiss were declared to be of "pure race" and, even more disappointingly, only 1.41 percent of these qualified as part of the desirable "Alpine race."

Racial overtones also characterized the notorious Swiss child-removal program called Kinder der Landstrasse ("children of the country-lanes"), which was carried out by the federal agency Pro Juventute from 1926 to 1972 and targeted Yenish families. The Yenish constitute the most significant group of travelers present in Switzerland (others being the Roma and Sinti). Yenish have traditionally lived a nomadic lifestyle in countries such as Switzerland, Germany, France, and Austria (and in smaller numbers, in Luxemburg, Belgium, Holland, and Italy), economically sustained by collecting and selling ironware, repairing pans, pots, and knives, and, in more recent times, recycling activities. Current estimates put the number of Yenish still living in Switzerland today at around 30,000 and at several hundred thousand in Europe as a whole.

Throughout the history of the Swiss state, regular persecution of "vagabonds" or "beggars" had been carried out by Swiss local authorities. The 1848 creation of the modern federal state additionally led to attempts at administrative control over all inhabitants of the Swiss national territory. The 1850 *Heimatlosat* law, which described nomadism as a "national scourge," allowed for the expulsion from the national territory of anyone who did not possess official identity papers demonstrating membership in a local commune. This was followed by the 1912 Intercantonal Conference of heads of police, which decided to imprison "Zigeuner" without identity papers in workhouses until they could be identified and expelled from the national borders. Switzerland was also an active member of the International Coordination of Policies Towards "Zigeuner," which was located in Berlin until World War II and in Paris from 1947.[12]

Against the backdrop of such earlier repressive policies, the stated aim of the Kinder der Landstrasse program was not to improve living conditions for the children of the "travelers" and "tinkers," but to eradicate the national "scourge of vagrancy" by "appropriate measures of placement and education," as Walter Leimgruber, Thomas Meier, and Roger Sablonier have reported.[13] The forced removal of the children of travelers was partly legitimized on eugenic grounds. Traveler children were considered racially inferior, following studies carried out at the psychiatric clinic Waldhaus in the Swiss-German canton of Chur. Psychiatrists there had been working for many years in the tradition of racial biology, carrying out anthropometric and genealogical research on Yenish individuals and families who were labeled as "amoral psychopaths," "nymphomaniacs," or "irredeemable alcoholics." In his influential 1919 work *Psychiatrische Familiengeschichte* (Psychiatric Family Histories), the psychiatrist Josef Joerger (1860–1933) thus came to describe "vagrancy, delinquency, immorality, feeble-mindedness and madness," as well as poverty, as hereditarily transmissible traits. However, Joerger also believed in the environmental theory of child development, according to which inherent hereditary flaws could be "corrected" by good racial hygiene, including placement in a "better" family or educational environment. The founder of the Kinder der Landstrasse operation and its director until 1959, Alfred Siegfried (1890–1972), shared Joerger's belief in the redeeming power of education, as did other eugenicists. When education failed to "improve" a Yenish child, sterilization and other measures (such as refusal to grant permission to marry) prevented further degenerate offspring—a view that Siegfried would promote until well into the 1960s.[14] In addition, Yenish were also placed in penal institutions when authorities argued that no other alternatives were available, or that there was a risk of flight.

Switzerland being a federal state, the legal bases for child removal practices were most often federal adoption and guardianship legislation. When parental authority was withdrawn from a married couple (unmarried parents having no legal parental rights anyway)—a practice that, incidentally, was not restricted to Yenish families alone—a child could be offered up for adoption without the knowledge of its biological parents. In addition, penal law could be drawn upon by the cantons, which were responsible for the local application of concrete removal measures, as well as by other institutions involved such as the government agency Pro Juventute and the Catholic charity Seraphisches Liebeswerk.

Despite the large scope for maneuver offered by the vagueness of such legal dispositions, several measures taken by the Kinder der Landstrasse clearly lacked legal basis, and some children were removed from their parents in the absence of any previous legal decision.[15] There is also documentary evidence of resistance. First, parents sometimes exercised their right to legal appeals, with occasional success. The large majority of victims, however, either did not have access to the necessary legal expertise, or lacked the financial means to take advantage of the possibility of appeal. Second, not all local authorities were equally enthusiastic participants in child-removal measures. Certain local authorities refused to cooperate with Pro Juventute, citing disagreement with its policies. Pro Juventute in turn bitterly complained that certain local police agents would "systematically forget" to deal with Yenish individuals in their territory.[16] The canton of Chur, which had the largest traveler population, seems to have been most active in implementing the removal of Yenish children. More generally, the Swiss-German cantons and the Italian-speaking canton of Ticino tended to be more cooperative than local authorities in French-speaking Switzerland, where only very few cases of child removal have been recorded, though in the absence of further archival research, reasons for this stark difference are as yet unclear.

Before taking up the directorship of Kinder der Landstrasse, which he held for several decades, Alfred Siegfried had been a schoolteacher in Basel. He had lost his post due to a conviction for a pedophile relationship with one of his young male students, which local authorities at the time chose to pass over in silence. His successor as director of Pro Juventute, Peter Döbeli, would later be removed from his post owing to a similar conviction for sexual abuse of his charges, replaced with Clara Reust.[17] Some Yenish victims of the child placements later reported that they had suffered sexual abuse from care personnel, as well as from Siegfried himself, echoing similar sexual abuse accusations in children's homes in Ireland and other countries.[18]

POLITICAL IDEOLOGY AND WELFARE

Eugenic concerns found support across the political spectrum. Whereas early research tended to amalgamate eugenics with conservative and extreme right-wing political ideologies, more recent studies have followed the lead of authors such as Michael Freeden and Diane Paul to document the links with different strands of leftist political thought.[19] For example, in France, socialists such as Georges Vacher de Lapouge (1854–1936), cofounder of the French Workers' Party and an anthropologist who had introduced Galton's eugenic ideas to France in the final decades of the nineteenth century, promoted the idea that male citizens should perform "selectionist breeding" as part of a "sexual service" to the nation, a duty which he compared to military service. In the United Kingdom and the United States, a movement of Bolshevist eugenics emerged in the 1930s, which looked to the Soviet Union as the only country where sufficient conditions were united for scientifically based policies to improve the quality of the population. Many figureheads of British socialism supported eugenic ideas. For the Fabians, socialism served the interests of nationalism: eugenic social policies would ensure greater control over the proletariat, thereby strengthening the internal cohesion of the nation and allowing the United Kingdom to fulfill its vocation as a "social-imperialist" state.

Despite widespread support for eugenics among many leading British intellectuals on the Left as well as the Right, the United Kingdom adopted relatively few concrete eugenic policies, certainly when compared to countries such as Sweden, Switzerland, or Germany. As Mathew Thomson documents in this volume and elsewhere, the British Mental Deficiency Acts of 1913 and 1927 reflected some eugenic aims, such as the right to impose involuntary institutionalization of certified mental "defectives," but diluted eugenic overtones (and avoided mentioning the term "eugenic" itself) in response to legislators' concerns about threats to individual liberties. A more ambitious campaign driven by the Eugenics Society for legislation involving sterilization of the "feeble-minded," marriage regulation, birth control, and segregation of the "unfit" in England and Wales resulted in the appointment of the 1931 Brock Committee to prepare a bill on voluntary sterilization, the closest the United Kingdom ever came to introducing a national sterilization law. However, the Committee's 1934 recommendation to pass legislation foundered for lack of public support. As Desmond King and Randall Hansen have pointed out, this failure resulted in particular from the political opposition of the Catholic Church and the labor movement, which judged the legislation to be anti-working class, as well as from the contested nature of the scientific data available.[20] Perhaps most influential was the fact that alarming reports about forced sterilization in Germany started to appear in the press, following the introduction of the 1933 German "Law for the Prevention of Genetically Diseased Offspring" which formed the basis for hundreds of thousands of forced sterilizations in Germany (and which the Brock Committee had praised).

Ultimately, the strong influence of liberal political thought in the United Kingdom, with its emphasis on the rights of individuals and attendant distrust of state intervention in private life, thus formed an ideological barrier against the translation of eugenic ideas into policy-making in that context. Political conditions were more favorable elsewhere in Europe. In the Nordic countries and Switzerland, ideological and political factors were particularly conducive to the merging of social democratic ideology and practice with eugenic science. Social democratic thought believed firmly in the responsibilities of the state toward its citizens. In addition, in contrast to political liberalism, it promoted the subordination of individual interests to the collective good. As a governmental technology of social engineering that aimed to alleviate poverty, social disorder, and public expenditure, eugenics was seen to be in the interest of the nation as well as the state. The Marxist heritage of a belief in the power of scientific explanations of the world was an additional factor that further encouraged the blending of social-democrat ideology with eugenics. Indeed, historical materialism shares its emphasis on scientific models of history with Darwinian and social Darwinist thought. In contrast to Darwinian analyses, however, Marx and Engels strongly rejected naturalistic explanations of social ills, to develop instead a materialist conception of history, which located the origins of social problems in the unequal material conditions of human existence. Merging socialist with eugenic ideas, the Swiss eugenicist Auguste Forel (1848–1931) thus called for "an intelligent, scientific (not dogmatic) social-democracy," in order to "solve the eugenic problem."[21] But political contingencies played a role too. In particular, the dramatic collapse of the socialist Second International in 1914 and the rise of militaristic nationalism in Europe since World War I led to an increasing conflation of the social with the national order in social democratic thought in Germany and Sweden as well as elsewhere.

This is not to say that eugenic policies were promoted only by the Left. Rather, social-democratic support for eugenics played a crucial political role in the translation of eugenic ideas into policy-making, especially in the context of expanding welfare policies. In Switzerland, as elsewhere, several key eugenicists were political conservatives, such as the psychiatrist Eugen Bleuler (1857–1939) best-known for having coined the concept of schizophrenia. Others were politically positioned on the far Right, most notoriously Ernst Rüdin (1874–1952), whose work was officially endorsed by the Nazi party in the 1930s. Rüdin had dual Swiss and German citizenship and was involved in the drafting of the German sterilization law. Prominent social-democrats such as Forel—internationally recognized as one of the founding fathers of modern sexology, member of the Advisory Board of the International Federation of Eugenic Organisations, and honorary president of the World League for Sex Reform in 1930—were, however, instrumental in promoting eugenic science, in pioneering and institutionalizing eugenic technologies, and in eugenic policy formulation in Switzerland.

In Sweden, the only Nordic country with a state eugenic society, eugenics became even more clearly intertwined with the construction of the social-democratic welfare state. Leftist strands of eugenic thought were preceded by earlier right-wing nationalist, racist, and anti-feminist eugenicists such as Herman Lundborg (1868–1943) (see also Tydén, chapter 21); however, the fact that Alva and Gunnar Myrdal, who had strong sympathies for non-racial versions of eugenics, played a key role in founding the Swedish welfare state created particularly favorable conditions for eugenic influence. Gunnar Myrdal's work also exercised a strong influence on the Finnish debates on eugenics. Karl Kristian Steincke (1880–1963), the chief architect of the Danish welfare state, was similarly a staunch supporter of eugenic policy-making. As he put it in his 1920 book, *The Social Welfare of the Future*: "we treat the nonentity with all kind of care and love, but forbid him, in return, only to reproduce himself."[22]

In Germany, the Social-Democrat Party (SPD), which had links with both the Swedish and the Swiss social democrats, played an important role in the development of left-wing versions of eugenics in the Weimar republic, long before the Nazis applied more radical measures. The SPD politicians Wolfgang Heine (1861–1944) and Alfred Grotjahn (1869–1931) (who also occupied the first Chair in Social Hygiene in Berlin) were involved in introducing the first eugenic measures, including the sterilization of disabled people in the social-democratic governed Prussia of the 1920s, where preference was given to negative over positive eugenics. A 1932 bill for the voluntary sterilization of hereditarily flawed individuals was drafted by the Prussian Health Council, though not passed under the Weimar Republic. It was the rise of the Nazi government that created the political conditions for the passing of the notorious 1933 law that introduced compulsory sterilization. The extent to which an authoritarian state such as Nazi Germany was able to implement forced sterilization was regarded with envy by many eugenicists from liberal countries, including the United States, as Stefan Kühl has pointed out.[23]

The emergence of modern welfare policies and the presence of a favorable political context offered an institutional framework for the translation of eugenic science into policy practice. The emerging welfare-state also added an additional motive to the eugenic aim of preventing degeneracy of the nation: limiting public expenditure. Indeed, the "inferior" categories of the national population were soon to become the main recipients of the expanding welfare institutions. Limiting the numbers of "weeds" in the national garden therefore appeared as a rational means of reducing welfare costs. Whereas many involved in the policy-making process did not agree with the eugenic emphasis on the influence of heredity rather than the social environment, civil servants, administrators, and medical personnel nevertheless supported measures such as the sterilization of indigent women on the grounds that it was cheaper for the state than long-term financial support.

It could be argued that while social-democratic politics was instrumental in promoting eugenics in many emerging European welfare states, it was not social-democratic thought as such, but the development of the welfare state and the attendant argument of cost reduction that was conducive to the implementation of eugenic measures. While not entirely without justification, such an argument would, however, fail to acknowledge the centrality of the welfare state to the social-democrat political project, as well as the ideological affinities between state intervention into citizens' reproductive sexuality and eugenic politics.[24] Far from constituting an "accident" in the history of social-democracy, the eugenic social experiments fit comfortably with core elements of social democratic ideology.

INSTITUTIONAL DESIGN AND POLICY IMPLEMENTATION

The specific institutional design of states affected both the ways in which eugenic policies were implemented, as well as the incentives for doing so. In Sweden, for example, eugenic sterilization of "asocial" and "work-shy" citizens such as prostitutes and vagrants, the mentally ill, and the mentally retarded came to be seen as a way of strengthening the social-democratic welfare state, since it limited the number of future welfare dependents. In turn, the presence of a strong centralized welfare state was seen as a guarantee against the risk of arbitrariness in the implementation of such measures, administered under the responsibility of the National Board of Health.[25]

In contrast, federalism led to variations in policy frameworks and practices between cantons or states. In the federalist system of the United States, important differences occurred in the scope of application of eugenic measures between different states, as studies by Wendy Kline, Johanna Schoen, and Alexandra Stern have revealed.[26] In the case of Switzerland, also a federal state, parallel differences can be observed between the different cantons. The main dividing line seems to have been religion: while Protestant cantons tended to engage in sterilization practices, Catholic cantons, on the whole, did not, reflecting more general differences in attitudes toward poverty, illness, and disability within Protestant and Catholic doctrine. Indeed, for Catholics, any form of life, no matter how "defective" or "flawed," is worthy of preservation, while Protestants have traditionally been more comfortable with ideas of human perfectibility.

More generally, eugenic thinking seems to have been more readily practiced as state policy in Protestant countries. This is certainly true for the European sterilization laws of the 1920s and 1930s. In liberal democratic regimes, sterilization laws were introduced exclusively in Protestant countries, including the Swiss canton of Vaud, as well as in Denmark, Norway, Sweden, Finland, Iceland, and Estonia. Eugenics did, nevertheless, develop with the support of Catholic forces in some contexts. In Nazi Germany, for example, the Catholic Church eventually sided with the authoritarian state, despite the condemnation of eugenics in the 1930 Papal Encyclical *Casti Connubii,* which argued that the family is more sacred than the state. However, eugenics tended to take different forms in Catholic contexts, generally privileging "positive" eugenics over "negative" eugenics. Religion alone was therefore significant but not decisive as a factor determining variations in eugenic practices both within and between states, its impact being moderated by the local constellations of political power.

Differences in institutional design of states produced further variations in policy implementation, depending on how welfare provision was organized. The Swiss state, again, constitutes a good example of this: local authorities, rather than the federal state, were responsible for the financial support of indigent members of local communes. This factor, first, increased the appeal of the argument of cost-reduction, since limiting the number of future "weeds" in the local gardens would have a direct effect on local budgets, which were modest compared to that of the federal state. Second, local authorities' financial responsibility for "their" citizens led to differences in welfare practices between communes with regard to marriage licenses, sterilization, or the granting of residence rights to travelers, again shaped by local economic concerns.

The implementation of eugenic policies was thus shaped by the specific design of Swiss political institutions, in particular, federalism and its attendant levels of autonomy of local agencies and authorities. Many eugenic practices, including coerced sterilization, were not carried out by the central state, but implemented by cantonal and local authorities, as well as para-state actors such as psychiatric clinics, on the basis of local legislation and administrative measures. Psychiatric clinics in particular offered practical opportunities for applying eugenic ideas and technologies to a population often already under tutelage or guardianship orders. Practices of direct intervention by the federal state were less widespread in Switzerland than in other countries, though they included the child-removal program which, while not driven by eugenic concerns alone, had eugenic overtones; as well as regulations in the criminal law aimed at curtailing sexual relations with the mentally deficient.[27] In addition, Switzerland was the first country in Europe to introduce eugenically motivated marriage interdiction legislation targeting the mentally ill in its Civil Code of 1907, which became effective in 1912.[28]

Article 97 of this federal law prohibited marriage to individuals who were "of unsound mind" or "mentally ill." Sterilization legislation, however, only existed at the cantonal level in the Swiss case.

GENDERING THE STATE

In 1928, the Swiss canton of Vaud, after public appeals from Forel, adopted the first European eugenic sterilization law, which would only be abrogated in 1985. It was followed by similar legislation in Denmark in 1929, Germany in 1933, Sweden and Norway in 1934, and Finland in 1935. In addition, the Vaud canton's Criminal Code of 1931 included a clause allowing for eugenically motivated abortions.

The Vaud law allowed for the sterilization without consent of the "mentally ill." However, it is important to emphasize that the general categories of mental illness and feeblemindedness were notoriously vague at the time. The famous eugenic psychiatrist Eugen Bleuler, for example, defined these terms "to include anything that deviates from the norm" in his influential 1916 *Textbook of Psychiatry*,[29] while his former student Hans W. Maier's 1908 dissertation on the term "moral idiocy" extended mental instability to moral flaws. The introduction of a legal basis for sterilization would, it was thought, allow for the regulation and curtailing of practices of sterilization that were already commonplace, an argument which played an important role in the debates around the adoption of the Vaud law. Indeed, many psychiatrists opposed legislation precisely for this reason. In practice, the law did appear to limit the number of sterilizations, since half the applications for sterilizations were rejected after the law came into effect.[30]

There were occasional attempts to introduce national legislation in Switzerland: psychiatrists petitioned for a federal law in 1910, and academics continued to press the case for legislation until well into the post-1945 period, including in the form of a legal dissertation by Hans-Rudolf Böckli in 1954 that was intended as a blueprint for a national sterilization law.[31] However, calls for the introduction of a federal sterilization law in the context of other ongoing legal reforms encountered opposition from the mid-1930s from doctors who resisted the legal restrictions upon their discretionary power that the legislation would entail. Swiss direct democracy added an additional barrier, since such legal reforms would have to be put to a vote from the cantons as well as the population. Legal experts feared that inclusion of a sterilization clause would cause Catholic cantons to reject the entire legal reform package, and were therefore reluctant to include this aspect. The Swiss Federal Council reported to parliament in 1944 that its family policies pursued three aims: demographic, pedagogic, and eugenic. Concerning the eugenic dimension of its family protection measures, the Council stated that "the state must help to prevent the founding of families which would produce hereditarily diseased offspring, and encourage the founding and stability of families who are hereditarily healthy."[32]

However, parliament and Council agreed that a federal law was unnecessary, since sterilization practices were already widespread.[33] For similar reasons, no other Swiss canton than Vaud ever adopted a sterilization law, preferring local guidelines such as in Bern (1931), or agreements between local authorities and doctors.

Exact figures on the number of sterilizations in all of Switzerland are not available to date. New archival research carried out in recent years by Swiss historians such as Geneviève Heller, Gilles Jeanmonod, Regina Wecker, Jacob Tanner, Roswitha Dubach, Beatrice Ziegler, and Gisela Hauss allows us, however, to understand practices in major urban centers.[34] Recent research reveals that sterilization practices were relatively common in the canton of Zürich, for example, where in the 1930s alone, between 1,700 and 3,600 sterilizations were carried out after approval from the local psychiatric policlinic.[35] The large majority of these were on women who had requested permission for an abortion, a procedure that was often made conditional on sterilization. The arguments used in Zürich were primarily social and psychiatric, including sexual promiscuity, the inability to financially support children, or illegitimacy of the children, while hereditary arguments appeared in around 30 percent of recommendations for sterilization.[36] In contrast, in the canton of Bern, doctors tended to apply explicit hereditary criteria, reflecting the preference of the director of the Bernese Women's Clinic, Hans Guggisberg, who refused to accept social indications for sterilization.[37] More generally, arguments for sterilization reflected the legal frameworks. For example, from 1931, local Bernese guidelines required psychiatric examination and no longer accepted either eugenic or social indications alone as grounds for sterilization. Psychiatrists from the Bernese psychiatric clinic Waldau thus amalgamated psychiatric, eugenic, and social arguments, including the prevention of pregnancies for "morally deficient" or "sexually pathological" women, welfare dependency of future children, or a family history of mental illness, suicide, or epilepsy; they recommended an average of 25 women per year for sterilization in the years 1935–1953.[38] As these examples illustrate, sterilization practices varied quite widely between different federal cantons, reflecting differences in local administrative and legal frameworks, but also in the scope for individual agency on the part of key officials in the implementation of such measures.

It is striking that, as in the Scandinavian countries, the vast majority of eugenic sterilizations in Switzerland were carried out on young female social deviants: unmarried women from lower social classes, who lived in poor conditions and had had children out of wedlock, labeled as "maladapted," "sexually promiscuous," of "low intelligence," "mentally ill," or "feebleminded." The policing of respectable female sexuality and of femininity more generally appears to have been a central motive in the practice of eugenic sterilization. Men labeled as sexually "abnormal," such as exhibitionists or homosexuals similarly risked being submitted to therapeutic castrations,[39] and sterilization and castration of men could also be applied in the context of the legal punishment of sex crimes.[40] However, most of these seem to have been carried out not on eugenic grounds, but with the therapeutic aim of moderating their "deviant" sexual drives, often under the pressure of long-term internment as the only alternative. The gendered nature of the Swiss figures is comparable to the Swedish context. Some 63,000 citizens were sterilized in Sweden between 1935 and 1975,[41] 93 percent of these women. Estimates of the number of sterilizations performed on eugenic and/or social grounds are around 18,600.[42] The only exception, Nazi Germany, where numbers of eugenic sterilizations and castrations seem to have been evenly divided between women and men, is perhaps explained by its aim to eradicate not just future, but also current generations of "degenerates." Sterilization policies were thus heavily gendered. More generally, they reflect states' concern with control over women—female bodies and female sexuality—as the reproducers of the nation, as well as the gendered nature of eugenic policy-making and implementation. Gender and sexuality are thus central categories in the history of eugenics, as authors such as Kline, Stern, and Schoen have emphasized in their work.[43]

And yet, it would be a mistake to assume that women were only the *victims* of eugenics: they were also important agents in the implementation of eugenic policies. Again, the Swiss case can serve to illustrate this point: in a country in which women did not obtain voting rights at the national level until 1971, educated women from the middle classes, in particular, claimed eugenic policy-making as an area for active political participation. In the slowly emerging Swiss welfare state, women's philanthropic organizations played a central role in the provision of early welfare services as well as in the exercise of social control. They provided personnel for the eugenic marriage advice clinics from the 1930s onward, where doctors and nurses—often female—increasingly focused on mothers as primary educators of the future generations, linking individual care with the collective obligation of "race improvement." More generally, among the health and welfare officials who coerced lower-class women into sterilization as a condition for allowing abortion or awarding welfare payments were many women from the bourgeoisie. These women not only shaped the implementation, but also influenced the formulation of eugenic policies; while women's social purity groups were instrumental in promoting eugenic ideas in the context of wider public debates on the regulation of sexuality between the 1890s and 1930s.[44]

CONCLUSION

The eugenic vision of the nation as an ordered system of exclusion and disciplinary regulation was central both to the formation of national identity and to the workings of modern welfare. The national order of the welfare state was founded on the notions of community and solidarity. However, entitlement to welfare provisions has always been conditional, and was initially restricted to a very limited number of categories of the population—especially so in the Swiss case where welfare provision was never as extensive as in the Scandinavian countries, the United Kingdom, or Germany. Against this backdrop, particular state configurations created different "political opportunity structures"[45] for eugenic influence on policy-making; that is, structural factors external to the eugenics movements themselves provided different possibilities for eugenic ideologues to see their ideas put into practice. Differences in institutional design, such as federalist or more centralist state formations, thus affected the implementation of eugenic practices, causing variations both within and between states. In the Swiss case, its political institutions—in particular, direct democracy—additionally discouraged national policy efforts such as a federal sterilization law.

Institutional factors alone, however, do not fully explain cross-national variations in eugenic policy trajectories. Political opportunity structures need to be examined in conjunction with the equally crucial role played by political ideology, as demonstrated by the case of the United Kingdom where, despite the promotion of eugenics by influential scientists and prominent figures from the Left, the introduction of a eugenic sterilization law foundered due to the strong influence of political liberalism.

Worldwide, eugenic rhetoric and practices have been intertwined with political ideologies ranging across the entire political spectrum, from anarchism, social democracy, and feminism to conservatism and fascism. Social democratic support for eugenics, operating in the context of emerging welfare states, created particularly favorable conditions for eugenic influence on welfare debates and policy-making in Scandinavian countries and parts of Switzerland, but this does not mean that social democracy was a *necessary* condition for eugenic policy-making, as the example of Nazi Germany demonstrates. In national contexts such as the Scandinavian countries and parts of Switzerland, the connections between eugenics, social democracy, and the welfare state are perhaps best seen in terms of an elective affinity between these political, scientific, and institutional elements: eugenic policy-making and strands of leftist thought were mutually conducive and shaped local and national welfare practices in these countries, especially in the 1920s–1940s. As a result of these particular political configurations, the original eugenic emphasis on the hereditary transmission of "defective" characteristics became diluted in more general state measures against "anti-social" behaviors that were not necessarily attributed to strictly hereditary factors. This has led some authors to argue for a stark distinction between Scandinavian-style welfare eugenics and Nazi-style racial eugenics.[46] An overly stark opposition between the two nevertheless seems problematic, since racial considerations did not disappear altogether from welfare practices in these contexts, as we have seen.

The rise of the Nazi regime provided the political opportunity to implement both more radical eugenic policies such as forced sterilization and euthanasia, and to do so on a dramatically wider scale than the liberal welfare states. The anti-liberal, authoritarian strands of nationalism that were at the heart of fascist ideology were marked by an obsession with the themes of purity and degeneracy. Fascism emphasized the subordination of individual rights to the collective interest of a strongly racialized nation, driven by the belief that the nation could only be strengthened by eliminating the weak and "degenerates." Despite the fact that many German social-democrat eugenicists, including the eminent sexologist Magnus Hirschfeld (1868–1935), later fell victim to the Nazis, or fled Germany, they did not, as a rule, oppose Nazi measures such as forced sterilization. Indeed, Hirschfeld described the practice as "an interesting experiment," adding the prudent qualification that "it will be a long while before the results can be judged on their merits."[47] Disapproval of eugenic policy implementation by the Nazi regime on the part of Hirschfeld as well as of British mainstream eugenicists centered, rather, on its obsession with race, in particular with (racialized) Jews, to the perceived neglect of other categories of "undesirable" citizens such as alcoholics or drug addicts. Interestingly, the *International Medical Bulletin,* which was edited in Prague by Jewish and social-democrat doctors who had fled the Nazi regime, attacked the German sterilization law on political rather than ethical grounds: "such a law is abused as an instrument of power in a capitalist state... only after a social revolution will it be possible to create the scientific and social conditions for 'true' eugenics."[48]

Whereas eugenic concerns with racial purity emerged in the United Kingdom and Germany against the backdrop of empire and the encounter with colonial "others," in non-colonial nations such as Switzerland and the Scandinavian countries, eugenic preoccupations turned primarily towards "internal others." The national order was seen to be under threat from various categories of "disorderly" citizens, including the mentally ill, the physically disabled, the "morally defective" or "anti-social" citizens, and "vagrants" or travelers (who were sometimes racialized, as in the case of the Yenish or the "Tattare"). Since it is through reproductive sexuality that the nation is biologically replaced, that domain became a concern of the state. The rational management of citizens' reproductive sexuality by the state, especially of female sexual morality and practices, was thus a central focus of the eugenic efforts to eradicate the "weeds" from the national gardens. Recognizing the importance of gender for the workings of the modern state is not to say, however, that the state exercises male power over its female citizens in any straightforward way. Women were often important agents in the implementation of eugenic measures, while men were sometimes its victims, as we have seen. The examples of the Kinder der Landstrasse operation and marriage bans on the mentally ill suggest, moreover, that gender was not the only category around which eugenic interventions were structured; some practices were linked to racialized differences and disability, while social class was a strongly differentiating factor in the application of eugenic measures, illustrating the importance of taking into account the intersectionalities between gender, sexuality, class, and other relevant categories. Welfare, political ideology, and state systems were structured by wider social relations of power around religion, class, "race," disabilities, gender, and sexualities, explaining further variations in eugenic policy-making within and between states.

Eugenic scientists generally promoted state intervention in citizens' private lives and contributed to the development of some of the technologies used in eugenics, including sterilization. Key eugenic experts were actively involved in the drafting of eugenic legislation in the Swiss, German, and Swedish case, for example, where they acted as consultants or as members of the legislative committees. Eugenic movements were thus able to exert important influence on these states' policy-making apparatuses. Against this backdrop, an important question to ask is: How much autonomy did the state have? While Marxist analyses have traditionally conceptualized states as privileging the political interests of a specific social class, new institutionalist perspectives developed by Theda Skocpol and others[49] have argued that state institutions do not just express the interests of actors from civil society but, to some extent, pursue their own logic and interests. Eugenic policy-making constitutes a good illustration of the institutionalist argument. Indeed, as we have seen, state actors at times supported and implemented eugenic measures without necessarily sharing eugenic aims, since in the context of the expanding welfare state systems, limiting the future numbers of indigent members of society appeared to have clear financial benefits. Moreover, individual bureaucrats' support for or resistance against eugenic practices could lead to wide variations in the scope of implementation, especially at the local administrative level.

More generally, the notion of the state itself needs unpacking. Comparative analysis of the connections between welfare, politics, and the state demonstrates, firstly, that states have not always acted in coherent, homogeneous ways, but in ways that were at times non-systematic and contradictory. Whereas eugenic ideologues often promoted ambitious national and international visions, concrete eugenic policies within liberal states did not, generally, reflect any grand "masterplan" on the part of the state, but were more often the product of accidental political opportunities and local compromise. Numerous, frequently incoherent, sometimes contradictory, eugenic discourses and practices sprang up from various institutional settings at the micro-level, and crosscut with other disciplinary motivations and practices that were not always intentionally eugenic. Eugenic intentions could, moreover, be resisted and subverted in practice: the Swiss marriage advice bureaus, for example, were much used by citizens; however, most consultations showed little interest in eugenic concerns and were driven by demands for contraceptive information and material. Eugenic discourses and practices also followed different institutional trajectories, with eugenically motivated sterilization practices fading away by the 1950s and 1960s in liberal countries; others, such as marriage advice bureaus, disappeared much earlier. Swiss child removal practices only came to an end in the early 1970s at much the same time as US states abandoned compulsory sterilizations.

Secondly, para-state actors such as psychiatric clinics, hospitals, prisons, local authorities, and local welfare boards played a key role in the implementation of eugenic practices, especially in the federal state systems, suggesting the need to differentiate between the level of the national state and that of local state, para-state, or private agencies. The often decentralized, scattered, and unsystematic nature both of the institutional design and of the implementation of eugenic policy-making generally demarcates eugenic practices in liberal states from those in authoritarian states.

Finally, a substantive number of eugenic measures seem to have been applied by local doctors or welfare workers, not only in the absence of any national legislation, but without any legal basis at all, as for example in the case of Swiss sterilization practices and child removal measures, which were, in part, eugenically driven. Caution must therefore be exercised in assuming that the scale of eugenics in national settings can be judged from the presence or absence of eugenic legislation by the state. In other, more unusual cases, eugenicists never appealed for state intervention in the first place, as illustrated by the Spanish anarchist versions of eugenics.[50] Eugenic practices thus occurred not only within, but also outside of and against the state.

ACKNOWLEDGMENTS

I am very grateful to Philippa Levine, Alison Bashford, Natalia Gerodetti, and Mattias Tydén for helpful suggestions.

NOTES

1. Karl Pearson, "The Scope and Importance to the State of the Science of National Eugenics," [1909] in *Sexology Uncensored: The Documents of Sexual Science*, eds. Lucy Bland and Laura Doan (Cambridge: Polity Press, 1998), 170.

2. Stefan Kühl, *Die Internationale der Rassisten. Aufstieg und Niedergang der Internationalen Bewegung für Eugenik und Rassenhygiene im 20. Jahrhundert* (Frankfurt: Campus Verlag, 1997).

3. Zygmunt Bauman, *Modernity and the Holocaust* (Cambridge: Polity Press, 1989).

4. Alexandra Minna Stern, *Eugenic Nation: Faults and Frontiers of Better Breeding in Modern America* (Berkeley, CA: University of California Press, 2005); Nancy Leys Stepan, *"The Hour of Eugenics": Race, Gender and Nation in Latin America* (Ithaca, NY: Cornell University Press, 1991).

5. The Swedish Sami from Lapland forming an important, though numerically relatively small, exception.

6. Gunnar Broberg and Mattias Tydén, "Eugenics in Sweden: Efficient Care," in *Eugenics and the Welfare State: Sterilization Policy in Denmark, Sweden, Norway, and Finland*, eds. Gunnar Broberg and Nils Roll-Hansen (East Lansing, MI: Michigan State University, 2005), 77–149.

7. Ibid., 85–87.

8. Ibid., 89.

9. Ibid., 127.

10. Alex Schwank, "Der Rassenhygienische (bzw. eugenische) Diskurs in der schweizerischen Medizin des 20. Jahrhunderts," in *Fünfzig Jahre danach: Zur Nachgeschichte des Nationalsozialismus*, eds. Sigrid Weigel and Birgit Erdle (Zürich: Hochschulverlag, 1996), 461–481.

11. Otto Schlaginhaufen, *Die Anthropologie der Eidgenossenschaft* (Zürich: Orell Füssli, 1946), 7 [my translation].

12. Walter Leimgruber, Thomas Meier, and Roger Sablonier, *Das Hilfswerk für die Kinder der Landstrasse* (Bern: Schweizerische Bundesarchiv, 1998).

13. Ibid., 29.

14. Ibid., 60.

15. Ibid., 49.

16. Ibid., 53.

17. Thomas Huonker, *Fahrendes Volk—verfolgt und verfemt. Jenische Lebensläufe* (Zürich: Limmat Verlag, 1990), 244; Thomas Huonker and Regula Ludi, *Roma, Sinti und Jenische. Schweizerische Zigeunerpolitik zur Zeit des Nationalsozialismus* (Zürich: Chronos, 2001), 45.

18. See Thomas Huonker's online Yenish archive, www.thata.ch. No systematic study of the scope of such abuse exists to date.

19. Michael Freeden, "Eugenics and Progressive Thought: A Study in Ideological Affinity," *The Historical Journal* 22, no. 3 (1979), 645–671; Diane Paul, "Eugenics and the Left," *Journal of the History of Ideas*, 45, no. 4 (1984): 567–590; see also Véronique Mottier and Natalia Gerodetti, "Eugenics and Social-democracy: Or, How the Left Tried to Eliminate the 'Weeds' from its National Gardens," *New Formations* 60 (2006–07): 35–49.

20. Desmond King and Randall Hansen, "Experts at Work: State Autonomy, Social Learning and Eugenic Sterilisation in 1930s Britain," *British Journal of Political Science* 29, no. 1 (1999): 103–104.

21. Auguste Forel, *La morale en soi* (Lausanne: Administration de la libre penseé, 1910).

22. Karl Kristian Steincke, *Fremtidens Vorsørgelsesvoesen* (Copenhagen: Fremad, 1920), 251.

23. Stefan Kühl, *The Nazi Connection: Eugenics, American Racism, and German National Socialism* (Oxford: Oxford University Press, 1994).

24. See also Mottier and Gerodetti, "Eugenics and Social-democracy;" Véronique Mottier, "From Welfare to Social Exclusion: Eugenic Social Policies and the Swiss National Order," in *Discourse Theory in European Politics*, eds. David Howarth and Jacob Torfing (Basingstoke: Palgrave, 2005), 255–274.

25. Broberg and Tydén, "Eugenics in Sweden."

26. Wendy Kline, *Building a Better Race: Gender, Sexuality, and Eugenics from the Turn of the Century to the Baby Boom* (Berkeley, CA: University of California Press, 2001); Johanna Schoen, *Choice and Coercion: Birth Control, Sterilization, and Abortion in Public Health and Welfare* (Chapel Hill, NC: University of North Carolina Press, 2005); Stern, *Eugenic Nation.*

27. Mottier and Gerodetti, "Eugenics and Social-democracy," 41.

28. Regina Wecker, "Eugenik—individueller Ausschluss und nationaler Konsens," in *Krisen und Stabilisierung. Die Schweiz in der Zwischenkriegszeit*, eds. Sebastien Guex, Brigitte Studer, Bernard Degen, Markus Kübler, Eduard Schade, and Beatrice Ziegler (Zürich: Chronos, 1998), 169.

29. Eugen Bleuler, *Lehrbuch der Psychiatrie* (Berlin: Julius Springer, 1916), 476.

30. Gilles Jeanmonod and Geneviève Heller, "Eugénisme et contexte socio-politique: l'exemple de l'adoption d'une loi sur la stérilisation des handicapés et malades mentaux dans le canton de Vaud en 1928," *Revue d'histoire suisse* 50 (2000): 20–44.

31. Thomas Huonker, *Diagnose: "moralisch Defekt." Kastration, Sterilisation und Rassenhygiene im Dienst der Schweizer Sozialpolitik und Psychiatrie 1890–1970* (Zürich: Orell Füssli, 2003), 152.

32. Bericht des Bundesrates an die Bundesversammlung über das Volksbegehren "Für die Familie," *Bundesblatt* 96, no. 1 (10 October 1944): 868.

33. Regina Wecker, "Vom Verbot, Kinder zu haben, und dem Recht, keine Kinder zu haben: Zu Geschichte und Gegenwart der Sterilisation in Schweden, Deutschland und der Schweiz," *Figurationen* 2 (2003): 108.

34. The main results of these recent studies are presented in Véronique Mottier and Laura Von Mandach, eds., *Pflege, Stigmatisierung und Eugenik. Integration und Ausschluss in Medizin, Psychiatrie und Sozialhilfe* (Zürich: Seismo, 2007).

35. Dubach, "Zur Sozialisierung," 189.

36. Ibid., 191.

37. Beatrice Ziegler, "Frauen zwischen sozialer und eugenischer Indikation: Abtreibung und Sterilisation in Bern," in *Geschlecht hat Methode: Ansätze und Perspektiven in der Frauen- und Geschlechtergeschichte*, eds. Veronika Aegerter, Nicole Graf, Natalie Imboden, Thea Rytz, and Rita Stöckli (Zürich: Chronos, 1999), 293–301.

38. Hauss and Ziegler, "Norm und Ausschluss in Vormundschaft und Psychiatrie: Zum institutionnellen Umgang mit jungen Frauen," in Mottier and Von Mandach, eds., *Pflege, Stigmatisierung und Eugenik*, 63–75.

39. Huonker, *Diagnose*, 232–233.

40. Roswitha Dubach, "Zur 'Sozialisierung' einer medizinischen Massnahme: Sterilisations praxis der Psychiatrischen Poliklinik Zürich in den 1930er Jahren," in *Zwang zur Ordnung. Psychiatrie im Kanton Zürich, 1870–1970*, eds. Marietta Meier, Brigitta Bernet, Roswitha Dubach, and Urs Germann (Zürich: Chronos, 2007).

41. See Maija Runcis, *Sterilisation in the Swedish Welfare state*, English summary (PhD diss., University of Stockholm, 1998).

42. Broberg and Roll-Hansen, eds. *Eugenics and the Welfare State*, 109–110. See also Tydén, chap. 21 in this volume. My thanks to Mattias Tydén for helpful suggestions.

43. On gender and sexuality in Swiss eugenics, see Véronique Mottier, "Narratives of National Identity: Sexuality, Race, and the Swiss 'Dream of Order,'" *Swiss Journal of Sociology* 26 (2000): 533–558; Véronique Mottier, "Eugenics and the Swiss Gender Regime: Women's Bodies and the Struggle against 'Difference,'" *Swiss Journal of Sociology* 32, no. 1 (2006): 253–267.

44. Natalia Gerodetti, "Lay Experts: Women's Social Purity Groups and the Politics of Sexuality in Late Nineteenth and Early Twentieth Century Switzerland," *Women's History Review* 13, no. 4 (2004): 585–610.

45. The concept of "political opportunity structures" was coined by political scientist Sidney Tarrow to refer to the structural factors that impact on the trajectories of social movements. While borrowing the term here, I make no claim to examine such factors exhaustively in the present essay. See Sidney Tarrow, *Power in Movement: Collective Action, Social Movements and Politics* (Cambridge: Cambridge University Press, 1994).

46. Alberto Spektorowski and Elisabet Mizrachi, "Eugenics and the Welfare State in Sweden: The Politics of Social Margins and the Idea of a Productive Society," *Journal of Contemporary History* 39, no. 3 (2004): 333–352.

47. Magnus Hirschfeld, *Racism* (London: Gollancz, 1938); see also Mottier and Gerodetti, "Eugenics and Social-democracy," 46.

48. Quoted in Sheri Berman, "Euthanasia, Eugenics and Fascism: How Close are the Connections? Review of Werner Brill: *Pädagogik im Spannungsfeld von Eugenik und Euthanasia*," *German Politics and Society* 17, no. 3 (1999): 147–152.

49. See Dietrich Rueschemeyer, Theda Skocpol, and Peter B. Evans, eds., *Bringing the State Back In* (Cambridge: Cambridge University Press, 1985).

50. See Richard Cleminson, "Eugenics Without the State: Anarchism in Catalonia, 1900–1937," *Studies in History and Philosophy of Biological and Biomedical Sciences* 39, no. 2 (2008): 232–239. Several British eugenicists similarly did not appeal to the state: see Freeden, "Eugenics and Progressive Thought."

FURTHER READING

Bleuler, Eugen. *Lehrbuch der Psychiatrie* (Berlin: Julius Springer, 1916).

Broberg, Gunnar, and Nils Roll-Hansen, eds. *Eugenics and the Welfare State: Sterilization Policy in Denmark, Sweden, Norway, and Finland* (East Lansing, MI: Michigan State University Press, 1996).

Forel, Auguste. *The Sexual Question: A Scientific, Psychological, Hygienic and Sociological Study for the Cultured Classes*, English adaptation by C. F. Marshall (London: Rebman, 1908).

Freeden, Michael. "Eugenics and Progressive Thought: A Study in Ideological Affinity," *The Historical Journal* 22, no. 3 (1979): 645–671.

Joerger, Josef. *Psychiatrische Familiengeschichte* (Berlin: Julius Springer, 1919).

King, Desmond, and Randall Hansen. "Experts at Work: State Autonomy, Social Learning and Eugenic Sterilisation in 1930s Britain," *British Journal of Political Science* 29, no. 1 (1999): 77–107.

Mottier, Véronique. "Eugenics, Politics and the State: Social Democracy and the Swiss 'Gardening State,'" *Studies in History and Philosophy of Biological and Biomedical Sciences* 39, no. 2 (2008): 263–269.

Mottier, Véronique. *Sexuality: A Very Short Introduction* (Oxford: Oxford University Press, 2008).

Mottier, Véronique, and Laura Von Mandach, eds. *Pflege, Stigmatisierung und Eugenik. Integration und Ausschluss in Medizin, Psychiatrie und Sozialhilfe* (Zürich: Seismo, 2007).

Paul, Diane. "Eugenics and the Left," *Journal of the History of Ideas* 45, no. 4 (1984): 567–90.

Spektorowski, Alberto, and Elisabet Mizrachi, "Eugenics and the Welfare State in Sweden: The Politics of Social Margins and the Idea of a Productive Society," *Journal of Contemporary History* 39, no. 3 (2004): 333–352.

Weingart, Peter. "Science and Political Culture: Eugenics in Comparative Perspective," *Scandinavian Journal of History* 24, no. 2 (1999): 163–177.

CHAPTER 8

INTERNATIONALISM, COSMOPOLITANISM, AND EUGENICS

ALISON BASHFORD

THE strong connection between eugenics and nationalism is now a clear interpretive strand in the historiography. From strident British "race patriotism," to "blood and homeland" arguments in central and southeast Europe, from anti-colonial nationalism in Latin America to nationalist race hygiene in Spain, eugenics was a key component of modern discourse on race and nations.[1] For all the local differences between these nationalist histories, the place of eugenics within them was remarkably similar. Eugenics was, in this sense, international. Proponents may have argued about Lamarckian and Mendelian theories, *puériculture* and hygiene-based approaches as opposed to interventionist sterilization, but the drive to shape national populations through an applied science of heredity was widely shared. Eugenic experts from across the globe understood each other, even if they disagreed. Indeed, eugenicists spoke an international language, perhaps more effectively than other internationalists of the period spoke Esperanto.

Early historical studies of eugenics emphasized a comparative and therefore international dimension. These, and the generation of work that followed, show how and why eugenic *ideas* might have been similar between nations, but eugenic *policies* completely different.[2] Other studies have traced circuits of exchange between influential scientific figures, linking a long-standing strand of analysis in the historiography of science with the more recent upsurge in transnational history. Important connections have been unearthed between eugenic scientists based in Germany and the United States, across the British Empire, and as Quine shows in this volume, between scientists based in southern Europe and their counterparts in Latin America.[3]

The long-standing historiographical interest in this aspect of eugenics stemmed partly from the availability of the proceedings of early international conferences. Twentieth-century eugenic societies and associations inherited a rich nineteenth-century tradition of international science meetings. The organizers were assiduous about publishing their proceedings widely and quickly, providing detailed papers for scientific and social analysis at the time, and for subsequent historical scrutiny. For the participants at these meetings, "international" meant first, and most simply, the gathering of experts from several nations, though unsurprisingly, perhaps, the range of national representation was limited. Substantive issues of internationalism and eugenics were also occasionally addressed: standardization of data was one key agenda item in this respect; migration and its regulation was another. This period's phenomenal uptake of migration law, and the eugenic clauses and powers therein, is arguably the most internationally consistent manifestation of eugenic ideas not just as policy, but also as practice. The various migration statutes themselves were remarkably similar across time and national contexts, in their fairly sudden appearance, in their drafting, and in their increasingly eugenic rationales.

If we know a good deal about the international eugenic congresses, we know far less about the place of eugenics in the two flagship international organizations of the twentieth century, the League of Nations (1919–1946) and its successor, the United Nations (1945–). Notwithstanding major efforts on the part of eugenic societies, it proved problematic for League of Nations' personnel to divorce eugenics from nationalism, to see it as a viably international issue. By contrast, eugenics *was* explicitly championed and harnessed by key players in the early postwar years of the United Nations. The twentieth-century chronology of the links between eugenics and the formal international organizations is thus surprising, and in many ways counterintuitive: avoided by the League in the 1920s and 1930s, eugenics was taken up by sections of the UN after World War II. Given that many scholars argue that eugenics became publicly indefensible in the post-Holocaust period,[4] this postwar uptake invites a reconsideration of the periodization of eugenics' decline.

The League and the United Nations were intergovernmental organizations, bound in many ways by nationalist politics that, as we shall see, came to determine just which issues could be deemed "international" and which could not. But there was a further intellectual and political tradition of internationalism driving certain elements within and behind the League and later the UN, which sought to diminish national agendas and even nations themselves. Deriving from a tradition of universalism and pacifism, historians have become interested in the influence of cosmopolitanism, the idea of a universal human community, a "supra-national" or world citizenship.[5] Especially the leftist "reform" eugenicists of the interwar and the post–World War II period should be interpreted partly within this tradition. Cosmopolitanism also shaped the links between eugenics and the problematization of world population growth, which intensified in the postwar decades, and which was one of the key trajectories of international eugenics over the twentieth century. As one population expert wrote to the long-standing Eugenics Society secretary C. P. Blacker (1895–1975) in 1954: "Narrow patriotism must go and one must become 'planet conscious.'"[6]

INTERNATIONAL CONGRESSES
AND ORGANIZATIONS

The first eugenic organizations were established in the very early twentieth century, initially in Germany. As its name suggests, the Internationale/Deutsche Gesellschaft für Rassenhygiene was intended to be international from the start.[7] A large International Eugenics Congress was held at the University of London in 1912, organized by the [British] Eugenics Education Society and presided over by Leonard Darwin (1850–1943), who argued explicitly for the national benefits of eugenics in a context of international competition.[8] This Congress divided eugenics into biological research, sociological and historical research, legislation and social customs, and the practical application of eugenic principles. In his review in the journal *Science,* U.S. biologist Raymond Pearl noted the "respectability" of the attendees, over 800 of them, with as many visitors in daily attendance.[9] The Congress established a Permanent International Eugenics Committee, which worked toward the second Congress. This Committee became, in 1925, the International Federation of Eugenics Organizations.[10]

If the first meeting bore the marks of eugenics' British origins (notwithstanding the congress's "international" claim), the second was a thoroughly North American affair, held at the American Museum of Natural History in New York in September 1921. It was organized by Henry Fairfield Osborn (1857–1935) of Columbia University; Madison Grant (1865–1937), chair of the Zoological Society; and Clarence Little (1888–1971), zoologist, neo-Malthusian, and at that point ending his assistant directorship in the Carnegie Institute's Department of Genetics, under Charles Davenport (1866–1944). The organizing committee arranged eugenics conceptually into four sections: pure genetics in animals, plants, and human heredity; the regulation of reproduction of "the human family;" human racial differences; and eugenics in relation to the state, society, and education.[11] Two large volumes resulted from this meeting: *Eugenics, Genetics, and the Family* (1923); and *Eugenics in Race and State* (1923).

A further international congress was held in New York in 1932, led this time by Charles Davenport, and distinctly reflecting his particular interest in race science. Speakers and papers were solicited and divided into: race differences and their measurement; "mate selection" and the birth rate; "the socially inadequate"; the physiology of reproduction; eugenics and society; and genetics.[12] And in 1940 there was a fourth international congress of eugenics led by the German Racial Hygiene Society, which gathered Axis experts together in Vienna.[13]

For population experts in Latin America, the pan-American political and geographic logic was more significant.[14] Extending prior pan-American medical and sanitary conferences, there was a series of equivalent "eugenic and homiculture" conferences, which linked with the Latin International Federation of Eugenics Societies, holding its first meeting in Mexico City, 1935.[15] At this meeting and at the

Paris meeting of Latin Eugenics in 1937, "Latinity" was constructed as an "oppositional identity to 'Anglo-Saxonism,'" as Nancy Stepan notes, and this manifested as resistance to the interventionist reproductive eugenics especially associated with the United States.[16]

In the manner of any number of international scientific congresses common from the later nineteenth century, the eugenics meetings gathered experts from several countries: the London and New York meetings were dominated by U.S. and British contributors, with typically sizable French, Italian, Scandinavian, and German contingents as well. The proceedings of the 1912 meeting lists only one eastern European participant and one East Asian delegate from the University of Kyoto, while the 1921 New York meeting included papers from Indian Gopalji Ahluwalia, and the Cuban Dr. D. F. Ramos, key organizer of the Pan-American Eugenics Committee and an important figure in the League of Nations' consideration of eugenics. In general, the eugenics meetings were less diverse than other comparable meetings, such as the various international birth control and population congresses of the period, which included much larger numbers of East and South Asian participants.

Ironically, the actual reach of eugenics was far wider and broader than the participation in these so-called "international" congresses. If one is guided by the proceedings of these meetings, or even the list of the formal members of the International Federation, the impact of eugenics appears falsely diminished. The contributing nations to the International Federation in 1934, for example, included the well-known US, British, and European organizations, as well as groups from Argentina, the Dutch East Indies, Estonia, South Africa, Switzerland, and Ramos's Pan-American Office of Homiculture in Cuba. But this list offers no sense of the extensive eugenic activity elsewhere: in Australia, Hong Kong, India, China, Japan, or New Zealand. Eugenics was in fact far more globally widespread than participation in, and the records of, the so-called "international" congresses would suggest, as chapters in part II of this volume demonstrate.

Social and biological scientists interested in eugenics also exchanged ideas at other international meetings: the International Congresses of Medicine, International Neo-Malthusian Conferences, and the International Congresses of Genetics. For example, at the fifth meeting of the latter (Berlin in 1927), Ruggles Gates (1882–1962) spoke on interracial inheritance, and the editors of the British *Eugenics Review* congratulated themselves: "eugenic science and heredity in man found itself . . . no longer a halting camp-follower of the progressive army of genetic studies."[17] Similarly, the 1931 International Congress for the Study of Population Problems held in Rome—with Benito Mussolini (1883–1945) as the honorary chair and demographer Corrado Gini (1884–1965) as the effective chair—had a section devoted to "Biology and Eugenics." Topics included "declining birth rate factors," and "effects of war on the rate, longevity, relation between intelligence and birth-rate." It should be noted that papers on "crossings in human races" were presented not to the eugenics section, but to the section titled "Anthropology and Geography."[18]

From the earliest international congresses, comparative national studies appeared. But occasionally the substantive topic of internationalism was put forward. Its least ambitious form involved plans for standardization of data, for example "International Biological Registration: the Norwegian System for Identification and Protection of the Individual" and "Plan for Obtaining an International Technique in Physical Anthropology."[19] The most ambitious consideration of eugenics and internationalism, to be discussed below, involved consideration of apparently universal principles of evolution and inheritance for humanity as a whole. Somewhere in between lay close consideration of the role of eugenics in regulating and monitoring international human movement.

EUGENICS AND IMMIGRATION RESTRICTION: INTERNATIONAL BIO-REGULATION

Historians of eugenics are typically concerned to assess the actual implementation of eugenic ideas, compared to their theoretical discussion. This is the common gap that Robert Nye notes between "the ambitions of the eugenicists and their real achievements in legal and institutional reform."[20] Indeed, eugenic movements were not infrequently unsuccessful by their own measures, failing dismally at the "application" end of applied science. In an under-recognized way, however, the remarkable proliferation of eugenic clauses in immigration laws across many nations in the first half of the twentieth century arguably constitute the single most internationally significant and consistent policy and legal application of eugenic ideas. U.S. historians in particular have shown the influence of eugenic arguments on the shape of the famous 1924 Immigration Act and more generally on linked histories of territorial governance, population management, and U.S. nationalism.[21] Yet this history needs to be understood as constituting a global trend.[22] Enacted and implemented as part of increasingly strident nationalisms in the interwar period, immigration law aimed to regulate intercontinental, interregional, and often interracial movement, which renders it an aspect of international eugenics of the first half of the twentieth century.

Beginning with Chinese exclusion acts in the 1850s, immigration restriction and regulation proliferated in a great number of countries in the 1920s and 1930s. These national statutes were a "new world" response to the massive global human movements of the nineteenth century, the Chinese and later Indian labor diasporas, and the economic migration of millions of Europeans to North and South America. National and colonial immigration laws were considered part of the management of the intergenerational biological character and health of domestic populations. Over time, the explicit nomination of race and nationality as grounds for exclusion (always problematic, especially within the British Empire and Commonwealth) declined and was increasingly replaced by racially coded health and eugenic clauses. By the 1920s, almost every statute in the global phenomenon of immigration regulation had a power of exclusion, deportation, or restriction of entry based on a eugenic rationale. And later in the century, new states like Israel and Singapore inherited this linked eugenic and migration history, introducing medical screening in bids to secure national health.[23]

Historians of eugenics and historians of migration regulation have generally pointed to the place of eugenics and eugenicists in arguing for race or nationality-based restrictions enacted in many laws. This is historically clear, not least in the multiple Chinese exclusion acts across the world, and in the 1924 U.S. Act that established national quotas for immigrants from various nations and ethnicities.[24] Indeed, from 1919 the leader of the U.S. Immigration Restriction League, Prescott F. Hall (1868–1921), called the proliferation of migration acts "world eugenics." To his mind, racial segregation of nations was an appropriate and effective response to the "yellow peril" of the Chinese diaspora and Chinese population growth.[25] But there needs to be an extension of our understanding of the eugenics of immigration restriction beyond a discourse of race difference. In the interwar period, many "new world" nations were hurriedly writing and rewriting the exclusion of the "unfit" from the old world into statutes, policy, and regulation. This was a means by which populations were to be improved, not necessarily on grounds of racial difference, but perhaps more commonly on grounds of the "unfitness" of individuals of the same "race." Thus, even more strictly eugenic than the race- or nationality-based exclusions were those clauses of immigration acts which sought to screen out the genetically dangerous from the population who, racially or ethnically speaking, *were* permitted entry: "whites" who were feeble-minded, syphilitic, criminally inclined, or alcoholic. This is the less familiar legacy of eugenics on the international regulation of global movement. Indeed, occasionally commentators would explicitly distinguish eugenic from racial exclusion. Anthropologist and geographer Griffith Taylor, for example, thought the obsession with blanket race-based exclusions should sensibly be dropped in favor of health and fitness criteria of entrants as individuals. "Eugenics rather than nationality," he wrote, "is the best criterion for those responsible for racial exclusion."[26]

In the U.S. 1917 Immigration Act, section 3 prohibited "all idiots, imbeciles, feeble-minded persons, epileptics, insane persons; persons who have had one or more attacks of insanity at any time previously; persons of constitutional psychopathic inferiority, persons with chronic alcoholism."[27] The process of health inspection on arrival by the U.S. Public Health Service (and in some circumstances at point of departure) was driven simultaneously by fiscal (the cost of welfare), health, and eugenic rationales, with the distinction between the latter increasingly imperceptible. The earlier Canadian laws were similar, the 1910 Act nominating in the "prohibited classes" "idiots, imbeciles, feeble-minded persons, epileptics, insane persons."[28] Even earlier again, the 1901 Australian Immigration Restriction Act had effectively ceased Chinese, Indian, Japanese, or Pacific Islander entry. This meant that the immigration powers to refuse entry on fitness grounds were far more commonly implemented against Britons, by design the most common migrants. In gaining a certificate of health to board a ship bound for Australia, would-be immigrants were questioned by representatives of the Australian government first on tuberculosis, second on whether they had ever been admitted to an insane asylum. As reported at the time, the most common grounds for rejection were "want of physical fitness, deficient height and weight, defective eyesight, deafness, mental deficiency, and tuberculosis."[29] In other contexts, immigration acts governed both race criteria and mental and physical health. The 1906 Newfoundland Act, for example, defined as undesirable any "Chinese who is...an idiot or insane."[30]

Considered collectively, as part of international eugenics, there is an arc to these legislative measures to manage global human movement through national statutes. The original twin legal rationales for exclusion and deportation—labor concerns on the one hand, quarantine and the management of acute epidemics on the other— increasingly merged and strengthened through a eugenic logic in the 1920s and 1930s in many receiving countries. Overall, the explicit nomination of race or nationality gave way to health and fitness (that is, eugenic) rationales for exclusion of individuals. Together, these were consistent and applied measures for the bio-regulation of future populations.

EUGENICS AND THE LEAGUE OF NATIONS

From its origins after World War I to its demise in 1946, the League of Nations considered many social, economic, and health issues raised by the member states of the Assembly and shaped them, via its various agencies and sections, into international issues: slavery, tariffs, the opium trade, infant welfare, labor conditions. If these did not naturally fit the League's brief to maintain peace through international cooperation, they were discursively made to do so. Over the 1920s and 1930s many eugenic advocates approached the Secretariat of the League and its various agencies, seeking to place eugenics officially on the agenda and attempting to "internationalize" eugenics for the League's consumption. Participants at the 1921 International Eugenics meeting in New York thought that a modest version of eugenics might have a "natural home" with the international health organization, for example, but this was not to be.[31] Perhaps surprisingly, eugenics was never authorized by the League as "international."

Notwithstanding this failure to formally internationalize eugenics, the various arguments put forward to the League illustrate the reach of eugenics, its links to any number of concerns in the period, and the flexibility it held, crossing social and biological issues. Charles Davenport argued his case first in terms of the global significance of human migration and its regulation:

> In view of the fact that racial differences are now recognized as matters of the greatest possible concern in a world organization, in view of the fact that they

played so important a part in the Peace Conference and in the delimitation of countries, and in view of the fact that they form so important a consideration in matters of immigration, it is thought that the progress of the world would be advanced by having a definite sub-section of the Health Section.[32]

Davenport received a firm decline. The honorary secretary of the International Eugenics Congress subsequently pressed Dame Rachel Crowdy (1884–1964), then secretary of the Social Questions and Opium Traffic Section of the League of Nations, on whether a Eugenics subsection had been considered. Progressive health policy, it was argued, demands that knowledge of human heredity, miscegenation, and vital statistics be disseminated rapidly and correctly to the health service of all countries. "The great Powers with their Colonial responsibilities cannot afford to neglect any opportunity of increasing the knowledge of such practical eugenic questions."[33] Although Crowdy's response was interested, neither the Social Questions section nor the Health Organization was persuaded.

When Davenport tried Crowdy again, later in 1920, his rationale rested specifically on race difference and its significance in world affairs. In Davenport's hands, eugenics was strategically rendered international by linking it to peace (resolving race tensions, as he saw it) through immigration regulation and through the constitution of nations. Eugenics promoted the "cause of the comity of nations and international good." In this case, the bid to argue eugenics into the League through race was foiled by Japanese Inazo Nitobé, one of the original undersecretaries-general of the League and founding director of the League's International Institute for Intellectual Cooperation (which became UNESCO).

> In view of the historical fact that races of all colors and grades have freely mingled all through the ages, I cannot share Dr Davenport's view that the progress of the world would be advanced by accentuating race differences. German scientists under the lead of Gobineau...tried to find scientific basis to demonstrate the absolute superiority of the "Hun." I hope America will not follow the German example—I hail all scientific researches: but I am doubtful of their hasty application to social politics as was done by [the] "Politische-Anthropologische Revue" set.[34]

C.B.S. Hodson, secretary of the British Eugenics Society, tried and failed again in 1924, identifying the Society's aims as "the more practical side of the Heredity work" and later urging the League's attendance at the 1927 World Population Conference, which Margaret Sanger and others organized in Geneva.[35]

It was not under the logic of race and race-mixing, or immigration regulation, but of infant health and protection, that eugenics came closest to consideration as a field for information and action. As a result of a resolution put forward by the Cuban delegation to the League's governing Assembly in 1926, the Health Organization was asked to what extent eugenics might shape its work on the protection of infants. The Secretariat's file, originally titled *Protection l'enfant* was significantly struck through to become *l'Eugénisme: Questions générale.* Dr. D. F. Ramos, representing the Cuban Ministry of Health and Welfare, presented eugenics as "homiculture," the French-influenced brand of hygiene and improvement.[36] He was a student of Pinard who, as

Ramos put it "undoubtedly has the honour, shared with the wise Englishman Francis Galton, of having founded the science for the betterment of the human species."[37] But the Health Organization of the League remained reluctant: "Avoiding all questions of a purely national character [the Health Organization would consider] only those problems which deserve international consideration."[38]

Part of the Secretariat's responsibility was carefully to adjudicate which issues were truly international and which might controversially breach national prerogatives. Even Ramos' *puériculture* version of eugenics touched too closely a range of sensitive population policies, and implicitly the ambition and competition of nations, effectively putting eugenics outside "internationalism" and inside "nationalism," as far as the League was concerned. Further, the close alignment of eugenics to birth control—in particular through common advocacy of sterilization—found no favor at all with Catholic nations, which constituted a significant lobby group in League politics.

EUGENICS AND UNESCO

While the League of Nations had very little to do with eugenics, one of the key postwar United Nations agencies was described by its director-general as having eugenics at its core. Famously, Julian Huxley (1887–1975), grandson of Charles Darwin's supporter T. H. Huxley and first director-general of United Nations Educational Scientific and Cultural Organization, placed eugenics front and center in his 1947 manifesto, *UNESCO: Its Purpose and Philosophy.* In his new international role, Huxley rendered globally urgent those projects which might improve "the average quality of human beings... accomplished by applying the findings of truly scientific eugenics."[39] Huxley was not in the least unaware of the race and even class implications of a science that had problematically assumed superiority and inferiority of certain groups,[40] advocating what scholars subsequently called a "reform eugenics," which rejected racism. He had delivered this message popularly in *We Europeans* in 1935, with anthropologist Alfred Cort Haddon (1855–1940) and social scientist (and eugenicist) Alexander Carr-Saunders (1886–1966). For Huxley, projects that delineated racial difference and that suggested action on the basis of hierarchized difference were unscientific, politically undesirable, and unconscionable. As a good evolutionary biologist, Huxley saw the significance of variation:

> It is therefore of the greatest importance to preserve human variety; all attempts at reducing it, whether by attempting to obtain greater "purity" and therefore uniformity within a so-called race or a national group, or by attempting to exterminate any of the broad racial groups... are scientifically incorrect and opposed to long-run human progress.[41]

But Huxley's opposition to what had been a significant strand of eugenics did not make him an opponent of eugenics per se. Other kinds of human difference *did* invite and require action, he thought: "There remains the second type of inequality. This has quite other implications; for, whereas variety is in itself desirable, the existence of weaklings, fools, and moral deficients cannot but be bad." This was, indeed, no longer a national issue, but a global one, "a major task for the world."[42] In other words, Huxley retained, fundamentally, a eugenic view not just of the possibility of, but the imperative for, the valuation of human difference.

It is instructive to note that at the time, Huxley's manifesto statements on birth control and world population were more controversial than his statements on eugenics. This was not because his milieu advocated or secretly harbored predilections for a eugenic race science. It is because Huxley and many of his contemporaries saw no *necessary* relation between eugenics and projects of racial purity with which eugenics later became so closely associated: indeed they were quite open advocates of eugenics' continuance and its social and scientific value.

It is similarly telling that eugenics was quite discussable in various quarters of the new United Nations. For example, Alva Myrdal (1902–1986), head of UNESCO's Social Science Division and later Nobel Prize winner, led a project in the early 1950s on the relationship between fertility and intelligence: "Differential fertility and its effects on the intelligence of the population stock" was to be UNESCO's main contribution to the 1954 UN-backed World Population Conference in Rome. The experts she invited to work through the issue were key representatives of postwar eugenics and genetics, and, importantly, unremarkably so. Dr C. O. Carter (1917-1984), secretary of the Eugenics Society (London) was nominated by the World Federation for Mental Health to participate in Myrdal's committee. Fraser Roberts (1900–1987) also advised the committee, a medical geneticist then deeply involved in establishing early genetic counseling. Frederick Osborn (1889–1981), who was about to launch the new journal *Eugenics Quarterly* was also invited, but could not attend.[43] The Committee returned to (or really represented a continuous link with) what was arguably the original eugenic project: class-based studies on differential fertility and intelligence.

Some of the experts present at this UNESCO meeting on fertility and intelligence were certainly more concerned than others about the term as well as the project of eugenics. Jan Böök (1915–1995) of the Swedish State Institute for Human Genetics and Race, said to his colleagues: "At our present state of knowledge I take a very sceptical attitude to any kind of recommendations of general eugenic measures." And Danish human geneticist Tage Kemp (1896–1964) thought that people receiving the report would be anxious to know what position the group had with respect to eugenics: "the most important task is to encourage and assist studies of medical and especially human genetics." A report should outline principles of voluntariness, he thought, the implementation of which he called a "negative eugenics programme" since a "positive" program would be "too controversial." It is unclear here whether Kemp was reversing the standard construction of negative and positive eugenics. It is possible that he was signaling that the key controversy of eugenics at that point concerned programs which favored the eugenically "fit," not those directed at the "unfit," as we might expect. The key to any acceptable eugenics, the

Committee agreed, was the voluntary principle,[44] consistent with (indeed, actively continuing) much interwar discussion on legitimate and illegitimate state powers.

It is important to note that discussion of eugenics within this UN agency was relatively unproblematic, and, in stark contrast to the League of Nations experience, was uncontroversially "international." In large part, this was because of the new discourse of economic development, closely linked to fertility studies. It was through the dominant notion of "development" that this classic eugenic topic became internationalized. And it was less the genetic counseling trajectory than demographic work on fertility rates and the measures to control and space births—all under demographic transition theories and development discourse—that most extended the momentum of eugenics as an international issue after 1945.

EUGENICS AND WORLD POPULATION CONTROL

Many historians and other commentators argue that after 1945, eugenics changed its name and to some extent its clothes, to become "global population control;" that this was a period in which eugenics operated "under new labels."[45] The creation of, and action around, the world population problem is often described as eugenics on a global scale, where the problematic population shifted from domestic "undesirables"—"the enemy within"—to the growing populations of South Asia, East Asia, and to some extent, Latin America. The quantitative global overpopulation problem was certainly used as a rationale for "qualitative" local population policies and eugenic practices of reproductive regulation. The technique of sterilization of both men and women was not the only method by which this was to be achieved, but was clearly inherited from interwar eugenics and came into favor with various international population-control organizations, as well as national campaigns, infamously in the so-called Indian Emergency of the mid-1970s. Historian Ian Dowbiggin's work reveals the connections between eugenic and sterilization organizations of the 1930s and the population control campaigns of the 1960s and 1970s, usefully nominating a twentieth-century-long "sterilization movement."[46] And Matthew Connelly has carefully detailed the marked continuity between anxious literature about overcrowded Asia from several twentieth-century generations, its links with post–World War II development theory, U.S. popular writing on world overpopulation, and the implementation of population control policies. These scholars join long-standing critics of population control, writing from Marxist, feminist, and postcolonial traditions.[47]

Yet both historians and sensationalist critics of "population control" deploy the link with eugenics as a kind of exposé of a movement that went underground after World War II. This is not to deny the case for criticism. But this exposé is slightly disingenuous: it overcomplicates at one level, and overlooks at another, several aspects of the history of eugenics. The connection should be unsurprising: this was one manifestation of standard prior links between eugenics and birth control. That is, many, even most interwar eugenic organizations intensified already existing family planning, birth control, or population control dimensions after the war. Further, as we have seen, many eugenicists on the international stage saw eugenics as neither controversial nor problematic, even if they understood the Nazi version of it to be so. They were not infrequently entirely open about their projects and interventions. And finally, eugenic and neo-Malthusian arguments about overpopulation (including global overpopulation) were not new, but had been entwined since the beginning of the twentieth century. What Pauline Mazumdar says of the British organization is widely applicable: "It is clear that population studies took their origin in and were developed through the eugenics movement."[48] There was not so much a shape-shifting of eugenics into a new global "population control movement" in the 1960s, as an intensification of overpopulation arguments long held by experts active also in eugenics research.[49]

To take one example, when anti-colonial nationalist demographer Sripati Chandrasekhar (1918–2001) prepared his *Population and Planned Parenthood in India* (1955), he was fully and openly engaged with eugenics. A key player in international and Indian sterilization programs, Chandrasekhar had thought through population questions in terms of eugenics for his entire professional life. Chandrasekhar undertook his doctoral training in neo-Malthusian economics and sociology under sometime American Eugenics Society, Planned Parenthood, and Population Association president Henry Pratt Fairchild (1880–1956). He published in the *Eugenics Review* in the late 1940s; he lectured to, and was elected Honorary Fellow by, the Eugenics Society in 1954; as late as 1965 he was writing to the Japanese embassy in Washington, seeking the best English translation of the 1948 Japanese Eugenics Law, for reference in his own work.[50] All this sat comfortably alongside his nationalism, especially given the Indian National Congress's own interest in population management, and indeed eugenics. Jawaharlal Nehru contributed the forward to Sripati Chandrasekhar's 1955 book, while Julian Huxley wrote the introduction. And for decades Chandrasekhar sought C. P. Blacker's editorial and substantive advice, both in the latter's Eugenic Society role and his International Planned Parenthood role. These postwar actors, and even the field of international population control as a whole, were entirely connected to earlier eugenics. Far from disavowing eugenics after the war, they often pursued it enthusiastically on a new global stage.

EUGENICS, COSMOPOLITANISM, AND ENVIRONMENTALISM

From the earliest part of the twentieth century, the idea of world overpopulation lent both to a race-based competitive model of the future (the "yellow peril" tradition on which Connelly focuses) but also to conceptions of humanity as a whole, emerging from cosmopolitan political traditions. As Huxley put it, arguing for evolutionary progress as a touchstone for the new world order, "A central conflict of our times is that between nationalism and internationalism, between the concept of many national sovereignties and one world sovereignty."[51] The "cosmopolitan" tradition of population expertise was certainly not free of racialized discourse on human difference and capacity, and colonial discourse on the right of certain populations to dominate and govern. Nonetheless, part of the interwar "retreat of scientific racism" which Elazar Barkan has traced,[52] and even the anti-nationalism and anti-colonialism of certain population scientists, lay in this cosmopolitan desire to think about humans as a whole, rather than as racially or nationally divided populations in the first instance. From the beginning of the twentieth century, some eugenicists partook in the politico-scientific project of "species" rather than "race," of world citizens rather than patriots.

While modern political cosmopolitanism is often traced to Immanuel Kant's *Perpetual Peace* (1795), for scientists, there was also a certain universalism in the claims of natural history. At the 1912 international eugenics conference in London, Leonard Darwin framed eugenics as his generation's work which extended "the practically universal acceptance of the principle of evolution in all fields of knowledge in the nineteenth century." This was, for him, the "great international achievement" of the Victorian period.[53] Once eugenics was accepted as part of a larger evolutionary principle, it would and should be understood to govern humans universally. In hands other than a strident patriot such as Leonard Darwin, this line of inquiry was sometimes used as scientific ground on which eugenics would become not just an international, but a cosmopolitan science, applicable to all humans. Legal writer C. E. A. Bedwell (1878–1950) pursued this aspect of science and the new world order when he presented "Eugenics in International Affairs" at the 1921 New York meeting. Scientists know, he argued, that national boundaries do not limit researches, that there is an "international character of knowledge" which needs to be incorporated. Bedwell approvingly quoted jurist Sir John Macdonell's (1846–1921) 1916 essay in the *Eugenics Review,* which raised the possibility that a dispassionate eugenic science might show that "unions between certain races" are possible, even "desirable and propitious." It might find that "certain stocks would be enriched and strengthened," and humans might thus, in his opinion, become "citizens of a better world."[54] For Macdonell, writing in the middle of World War I, and for Bedwell, writing in its aftermath, "eugenics in international affairs" could potentially lead the way by showing the "unity of humanity" a "rational *jus connubii* as yet undreamed of."[55]

Such statements were certainly not mainstream eugenics. Indeed, Bedwell's audience in New York was made up of the architects of the 1924 Immigration Act, whose eyebrows and ire would have been raised by his arguments. Yet these ideas did align with the cosmopolitanism of the adjacent and often interconnecting neo-Malthusians, the tradition in which economist J. M. Keynes (1883–1946) was at that point thinking and writing. No stranger to the rapidly rising popularity of Galton and Pearson's eugenics, Keynes wrote on the supra-national significance of "population" in 1912:

Racial and military feeling now runs high, and every patriot urges his country forward on a course of action in the widest sense anti-social... The problem therefore, is made much worse and far harder of solution by having become, since Malthus's time, cosmopolitan. It is no longer possible to have a *national* policy for the population question.[56]

The idea of a connected humanity, a "rational *jus connubii*," was a legal rendition of ideas that later experts rendered scientific—both anthropological and genetic—in the UNESCO statements on race.[57]

Huxley wanted the scientists under his employ at UNESCO to think about the planet as an ecological whole. "The spread of man must take second place to the conservation of other species," he wrote.[58] These concerns signal a further dimension to the link between eugenics and internationalism. While historians have detailed the long twentieth-century trajectory of eugenics into reproductive population control on the one hand, and to a lesser extent individual genetic counseling on the other, the links with conservationist and environmentalist politics and sciences at a global level are more surprising, and only beginning to be studied.[59] Yet, for many eugenicists, the connection between population quality and quantity, between differential fertility rates and overall population growth rates, found clear expression as critique of resource depletion and destruction. Leading U.S. conservationist William Vogt (1902–1968), for example, linked population and resource questions in the influential *Road to Survival* (1948), eliding his work as president of the Family Planning Association, participation in the Human Betterment Association's scientific work, as well as that of the Association for Voluntary Sterilization.[60] The formidable Osborn cousins—Fairfield the conservationist and Frederick the eugenicist—together represented the way in which the population growth issue drew in both "quantity" and "quality" arguments, connecting politics and sciences of reproduction, with politics and sciences of environmentalism. As Frederick Osborn, founding member and later re-organizer of the American Eugenics Society, commented: "I found that the quantitative aspect of the population could not really be separated from the qualitative aspects."[61] And Fairfield raised the stakes in *Our Plundered Planet*, in a classic ecological statement: "Each part is dependent on another, all are related to the movement of the whole. Forests, grasslands, water, animal life—without one of these the earth will die—will become dead as the moon."[62]

In her examination of the underresearched conservationist-eugenicist alliance, Alexandra Minna Stern understands Fairfield Osborn and his ilk to have repackaged conservation "in terms of overpopulation and its frightening consequences."[63] But at another level, the Osborns and Vogt, so vocal in the post–World War II period, so influential on the subsequent generation of environmentalists, had inherited a planet-level problematization of population and resources presented at the very least by the World War I generation of population experts. As early as 1917, for example, one statistician linked eugenics with an early ecological conception of the planet and the human race. He listed the critical planetary problems deriving from population growth, including "The multiplying power of the human race; The organic constitution of Nature and the means at human disposal for avoiding the incidence of its unfavorable aspects; i.e. eugenics in its wider sense… Internationalism and the solidarity of humanity."[64] Thus, when Huxley declared, as director-general of UNESCO, that "population is really a world problem, involving potentialities of good or evil for the whole human species,"[65] he was developing links between eugenics, population studies, and internationalism that were already several generations old.

It was the pacifism authorizing this version of internationalism and providing such a powerful moral claim, which postwar eugenicists like Blacker, Huxley, and Faifield Osborn seized upon, and which did a good deal of work to rescue eugenics from its connections with illiberal authority. As historian of Spanish eugenics, Richard Cleminson notes, the lineage connecting controlled reproduction, the perfection of humanity, and utopian thought, is long.[66] "World, Globe, Orb, Whole, One," Blacker wrote floridly in the late 1940s about "the planetary problem." "U.N.O. Is it not the perfect word? The last of the three letters denotes our spherical planet; the first two sound the call to unite."[67] Such purple language may indicate how far from science eugenics had strayed. And the call to unite, indeed the entire field of what I am calling here cosmopolitan eugenics, need only be scratched lightly to reveal underlying divisions and inequities (the more familiar history). But understanding this particular strand of internationalism and cosmopolitanism is necessary to analyze eugenicists' own comprehension of their project, especially but not only in the postwar period. In other words, it is necessary to understand internationalism at various points in the modern period, to properly comprehend the historical development of eugenics. Strangely, then, given that the history of eugenics is fundamentally about the devastating implications of a science of human differentiation, it is also part of, and needs to be understood through, the modern history of universalism, internationalism, and cosmopolitanism.

ACKNOWLEDGMENTS

My thanks to Marius Turda and Philippa Levine for comments on drafts of this chapter.

NOTES

1. Dan Stone, "Race in British Eugenics," *European History Quarterly* 31, no. 3 (2001): 397–425; Marius Turda and Paul J. Weindling, eds., *"Blood and Homeland:" Eugenics and Racial Nationalism in Central and Southern Europe, 1900–1940* (Budapest: Central European University Press, 2007); Laura Briggs, *Reproducing Empire: Race, Sex, Science, and*

U.S. Imperialism in Puerto Rico (Berkeley, CA: University of California Press, 2002); Mary Nash, "Social Eugenics and Nationalist Race Hygiene in Early Twentieth Century Spain," *History of European Ideas* 15, nos. 4–6 (1992): 741–748.

2. Daniel Kevles, *In the Name of Eugenics* (New York: Knopf, 1985); Nancy Leys Stepan, *"The Hour of Eugenics": Race, Gender and Nation in Latin America* (Ithaca, NY: Cornell University Press, 1991); Mark B. Adams, ed., *The Wellborn Science: Eugenics in Germany, France, Brazil, and Russia* (Oxford and New York: Oxford University Press, 1990); Randall Hansen and Desmond King, "Eugenic Ideas, Political Interests and Policy Variance: Immigration and Sterilization Policy in Britain and the US," *World Politics* 53, no. 2 (2001): 237–263; Mark B. Adams, Garland E. Allen, and Sheila F. Weiss, "Human Heredity and Politics," *Osiris* 20 (2005): 232–262.

3. For example, Paul Weindling, "International Eugenics: Swedish Sterilization in Context," *Scandinavian Journal of History* 24, no. 2 (1999): 179–197; Stefan Kühl, *The Nazi Connection: Eugenics, American Racism and German National Socialism* (Oxford and New York: Oxford University Press, 1994); Nils Roll-Hansen, "Scandinavian Eugenics in the International Context," in *Eugenics and the Welfare State: Sterilization Policy in Denmark, Sweden, Norway, and Finland*, eds. Gunnar Broberg and Nils Roll-Hansen (East Lansing, MI: Michigan State University Press, 1996); David Mitchell and Sharon Snyder, "The Eugenic Atlantic: Race, Disability, and the Making of an International Eugenic Science, 1800–1945," *Disability and Society* 18, no. 7 (2003): 843–864; Stefan Kühl, *Die Internationale der Rassisten. Der Aufstieg und Niedergang der internationalen Bewegung für Eugenik und Rassenhygiene im 20. Jahrhundert* (Frankfurt/Main: Campus Verlag, 1997).

4. For example, Deborah Barrett and Charles Kerzman, "Globalizing Social Movement Theory: The Case of Eugenics," *Theory and Society*, 33, no. 5 (2004): 487–527.

5. See for example, essays in *Perpetual Peace: Essays on Kant's Cosmopolitan Ideal*, ed. James Bohman and Matthias Lutz-Bachmann (Cambridge, MA: MIT Press, 1997), 25–57.

6. V. H. Wallace to C. P. Blacker, 27 June 1954, SA/EUG/E.3/1, Eugenics Society Papers, Wellcome Library, London.

7. Weindling, "International Eugenics," 182.

8. Leonard Darwin, "Presidential Address," in *Problems in Eugenics. Papers Presented. 1st International Eugenics Congress*, vol. 1 (Adelphi: The Eugenics Education Society, 1912), 6. *Problems in Eugenics*, volume 1, was published prior to the Congress, for participants' reference; volume 2, *Proceedings*, was published in 1913.

9. Raymond Pearl, "The First International Eugenics Congress," *Science* 36, no. 926 (1912): 395.

10. "The Third International Congress of Eugenics," *Science* 73, no. 182 (1931): 357–358.

11. "The Second International Congress of Eugenics," *The Scientific Monthly* 13, no. 2 (1921): 186–187.

12. "Third International Congress of Eugenics," *Man* 33 (1932): 51.

13. Paul Weindling, *Health, Race and German Politics between National Unification and Nazism* (Cambridge: Cambridge University Press, 1989), 505.

14. Stepan, *"The Hour of Eugenics,"* 170.

15. Ibid., 185.

16. Ibid., 190.

17. "The 5th International Congress on Genetics," *Eugenics Review* 20 (1928–29): 34.

18. Population Problems—International Congress for Studies Regarding Population, Rome, 7–10 September 1931, Box R2872 Economic Section, League of Nations Archives, Geneva [LNAG].

19. Jon Alfred Mjøen and Jan Bö, "International Biological Registration," *Eugenics Review* 16, no. 3 (1924): 183–188; R. Ruggles Gates, "Plan for Obtaining an International

Technique in Physical Anthropology," in *A Decade of Progress in Eugenics: Scientific Papers of the Third International Congress of Eugenics* (Baltimore, MD: Williams and Wilkins, 1934), 47.

20. Robert A. Nye, "The Rise and Fall of the Eugenics Empire," *The Historical Journal* 36, no. 3 (1993): 695.

21. Alexandra Minna Stern, *Eugenic Nation: Faults and Frontiers of Better Breeding in Modern America* (Berkeley, CA: University of California Press, 2005).

22. Marilyn Lake and Henry Reynolds, *Drawing the Global Colour Line: White Men's Countries and the International Challenge of Racial Equality* (Cambridge: Cambridge University Press, 2008).

23. See Shifra Shvarts, Nadav Davidovitch, Rhona Seidelman, and Avishay Goldberg, "Medical Selection and the Debate over Mass Immigration in the New State of Israel (1948–1951)," *Canadian Bulletin of Medical History / Bulletin canadien d'histoire de la médecine,* 22, no. 1 (2005): 5–34.

24. Kevles, *In the Name of Eugenics,* 97; Mae M. Ngai, *Impossible Subjects: Illegal Aliens and the Making of Modern America* (Princeton, NJ: Princeton University Press, 2004), 24–25.

25. Matthew Connelly, "To Inherit the Earth: Imagining World Population, from the Yellow Peril to the Population Bomb," *Journal of Global History* 1, no. 3 (2006): 299–319.

26. Griffith Taylor, *Environment and Race: A Study of the Evolution, Migration, Settlement and Status of the Races of Man* (Oxford: Oxford University Press, 1927), 341.

27. *Immigration Act* (1917), United States of America, Section 3.

28. *Immigration Act* (1910), Canada, Section 3(a).

29. W. E. Agar, "Some Eugenic Aspects of Australian Population Problems," in *The Peopling of Australia,* eds. P. D. Phillips and G. L. Wood (Melbourne: Macmillan, 1928), 142.

30. *Chinese Immigration Act* (1906), Newfoundland, Section 4 and section 5(b).

31. C. E. A. Bedwell, "Eugenics in International Affairs," in *Eugenics in Race and State: Scientific Papers of the Second International Congress of Eugenics,* vol. 2 (Baltimore, MD: Williams and Wilkins, 1923), 428.

32. Davenport to Crowdy, 23 November 1920, Box R642, International Eugenics, Social Section, LNAG.

33. Rolfe to Crowdy, 28 September 1920, Section 12 7260/7260, LNAG.

34. Handwritten Note by Inazo Nitobé, 24 December 1920, Box R642, International Eugenics, Social Section, LNAG.

35. C. B. S. Hodson to Dr. Norman White, 29 February 1927, Box 1602, Dossier Concerning World Population Conference 1927, LNAG.

36. Alejandra Bronfman, *Measures of Equality: Social Science, Citizenship and Race in Cuba, 1902–1940* (Chapel Hill, NC: University of North Carolina Press, 2004), 120–23.

37. D. F. Ramos to director of the Department of Hygiene of the Office of the League of Nations, 21 September 1926, Box R975, Infant Welfare Enquiry Dossier respecting Cuba, LNAG.

38. Report on the Work of the Health Committee, 8th Session October 1926, Box R912, Health Section, LNAG.

39. Julian Huxley, *UNESCO: Its Purpose and Philosophy* (Washington, DC: Public Affairs Press, 1947), 37–38.

40. Ibid., 37.

41. Huxley, *UNESCO,* 19. For analysis of Huxley on variation and diversity, see chapters by Garland Allen, Diane Paul, and Elazar Barkan in *Julian Huxley: Biologist and Statesman of Science,* eds. C. Kenneth Waters and Albert Van Helden (Houston, TX: Rice University Press, 1992).

42. Huxley, *UNESCO,* 20.

43. "Contribution of UNESCO to the World Population Conference," 1 September 1953, and correspondence with Alva Myrdal, Fertility Studies, July 1953–January 1954, 312.A 53, UNESCO Archives, Paris.

44. UNESCO/SS/POP.M/Conf.1/1/S.R.1, UNESCO Archives.

45. Dowbiggin, *The Sterilization Movement*, 6; Garland Allen, "From Eugenics to Population Control," *Science for the People* 12, no. 4 (1980): 22–28.

46. Dowbiggin, *The Sterilization Movement*.

47. See Mohan Rao, *From Population Control to Reproductive Health: Malthusian Arithmetic* (New Delhi: Sage, 2004); Matthew Connelly, *Fatal Misconception: The Struggle to Control World Population* (Cambridge, MA: Harvard University Press, 2008); see also Ines Smyth, "Gender Analysis of Family Planning: Beyond the Feminist vs. Population Control Debate," in *Feminist Visions of Development: Gender Analysis and Policy*, eds. Cecile Jackson and Ruth Pearson (London: Routledge, 1998).

48. Pauline M. H. Mazumdar, "Essays in the History of Eugenics [review]," *Bulletin of the History of Medicine* 74, no. 1 (2000): 180–183.

49. Alison Bashford, "Nation, Empire, Globe: The Spaces of World Population in the Interwar Years," *Comparative Studies in Society and History* 49, no. 1 (2007): 170–201.

50. S. Chandrasekhar to Ambassador, Japanese Embassy (Washington, DC) 12 October 1965, Box 14, Chandrasekhar Papers, Ward M. Canaday Center for Special Collections, University of Toledo Library.

51. Huxley, *UNESCO*, 13.

52. Elazar Barkan, *The Retreat of Scientific Racism* (Cambridge: Cambridge University Press, 1992).

53. Darwin, "Presidential Address," 1.

54. Sir John Macdonell, *Eugenics Review* (1916) cited in Bedwell, "Eugenics in International Affairs," 428.

55. Bedwell, "Eugenics in International Affairs," 428.

56. John Maynard Keynes, "Population [1912]," in John Toye, *Keynes on Population*, (Oxford and New York: Oxford University Press, 2000), 66.

57. Michelle Brattain, "Race, Racism, and Antiracism: UNESCO and the Politics of Presenting Science to the Postwar Public," *American Historical Review* 112, no. 5 (2007): 1386–1413.

58. Huxley, *UNESCO*, 45.

59. Jonathan Peter Spiro, *Defending the Master Race: Conservation, Eugenics, and the Legacy of Madison Grant* (Burlington, VT: University of Vermont Press, 2009).

60. Dowbiggin, *The Sterilization Movement*, 111–114.

61. Frederick Osborn, National Academy of Sciences, Conference on Population Problems, June 20, 1952, Rockefeller Archive Center, Rockefeller Family Papers, Record Group 5, Series 1, Sub-Series 5, Box 85, Folder 720, 15.

62. Fairfield Osborn, *Our Plundered Planet* (London: Faber and Faber, 1948).

63. Stern, *Eugenic Nation*, 126.

64. Sir George Knibbs, *Mathematical Theory of Population, of Its Character and Fluctuations, and of the Factors Which Influence Them*, Appendix A, *Census of the Commonwealth of Australia, 1911* (Melbourne: Government Printer, 1917), 456.

65. Julian Huxley, "Statement by the Representative of UNESCO on the Desirability of Convening a UN Conference on World Population Problem," 13 May 1948, GX 6/1/7, LNAG.

66. Richard Cleminson, "'A Century of Civilization under the Influence of Eugenics:' Dr. Enrique Diego Madazo, Socialism and Scientific Progress," *Dynamis* 26 (2006): 222.

67. C. P. Blacker, "Population," *Eugenics Review* 39 (1947–48): 27.

FURTHER READING

Adams, Mark B., ed. *The Wellborn Science: Eugenics in Germany, France, Brazil, and Russia* (Oxford and New York: Oxford University Press, 1990).

Barrett, Deborah, and Charles Kerzman. "Globalizing Social Movement Theory: The Case of Eugenics," *Theory and Society* 33, no. 5 (2004): 487–527.

Bashford, Alison. "Nation, Empire, Globe: The Spaces of World Population in the Interwar Years," *Comparative Studies in Society and History* 49, no. 1 (2007): 170–201.

Cocks, Geoffrey. "The International Eugenics Community," *Reviews in American History* 22 (1994): 674–678.

Connelly, Matthew. *Fatal Misconception: The Struggle to Control World Population* (Cambridge, MA: Harvard University Press, 2008).

Dowbiggin, Ian. *The Sterilization Movement and Global Fertility in the Twentieth Century* (Oxford and New York: Oxford University Press, 2008).

Kevles, Daniel J. "International Eugenics," in *Deadly Medicine: Creating the Master Race,* eds. Dieter Kuntz and Susan Bachrach (Washington, DC: US Holocaust Memorial Museum, 2004), 41–60.

Kühl, Stephan. *The Nazi Connection: Eugenics, American Racism and German National Socialism* (Oxford and New York: Oxford University Press, 1994).

Spektorowski, Alberto. "The Eugenic Temptation in Socialism: Sweden, Germany, and the Soviet Union," *Comparative Studies in Society and History* 46, no. 1 (2004): 84–106.

Weindling, Paul. "International Eugenics: Swedish Sterilization in Context," *Scandinavian Journal of History* 24, no. 2 (1999): 179–197.

CHAPTER 9

....

GENDER AND SEXUALITY: A GLOBAL TOUR AND COMPASS

....

ALEXANDRA MINNA STERN

EUGENICS was a plastic and sprawling phenomenon that attracted a motley crew of supporters, hailing from many professional corners and political persuasions. This malleability helps to explain why eugenics attained popularity in so many different places around the globe. From Berlin to Buenos Aires, and Tehran to Tokyo, eugenics found fertile ground in the first half of the twentieth century. Yet eugenics followed distinct paths, depending on the particular national and cultural milieu in which it took hold. In some places, such as Mexico, eugenics had much more to do with better baby care than immigration bans or compulsory sterilization, and continued in this vein with little disruption until the 1960s.[1] In others, including most European countries, the tarnished status of eugenics after 1945 resulted either in eugenicists inconspicuously moving into the domains of human genetics, demography, or sociology, or furthering less controversial endeavors such as maternal and infant hygiene.[2] In some places, like India and Puerto Rico, eugenics movements that had emerged in earnest in the 1920s and 1930s transmogrified into population control efforts that endorsed family planning and birth control.[3]

Just as the elasticity and multidimensionality of eugenics makes it a fascinating historical puzzle, they also make it very challenging to conceptually contain eugenics as a coherent social and scientific phenomenon. Two of the most illuminating lenses through which we can productively explore the global history of eugenics are gender and sexuality. From its beginnings in the late nineteenth century, eugenics was intimately entangled with reproduction, sex, the family, as well as human physiology and form. Framed by the adjacent analytics of gender and sexuality, this chapter explores the emergence, consolidation, splintering, and persistence of eugenics over the twentieth century with keen attention to transnational variations and networks. It seeks to synthesize the growing body of literature on gender, sexuality, and eugenics and is leavened with examples from the author's archival research into hereditarian ideas and practices in the United States and Latin America.

Following a discussion of gender and sexuality studies, I delve into three substantive areas: (1) women's ambivalent relationship to eugenics, with emphasis on how female reformers navigated the tensions between breeding as an act of empowerment versus a biological burden; (2) how the men who spearheaded eugenics movements across the globe approached and articulated gender norms, including how they sought to embody rational masculinity and obsessed about male sterility and sexual prowess (often their own); and (3) the complicated relationship between sexology and eugenic thought, which ultimately supported an overwhelmingly hetero-normative interpretation of the family, despite scattered subversive possibilities. A brief conclusion considers eugenic continuities into the twenty-first century, especially in regard to debates over the "gay gene" and the demonization of same-sex relationships and families.

GENDER AND SEXUALITY STUDIES

Gender and sexuality are separate but intimately related categories of analysis and human experience that broadly relate to issues of reproduction, biology, identity, and community. Both are concerned with the social organization of power and can be understood as systems or regimes that help to order society, even as they can be contested and transformed. Gender refers most directly to sexed identity (male or female), and in this sense, gender studies has concerned itself with how experiences can be gendered male or female, acquire or exhibit masculine or feminine traits, or how subjects can perform gender. Gender studies traces its matrilineage to feminist and women's studies, fields with long political trajectories that exploded onto the academic scene in the 1960s.

Sexuality studies overlaps with gender studies, but pertains more directly to how subjects have expressed and embodied sexual identities, above all in terms of sexual orientation and desire. If gender studies evolved out of feminist studies and an interest in women as agents, then the foundational subjects of sexuality studies were gay men. Increasingly, as sexuality studies became a close companion of queer studies, the focus on gay men has broadened to encompass histories, experiences, and issues related to lives and labels of lesbian, transexual, bisexual, and intersex people.[4]

Both gender and sexuality studies are firmly grounded in what is broadly termed "critical studies," and both pivot on the premise that social meanings and situations can not be taken for granted, but must be interrogated using the tools of humanistic and sociological analysis. The incisive inquiry that propels gender and sexuality studies gives them strong family resemblances to other interdisciplinary fields such as ethnic, science, liberal, and environmental studies.

Exploring eugenics with the conceptual tools offered by gender and sexuality studies has tremendous possibilities but also brings unique exigencies. To begin, it is crucial to recognize that the emergence of gender and sexuality studies are themselves threads in the history of eugenics. Perhaps surprising to some, a minority of eugenicists can be placed on the pathway that led eventually to contemporary sexuality and queer studies. For example, during the Weimar era, German sexologist Magnus Hirschfeld (1868–1935) embraced key tenets of eugenics, evincing hereditarian precepts to assert that homosexuals deserved rights because they embodied natural evolutionary variation.[5] However, Hirschfeld's egalitarian message and unabashed visibility as a gay man were soon condemned by an increasingly reactionary political regime. In 1933 the Nazis shut down his sexology institute, burning many of its tomes, and Hirschfeld took up exile in France where he died of natural causes two years later.

Indeed, the broader historical record demonstrates that radical sexology and eugenics were fickle friends. Much more resoundingly, gender and sexuality studies constituted pointed replies to the rigid gender and sex binaries integral to most eugenic thought, much of which sanctioned top-down reproductive and erotic control. The now classic 1984 anthology *When Biology Became Destiny: Women in Weimar and Nazi Germany*, edited by Renate Bridenthal, Atina Grossman, and Marion Kaplan, was instrumental in demonstrating that eugenics and its myriad implications could not be understood without the frameworks of women's and gender studies.[6] This book and similar studies by women's historians showed how hereditarian theories and practices worked to construct gender identity and sexed categories under patriarchal regimes, providing a model for scholars eager to probe eugenics with the tools of gender (and to a lesser extent, sexuality) studies.

Since the 1980s, the basic contours of a gendered analysis of eugenics have remained intact, inspiring a steady stream of rich research into the ways in which women contributed to and were constrained by eugenics. These studies have delved into representations of femininity and motherhood and traced the stratification of reproductive health technologies, showing, for example, how white women in North America and Europe organized for abortion rights while women of color mobilized against forced sterilization or birth control.[7] In addition, many gender studies scholars have incorporated the frames of (post)colonial studies and critical race theory, producing scholarship that, at its most dynamic, elucidates the interplay among eugenics, race, gender, class, and other contextually relevant variables.[8] At the same time, sexuality studies has shaken up eugenics scholarship, uncovering new links between genetic science and stigmatization that remained largely hidden in the initial wave of literature. At its most intellectually daring, sexuality studies has upended the assumptions of biological fixity behind the distinction between gender (expressed identity) and sex (anatomical identity), thus destabilizing some of the stock characters in eugenics' history and posing intriguing questions about the family, sexuality, and the outer limits of reproductive and genetic technologies in our current biotechnological century.[9]

WOMEN AND THE BREEDING BIND

A significant body of scholarship, which is situated primarily in women's and gender studies, emphasizes women's potent and ambivalent relationships to eugenic ideas and organizations. These affiliations have taken many forms, ranging from women who served as leaders in national eugenics movements, to the female foot soldiers who carried out thousands of family studies and ran "fitter families" contests, and finally to those women and girls whose lives were irrevocably damaged by eugenic policies of institutionalization, sterilization, and coercive family planning.[10] From the late nineteenth century, women across the world were drawn to or targeted by eugenics because of their status as mothers of the family, nation, and future.[11]

In some countries, eugenic ideologies left little room for female agency. In Iran, for example, worries about demographic decline prompted social reformers to advocate a pronatalist platform that exalted motherhood. Yet in the context of a legal model of male guardianship, acting as beacons of the country's well-being translated not into empowerment for Iranian women, but rather into shouldering the burden and blame for an array of national health and hygiene problems.[12] In China and Romania, feminists who initially saw in eugenics a possible avenue for greater reproductive autonomy quickly had their hopes dashed by a male medical and scientific establishment that placed better breeding for national progress far above female reproductive autonomy.[13] In the colonial domain of South Africa, physicians championed white women as upholders of the race and placed the burden of racial segregation in their wombs. As one doctor wrote in the *South African Medical Record*, we "want to make baby culture, breast-feeding and mother-craft popular and fashionable; secure full recognition of the truth that there is no nobler ideal, no more useful career, for women than making and keeping real homes and the rearing and bringing up of families and robust children."[14]

In nation-states founded on ideals of equal rights and citizenship—even as these remained unrealized for all but propertied white men—women frequently found common cause between feminism and eugenics. Women's historians have produced excellent research on the complex approaches to heredity and reproduction taken by feminists such as Margaret Sanger (1879–1966), Sarah Grand (1853–1943), Olive Schreiner (1855–1920), and Victoria Woodhall (1838–1927), in their respective countries and on the global stage.[15] If feminist eugenicists could exploit the liberatory potential of eugenics as a social movement, disenfranchised or vulnerable women could not. Atop the list of those persecuted by eugenically informed policies were prostitutes, and women seen as too public or oversexed. Indeed, early-twentieth-century campaigns to regulate prostitution, which entailed spatial and medical regulation, often included well-known eugenicists.[16] For instance, in the only part of Latin America to pass a eugenic sterilization law—Mexico's eastern state of Veracruz—the targets were prostitutes whom municipal physicians and legislators sought to round up for venereal disease testing and ongoing moral and medical surveillance.[17] Nonetheless, in multiple countries, the group of women consistently considered the greatest threat to a country's biological worth and integrity were "feebleminded" females, who ostensibly threatened the social order with their irresponsible sexual proclivities and bad moral judgment.[18] This loose category included women we would identify today as developmentally or mentally disabled, as well as poor and undereducated girls and women, many of whom became caught in the net of public or juvenile agencies after fleeing a broken home or domestic sexual abuse.[19] Not only did the feebleminded woman often become the quintessential symbol of degeneracy, she was subjected to institutional segregation and high rates of sterilization. In Switzerland, those sterilized were preponderantly women stamped with the label of "feebleminded." In practice, and following the circular logic typical of eugenicists, this often meant that so-called feebleminded women simply deviated in perceptible ways from what was deemed normal femininity. As Natalia Gerodetti explains, Swiss eugenics entailed the widespread pathologization of female sexuality, which followed from earlier perceptions that held that women's uncontrollable bodies made them prone to inadequate sexual activities, excitation, or hysteria. Thus, while women in general were usually perceived in passive terms, feebleminded women were construed in terms of reckless promiscuity, unable to reject advances from unfit men, "easy game," and seductresses of married men. Akin to prostitutes, they were depicted as dangerous women who expressed their gender inappropriately and who could destroy the lives of respectable married men and, if not spatially contained or surgically fixed, spawn defective progeny.[20] Canadian eugenicists, for example, overtly linked the two, claiming that 75 percent of all prostitutes were feebleminded, and moreover, that their breeding needed to be curtailed.[21]

Although British and American feminist eugenicists have received the most press, across the globe biological betterment became integral to many a platform of women's emancipation.[22] Scholars interested in the interplay of gender, sexuality, and eugenics have shown over and over again how early-twentieth-century female reformers evoked the mantra of eugenics to police the boundaries of class, race, and disability. For example, Angela Wanhalla has shown that New Zealand women's groups, affiliated with the National Council of Women and the Women's Christian Temperance Union, were some of the noisiest proponents of race betterment. These elite women provided evidence before New Zealand's 1924 Inquiry into Mental Defectives and Sexual Offenders and helped to create an association between feeblemindedness, degeneracy, and working-class women. Like their counterparts in other parts of the world, New Zealand's feminist eugenicists concentrated first and foremost on finding the means to restrict "unfit" births among the lower classes while encouraging "better breeding" among the middle class.[23]

Throughout Europe and the Americas, female eugenicists regularly worked to bolster their own authority and professional stature by drawing a stark line between themselves—the "fit"—and those they considered "unfit." Emblematic of this impulse was Margaret Sanger, whose tireless advocacy of contraception was tied always to a desire to lower birthrates among the laboring classes, immigrants, and racial minorities, whom she deemed to be biologically inferior.[24] Yet beyond high-profile actors like Sanger, there were hundreds if not thousands of professional, usually white, women who represented the early-twentieth-century eugenic creed by participating in local eugenics societies and mental hygiene campaigns and discouraging rural and urban poor women from reproduction.

In sum, a gendered analysis of the intersections of eugenics and feminism demonstrates that if middle-class women accepted biology as destiny, they could often wield otherwise unattainable political power and claim moral authority. Such empowerment was, of course, highly conditional, and came at the high price of reinscribing the essentialist meanings of motherhood and womanhood that many of these reformers actively disputed and defied in their writing and activism. At the same time, gender dynamics—between men and women and among women—profoundly shaped eugenics movements across the globe. Again and again, middle-class degreed women armed with the instruments of hereditary science sought to sharply delineate the lines between "us" and "them" and concomitantly to advance their professional standing. In any case, recent scholarship based in women's and gender studies poignantly elucidates the complex and shifting relationship of eugenics to the politics of feminism, motherhood, and intragender differences.

Male Eugenic Fantasies

Even as scholars have highlighted the fraught marriage between feminism and eugenics, there has been little curiosity about how male eugenicists viewed and strove to embody masculinity and fatherhood. Most male eugenicists defined femininity in Manichean terms, contrasting wholesome middle-class women who must breed more (positive eugenics) with degenerate lower-class women whose procreative capacity must be curtailed (negative eugenics). Yet how did they map normal and abnormal, fit and unfit, when it came to their lives and conceptions of masculinity? To begin, male eugenicists did not hesitate to proclaim themselves and their ilk as specimens begat of superlative family lines, usually in opposition to working-class, immigrant, and racial minority men they disparaged as likely alcoholics, criminals, or sex deviants. For instance, gesturing toward Galton's aristogenesis thesis, namely that the best and brightest indubitably will propagate more of the same, *Eugenical News* (the organ of the U.S. Eugenic Records Office) regularly featured pedigree charts of great white forefathers, such as Woodrow Wilson and Henry Cabot Lodge.[25] Most male eugenicists, no matter their location, glibly assumed and gladly asserted their superior patrilineage. For example, at the Second International Congress of Eugenics, held in New York City in 1921, J. Joaquin

Izquierdo (1893–1974) a renowned Mexican physiologist and strong supporter of the child hygiene doctrine of *puériculture* popular in Latin countries, presented his illustrious family tree, narcissistically tracing how it reached back to the Spanish conquistadores.[26]

In addition to heralding their own genealogies, many male eugenicists, such as Galton and Teddy Roosevelt, fancied themselves swashbuckling colonists who embarked on hair-raising adventures to colonial territories, above all, Africa.[27] Indeed, a brand of colonizer masculinity was integral to eugenics movements across the globe. In Japan, eugenicists idealized the Greco-Roman male form and promoted calisthenics in the army, schools, and local communities in the name of empire and territorial expansion.[28] Throughout the twentieth century, analogous versions of masculinized nationalism thrived in countries with strong socialist or fascist movements, where leaders often expounded on the need for "new men" for a new century. The worship of the strapping and soldierly male form gained great traction in Germany, Mexico, Italy, and Cuba. Fidel Castro's brawny and bearded *revolucionario* was heralded not just as a political hero but as the carrier of superior heredity. In 1980, Castro described the Mariel boat lift, in which thousands of Cubans—including many previously imprisoned gay men—were allowed to leave Cuba for the United States as the purging of those without "revolutionary genes" and "revolutionary blood" from the island.[29]

Galton, too, dreamed of supreme men in his last substantial piece of writing, the utopian novel *Kantsaywhere*. Penned several months before he died and never published, this story envisaged a race of men "well built, practiced both in military drills and athletics, very courteous, but with a resolute look that suggests fighting qualities of a high order." Explaining their role vis-à-vis women, Galton wrote "both sexes are true to themselves, the women being thoroughly feminine, and I may add, mammalian, and the men being as thoroughly virile."[30] Extreme gender polarity characterized eugenics around the world, although the apotheosis of super-masculinity did not come without its own paradox. Male eugenicists regularly sought to ensure that their deep reverence for either Adonis or Apollo did not lapse into overt expressions of homoeroticism and same-sex love.[31] This tension played out brutally in Nazi Germany, where SA chief Ernst Röhm (1887–1934) was lauded for his masculinity, same-sex solidarities, and devotion to the Fuehrer. Yet once the contradictions between his homosexuality and fascist family values became too conspicuous, he paid the ultimate price—he was murdered by his Nazi brethren.

Enamored by science and medicine, male eugenicists readily applied emergent biotechnologies and therapies in attempts to boost their manly vigor. During the 1920s and 1930s, this often meant experimentation with, and the popularization of, male hormones. As Sabine Frühstück has shown for Japan, these decades saw the intertwined rise of racial hygiene and the commercialization of hormonal treatments, which men were urged to take in order to heighten their sexual drive and combat modernity-induced neurasthenia.[32] Dabbling in their labs or working with subject patient populations, eugenically minded scientists intent on sexual rejuvenation or the treatment of putative sexual problems launched endocrinology experiments.[33] For example, Leo Stanley (1886–1976), the medical superintendent at California's San Quentin prison, grafted the testes and scrota of dozens of male prisoners with testicular tissue derived from deceased fellow prisoners, goats, rams, boar, and deer in an attempt to cure hypersexuality and excessive onanism. As Ethan Blue has shown, Stanley viewed his testicular grafting procedures as one component of a larger eugenic program that included segregation and sterilization of the prisoners he identified as mentally deficient and sexually depraved.[34] Spain's leading eugenicist and an outspoken pronatalist, Gregorio Marañon (1887–1960), also founded endocrinology in that country. He believed that sex glands controlled the body's entire metabolic and physiological system and that "all differentiation between males and females could ultimately be explained by gonadal differentiation."[35] Based on this premise, Marañon placed reproductive and sex endocrinology at the crux of his plan for national biological betterment. Finally, as Angus McLaren has shown, during the 1920s and 1930s many European and North American physicians who became sold on the prospect of sexual rejuvenation developed synthetic male hormones to mimic the physiological effects of testosterone.[36]

For some male eugenicists, an interest in regeneration led to fantasies of immortality. For instance, the close friendship of the Nazi sympathizer, Charles Lindbergh (1902–1974), and the French surgeon, Alexis Carrel (1873–1944), was based in large part on their mutual interest in life extension. Notably, one of Carrel's many lab experiments was to create "heroic" male mice resistant to disease and endowed with greater strength and longevity. Carrel incited mice to fight each other, and the winners were given females to impregnate, the losers autopsied. Carrel declared, "If I could do the same tests on humans, I might produce a man who could jump in the air twenty feet and live to be two hundred."[37] Except for their own female relatives, improving the lives of women never was entertained by Carrel and Lindbergh, whose goal rather was to establish an "Institute of Man" where a "nucleus" of men of unquestioned achievement and "universalist minds" would direct a small, elite group of specialists entrusted with amassing data and studying all the issues paramount to the establishment of a "civilized" society.[38]

In this same vein, some male eugenicists imagined ways to spread their seed—or that of their exalted brotherhood—in order to produce exceptional offspring. This is particularly ironic, given that many male eugenicists in Europe and the Americas were either sterile or chose not to have children, perhaps making the question of eugenic progeny more pressing than ever to them. It was not uncommon for doctors treating couples with infertility problems to try to impregnate an unknowing wife with ejaculate generously donated by the physician or one of his heartier residents.[39] By the 1970s, plans for managed breeding merged with new storage and insemination techniques to support the establishment of the first sperm bank in the United States. In 1980 the inventor and unusual visionary Robert Graham (1906–1997) founded the Repository for Germinal Choice in Escondido, California. Graham's aim was to disseminate the genes of Nobel Laureates through an elite sperm-banking enterprise, which attracted notoriety and controversy when journalists revealed that William Shockley (1910–1989), the vociferous raciologist and Nobel Prize recipient, had agreed to donate his semen to the facility.[40] As David Plotz has shown, even if Graham ultimately was not successful in acquiring or spreading the genius sperm he so coveted, his eugenically minded experiment provided the prototype for sperm banks in the United States, which started in southern California and subsequently multiplied across the nation and the globe.

As androcentric eugenics highlighted male desire and bodies in pursuit of perfection, it frequently demoted or symbolically—and literally—erased women. For example, Aldous Huxley's novel *Brave New World* (1932) features a universe in which female reproduction has been thoroughly technologized, and its emotional counterpart, motherhood, is regarded with cynicism and contempt. Although the female characters in this novel provide men with fleeting sexual gratification and shore up the semblance of a binary male-female social structure, they are not essential.[41] Quite presciently, similar themes appeared over one decade earlier in *Eugenia* (1919), a science fiction story recently rediscovered by historians and literary scholars. Written by Eduardo Urzaiz (1876–1955), a Mexican psychiatrist living in the state of Yucatan, this novel portrays a dystopian twenty-third-century realm called Villautopia in which technology and gender reversal have removed most women from the reproductive process. Procreation, now controlled entirely by the Bureau of Eugenics, is undertaken by a handful of women who have been chosen because of their fitness and fecundity or by an exceptional subset of men entrusted to serve as gestational surrogates. The Bureau of Eugenics requires that these male reproducers serve as official breeders for one year and fertilize at least 20 embryos. In this futuristic tale, the new reproductive regime of Villautopia has guaranteed that "the earth's resources are not exhausted, economic equilibrium is maintained, and the process of genetic degeneration is ultimately reversed."[42] As in *Brave New World* and the popular film *Gattaca*, several creative and passionate individuals manage to escape biotechnological tyranny, either by passing as genetically acceptable humans or escaping to the wild corners of what is left of planet Earth.[43] *Eugenia* concludes with the protagonist, Ernesto, fleeing for the countryside, where he raises a naturally born child with his lover, Eugenia, and eventually realizes the profound corruption and perverse anti-humanistic values of Villautopia.

It is impossible to understand the content and contours of eugenics movements across the globe without considering how male eugenicists, who directed most official eugenic organizations and institutions, approached gender and sexuality. Beyond a general concern with female procreation, many male eugenicists expressed their fears and hopes about genetic betterment through conceptualizations of masculinity that tested the limits of the physical body, the aging process, and reproductive biology. Today the pursuit of immortality and biological enhancement continues with transhumanism, whose adherents are confident that newfangled cybernetic, genetic, and pharmacological technologies can and inevitably will dramatically extend life expectancy, stave off decrepitude, and make humans smarter, healthier, and stronger. Notably, it was Julian Huxley (1887–1975) who first used the term "transhumanism" in 1957, defining it as "man remaining man, but transcending himself, by realizing new possibilities of and for his nature."[44]

Sexology and the Eugenic Quest
for Normality

One of eugenics' central icons and analytical objects was the family. In the United States, studies of ostensibly unfit clans, such as the Jukes or the Kallikaks, constituted foundational tracts of the eugenics movement.[45] These morality tales usually followed a predictable plot: a man or woman married, often unwittingly, a degenerate partner, forever contaminating generations of individuals who suffered hereditary antisocial afflictions, which in turn caused societal deterioration. In the United States and beyond, the genre of family studies encapsulated eugenicists' deep anxiety over the prospect that deleterious genes could lurk in family lines and, in keeping with recessive inheritance patterns, skip across generations.

In fixating on the family—its formation, mating patterns, and supposed genetic worth—eugenicists across the globe often linked social biology to nationalist ideas and campaigns. For example, in France in the 1940s, working-class couples regarded as positive examples of national stock were provided housing and incentives to reproduce larger numbers of children.[46] In Germany, the Soviet Union, and the United States, families judged superior due to large size, robust appearance, or mental and physical test scores won medals and special recognition. Of course, the reverse side of the coin was that families labeled dysgenic faced interventions ranging from marriage counseling to forced sterilization (sometimes of entire sibling groups). As Jennifer Robertson has demonstrated, one of the cornerstones of Japanese eugenics was marital advice aimed to match-make couples and eliminate "blood marriages" considered to be incestuous. In Japan, the ideal couple was supposed to marry early in life (21 for women and 25 for men), discard superstitious beliefs and customs, and reproduce prolifically for the sake of the nation.[47]

In almost every setting, the family was central to eugenics movements. Furthermore, it retained its importance over the course of the twentieth century. As early as the 1920s, well-regarded biologists began to express skepticism that genes (or unit characters, as they were often called) could be solely responsible for complex human traits. In addition, geneticists inspired both by Galtonian biometrics and Mendelian inheritance theories increasingly came to believe that any attempt to control breeding was futile; such regulations would have little to no medium- or long-term impact on the hereditary composition of the population.[48] Over time, the incongruence between eugenic policies and ideologies and the growing sophistication of human and plant genetics prompted some scientists to leave the fold, others to embrace related fields such as population genetics and demography, and yet others to cling ever more stridently to simplistic biological explanations. For the most part, however, after World War II, if they had not already, eugenicists around the world deliberately disassociated themselves from the eugenic racism that had supported anti-Semitism, xenophobic nativism, and apartheid-style segregation. If anything, this reconfiguration of eugenics made the spotlight shine even brighter on the family, the essential social hub when it came to matters related to sexuality, reproduction, and population planning.

At the heart of eugenicists' focus on the family lay strong opinions about normative sexuality and gender identity and expression. As suggested in the two earlier sections, even if eugenicists, as a loose-knit and heterogeneous group, had different ideas about the relationship of heredity and reproduction to femininity and masculinity, they almost all accepted gender dimorphism. In general, this translated into the belief that men and women had distinct yet complementary functions in the family, whose primary purpose was to serve as the sanctioned vehicle for enlightened reproduction and well-adapted socialization. In practice, this meant that the person who failed to create or sustain a normative heterosexual family through marriage (and its presumed corollary, procreation) was at best a redeemable misfit and at worst a social and sexual deviant with little chance of rehabilitation.

Because eugenics has often been interpreted as a principally regressive and exclusionary movement, scholars have discounted the degree to which eugenicists, in their enthusiasm to encourage marriage and breeding, produced sex talk and knowledge. Eugenicists broke barriers, especially when it came to discussing female bodies and sexuality. Eschewing prudery and sympathetic to women's erotic enjoyment as long as it occurred in the missionary position, eugenicists in many countries found themselves openly devising and recommending methods to spice up the sexual activities of spouses. As Sarah Arvey has shown, in the 1930s Cuban eugenicists became concerned about the felicity of married couples given a marked rise in divorce, separation, and reports of marital discord. In print and on the radio, Cuban eugenicists addressed sexuality with great gumption, presenting salacious topics to an audience largely unaccustomed to such frankness. Nevertheless, like their counterparts across the globe, Cuban eugenicists did so while maintaining very traditional assumptions about femininity and masculinity, presuming for example that most men came to marriage endowed with sexual prowess, whereas women remained virgins until their wedding night.[49]

During the same period, Paul Popenoe (1888–1979)—a vocal sterilization advocate and well-known American eugenicist—counseled thousands of white middle-class couples at the Institute for Family Relations, which he founded in Los Angeles, California. From the 1930s until the 1960s, Popenoe practiced a family-centered eugenics that sought to coach couples and individuals about gender norms and procreative sexuality. Like most of his contemporaries, Popenoe conflated gender and sexuality, presupposing that anatomy determined gender identity and sexual expression. He relied on a model of strict gender dimorphism in which men were dominant husbands who provided for their passive and subservient wives.[50] As long as these rules were met, the fulfillment of female sexuality was a viable and wanted option. Popenoe and his counseling team urged husbands to ensure that their wives receive sexual gratification in marriage, instructing them on the attainment and importance of female orgasms. Toward this end, Popenoe collaborated with the sexologist Ernest Kegel, who conducted a study with female clients. His objective was to pinpoint women's erogenous zones, a project that resulted in the theory of the "G spot" and the admonition to husbands that this special vaginal area needed regular and sensitive stimulation.

If many heterosexual women found Popenoe's advice helpful and even liberatory, individuals who did not fit the sex-gender model were not so lucky. One significant area of the history of eugenics, which deserves additional research and analysis, is the extent to which hereditary theories and practices stigmatized and mistreated those self-identified or classified as gay or lesbian. On every continent, gays and lesbians categorized as sexual deviants, perverts, or mentally deficient were frequently institutionalized and sterilized. Over the past decade, German researchers have begun to bring to light the extent to which gay men were persecuted during the Nazi regime, showing that they faced unfavorable outcomes no matter how their identity was interpreted by the experts of the day. One strand of Nazi homophobia held that sexual orientation was not hereditarily fixed, but largely in accordance with Freudian quasi-evolutionary theories, a developmental phase through which most "normal" individuals passed and out of which they matured.[51] In practice, this resulted not necessarily in the sterilization of gay men but in extended duty at forced labor camps, where arduous physical work was seen as a potentially masculinizing and appropriately punitive cure.[52] On the reverse side of the nature-nurture spectrum, gay men were used as subjects in some of the most heinous and scientifically flawed twin studies conducted by Nazi researchers to prove the genetic origins of homosexuality.[53]

Similar patterns were at play in the United States. Looking closely at the nearly 20,000 sterilizations ordered at California state institutions from 1909 to 1979 (when the sterilization law was in effect) corroborates what Wendy Kline has asserted, namely that girls and women were typically sterilized after being labeled feebleminded, morons, or promiscuous.[54] These sterilization orders also show that vasectomies were performed on many men apprehended for same-sex encounters. For example, in 1943, Fred Butler, the superintendent of the Sonoma State home, recommended that a young man sentenced for "fellatio and possibly other sexual perversions with a number of men" be sterilized. As Butler explained to his supervisor in Sacramento, "it was unanimous that he should be sterilized and since there is no known guardian we are asking authorization from the Director of Mental Hygiene to sterilize this man on account of his history of sexual misbehavior and his I.Q. of 61."[55] Again and again, men perceived as effeminate or who engaged in same-sex relations in or outside the institution were categorized as sexual deviants and sterilized, sometimes with their own consent or that of a family member, and sometimes against their will.

Given their shared concerns, eugenics and sexology developed in tandem at the outset of the twentieth century. Sometimes they overlapped to such a degree that they were virtually indistinguishable. More often, they converged on a specific topic, for instance when psychologist Lewis Terman (1877–1956) worked with Popenoe's institute to design his Male-Female Test to measure gender normativity (and with the added bonus of identifying "passive" versus "active" homosexuals), or when the European sexologists who drafted the program for the inaugural meeting of the Third World League for Sexual Reform Congress in London in 1929 agreed that eugenics should be pursued in "the Nietzschean sense of not merely the perpetuation of the race, but its improvement."[56] Yet in other contexts, the alliance between sexology and eugenics was transient and conflicted. In Germany and Japan, for example, sex research played an instrumental role in laying the intellectual foundations for eugenics. Yet, in their quest for professional recognition and as they promoted nationalist projects, Japanese and German eugenicists often marginalized sexology, particularly when its proponents backed women's sexual autonomy, freer marriage arrangements, and a nonjudgmental stance toward homosexuality.[57]

Ironically, eugenics helped to generate the conceptual architecture and lexicon that underpins contemporary epistemologies of gender and sexuality. The obsession of many eugenicists with the question of the origins—whether genetic, familial, or social—of homosexuality and non-normative heterosexuality opened a wedge for the conceptual separation of sex (as biology and anatomy) from gender (as expression and identity). As Joanne Meyerowitz and Jennifer Terry have argued in their respective studies of transsexuality and homosexuality, the bifurcation of these two interrelated yet distinct terms was absolutely critical to the development of our current understanding of gender and sexuality.[58]

Examining mid-twentieth century eugenicists through the lenses of gender and sexuality demonstrates Michel Foucault's claim that biopolitics often produced, rather than silenced, discourses about sex, sexuality, and the body. Of course, eugenicists hoped, somewhat naively, that their idealized sex-gender-family system could contain, and even neutralize, such discourse.[59] Yet their wishes were not granted, and by the 1950s and 1960s, sexology and the sex research that had been supported partly by eugenics supplied tropes and identity terms for the emergent feminist and gay rights movements.[60] Thus, in the end, eugenics sowed many of the seeds of its own demise, which began in earnest in the 1960s and unfolded unevenly over the following decades.

Remnants of twentieth-century eugenics remain and resonate today. Popenoe's story, for example, illustrates how the eugenic focus on the family transferred quite neatly to the socially conservative, often evangelical, family values of the late twentieth and early twenty-first centuries. By the 1960s, Popenoe was finding less reception and more hostility than ever toward his ideas about the hard-wiring of gendered behavior and procreative sexuality. In response, he found new allies in evangelical Christianity. Indeed, the temperament test that Popenoe and his colleagues designed to measure degrees of masculinity and femininity and put to extensive use at the Institute for Family Relations provided the prototype for the Taylor-Johnson Temperament test, a favorite today among marriage counselors in fundamentalist ministries.[61]

CONCLUSION

Taken as a trio, gender, sexuality, and eugenics offer a fascinating kaleidoscope through which to trace broader themes of science, society, the state, and the politics of differences from the late nineteenth century to the present. This chapter has explored three key arenas where eugenics, sexuality, and gender intersected in critical ways. First, it has shown how women affiliated with and affected by eugenics imagined the relationship between heredity and motherhood, and how middle-class professional women were often invested in policing motherhood and reproduction, primarily in terms of working-class, immigrant, and racial minority populations. It has also delved into the ways in which male eugenicists articulated and strove to embody masculinity, usually in a quite egocentric fashion. This analysis helps to reveal the patriarchal and anti-feminist dimensions of eugenics and to appreciate the enormous energy that male eugenicists devoted to contemplating their illustrious lineages and magnificent futures. More often than those, the male eugenic imagination denigrated or erased women, whose function easily devolved into breeding vessel. Finally, this chapter has explored the fractious relationship between eugenics and sexology, demonstrating that these humanistic sciences developed in tandem with one another, and sometimes came together in significant and portentous ways. They both sought to study and categorize the normal and the pathological within the parameters of gender, sexuality, and reproduction, an exercise that involved sustained attention to the family as a social and biological unit.

Even as this synthetic chapter has surveyed a wide range of scholarship, it is clear that much research and analysis on the historical dynamics of gender, sexuality, and eugenics remains to be done. For example, debates continue to rage about the potential existence of, and the underlying motivations to identify, a gene that determines sexual orientation. Many gay people, including prominent gay scientists, believe that identifying such a fixed biological marker and proving that sexual orientation is not a choice will be politically and personally liberating. Yet, time and time again, human geneticists have shown that behavioral and personality traits are too complex to be attributed to one allele or even one set of interacting genes, and that the role of environment, even if it can not be quantified, must be considered.[62] Thus, the quixotic quest for the "gay gene" should be put in the historical context of eugenics and weighed against the dangerous and persistent allure of genetic determinism.

Over the past decade, approximately 30 U.S. states have passed laws limiting marriage to a union between a man and woman. Marriage equality advocates often compare their struggle to the fight against anti-miscegenation laws, most poignantly represented by the 1967 U.S. Supreme Court decision *Loving v. Virginia,* in which restrictions on interracial marriage were ruled unconstitutional. However, a more apt analogy might be eugenic marriage laws, quietly passed in over 30 states in the early to mid-twentieth century, and the model for such laws in other countries. Framed by the eugenic idealization of fit families and the excoriation of those who failed to satisfy sexual, gender, and social norms, these statutes decreed that those deemed "unfit" and classified as mentally and physically defective could not wed. As this chapter has shown, eugenic reformers and ideas usually worked to police the boundaries of morality through ensuring that dichotomies and differences—of race, class, gender, sexuality, and disability—were emphasized and upheld. For those who believe that science should inform democracy, and vice versa, there are multiple lessons from eugenics, in its myriad global manifestations, that are relevant in today's political age and for tomorrow's genomic future.

ACKNOWLEDGMENTS

I thank Cookie Woolner for superb research assistance for this chapter, and Philippa Levine, Alison Bashford, Jennifer Robertson, and Patience Schell for their critical insightful comments on earlier drafts.

NOTES

1. Nancy Leys Stepan, *"The Hour of Eugenics": Race, Gender, and Nation in Latin America* (Ithaca, NY: Cornell University Press, 1991); Alexandra Minna Stern, "Responsible Mothers and Normal Children: Eugenics, Nationalism, and Welfare in Post-revolutionary Mexico, 1920–1940," *Journal of Historical Sociology* 12, no. 4 (1999): 369–397; and Patience Schell, chap. 28 this volume.

2. See for example, William H. Schneider, *Quality and Quantity: The Quest for Biological Regeneration in Twentieth-Century France* (Cambridge and New York: Cambridge University Press, 1990); Alisa Klaus, *Every Child a Lion: The Origins of Maternal and Infant Health in the United States and France, 1890–1920* (Ithaca, NY: Cornell University Press, 1993).

3. Laura Briggs, *Reproducing Empire: Race, Sex, Science and US Imperialism in Puerto Rico* (Berkeley, CA: University of California Press, 2002); Matthew Connelly, *Fatal Misconception: The Struggle to Control World Population* (Cambridge, MA: Harvard University Press, 2008).

4. Chris Beasley, *Gender and Sexuality: Critical Theories, Critical Thinkers* (London: Sage, 2005); and Robert A. Nye, ed., *Sexuality* (Oxford: Oxford University Press, 1999).

5. James D. Steakley, *"Per scientiam ad justitiam:* Magnus Hirschfeld and the Sexual Politics of Innate Homosexuality," in *Science and Homosexualities,* ed. Vernon A. Rosario (New York: Routledge, 1997), 133–154; Chandak Sengoopta, "Glandular Politics: Experimental Biology, Clinical Medicine, and Homosexual Emancipation in Fin-de-Siècle Central Europe," *Isis* 89 (1998): 445–473.

6. Renate Bridenthal, Atina Grossmann, and Marion Kaplan, eds., *When Biology Became Destiny: Women in Weimar and Nazi Germany* (New York: Monthly Review Press, 1984).

7. Alexandra Minna Stern, *Eugenic Nation: Faults and Frontiers of Better Breeding in Modern America* (Berkeley, CA: University of California Press, 2005); Jennifer Nelson, "'Abortions under Community Control:' Feminism, Nationalism, and the Politics of Abortion among New York City's Young Lords," *Journal of Women's History* 13, no. 1 (2001): 157–180.

8. Ann Stoler, *Carnal Knowledge and Imperial Power: Race and the Intimate in Colonial Rule* (Berkeley, CA: University of California Press, 2002); Alison Bashford, *Imperial Hygiene: A Critical History of Colonialism, Nationalism and Public Health* (Basingstoke: Palgrave, 2004).

9. See for example, Anne Fausto-Sterling, *Sexing the Body: Gender Politics and the Construction of Sexuality* (New York: Basic Books, 2000).

10. Amy Sue Bix, "Experiences and Voices of Eugenics Field-Workers: 'Women's Work' in Biology," *Social Studies of Science* 27, no. 4 (1997): 625–668.

11. Seth Koven and Sonya Michel, eds., *Mothers of a New World: Maternalist Politics and the Origins of the Welfare State* (New York: Routledge, 1993); Faye D. Ginzburg and Rayna Rapp, eds., *Conceiving the New World Order: The Global Politics of Reproduction* (Berkeley, CA: University of California Press, 1995).

12. Cyrus Schayegh, "Hygiene, Eugenics, Genetics, and the Perception of Demographic Crisis in Iran, 1910s–1940s," *Critique* 3, no. 3 (2004): 335–361.

13. Yuehtsen Juliette Chung, *Struggle for National Survival: Chinese Eugenics in a Transnational Context, 1896–1945* (New York and London: Routledge, 2002). See Maria Bucur, *Eugenics and Modernization in Interwar Romania* (Pittsburgh, PA: University of Pittsburgh Press, 2001).

14. Quoted in Susanne Klausen, "'For the Sake of the Race:' Eugenic Discourses of Feeblemindedness and Motherhood in the South African Medical Record, 1903–1926," *Journal of Southern African Studies* 23, no. 1 (1997): 46.

15. Angela Franks, *Margaret Sanger's Eugenic Legacy: The Control of Female Fertility* (New York: McFarland, 2005); Angelique Richardson, *Love and Eugenics in the Late Nineteenth Century: Rational Reproduction and the New Woman* (Oxford: Oxford University Press, 2003).

16. On this pattern in Argentina, see Natalia Milanesio, "Redefining Men's Sexuality, Resignifying Male Bodies: The Argentine Law of Anti-Venereal Prophylaxis, 1936," *Gender and History* 17, no. 2 (2005): 463–491; on Mexico, see Katherine Bliss, "The Science of Redemption: Syphilis, Sexual Promiscuity and Reformism in Revolutionary Mexico," *Hispanic American Historical Review* 79, no. 1 (1999): 1–40; on intersections of eugenics and anti-vice movements in British colonial domains, see Philippa Levine, *Prostitution, Race and Politics: Policing Venereal Disease in the British Empire* (New York and London: Routledge, 2003).

17. Stepan, *"The Hour of Eugenics"*; and Schell, chap. 28 of this volume. For a reprint of Ley 121 (Law 121), which was passed in Veracruz in 1932 and the creation of the "Sección de Eugenesia e Higene Mental" signed by Veracruz's Socialist governor Adalberto Tejeda, see *Eugenesia* 2, no. 4 (August 25, 1932): 4.

18. Wendy Kline, *Building a Better Race: Gender, Sexuality, and Eugenics from the Turn of the Century to the Baby Boom* (Berkeley, CA: University of California Press, 2002); Angie C. Kennedy, "Eugenics, 'Degenerate Girls,' and Social Workers During the Progressive Era," *Affilia: Journal of Women and Social Work* 23, no. 1 (2008): 22–37.

19. Paul Weindling, "International Eugenics: Swedish Sterilization in Context," *Scandinavian Journal of History* 24, no. 2 (1999): 179–197; Anna Stubbefield, "'Beyond the Pale': Tainted Whiteness, Cognitive Disability, and Eugenic Sterilization," *Hypatia* 22, no. 2 (2007): 162–181; Pamela Block, "Sexuality, Parenthood, and Cognitive Disability in Brazil," *Sexuality and Disability* 20, no. 1 (2002): 7–28; Richard Sonn, "'Your Body is Yours':

Anarchism, Birth Control, and Eugenics in Interwar France," *Journal of the History of Sexuality* 14, no. 4 (2005): 415–432.

20. Natalia Gerodetti, "From Science to Social Technology: Eugenics and Politics in Twentieth-Century Switzerland," *Social Politics* 13, no. 1 (2006): 58–88; Véronique Mottier, "Narratives of National Identity: Sexuality, Race, and the Swiss 'Dream of Order,'" *Swiss Journal of Sociology* 26, no. 3 (2000): 533–556.

21. Joan Sangster, *Regulating Girls and Women: Sexuality, Family and the Law in Ontario, 1920–1960* (Oxford: Oxford University Press, 2001).

22. Ann Taylor Allen, "Feminism and Eugenics in Germany and Britain, 1900–1940: A Comparative Perspective," *German Studies Review* 23, no. 3 (2000): 477–505.

23. Angela Wanhalla, "'To Better the Breed of Man:' Women and Eugenics in New Zealand, 1900–1935," *Women's History Review* 16, no. 2 (2007): 163–182.

24. Franks, *Margaret Sanger's Eugenic Legacy*.

25. Eugenic Records Office, *Eugenical News* 1 (July 1916; August 1916).

26. International Eugenics Congress,, *Scientific Papers of the Second International Congress of Eugenics, September 22–28, 1921, vol. 1, Eugenics, Genetics, and the Family*(Baltimore, MD: Williams & Williams, 1923).

27. Nicholas Wright Gillham, *A Life of Sir Francis Galton: From African Explorer to the Birth of Eugenics* (Oxford and New York: Oxford University Press, 2001); and the now classic essay by Donna Haraway, "Teddy Bear Patriarchy: Taxidermy in the Garden of Eden, New York City, 1908–1936," *Social Text* 11 (1984): 20–64.

28. Jennifer Robertson, "Blood Talks: Eugenic Modernity and the Creation of New Japanese," *History and Anthropology* 13, no. 3 (2002): 191–216.

29. Adrian Sainz, "Mariel, 25 Years Later: 125,000 Migrants Filled the Straits Bound for Keys," *Associated Press*, April 5, 2005.

30. Gillham, *Galton*, 343.

31. George Mosse, *The Image of Man: The Creation of Modern Masculinity* (Oxford and New York: Oxford University Press, 1996).

32. Sabine Frühstück, *Colonizing Sex: Sexology and Social Control in Modern Japan* (Berkeley, CA: University of California Press, 2003).

33. Howard Markel, "The Billy Goat War: Morris Fishbein and the AMA's Crusade against America's Consummate Quack, John Brinkley," *Journal of the American Medical Association* 299, no. 18 (2008): 2217–2219; Christer Nordlund, "Endocrinology and Expectations in 1930s America: Louis Berman's Ideas on New Creations in Human Beings," *British Journal for the History of Science* 40, no. 1 (2007): 83–104.

34. Ethan Blue, "The Strange Career of Leo Stanley: Manhood and Medicine at San Quentin State Penitentiary, 1913–1951," *Pacific Historical Review* 78, no. 2 (2009): 210–241.

35. Thomas F. Glick, "Sexual Reform, Psychoanalysis, and the Politics of Divorce in Spain in the 1920s and 1930s," *Journal of the History of Sexuality* 12, no. 1 (2003): 78.

36. Angus McLaren, *Impotence: A Cultural History* (Chicago, IL: University of Chicago Press, 2007).

37. David M. Friedman, *The Immortalists: Charles Lindbergh, Dr. Alexis Carrel, and Their Daring Quest to Live Forever* (New York: Harper Collins, 2007), 9.

38. Ibid., 168.

39. Cynthia R. Daniels and Janet Golden, "Procreative Compounds: Popular Eugenics, Artificial Insemination, and the Rise of the American Sperm Bank," *Journal of Social History* 38, no. 1 (2004): 5–27.

40. David Plotz, *The Genius Factory: The Curious History of the Nobel Sperm Bank* (New York: Random House, 2006).

41. Joanne Woiak, "Designing a Brave New World: Eugenics, Politics, and Fiction," *The Public Historian* 29, no. 3 (2007): 105–129; Aldous Huxley, *Brave New World* (1932; New York: Perennial Classics, 1998).

42. Aaron Dziubinskyj, "Eduardo Urzaiz's *Eugenia*: Eugenics, Gender, and Dystopian Society in Twenty-Third-Century Mexico," *Science Fiction Studies* 34, no. 3 (2007): 436–472.

43. Laura Briggs and Jodi I. Kelber-Kaye, "'There Is No Unauthorized Breeding in Jurassic Park': Gender and the Uses of Genetics," *NWSA Journal* 12, no. 3 (2000): 92–113.

44. Julian Huxley, *New Bottles for New Wine* (London: Chatto & Windus, 1957), 13–17.

45. Nicole Hahn Rafter, *White Trash: The Eugenic Family Studies, 1877–1919* (Boston, MA: Northeastern Press, 1988).

46. Schneider, *Quality and Quantity*.

47. Jennifer Robertson, "Biopower: Blood, Kinship, and Eugenic Marriage," in *The Companion Volume to Japanese Anthropology*, ed. Jennifer Robertson (London: Blackwell, 2007).

48. For an excellent discussion of this, see Diane B. Paul, *The Politics of Heredity: Essays on Eugenics, Biomedicine, and the Nature-Nurture Debate* (Albany, NY: State University of New York Press, 1998).

49. Sarah R. Arvey, *"Labyrinths of Love:" Sexual Propriety, Family, and Social Reform in the Second Cuban Republic, 1933–1958* (PhD diss., University of Michigan, 2007).

50. Stern, *Eugenic Nation;* Kline, *Building a Better Race*; Molly Ladd-Taylor, "Eugenics, Sterilisation, and Modern Marriage in the USA: The Strange Career of Paul Popenoe," *Gender and History* 13, no. 2 (2001): 298–327.

51. Elizabeth D. Heineman, "Sexuality and Nazism: The Doubly Unspeakable?" *Journal of the History of Sexuality* 11, no. 1–2 (2002): 22–65; Dagmar Herzog, "Hubris and Hypocrisy, Incitement and Disavowal: Sexuality and German Fascism," *Journal of the History of Sexuality* 11, no. 1–2 (2002): 3–21.

52. Andreas Pretzel, "Biopolitics, Homosexuality, Castrations and the Politics of Reparations and Restorative Justice after 1945," paper presented at the Eugenics and Restorative Justice Workshop, Hanover, Germany, July 5, 2008.

53. Garland E. Allen, "The Double-Edged Sword of Genetic Determinism: Social and Political Agendas in Genetic Studies of Homosexuality, 1940 to 1980," in Rosario ed., *Science and Homosexualities*, 242–270.

54. Kline, *Building a Better Race*.

55. Fred O. Butler, to Mrs. Dora Shaw Heffner, Director, California Department of Mental Hygiene, July 20, 1948, California Sterilization Orders, microfilm, cited without revealing any sensitive patient information and with IRB approval from the California Office of Human Subjects Protection.

56. Ivan Crozier, "Becoming a Sexologist: Norman Haire, the 1929 London World League for Sexual Reform Congress, and Organizing Medical Knowledge about Sex in Interwar England," *History of Science* 39 (2001): 299–329, 317; on Terman, see Stern, *Eugenic Nation* and Jennifer Terry, *An American Obsession: Science, Medicine, and Homosexuality in Modern Society* (Chicago, IL: University of Chicago Press, 1999).

57. Frühstück, *Colonizing Sex,* and Herzog, "Hubris and Hypocrisy."

58. Joanne Meyerowitz, *How Sex Changed: A History of Transsexuality in the United States* (Cambridge, MA: Harvard University Press, 2002); Terry, *An American Obsession.*

59. See Michel Foucault, *The History of Sexuality*, vol. 1 (New York: Vintage, 1990).

60. Eugenic themes, alternately endorsed and rejected, were regularly discussed in the early gay rights publications of the 1950s, usually associated with what was called the homophile movement. See, for example, Alfred Craig, "Does Homosexuality Have a Biological Basis," *Homophile Studies: One Institute Quarterly* 5, no. 1 (1962): 32–35.

61. See Stern, *Eugenic Nation*.

62. For an excellent discussion of the complexities of genetic determinism in regard to the "gay gene" see Nancy Ordover, *American Eugenics: Race, Queer Anatomy, and the Science of Nationalism* (Minneapolis, MN: University of Minnesota Press, 2003); also Marcy Darnovsky, "Homo Genesis," *Bitch* 40 (Summer 2008): 61–63.

FURTHER READING

Broberg, Gunnar, and Nils Roll-Hansen, eds. *Eugenics and the Welfare State: Sterilization Policy in Denmark, Sweden, Norway, and Finland* (East Lansing, MI: Michigan State University Press, 1996).

Bucur, Maria. *Eugenics and Modernization in Interwar Romania* (Pittsburgh, PA: University of Pittsburgh Press, 2001).

Chung, Yuehtsen Juliette. *Struggle for National Survival: Chinese Eugenics in a Transnational Context, 1896–1945* (New York and London: Routledge, 2002).

Kevles, Daniel J. *In the Name of Eugenics: Genetics and the Uses of Human Heredity*, 2nd ed. (Cambridge, MA: Harvard University Press, 1995).

Kühl, Stefan. *The Nazi Connection: Eugenics, American Racism, and German National Socialism* (Oxford and New York: Oxford University Press, 1994).

Ladd-Taylor, Molly. "The 'Sociological Advantages' of Sterilization: Fiscal Politics and Feebleminded Women in Interwar Minnesota," in *Mental Retardation in America: A Historical Anthology*, eds. Steven Noll and James Trent (New York: New York University Press, 2004), 281–299.

McClaren, Angus. *Our Own Master Race: Eugenics in Canada, 1885–1945* (Toronto: McClelland and Stewart, 1990).

Proctor, Robert N. *Racial Hygiene: Medicine under the Nazis* (Cambridge, MA: Harvard University Press, 1988).

Schoen, Johanna. *Choice and Coercion: Birth Control, Sterilization, and Abortion in Public Health and Welfare* (Chapel Hill, NC: University of North Carolina Press, 2006).

CHAPTER 10

....

EUGENICS AND GENOCIDE

....

A. DIRK MOSES AND DAN STONE

THE relationship between eugenics and genocide is widely presumed to be intimate and logical because of the well-known involvement of German biomedical sciences and practitioners in the crimes of the Nazi regime. German scientists and physicians participated in the sterilization and euthanasia programs, carried out human experiments in concentration camps, and assessed the "racial value" of central and eastern European populations under German occupation.[1] Notoriously, German doctors were the largest professional group in the Nazi party—45 percent of doctors joined up—while they comprised 7 percent of SS members, outnumbering lawyers.[2] Adding to the shock of their crimes is the fact that the vast majority of guilty doctors continued to practice after the war, even publishing findings based on their former human experimentation. It was no coincidence that the first three leaders of the West German Federal Physicians' Chamber (Bundesärztekammer) had been active Nazis, or that 20 of the 23 defendants indicted by War Crimes Tribunal No. 1 were doctors.[3]

The association between the Nazi regime and eugenics was strengthened by historiographical trends in the 1980s. Feminist historians began to explore the relationship between medical science and the sterilization programs, which affected mostly women,[4] while others reconstructed the social history of the medical profession under Nazism and its involvement in its various schemes. The paradigm of generic racism dominated the literature on Nazi Germany and its exterminatory polices, signified by book titles like *The Racial State*, *Murderous Science*, and *Racial Hygiene*.[5] The relationship between eugenics and the Holocaust itself was made in an influential book by Henry Friedlander, *The Origins of the Nazi Genocide*, which argued that the killings of mentally disabled people prefigured the genocide of European Jewry, because the same euthanasia experts had been sent to establish the gas chambers in the death camps.[6]

This fascination with the Nazi doctors had two important consequences for our topic. One was that the literature linking eugenics and genocide fixated on sterilization, drawing attention eventually also to Scandinavian, British, and North American cases, but giving the impression that eugenics was uniformly Mendelian, with its insistence on the continuity of genetic inheritance and consequent fear of group degeneration. The other consequence was the conflation of eugenics with racial hygiene, birth control, and population policy advocacy. In the rest of the world, however, Lamarckian traditions, which postulated the inheritability of environmentally acquired characteristics, persisted and led to a range of non-eliminationist eugenic policies toward majority and minority peoples.

Closer inspection of the record also shows that eugenics did not necessarily lead to genocide, indeed that the relationship was highly contingent. Only those German racial hygienists who also subscribed to the "Aryan myth" targeted Jews, while others could find no scientific grounds for anti-Semitism. In other words, eugenics and anti-Semitism were not necessarily related, and the Holocaust was motivated more by the latter than the former.[7] Moreover, as Alison Bashford and others have argued, eugenics needs to be analytically distinguished from racism and even racial hygiene in order properly to understand historically significant transformations. Thus the preoccupation with racial difference, so characteristic of the lead-up to World War I, was superseded or overlain by a policy focus on supposedly inferior members of one's *own* "racial" population during the interwar period.[8] Indeed, while German eugenicists began to advance arguments in favor of peace because they perceived World War I to have been "contra-selective" or "dysgenic," they became obsessed with the quality of their German stock. The problem was, according to the Social Democrat Alfred Grotjahn (1869–1931), "the army of beggars, alcoholics, criminals, prostitutes, psychopaths, epileptics, mental invalids, feebleminded, and cripples," who were hindering the regeneration of the German people.[9]

To assess whether the sterilization and murder of such people can be understood as genocide, it is also necessary to examine that concept carefully. Neither in the thought of Raphael Lemkin (1900–1959), who coined the term during World War II, nor in the United Nations Convention on the Prevention and Punishment of the Crime of Genocide (1948), has genocide ever been synonymous solely with mass murder. Lemkin himself identified eight types of genocidal policies, of which two have eugenic overtones: first, the "biological" policy intended "to decrease the birthrate of the national groups of non-related blood," while encouraging the birthrate of the related blood group, for example, marriage restrictions, the separation of males and females, and calculated undernourishment of parents. Second, Lemkin referred to the "physical" policy that consciously endangered the health of subject peoples.[10]

The UN Convention adopted some of Lemkin's ideas, defining genocide in Article II thus:

genocide means any of the following acts committed with intent to destroy, in whole or in part, a national, ethnical, racial or religious group, as such:

(a) Killing members of the group;
(b) Causing serious bodily or mental harm to members of the group;
(c) Deliberately inflicting on the group conditions of life calculated to bring about its physical destruction in whole or in part;
(d) Imposing measures intended to prevent births within the group;
(e) Forcibly transferring children of the group to another group.

If sections (d) and (e) possess eugenic dimensions, it is important to note that genocide only occurs when such policies are motivated by an intention to destroy, in whole or in part a "racial, ethnical, national or religious group," in the now outdated vocabulary of the Convention.

Eugenics thus does not necessarily entail genocide, because eugenics was typically conceptualized and practiced with respect to the same group; that is, it was not normally directed against other groups, let alone intended to bring about their destruction, notwithstanding immigration restrictions against or deportations of "unfit" members of other groups.

Is, then, the relationship between eugenics and genocide tenuous, contingent, or even non-existent? In this chapter, we argue that these phenomena can be related at a deeper, contextual and discursive level. A historical consideration of the relationship entails viewing eugenics as part of a broader "biologization of the social" which characterized modernizing societies since the eighteenth century. This social imaginary became hegemonic in the "racial century," that is, the one hundred years since the 1870s, when preoccupations with "degeneration," "racial fitness" and "social hygiene" became paramount.[11] The imperative was collective survival and assertion, driven by anxiety about possible "extinction" in the competition between rival "races" and "nations." This imaginary manifested itself in a "political biology" that justified both positive and negative eugenics to increase a society's "efficiency" and "vitality," often understood as reproductive potential and military viability.[12] Genocidal, or at least eliminationist, thinking tended to arise when societies were subject to pressures on resources and when their leaders felt that their survival was at stake. Thus the sterilization of the "feebleminded" in Sweden—as in Germany—in the 1930s was justified by a Social Democratic politician with the argument that without such measures "our people's imminent disappearance" was at hand.[13] The context of crisis radicalized—and actualized—policy potentials in the logic of eugenic thinking.

This chapter examines the historical relationship between biopolitics, eugenics, racial hygiene, and genocide globally in this period. Just as the historiography of eugenics has broadened out from its Anglo-American core to an international and transnational perspective, so the focus of genocide studies has shifted from the Holocaust as the paradigmatic case to other, often extra-European, genocides.[14] In the following sections, we examine various policy modalities developed to solve the "problem" of minority and "useless" populations. We will see that "mixed-race" children posed particular challenges to eugenicists in thrall to ideals of cultural homogeneity, in which case eliminationist policies of assimilation, absorption, or sterilization might be pursued. We do not suggest that these policies or discourses were genocidal per se, but that they could, in certain circumstances, escalate in a genocidal direction.

ASSIMILATION AND ABSORPTION

If eugenicists in all countries shared assumptions about the importance of "selective breeding" and "biological laws" in determining the health and fitness of later generations, they were operating in very different environments and intellectual contexts. The striking variety of eugenically justified public policies testifies not only to the heterogeneity of the eugenic movement but also to the fact that, as Frank Dikötter has observed, "eugenics belonged to the political vocabulary of virtually every significant modernizing force between the two world wars."[15]

Nowhere were the distinctions between eugenic projects more evident than in Latin America between the world wars. In a series of Pan-American Congresses, Latin American doctors, eugenicists, and feminists consistently resisted the entreaties of their North American counterparts to support coercive policies of racial population categorization, selective marriage, and sterilization.[16] As Maria Sophia Quine and Patience Schell's chapters in this volume show, they felt an affinity with French and Italian colleagues, making for a "Latin" brand of eugenics that was geared to the demographic challenges of their societies. Neo-Lamarckian notions of the inheritability of acquired traits led to an emphasis on improving the environment of parents and children, especially since very high rates of child mortality prompted the medical profession to call for state intervention to "modernize" society.[17] Policies of sanitation and public health trumped North American calls for strict reproductive regulation. The scrutiny of marriage was limited to counseling, prenuptial testing, mandatory prenatal care, and eugenic identification cards.[18] In general, then, neo-Larmarckianism was suited to contending with Latin America's Catholic, racially diverse, poor, and rural population.

Mendelianism, by contrast, with its anti-environmental, hereditary fundamentalism, reflected the embattled sense of superiority possessed by Anglo-Saxon Protestant populations. For them, racial mixing often entailed what the U.S. senator Samuel Shortridge in 1930 called "mongrel or hybrid races." Perhaps the most famous North American representative of this dogmatic Mendelianism was the eugenicist Madison Grant (1865–1937). A conservationist as well as a eugenicist—he was concerned with threatened species, whether they were white people or rare animals and plants—he held miscegenation to be "a social and racial crime of the first magnitude," and therefore opposed marriages based on individual preference rather than eugenic criteria.[19]

Such notions found their way into social policy. Segregationist laws preventing the intermarriage of whites and blacks, and sometimes with Native Americans and Asians, were passed in dozens of U.S. states in the interwar years.[20] Since black Americans ostensibly could not be absorbed by intermarriage, some—such as Edward Eggleston in his *The Ultimate Solution of the American Negro Problem* in 1913—speculated that they might die out in competition with superior whites.[21] In general, the prejudice against miscegenation meant that Native American children were to be assimilated by attending separate boarding schools, where they would be taught "civilization." Other commentators, however, were confident that Native American "blood" would not "damage" the majority white gene pool, and hoped that Native Americans would eventually disappear via incremental "amalgamation"—that is, "inter-breeding"—with the majority white population.[22] Whether a strict Mendelian approach was invoked depended on the population group in question.

For the minority white population of South Africa, there was no question of absorbing or assimilating the majority Africans. In keeping with Anglo-American eugenics, the discourse of degeneration was turned inward, as poor whites were thought to be endangered by contact and competition with Africans. As one writer put it in 1911, the policy should be "the segregation of the races as far as possible, our aim being to prevent race deterioration, preserve race integrity, and to give both opportunity to build up and develop their race life."[23] If this brand of segregationism, based on Mendelian premises, seemed to respect difference, it was only because the large majority status of Africans told against eliminatory fantasies, let alone absorptionist possibilities.

What if the population balance was reversed? In central and southeastern Europe, where the foundation of nation-states after the disintegration of the Austro-Hungarian Empire coincided with the establishment of eugenics associations, bourgeois elites understood the state as the instrument of the dominant ethnicity—at the expense of national minorities. Such "racial nationalism" sought to raise the level of the majority population with the usual array of positive eugenic measures while actively discouraging minorities, although calls for outright sterilization and population transfer were not realized until the Nazi occupation decades later. As in Germany, all these racial nationalisms regarded Jews as an inassimilable and dangerous minority. Whether a minority was assimilated and absorbed or subject to discrimination and segregation depended on its perceived "cultural level" in relation to the majority. Thus Romanian eugenicists hoped to absorb ethnic Hungarians in Transylvania by proving they were really Romanian, while the Polish state thought it could "Polonize" Ukrainian peasants living within its borders. Ethnic Germans and Jews, however, were not considered absorbable and were subject to policies of dissimilation.[24]

The same, frankly colonial, considerations about cultural level were entertained by Zionists with regard to "Oriental" or Arab Jews (also known as Sephardim and Mizrachim) who came to Palestine and later Israel.[25] Prominent Ashkenazi (European Jewish) theorists of Zionism like Arthur Ruppin (1876–1943) were greatly influenced by German *völkisch* and even Nazi race theorists and were contemptuous of the cultural and ethnic status of Jews living in the Middle East. Yemenite Jews, for instance, were at best "human material" to be imported as "natural workers" to compete with Arabs, who comprised the overwhelming majority in mandate Palestine.[26]

As might be expected given these assumptions, the immigration of almost half a million Arab Jews to Israel after 1948—the population of the country virtually doubled in a few years—prompted anxiety about the Zionist character of the new state because the newcomers were widely regarded, as the first president David Ben-Gurion (1886–1973) put it, as a "melange and human dust without a language, without education, without roots and without drawing on the tradition and vision of the nation."[27] They also came with many illnesses, overwhelming the medical system, and sparking an intense debate about the medical selection of immigrants. There was also considerable concern about "negative selection," because the wealthiest Jewish families migrated to the United States, France, Australia, and Canada rather than Israel.[28] The Arab Jews, especially those from Yemen, were to be absorbed—the name of the government agency responsible for assimilating immigrants was the "Absorption Department of the Jewish Agency"—inter alia by an authoritarian regime of hygiene that would inculcate European civilization by teaching modern practices of washing, child-rearing, and even sexual intercourse. In the enormous camps established in 1949 to accommodate the immigrants, babies were routinely taken from their mothers for medical treatment, and hundreds disappeared into the health system, pronounced dead, though apparently adopted to Ashkenazi families "for their own good."[29]

Because this heavy-handed policy of assimilation and absorption aimed to efface the Arab cultural heritage of these Jewish immigrants, the question of "cultural genocide" might be raised.[30] Not only does the UN Convention omit "cultural genocide" from its provisions, Lemkin himself did not think that assimilation amounted to genocide. Referring to the terms used in the interwar period, he wrote that "Germanization," "Magyarization," and "Italianization," which connoted "the imposition by one stronger nation (Germany, Hungary, Italy) of its national pattern upon a national group controlled by it," did not constitute genocide because they left "out the biological aspect, such as causing the physical decline and even destruction of the population involved."[31] Arab Jews were still regarded as Jews, after all, sometimes even more "authentic" (if uncivilized).[32] Yet if, according to Lemkin, a policy of genocide aims, by a range of coercive measures, to tip the demographic balance in favor of the occupier, then the function of "Oriental" Jewish immigration in countering Arab labor in the interwar period needs to be brought into the equation. The eugenically inspired Zionist project of regenerating the Jewish people did not occur in a vacuum; as a setter colonial project, it necessarily entailed the supplanting and large-scale destruction of Palestinian society, which some have called "politicide."[33]

The settler colonial model clearly applies to Australia, where geographically and racially diverse contexts issued in absorptionist, assimilationist, as well as segregationist policies. Generally, the more anxious that whites felt about the viability of their society, the more likely they were to implement authoritarian measures. Asians, for instance, who resided in northwest Australia and the Northern Territory, were almost always classed as a dangerous "alien" race, and were treated much like ethnic Germans and Jews in interwar Poland. The colonial gaze fixed upon the supposedly weaker indigenous populations. The situation with children of European-Aboriginal unions—so-called "half-castes"—varied according to location. "Half-castes" outnumbered "full-bloods" in the southern states, while the reverse pattern obtained in Western Australia, the Northern Territory, and Queensland. "Full-bloods" were generally thought to be "dying out" of their own accord, in view of their catastrophic decline in the nineteenth century, and were therefore not a policy priority, although the question whether the authorities engaged in willful blindness and calculated neglect in their treatment of remote indigenous communities warrants further consideration.[34]

Race anxiety was especially acute in the Northern Territory where the white population was outnumbered by full-bloods, half-castes, and Asians. Its Chief Protector of Aborigines, Dr. Cecil Cook (1897–1985), indulged in dire predictions about the fate of white civilization there, as "the preponderance of colored races, the prominence of colored alien blood and the scarcity of white females to mate with the white male population, creates a position of incalculable future menace to purity of race." It was possible, he continued, that one day there might be "a large black population which may drive out the white."[35] He and his counterpart in Western Australia, A. O. Neville (1875–1954), were particularly concerned about the "mating" of "half-caste" women and Asian men—a concern first expressed in nineteenth-century Queensland[36]—who they thought abused their concubines and, more significantly, introduced an alien, unabsorbable bloodstream into the Australian population.

To combat these threats, they systematized and integrated a number of existing policies during the 1930s: the prohibition of marriages between Asians and Aborigines and the removal of "half-caste" children from their families and their placement in institutions, where they could be raised as whites and the girls married off to white men. Such interbreeding would "stamp out"—a widely used term at the time—the black blood over the course of three or four generations. With the remaining "full-bloods" either dying out or themselves yielding half-caste children, so the thinking went, the presence of indigenous people could be eliminated within fifty years by a guided process of "breeding out the black."[37]

The Protectors of Aborigines in each state and some academic anthropologists, who theorized that Aborigines were in fact "Caucasian" and not "Negroid," developed similar policy solutions to the perceived "half-caste" problem. By the 1930s, the unexpected appearance and expansion of the "half-caste" population threatened "White Australia." Even if the "full-bloods" were thought to eventually wither away in accordance with the widespread "dying race theory," the racial ideal to which all mainstream political parties and policy-makers were committed was now endangered by the mixed-race "half-caste."[38] At a national conference in 1937, the

Protectors of the other states agreed, particularly in the child removal provisions, affirming the motion "that the destiny of the natives of aboriginal origin, but not of the full-blood, lies in the ultimate absorption by the people of the Commonwealth." The policy should ensure, as Neville rhetorically asked, that "we...forget that there were ever any aborigines in Australia?"[39]

The accusation of genocide was made by a government inquiry in 1997, occasioning a vitriolic public debate in Australia about the applicability of the term. Even if the inquiry controversially labeled the postwar assimilation policies as genocide—biological absorption effectively ceased as a policy ideal with the retirements of Cook and Neville in 1939 and 1940, respectively, although child removal continued under different legal aegis until the 1960s—contemporaries in the 1930s were in no doubt that the policy aimed to eradicate Aborigines over time.[40] Whether policies were driven by eugenics, which was concerned with the "fitness" of immigrating whites in this period, is another question. Indeed, some eugenicists opposed Neville's absorption policy on Mendelian grounds, alleging that such miscegenation would corrupt the purity of "White Australia." This was also the stance taken by the state of Queensland, which declined to follow the absorptionist line, holding fast to its segregationist regime.[41]

The Nazis, too, engaged in the absorption of those considered racially proximate. The offspring of German soldiers and Slavic women, and the children of eastern Europeans considered potentially "racially valuable" were "racially screened" and successful candidates adopted out to German families. Though the eugenic rationale of absorbing "related" blood is the same as in the Slavic, Zionist, and Australian cases discussed above, the Nazis took this logic to its extreme conclusion, hoping to denude Slavic countries of their "best" (i.e., "Aryan") racial stock while strengthening their own. The policy was not justified by individualist rhetoric of "rescuing" the half-caste child—"for their own good," as one book about the Australian case is called. The survivalist imperatives of the race trumped any such considerations.[42]

EUGENIC STERILIZATION

Central to the eugenic project in many countries—in the days before gene therapy and fetal screening—was the question of sterilization. Categorizing the "unfit" and then preventing them from breeding was the greatest ambition of eugenicists, who argued that modern civilization—with its poor laws, welfare legislation, and Christian ethics—had brought about a dysgenic condition in which the "inferior stocks" of human beings were out-breeding the "superior." In the Anglo-American context, this fear was largely class-driven, though it intersected with anxieties about race in many ways—from worries about the outcome of miscegenation to broader fantasies about biological "pollution."[43] Fantasies about "interbreeding," fears of the deleterious effects of the tropics on the health of the "white race," or of the sexual proclivities of "natives" are especially significant here; they provide links between the metropoles and the colonies that suggest an increasing "racialization" of eugenics as one moves further from the metropole. However, the focus of such "race thinking" was the dominant racial group rather than colonized "others." Eugenics was not inherently racist but, in practice, tended toward a racial view. As Arthur Keith (1866–1955), one of Britain's leading social Darwinists put it during a Eugenics Society discussion just after the Great War, "National spirit is really a modified form of racial feeling, which becomes stronger still when peoples have dealings with one another who are altogether different in feature and colour."[44] This claim is hardly surprising, given that racial categories were part of the normal mental tool kit of the nineteenth and twentieth centuries. But it implies that the connection between eugenics as science and racial phobias was more than contingent. We will return to this in the section on population management and modernity.

In Britain, despite the efforts of civil servants and experts—who often pushed their arguments in favor of sterilization further than the scientific evidence warranted[45]—no major eugenic legislation was enacted between the wars, with the exception of some aspects of the Mental Deficiency Acts of 1913 and 1927.[46] Nevertheless, as the birthplace of eugenics, British eugenicists enjoyed cultural capital at home and on the international stage that was incommensurate with their numbers or power.[47] In the early-twentieth-century "white settler colonies," eugenics societies often looked to London for scientific approval, and there was considerable interchange of ideas and personnel between the metropole and its former colonies, for example, correspondence between eugenics societies in Britain, the United States, Australia, and New Zealand, or the influence of individuals, such as Lancelot Hogben (1895–1975), who developed his critique of eugenics and distaste for racism in the period (1927–1930) he spent as professor of zoology at the University of Cape Town. With the rise of Nazism, the Eugenics Society in London straddled an awkward line between tentative admiration for Nazi resolve in pushing ahead with sterilization and anxiety that the illiberal context of the legislation was not to be emulated.

Thus, although Britain retained its status as central to debates and research on eugenics, it was overtaken between the wars—first, by the United States and, second, by the far-reaching implementation of eugenics-inspired legislation across the world, legislation that saw hundreds of thousands of people sterilized without consent and with eugenic intent. The question here is whether this attempt to control people's right and ability to reproduce constitutes, or in some senses led to genocide.

Sterilization legislation was enacted across the globe, aimed, as Thomson's chapter in this volume documents, at the "feebleminded," inmates of state institutions, and criminals. It did not usually target "racial" or ethnic groups, as such, even if particular racial groups (for example, Aboriginal people in Canada) were often vastly overrepresented in those institutions. If the American example is the best known, many chapters in this volume show that sterilization was debated and in some cases implemented throughout the world. In Scandinavia, sterilizations were carried out by technocratically minded Social Democratic governments until the 1970s.[48] Even in France, where it is not surprising to discover that Catholic sensibilities prevented the adoption of sterilization laws, vigorous debates on the subject nonetheless took place.[49] In Italy, despite the Fascist regime, religion prevented the adoption of sterilization, as well. After World War II, one finds cases of poor women in the United States demanding to be sterilized as a means of obtaining permanent birth control, even if this meant being stigmatized as "feeble-minded."[50] Thus, eugenic sterilization was not always carried out with a racial intent, even if it had a racial effect. Where eugenics has been condemned as genocidal, this is largely as a consequence of this racial effect, but the reality is more complex.

Eugenics was, as Bashford's chapter details, an international affair, complete with international conferences, journals, and scholarly networks. American and Danish (1929) sterilization legislation influenced the Nazis' sterilization law of 1933, and the 1935 amendment was justified partly on the basis of the rising numbers of sterilizations taking place in the United States, even as eugenicists were beginning to acknowledge that such surgery could do little to prevent the appearance of undesirable recessive genes in the population. But no other country carried out the law so vigorously as Germany; by the outbreak of World War II, some 300,000 people had been subjected to sterilization, and a further 100,000 by May 1945—one percent of the German population aged between 14 and 50.[51] The figure includes some 30,000 women who underwent eugenic abortions with compulsory sterilization.[52] Paul Weindling suggests that with the drift from sterilization to "euthanasia," and with the specific targeting of ethnic groups, such as the so-called "Rhineland bastards" (children born of German mothers and French-Moroccan occupation soldiers in the early 1920s), Jews, and Romanies, "medicine became part of genocidal policies of extermination and resettlement."[53]

It is clear, then, that if the attempt to control reproductive sex by the state, primarily through sterilization, was not usually in itself genocidal, it certainly encouraged the proliferation of a eugenic vocabulary of "inferior" and "superior" stocks. The proliferation of organic metaphors, like that of the state as a "garden" that needs to be "weeded," was commonplace in these debates.[54] Nevertheless, in Britain one can argue that advocates of sterilization actually contributed to the *decline* of mainstream eugenics (because they represented a more progressive, more technocratic, and less dogmatically hereditarian mindset than the first generation of eugenicists).[55] And in general, one sees that sterilization was implemented less to eradicate people considered as external racial pollutants or otherwise biologically dangerous than to "cleanse the racial self." In the United States, Kline documents that the vast majority of sterilizations before World War II were performed on "feebleminded" white women with the aim of purifying the "white race" by eliminating "racial poisons," sexual perversions, and other negative traits[56] (although after 1945, non-consensual sterilization continued to be practiced on Hispanic women in the

Western states). And in South Africa, Klausen shows that eugenicists worried far more about "lower class whites," mostly Afrikaners, than they did about non-whites, at least until the late 1920s.[57]

This is also how we should understand the Nazi "euthanasia" program, whose focus was the removal of undesirable traits from the "Aryan" gene pool. It was not central to the "Jewish Question." If there were continuities of personnel and technology from the euthanasia killing centers to the Operation Reinhard death camps (Bełżec, Sobibór, and Treblinka), those links are insufficient to explain the killing of the Jews as a solely eugenic undertaking.[58] By contrast, when it came to the occupation of eastern Europe and the Holocaust, genocide was committed against Slavic nations such as the Poles primarily because of the desire for *Lebensraum* (living space). And against the Jews, genocide was committed out of fear that the "international Jew" would destroy "Germandom." These genocides were justified on the basis of vague eugenic slogans about the inferiority of the Poles (hence it was necessary to send out racial experts to identify children who could be "re-Germanized") and, in the case of the Jews, the strange mix of their alleged racial inferiority alongside fear of their perceived worldwide power. In other words, we see in Nazi genocide the sharing of a mental space with eugenic language, but more a paranoid racist than a strictly eugenic program per se.[59] Hence in the Warthegau, the area of western Poland incorporated directly into the Third Reich after 1939, racial politics was less strictly enforced than one might expect, and Poles could be tolerated as long as they knew their place in the racially determined hierarchy. If Nazi Germany enacted the most radical program of sterilization seen in the twentieth century—more people were sterilized in Germany than in all other countries combined—this should be confused neither with the Holocaust nor with the genocidal occupation of eastern Europe.

Nevertheless, this distinction between Nazi sterilization and Nazi genocide should not blind us to the fact that there were of course significant historical links between them, especially on the general level of racial fantasies and dreams. The idea of purifying the race (which cannot legally be defined as genocide) clearly drew on the same reservoir of racial visions and blueprints as the elimination of racially defined "enemies" (which is genocide). The two went hand in hand.

Despite this apparent path from eugenics to genocide through sterilization and euthanasia, it is vital to remember that, in the 1920s and 1930s, sterilization was considered a progressive measure, akin to preventive medicine, and was presented as cost-saving in comparison with long-term institutionalization and even, in some quarters, as "'liberating' women from the biological determinism of the past" because it left women's sexual feelings intact.[60] Those advocating it would have been astonished to learn that they have been labeled *génocidaires*. The issue we must turn to, then, is the relationship between science, the state, and population management in the context of modernity.

Conclusion: Science, the Modern State, and Population Management

We have learned that eugenics was not tied in a neat correlation to the emergence of Mendelian genetics or to the hardening of the distinction between nature and nurture; and we have learned that eugenics was not necessarily racist, reactionary, or tied to the political Right.[61] Although genocide claims are sometimes made at a popular level, one could not argue that the sterilization of 2,834 people in Alberta, Canada, under the aegis of the Alberta Eugenics Board between 1929 and 1972, constitutes genocide.[62] The same is true even of the more extreme cases of Native American women in the 1970s or Puerto Rico, in which about a third of all women were sterilized until the 1980s. These cases have historically and recently been linked to genocide,[63] but all, though racist, were not genocidal, for one sees not an intention to eliminate the group as such but to "improve" it.

In many instances, this was a policy that was authoritarian, yet Janus-faced, for it often met with the approval of relatives and even the "patients" themselves. For example, it is perhaps no surprise that "eugenicists' desire to control women's sexuality and prohibit the 'degenerate' from having children may have converged with the interests of some impoverished women to control childbearing and improve their health."[64] And even, in the case of Puerto Rico, one should add, some wealthy women. In Japan, eugenic legislation from 1940 to as recently as 1996 has been understood in terms of protecting the reproductive health of mothers.[65] This is a long way from genocide. Where, then, does the relationship lie?

What eugenics shares with genocide is state intervention at the level of the population, whether actualized or desired. One does not need a state for genocide to take place—a common misconception about the UN Genocide Convention— but, historically speaking, one sees in the twentieth century the convergence of state-directed eugenic assimilation and sterilization policies with the targeting of ethnic and racial groups, as they were defined by the authorities. From Alberta to Puerto Rico, and Denmark to Japan, the modern state operated to control its population's freedom to reproduce.

Is there a connection between this state ambition and the Holocaust and therefore between eugenics and genocide? Not for nothing have theorists of biopolitics like Michel Foucault and, especially, Giorgio Agamben, seen in the Nazi state the apogee not only of racial thinking (a notion common in liberal historiography for decades), but also of the racist constitution and illiberal nature of the nation-state per se.[66] But whereas Foucault saw Nazism as the ultimate expression of modern biopolitics, Agamben goes further and sees Nazism—in particular, the concentration camp—not only as exemplifying modern biopolitics, but as "the *nomos* of the modern" and "the bare essence of politics as such."[67] Our analysis of the relationship between eugenics and genocide would tend to support Foucault's position more than Agamben's, for it is clear that while modern states have developed (and continue to develop) technologies for intervening at the level of the population, it would be too reductive of the multiple variations of eugenic practice to claim that their intersection with genocide represents their logical or necessary telos.[68]

Equally, in the colonial context, there was no necessary connection between eugenics and genocide. Colonial genocide was not a rare occurrence, but it usually resulted from more immediate short-term crises, even if long-term background ideas of racial superiority were vital ingredients; and colonial eugenics was, as we have seen, often aimed at segregating settler and indigenous populations or "purifying" the settler community from "enemies within," such as the feebleminded, alcoholic, or syphilitic colonists (or prospective migrants from the metropole). Eugenics and genocide have thus never been synonymous, but eugenics (indeed, biopolitics as such) has fed genocidal programs in nations where biopolitics has not been one aspect of state management but central to the self-conception of the regime. In other words, the eugenic concern with the "fitness" of its own population was conjoined with a discourse of racial hygiene about perceived dangerous "racially alien" others. This is the genocidal conjuncture, and what historians need to ask is in what circumstances it develops. This is not a question that can be answered by studying the history of eugenics alone. The answer lies in the geopolitics of national and imperial competition and racial anxieties about "extinction." Take the case of Japanese imperial schemes in the early twentieth century. Here eugenic ideas were promoted among the Japanese themselves for the reason that "the popularization of eugenics, race hygiene, and eugenic endogamy as elements of quotidian life was a (bio) powerfully effective method of national mobilization."[69]

The Holocaust has not only overshadowed the discussion of eugenics and genocide.[70] It has helped dissociate eugenics and race science from cases of genocide where it was more profoundly involved. In other words, while eugenics should not be equated solely with Nazism or the Holocaust, one can see that eugenics is in fact deeply implicated in the history of genocide once it is placed in a wider context. Furthermore, linking eugenics solely or primarily with Nazism prevents one from seeing the continuities in worldwide eugenic thought from the late nineteenth century through to the twenty-first, as can be shown, for example, by the ways in which eugenicists in the United States in the 1940s diverted their attentions "away from public and legislative arenas and into the intimate domain of domesticity and the family."[71] Looking beyond Nazism, we need to rethink the standard periodization of eugenics that sees a collapse of "mainline" hereditarianism in the wake of the Third Reich's radical biopolitics.[72] The history of sterilization, reproductive practices, and assimilation policies across the world, and especially in colonial settings, was not necessarily genocidal, and we are not arguing for a strong or overdetermined link between them. Yet, where such practices were aimed at particular "racial" groups, as in Australia or North America, there is indeed a good prima facie case for arguing that, even if those implementing the policies thought that they would ultimately benefit the "natives" and/or the nation as a whole, the race-science that underpinned those policies led logically to genocide: the nullification of peoples.

NOTES

1. Stefan Kühl, *The Nazi Connection: Eugenics, American Racism, and German National Socialism* (Oxford and New York: Oxford University Press, 1994), 105.

2. Michael Kater, "Criminal Physicians in the Third Reich: Towards a Group Portrait," in *Medicine and Medical Ethics in Nazi Germany: Origins, Practices, Legacies,* eds. Francis R. Nicosia and Jonathan Huener (New York: Berghahn Books, 2002), 77–92.

3. William Seidelmann, "The Pathology of Memory," in Nicosia and Huener, *Medicine and Medical Ethics in Nazi Germany,* 92–111; Alexander Mitscherlich and Fred Miekle, *Doctors of Infamy: The Story of the Nazi Medical Crimes* (New York: Henry Schuman, 1949).

4. Gisela Bock, "Racism and Sexism in Nazi Germany: Motherhood, Compulsory Sterilization, and the State," in *When Biology Became Destiny: Women in Weimar and Nazi Germany,* eds. Renate Bridenthal, Atina Grossmann, and Marion Kaplan (New York: Monthly Review Press, 1984), 271–296.

5. Michael Burleigh and Wolfgang Wippermann, *The Racial State: Germany, 1933–1945* (Cambridge: Cambridge University Press, 1991); Benno Müller-Hill, *Murderous Science: Elimination by Scientific Selection of Jews, Gypsies, and Others in Germany, 1933–1945* (Oxford: Oxford University Press, 1988); Robert N. Proctor, *Racial Hygiene: Medicine under the Nazis* (Cambridge, MA: Harvard University Press, 1988).

6. Henry Friedlander, *The Origins of Nazi Genocide: From Euthanasia to the Final Solution* (Chapel Hill, NC: University of North Carolina Press, 1995).

7. Dan Stone, *Constructing the Holocaust: A Study in Historiography* (London: Mitchell Vallentine, 2003).

8. Alison Bashford, *Imperial Hygiene: A Critical History of Colonialism, Nationalism and Public Health* (Basingstoke: Palgrave, 2004), 141.

9. Stefan Kühl, "The Relationship between Eugenics and the So-Called 'Euthanasia Action' in Nazi Germany: A Eugenically Motivated Peace Policy and the Killing of the Mentally-Handicapped During the Second World War," in *Science in the Third Reich,* ed. Margit Szöllösi-Janze (Oxford: Berg, 2001), 185–211.

10. Raphael Lemkin, *Axis Rule in Occupied Europe* (Washington, DC: Carnegie Council, 1944), 86–98. Lemkin also placed mass killing under the heading of "physical" policy of genocide.

11. A. Dirk Moses, "Conceptual Blockages and Definitional Dilemmas in the 'Racial Century': Genocides of Indigenous People and the Holocaust," *Patterns of Prejudice* 36, no. 4 (2002): 7–36.

12. The term "political biology" is taken from Marius Turda and Paul J. Weindling, "Eugenics, Race and Nation in Central and Southeast Europe, 1900–1940," in *Blood and Homeland: Eugenics and Racial Nationalism in Central and Southeast Europe, 1900–1940,* ed. Turda and Weindling (Budapest: Central European University Press, 2007), 13.

13. Alberto Spektorowski, "The Eugenic Temptation in Socialism: Sweden, Germany, and the Soviet Union," *Comparative Studies in Society and History* 46, no. 1 (2004): 93–94.

14. A. Dirk Moses, ed., *Empire, Colony, Genocide: Conquest, Occupation and Subaltern Resistance in World History* (New York: Berghahn Books, 2008).

15. Frank Dikötter, "Race Culture: Recent Perspectives on the History of Eugenics," *American Historical Review* 103, no. 2 (1998): 467.

16. Donna J. Guy, "The Pan American Child Congresses, 1916 to 1942: Pan Americanism, Child Reform, and the Welfare State in Latin America," *Journal of Family History* 23, no. 3 (1998): 272–291.

17. Anne-Emanuelle Birn, "'No More Surprising Than a Broken Pitcher'? Maternal and Child Health in the Early Years of the Pan American Sanitary Bureau," *Canadian Bulletin of Medical History/Bulletin Canadien d'histoire de la médecine* 19, no. 1 (2002): 17–46.

18. Nancy Leys Stepan, *"The Hour of Eugenics": Race, Gender, and Nation in Latin America* (Ithaca, NY: Cornell University Press, 1992).

19. Jonathan Spiro, *Defending the Master Race: Conservation, Eugenics, and the Legacy of Madison Grant* (Burlington, VT: University Press of Vermont, 2009).

20. Peggy Pascoe, *What Comes Naturally: Miscegenation Law and the Making of Race in America* (Oxford and New York: Oxford University Press, 2009).

21. James A. Tyner, "The Geopolitics of Eugenics and the Exclusion of Philippine Immigrants from the United States," *The Geographical Review* 89, no. 1 (1999): 54–73.

22. Katherine Ellinghaus, "Indigenous Assimilation and Absorption in the United States and Australia," *Pacific History Review* 75, no. 4 (2006): 563–585.

23. Saul Dubow, *Scientific Racism in Modern South Africa* (Cambridge: Cambridge University Press, 1995), 166–170.

24. See the essays in Turda, and Weindling, eds., *Blood and Homeland*; Rogers Brubaker, *Nationalism Reframed: Nationhood and the National Question in the New Europe* (Cambridge: Cambridge University Press, 1996), 100–102.

25. On the concept of Arab Jews, see Lital Levy, "Historicizing the Concept of Arab Jews in the *Mashriq*," *Jewish Quarterly Review* 98, no. 4 (2008): 452–469.

26. See Raphael Falk's chapter in this volume. Etan Bloom, "What 'the Father' Had in Mind? Arthur Ruppin (1876–1943), Cultural Identity, Weltanschauung, and Action," *History of European Ideas* 33, no. 3 (2007): 330–349.

27. Nadav Davidovich and Shifra Shvarts, "Health and Hegemony: Preventive Medicine, Immigrants and the Israeli Melting Pot," *Israel Studies* 9, no. 2 (2004): 150–179.

28. Shifra Shvarts, Nadav Davidovitch, Rhona Seidelman, and Avishay Goldberg, "Medical Selection and the Debate over Mass Immigration in the New State of Israel (1948–1951)," *Canadian Bulletin of Medical History/Bulletin Canadien d'histoire de la médecine* 22, no. 1 (2005): 5–34.

29. Meira Weiss, "The Immigrating Body and the Body Politic: The 'Yemenite Children Affair' and Body Commodification in Israel," *Body and Society* 7 (2001): 93–109.

30. Cf. Ella Shohat, "Sephardim in Israel: Zionism from the Standpoint of Its Victims," *Social Text*, nos. 19/20 (1988): 1–35.

31. Lemkin, *Axis Rule*, 80.

32. John M. Efron, "Scientific Racism and the Mystique of Sephardic Racial Superiority," *Leo Baeck Institute Year Book* 38 (1993): 75–96.

33. Baruch Kimmerling, *Politicide: Ariel Sharon's War against the Palestinians* (London: Verso, 2003), 4; Lorenzo Veracini, *Israel and Settler Society* (London: Pluto Press, 2006).

34. Pat O'Malley, "Gentle Genocide: The Government of Aboriginal Peoples in Central Australia," *Social Justice* 21, no. 4 (1994): 46–65.

35. Quoted in Robert Manne, "Aboriginal Child Removal and the Question of Genocide, 1900–1940," in *Genocide and Settler Society: Frontier Violence and Stolen Indigenous Children in Australian History*, ed. A. Dirk Moses (New York: Berghahn Books, 2004), 229, 237.

36. Raymond Evans, Kay Saunders, and Kathryn Cronin, *Exclusion, Exploitation, and Extermination: Race Relations in Colonial Queensland* (Sydney: Australia and New Zealand Book, 1975).

37. Katherine Ellinghaus, "Absorbing the 'Aboriginal Problem': Controlling Interracial Marriage in Australia in the Late 19th and Early 20th Centuries," *Aboriginal History* 27 (2003): 183–207.

38. Russell McGregor, *Imagined Destinies: Aboriginal Australians and the Doomed Race Theory, 1880–1939* (Carlton: Melbourne University Press, 1997); Warwick Anderson, *The Cultivation of Whiteness: Science, Health and Racial Destiny in Australia* (New York: Basic Books, 2003).

39. Manne, "Aboriginal Child Removal," 219.

40. Robert van Krieken, "The Barbarism of Civilization: Cultural Genocide and the 'Stolen Generations,'" *British Journal of Sociology* 50, no. 2 (1999): 295–313.

41. Bashford, *Imperial Hygiene;* Russell McGregor, "'Breed Out the Colour' or the Importance of Being White," *Australian Historical Studies* 33 (2002): 286–302.

42. Isabel Heinemann, "'Until the Last Drop of Good Blood': The Kidnapping of 'Racially Valuable' Children and Nazi Racial Policy in Occupied Eastern Europe," in Moses, *Genocide and Settler Society,* 244–266; Anna Haebich, *"For Their Own Good": Aborigines and Government in the Southwest of Western Australia, 1900–1940* (Perth: University of Western Australia Press, 1988).

43. Dan Stone, "Race in British Eugenics," *European History Quarterly* 31, no. 3 (2001): 397–425; Lucy Bland, "White Women and Men of Colour: Miscegenation Fears in Britain after the Great War," *Gender and History* 17, no. 1 (2005): 29–61.

44. "Eugenics and Imperial Development," *Eugenics Review* 11, no. 3 (1919): 129.

45. Desmond King and Randall Hansen, "Experts at Work: State Autonomy, Social Learning and Eugenic Sterilization in 1930s Britain," *British Journal of Political Science* 29, no. 1 (1999): 77–107.

46. Edward J. Larson, "The Rhetoric of Eugenics: Expert Authority and the Mental Deficiency Bill," *British Journal for the History of Science* 24, no. 1 (1991): 45–60; Mathew Thomson, *The Problem of Mental Deficiency: Eugenics, Democracy and Social Policy in Britain, 1870–1959* (Oxford: Oxford University Press, 1998), chap. 5.

47. Dan Stone, *Breeding Superman: Nietzsche, Race and Eugenics in Edwardian and Interwar Britain* (Liverpool: Liverpool University Press, 2002); Gavin Schaffer, *Racial Science and British Society 1930–1962* (Basingstoke: Palgrave, 2008).

48. Gunnar Broberg and Nils Roll-Hansen, eds., *Eugenics and the Welfare State: Sterilization Policy in Denmark, Sweden, Norway, and Finland* (East Lansing, MI: Michigan State University Press, 1996).

49. William H. Schneider, *Quality and Quantity: The Quest for Biological Regeneration in Twentieth-Century France* (Cambridge: Cambridge University Press, 1990).

50. Alexandra Minna Stern, *Eugenic Nation: Faults and Frontiers of Better Breeding in Modern America* (Berkeley, CA: University of California Press, 2005), 210.

51. Gisela Bock, "Nazi Sterilization and Reproductive Policies," in *Deadly Medicine: Creating the Master Race,* eds. Dieter Kuntz and Susan Bachrach (Chapel Hill, NC: University of North Carolina Press, 2004), 62.

52. Bock, "Nazi Sterilization," 80.

53. Paul Weindling, "International Eugenics: Swedish Sterilization in Context," *Scandinavian Journal of History* 24, no. 2 (1999): 192.

54. Zygmunt Bauman, *Modernity and the Holocaust* (Cambridge: Polity Press, 1989); Amir Weiner, ed., *Landscaping the Human Garden: Twentieth-Century Population Management in a Comparative Framework* (Stanford, CA: Stanford University Press, 2003).

55. Thomson, *The Problem of Mental Deficiency,* 192.

56. See Kline, chap. 30, this volume; Wendy Kline, *Building a Better Race: Gender, Sexuality, and Eugenics from the Turn of the Century to the Baby Boom* (Berkeley, CA: University of California Press, 2001).

57. Susanne Klausen, "'For the Sake of the Race': Eugenic Discourses of Feeblemindedness and Motherhood in the South African Medical Record, 1903–1926," *Journal of Southern African Studies* 23, no. 1 (1997): 49.

58. Friedlander, *The Origins of Nazi Genocide*.

59. See Eric Ehrenreich, "Otmar von Verschuer and the 'Scientific' Legitimization of Nazi Anti-Jewish Policy," *Holocaust and Genocide Studies* 21, no. 1 (2007): 55–72.

60. Weindling, "International Eugenics," 186; Kline, *Building a Better Race*, 68.

61. Philip J. Pauly, "The Eugenics Industry—Growth or Restructuring?," *Journal of the History of Biology* 26, no. 1 (1993): 133.

62. Jana Grekul, Harvey Krahn, and Dave Odynak, "Sterilizing the 'Feeble-minded': Eugenics in Alberta, Canada, 1929–1972," *Journal of Historical Sociology* 17, no. 4 (2004): 358–384.

63. Laura Briggs analyzes these claims in *Reproducing Empire: Race, Sex, Science, and U.S. Imperialism in Puerto Rico* (Berkeley, CA: University of California Press, 2004), 143; Sally J. Torpy, "Native American Women and Coerced Sterilization: On the Trail of Tears in the 1970s," *American Indian Culture and Research Journal* 24, no. 2 (2000): 1–22.

64. Molly Ladd-Taylor, "Saving Babies and Sterilizing Mothers: Eugenics and Welfare Policies in the Interwar United States," *Social Politics* 4, no. 1 (1997): 149; Katherine Castles, "Quiet Eugenics: Sterilization in North Carolina's Institutions for the Mentally Retarded, 1945–1965," *Journal of Southern History* 68, no. 4 (2002): 849–878.

65. Briggs, *Reproducing Empire*, 156; Jennifer Robertson, "Biopower: Blood, Kinship, and Eugenic Marriage," in *A Companion to the Anthropology of Japan*, ed. Robertson (Oxford: Blackwell, 2005), 337.

66. Martin Stingelin, ed., *Biopolitik und Rassismus* (Frankfurt a/M: Suhrkamp, 2003).

67. Mark Mazower, "Foucault, Agamben, Theory and the Nazis," *boundary 2* 35, no. 1 (2008): 34.

68. See especially Michel Foucault, *The History of Sexuality*, vol. 1, *An Introduction* (London: Penguin, 1984); Giorgio Agamben, *Homo Sacer: Sovereign Power and Bare Life* (Stanford, CA: Stanford University Press, 1998). See the discussion in Dan Stone, "Biopower and Modern Genocide," in *History, Memory and Mass Atrocity: Essays on the Holocaust and Genocide* (London: Vallentine Mitchell, 2006), 217–235.

69. Robertson, "Biopower," 344.

70. Dubow, *Scientific Racism*, 1–2; Falk, "Zionism and the Biology of the Jews," *Science in Context* 11, no. 3–4 (1998): 587; Stern, *Eugenic Nation*, 209–210.

71. Stern, *Eugenic Nation*, 114.

72. Robert Carter, "Genes, Genomes and Genealogies: The Return of Scientific Racism?," *Ethnic and Racial Studies* 30, no. 4 (2007): 546–556.

FURTHER READING

Anderson, Warwick. *The Cultivation of Whiteness: Science, Health and Racial Destiny in Australia* (New York: Basic Books, 2003).

Ehrenreich, Eric. *The Nazi Ancestral Proof: Genealogy, Racial Science, and the Final Solution* (Bloomington, IN: Indiana University Press, 2007).

Haebich, Anna. *Broken Circles: Fragmenting Indigenous Familsies, 1800–2000* (Fremantle: Fremantle Arts Centre Press, 2000).

Hutton, Christopher M. *Race and the Third Reich: Linguistics, Racial Anthropology and Genetics in the Dialectic of Volk* (Cambridge: Polity, 2005).

Moses, A. Dirk, ed. *Empire, Colony, Genocide: Conquest, Occupation, and Subaltern Resistance in World History* (New York: Berghahn Books, 2008).

Moses, A. Dirk, and Dan Stone, eds. *Colonialism and Genocide* (London and New York: Routledge, 2007).

Reggiani, Andrés Horacio. *God's Eugenicist: Alexis Carrel and the Sociobiology of Decline* (New York: Berghahn Books, 2007).

Spiro, Jonathan. *Defending the Master Race: Conservation, Eugenics, and the Legacy of Madison Grant* (Burlington, VT: University Press of Vermont, 2009).

Stone, Dan. *Breeding Superman: Nietzsche, Race and Eugenics in Edwardian and Interwar Britain* (Liverpool: Liverpool University Press, 2002).

Stone, Dan, ed. *The Historiography of Genocide* (Basingstoke: Palgrave, 2008).

Stone, Dan, *Histories of the Holocaust* (Oxford: Oxford University Press, 2010).

Turda, Marius, and Paul J. Weindling, eds. *Blood and Homeland: Eugenics and Racial Nationalism in Central and Southeastern Europe 1900–1940* (Budapest: Central European University Press, 2007).

Weikart, Richard. *From Darwin to Hitler: Evolutionary Ethics, Eugenics, and Racism in Germany* (Basingstoke: Palgrave, 2004).

PART II

NATIONAL/COLONIAL FORMATIONS

CHAPTER 11

EUGENICS IN BRITAIN: THE VIEW FROM THE METROPOLE

LUCY BLAND AND LESLEY A. HALL

THE RISE AND APPEAL OF BRITISH EUGENICS

The concluding summary of Charles Darwin's *Descent of Man* (1871) contains the following passage: "As Mr Galton has remarked, if the prudent avoid marriage, whilst the reckless marry, the inferior members tend to supplant the better members of society."[1] Darwin was referring to what his cousin Francis Galton was later to term "eugenics," a set of ideas that gained much of its force from its association with Darwinism.[2] By the turn of the century, the appeal of eugenics in Britain had spiraled, largely because it tapped into British middle- and upper-class anxieties of the period. Britain faced challenges to the economic supremacy of its empire from Germany, the United States, and Japan, colonial resistance from Ireland, India, and Egypt, and internal disruptions in the form of organized labor unrest, socialist revival, and the women's suffrage movement. The falling birthrate (a differential fall, far higher among the middle and upper classes), coupled with high infant mortality, the extent of poverty revealed in the Booth and Rowntree social surveys,[3] and the significant rejection level (37 percent) of British volunteers for the 1899–1902 South African (Anglo-Boer) War,[4] all contributed to a widespread concern with British "unfitness." There was also concern that public health and sanitation were interfering with natural selection, thereby allowing "undesirables" to survive, in particular the casual poor or "residuum" of the city slums.[5] As Richard Soloway succinctly expresses it: "More than anything else, eugenics was a biological way of thinking about social, economic, political, and cultural change…it gave scientific credibility…to…prejudices, anxieties, and fears that…were prevalent primarily…among the middle and upper classes."[6]

Eugenists did not call for a return to unfettered natural selection, but for "rational" selection through "race building" and "race cleansing." The former was to be achieved primarily through education and financial incentives; the latter also through education, alongside marriage restriction, segregation, sterilization, and birth control. The heart of the problem, as far as eugenists were concerned, was the inverse correlation between fertility and social class: on the one hand the restricted breeding of the middle classes, especially the professionals (where women were "shirking" their "racial" duty), and on the other, the relatively prolific breeding of the poor, with their "feeble and tainted" constitutions. The birthrate was also thought to be differential in terms of race and ethnicity. Eugenist and Fabian Sidney Webb (1859–1947), for example, feared that "this country [is] gradually falling to the Irish and the Jews" due to their high rate of reproduction.[7] There was wild talk of "race suicide"—"race" in this context referring to the white "race" and implicitly to the white middle classes. Although from the eighteenth century on into the early twentieth century, the word "race" had a variety of meanings (as historian Nancy Stepan points out, it was "used to refer to cultural, religious, national, linguistic, ethnic, and geographical groups of human beings"),[8] there was a dominant idea of "primary races," thought to be between three and five in number, frequently color-coded, and positioned on an evolutionary hierarchy.[9]

It was in the years around World War I that the concept of eugenics began to have an impact in Britain. That the newly founded Sociological Society debated eugenics at length at a meeting at the London School of Economics in 1904 indicated its arrival in academic and intellectual circles.[10] The same year saw the establishment of the Eugenics Record Office (later renamed the Eugenics Laboratory) at University College, London, followed the next year by the first fellowship in National Eugenics, funded by Galton, and taken up by his disciple and friend the mathematician Karl Pearson (1857–1936). Pearson, along with zoologist Walter Raphael Weldon (1860–1906), had recently formed a group of researchers to focus on biometry. Pearson's biometricians were adamantly anti-Mendelian, following Galton's theory of inheritance through continuous blending and variation, a position that became increasingly untenable with the rise of genetics in the interwar years.[11] On Galton's death in 1911, Pearson became the first Professor of Eugenics, paid for by a bequest in Galton's will. In 1907 the Eugenics Education Society was founded (renamed the Eugenics Society in 1926) and although most active eugenists joined, Pearson remained aloof, seeing its work as "rank propaganda."[12] The two organizations had different objectives—the Society, as its name suggested, being committed to education and popularization, the Laboratory to scientific research. The Society was quickly approached for evidence by a number of Royal Commissions, most notably, in terms of its influence on their findings, the Royal Commissions on the Care and Control of the Feeble-Minded (1904–1908) and on Venereal Diseases (1913–1916).

The Society was never large (at its highest its membership was under 800),[13] yet it would be wrong to reduce the eugenics movement to the Society alone, for its influence stretched beyond organizational confines. Those who joined the Society were largely middle-class professionals, and in particular doctors, scientists, lecturers, teachers, clerics, and politicians. Fabians such as Sidney and Beatrice Webb (1858–1943), H. G. Wells (1866–1946), and George Bernard Shaw (1856–1950) became members, as did several leading politicians, including Winston Churchill (1874–1965), Arthur Balfour (1848–1930), and Neville Chamberlain (1869–1940). Many women, including a number of feminists, were initially drawn to eugenics. Indeed women formed a majority in the Society's London branch (the parent body) in its first years, as well as among the Society's visiting lecturers; nearly half of the Society's Council were women, the Society having made a formal commitment to women's eligibility for election. What was the attraction for women? Women were central to the eugenic agenda, through its focus on the female reproductive body: the feckless over-fertile working-class woman, or the selfish, birth-restricting, middle-class woman. Despite such stereotypes, women could read this centrality as empowering: "fit" women were the "carriers and regenerators of the race," with "race" implicitly carrying several simultaneous meanings—the "human race," the "Anglo-Saxon race," and the "British race."[14]

Within the eugenic program, women were also seen as the ideal educators on the need for "responsible motherhood," and several feminist doctors, including Mary Scharlieb (1845–1930) and Elizabeth Sloan Chesser (1878–1940), were prominent in promoting education in "mothercraft."[15] Eugenics had additional appeal to social purists, including the feminists among them, because it offered apparently scientific validation to moral purity. Feminist eugenists appropriated the idea of rational selection and recast it in a feminist light, with women as the key agents of change. Neo-Malthusian Alice Vickery (1844–1929) asserted that "true" sexual selection (females selecting their mates) was inherently eugenic, but had been hindered by "matrimonial social selection determined by the economic dependence of women."[16] With economic independence, women's "right to selection" would be restored. But not all Society members were sympathetic to this view. While female correspondents and organizations pleaded the case for lifting the marriage bar in the professions, which forced women to choose between a career or marriage with motherhood, some Society members emphasized the need to encourage women back into domestic service, since lack of domestic help was held partly responsible for "the very great limitation of families of educated and responsible people"[17]—a view that related to anxieties about the changing role of women.

There were not only anxieties about women; concern also focused on men, especially after World War I, when it was feared that the best of a generation had been lost, leaving only a substandard residue.[18] Many male British eugenists during the interwar period were childless, or had smaller than average families even by the standards of the professional middle classes, well under the size that they were advocating. One leading figure in the Society politely turned down a request to become a eugenic father via artificial insemination, pleading his "five degrees of myopia" in spite of having three children by more traditional means.[19] Men too had concerns about their fitness to breed.

DIVISIONS WITHIN THE SOCIETY

Despite its small size, the Society was subject to much internal wrangling, as well as undergoing significant changes in orientation and policy over time. The tensions between "classic" and "reform" eugenists have been delineated by Daniel Kevles and Richard Soloway,[20] although this is only one modality along which to align the complex factors that polarized the Society—some of them ideological, some of them about tactics, and some based on personalities. The classic (also defined as orthodox or mainline) eugenists (whose archetype is perhaps the figure of Major Leonard Darwin (1850–1943), the Society's president, 1911–1928, not himself a scientist but bearing the proud Darwin name) believed that heredity was overwhelmingly predominant and therefore that health and welfare measures based on environmental interventions against mortality and morbidity would merely encourage the proliferation of the "unfit." Reform eugenists, however, wanted to dissociate eugenics from the often highly transparent class bias of earlier proponents and to suggest that socially valuable qualities might be found throughout all social groups. They were also associated with the effort to shift the Society from being merely a propagandist organization to one that also supported research as the basis for any future programs. They were far more sympathetic to improving the environment through public health measures, on the grounds that this would enable a much clearer identification of specifically genetic problems so that appropriate measures to deal with them could be devised. As embodied in C. P. Blacker (1895–1975), general secretary of the Society (1930–1952), the Society became increasingly open to the formation of coalitions with other organizations and campaigns for strategic purposes, to the point where members of the Old Guard wondered if it still had anything to do with eugenics as they understood it.

Eugenics is too often discussed as if it were a clearly understood ideology, stable over time, and predictive of particular attitudes and sympathies in its adherents. It is more plausible to argue that there was no one monolithic eugenics, either in beliefs or policy implications. Eugenics was sufficiently protean to be harnessed to different ideological beliefs, ranging from the ultraconservative to the social-reformist and socialist.[21] There was little common ground, for example, between the extreme right-wing thinker Captain Anthony Ludovici (1882–1971), who had radical notions about improving the race, including postnatal selection through tolerated infanticide of "faulty, abnormal and unsavoury" offspring,[22] and the Communist doctor Eden Paul (1865–1944), who regarded capitalism itself as profoundly dysgenic.[23]

Dr. Caleb Saleeby (1878–1940), a qualified doctor who turned to freelance journalism and writing on health and social issues, had a leading role as propagandist in the early days of the Society. His belief in the role of environmental factors, expressed particularly in his interest in infant welfare and issues such as alcoholism, made him a somewhat suspect figure to the true believers of the "better dead" school of eugenic thought. But his role as a popularizer through his widely read books and articles on eugenics intimates that many people gained their ideas of what eugenics was, and how it fitted in with a range of other contemporary health reform movements, via this maverick figure.[24] A similar maverick popularizer was the writer on marriage and birth control, Marie Stopes (1880–1958), often characterized as a rabid eugenist. There was certainly a strong eugenic strain in her views, but it was modified by her feminist convictions. She argued that much of the "C3 problem" (a popular contemporary expression tellingly derived from the classification of substandard military recruits) could be eradicated by enabling working-class women to limit and space pregnancies, with beneficial effects on their own and their progeny's health; but, as a high-achieving professional woman herself, she also vigorously derided the sacrifices involved in the "perpetual sinking of woman's personality in a mistaken interpretation of her duty to the race."[25]

THE INFLUENCE OF EUGENICS

For many people, including several active in the Eugenics Society, eugenics was part of a general bundle of "modern" ideas about the reform of society. It is far from clear that eugenics had a fixed meaning for individuals in Britain during the interwar period, and the vast majority simply did not know what the term meant—Blacker even suggesting that for many people " 'eugenics' is confused with 'eurythmics.' "[26] There was definitely a pervasive form of "popular" or "folk" eugenics, or at least ideas of good and bad breeding. However, the extent of confusion about what was and was not hereditary and what fell within the purlieu of eugenics can be seen in inquiries received by the Eugenics Society, and in the questions asked after talks by Society lecturers. Anxieties were expressed about the potential hereditability of various non-genetic conditions, the effects of maternal impressions, and "telegony" (the hypothetical influence of a previous sire on the progeny from the same mother by a subsequent sire). In some cases there was a complete misunderstanding of what eugenics was about, as in the instance of the psychologist looking for assistance with individuals troubled by flagellatory fantasies: "I just wondered if Eugenics wasn't the thing they were needing."[27] Soloway has noted that the desire of eugenists to encourage marriage with war-wounded "broken soldiers," still capable of fathering "fit" offspring, encountered counterproductive popular beliefs in the inheritance of acquired characteristics such as wartime mutilations.[28]

Evidence suggests that "negative" eugenic ideas did not generally affect the people for whom they were intended, but were taken up by the more "desirable" types, who rather than being encouraged to have larger families, were influenced by concerns that they themselves might be perpetuating hereditary problems. The extent to which conscientious couples were concerned about relatively minor issues of potential hereditary defects can be discerned not only in letters received by the Society,[29] but also in letters to Marie Stopes, from those who had read her popular manuals on marriage, motherhood, and birth control.[30]

The polyvalent quality of eugenics may be one of the reasons why the Society never found a political place and was unable to map its interests onto conventional political divisions. Its agenda of intervention into the "natural" sphere of human breeding was potentially antipathetic to Tories (although there were Conservative members and sympathizers), while the labor movement traditionally thought of the Eugenics Society (in spite of the efforts of socialist eugenists) as essentially anti-working-class. The Society had little interaction with the Far Right, although it provided a forum for Ludovici of the Far Right splinter group English Mistery, and its members included admirers of Hitler and Mussolini, such as Sir Arnold Wilson (1884–1940), MP, and Sir Josiah Stamp (1880–1941). It was certainly impressed by the successes of pronatalist interventions in Germany and Italy, and initially welcomed Germany's 1933 compulsory sterilization of the physically and mentally dysgenic, although it was strongly opposed to the sterilization of Jews: "Herr Hitler has still not realised . . . that in declaring that the small number of Jews in Germany have achieved an altogether disproportionate measure of success . . . he has publicly acknowledged their superiority."[31] And on a prompt from Julian Huxley (1887–1975), the Society officially dissociated itself from Nazi Race Hygiene policies—"so-called eugenic policy. . . . pseudo-science"—in a letter to *The Lancet*.[32] There was an influential contingent in the Society, growing throughout the 1930s under Blacker's tenure as general secretary, who represented a liberal/leftist progressive tendency, for whom eugenics formed part of a wider vision of a scientific approach to the management of society as a whole—one in which meritocracy and/or technocracy were central.

In 1929 the Eugenics Society was placed on a firm financial footing by a substantial bequest from eccentric Australian sheepfarmer Henry Twitchin (1867–1930). This meant that the Society was able to pursue a much more active policy and became a more attractive partner to potential allies unlikely to be impressed merely by its ideological position. The National Birth Control Association readily accepted funding for research into improved, cheaper, and easier to use contraceptives from the Eugenics Society, as well as free office space and contributions to its running costs, but adroitly evaded any closer union and, on its rebranding as the Family Planning Association in 1939, failed to include any mention of eugenics among its new objectives.[33]

AIMS AND OBJECTS

In the mid-1930s the Eugenics Society's "Aims and Objects" no longer mentioned propaganda or education, although propaganda efforts were still active: paid Society lecturers spoke to a wide range of local organizations across the country, and the Society set up a stall at Health Exhibitions. It also made a film, "From Generation to Generation," presented by Julian Huxley, giving simple explanations of the mechanisms of heredity and illustrating both gifted and problem human families. In its Aims and Objects, the Society differentiated its activities into Study and Practice. Under "Study" were included the social problem group; research into contraceptive methods; family allowances; race mixture; and immigration. The "Practices" were divided into negative and positive. Under the "negative" were included birth control (the Society wanted to extend the grounds for giving birth control by local authorities beyond the rather restricted terms of the Ministry of Health circular 153/MCW), sterilization (voluntary, but appended to this was the aim of "awakening throughout the community an enlightened eugenic conscience"), segregation, and the legalization of termination of pregnancy. The legal prohibition of marriage was mentioned but as ineffective and undesirable. "Positive" practices included family allowances on a graded rather than a flat rate; taxation allowances; scholarships and other interventions to ease the financial burdens of education; birth control for spacing pregnancies within the desirable family; and health examinations before marriage.[34]

"Race Mixture"

It may surprise students of British eugenics that "race mixture" was listed as a study area, for Kevles is correct in claiming that relative to American eugenics, "British eugenics was marked by a hostility decidedly more of class than race."[35] However, it would be wrong to underestimate British eugenists' interest in race; after all, Galton had argued in 1883 that the improvement of stock involved not simply selective breeding, but "cognisance of all influences that tend...to give *more suitable races* or strains of blood a better chance of prevailing speedily over the less suitable."[36] At the Eugenics Society's annual general meeting in 1919, Leonard Darwin announced that "what is urgently needed is a thorough scientific study of the mental and physical characteristics of mixed races."[37] Four years later, at the Imperial Conference, he expressed a view held by many British eugenists that "interbreeding between widely divergent races may result in the production of types inferior to both parent stocks."[38] Later that year the Society employed Professor Herbert Fleure (1877–1969) and his assistant, Rachel Fleming (1881–1968), both from University College, Aberystwyth, in a "race crossing" project: the investigation of mixed-race children (with Chinese or black fathers) in Liverpool, Cardiff, and East London.[39] The two anthropologists took typical anthropometric measurements involving the proportions of the skull and the shape of the head (craniometry), the shape of the nose, ear, and eye, and the fold of the upper eyelid. They also noted the color of skin, eyes, and hair, operating with assumptions as to such specific racial markers as the "Negroid nose" or the "Mongolian eye."

For many eugenists, including Galton and Pearson, anthropometry was a key methodology in their attempt to measure human heredity. Galton had set up an anthropometrical laboratory in 1884, and within a year the laboratory had measured 9,000 people.[40] Pearson, with one of his female research assistants, undertook an extensive anthropometric survey in the 1920s of Russian and Polish Jewish children domiciled in Britain, concluding that these children were slightly inferior to their native equivalents, and in future should only be admitted to the country if demonstrably superior, mentally and physically.[41] By the 1920s, Pearson's work aside, anthropometry was in decline, because of the rise of mental over bodily measuring on the one hand,[42] and the replacement of physical anthropology by social anthropology on the other.[43] The latter, as Elazar Barkan points out, related to British anthropology's "growing confusion about the ontological status of race" in the face of the development of population genetics.[44] Mendelianism, by now the dominant theory of human heredity, was not interested in observational data but in unseen (to the naked eye) genetic structures.[45]

In Fleming's "interim report" of 1927 she claimed that only 5 percent of the children "might have passed as English."[46] Not only was there an implicit assumption that "Englishness," like "negritude," was a recognizable ethnicity, but the term "passing" had the connotation of deceit and disguise, and implied that the offspring of mixed heritage could never be truly English, despite their birth in England and their English mothers. Just as nineteenth-century anthropometry had been comparative, so too in effect was Fleming's study—not between white and non-white this time, but between different categories of mixed race, resulting in a hierarchy of "race crossings." Fleming claimed that some of the half-Chinese children were exceptionally talented. She appears to have made such comments not on the basis of anthropometric measurements or mental testing, but with reference to social/sociological observation. Comparing the two categories of mixed race, Fleming argued that the children with white mothers and black fathers were more disadvantaged than those termed the "yellow/white hybrids," although she did not explain how she was measuring "disadvantage."[47]

Fleming's work led to the establishment of the Liverpool Association for the Welfare of Half-Caste Children, which held that "mixed parentage" was "a handicap comparable to physical deformity."[48] But rather than confronting racism, it was eager to discourage racial intermarriage.[49] By the time Fleming came to produce her final report in 1939, which entailed detailed measurements of over 200 mixed-race children but offered neither a conclusion nor a commentary,[50] the anthropometric methodology had been finally discredited. The Society's concern with race issues did not go away, however. The Society awarded a Leonard Darwin research fellowship to focus on "race crossing" in the 1930s; the recipient surveyed existing anthropological studies of hybridity.[51] In the 1950s and 1960s, further studies were undertaken, including an investigation of immigrants' fertility in Sparkbrook, Birmingham.[52]

Mixed-race children were not simply the concern of researchers or policymakers; members of the public also had their own anxieties on this score, evident in

EUGENICS IN BRITAIN   221

letters to the Society. In May 1937, for example, on the prompting of her doctor, a Mrs. Burton wrote of her fear that a child of her marriage might be "born dark." Her husband, although looking "English" (and here again was the commonsense assumption that English meant white), had a father who was "dark brown skinned." The following year a Dr. Galton wrote to the Society on his patient's behalf, telling of how she was holding back on marrying her boyfriend for fear that his "black father" would lead to her "having a black child." Blacker's reply to both letters was identical, namely that skin color was hard to predict, but that "the smaller the contribution made by dark-skinned ancestors, the smaller are the chances of pigmentation in their descendants."[53]

The Feebleminded, Segregation, Sterilization, and Artificial Insemination by Donor

Not only did eugenists influence the Royal Commission on the Care and Control of the Feeble-Minded, but they were also instrumental in the drafting of the 1913 Mental Deficiency Act.[54] The Act allowed for the incarceration in mental-defective establishments of those labeled "feebleminded." There was no accepted definition of "feeblemindedness"[55]—a blanket term for a cluster of conditions—but it was supposedly "knowable" on the basis of the antisocial behavior it induced, such as vagrancy, promiscuity, illegitimacy, and immorality. Many young women designated morally wayward were thereby incarcerated.[56] Eugenists saw feeblemindedness as hereditary, emblematic of degeneracy, and contributing to numerous social problems, such as poverty and unemployment, not least because feebleminded women were deemed among the most prolific breeders. The idea of segregation was neither new nor exclusive to eugenists: since the 1880s, social investigators and others had proposed labor colonies for the "residuum."[57]

With World War I, recruitment, and high employment, the panic over the residuum or "submerged tenth" dissipated. But by the early 1930s, in the context of the Depression, massive cuts in public spending, and the less employable being the first to be "let go," the concern reappeared, now centering on voluntary sterilization as a solution—eugenics' "leading edge," according to John Macnicol,[58] and a cheaper alternative to long-term custody. A Departmental Committee Report of 1934 supported the view that mental deficiency was largely inherited, and recommended legalizing voluntary sterilization of mental defectives and those with a hereditary physical or mental disability. The government, however, held that public support was insufficient, and the case for inherited mental deficiency unproven.[59] The topic was also regarded, like most issues to do with sex and reproduction, as a political minefield best avoided.[60]

Geneticists did not support voluntary sterilization. There was a distinct lack of dialogue between them and the Eugenics Society. Genetics as a science was flourishing in the wake of the rediscovery of Mendel's work, the development of the use of the fruit fly *Drosophila* to establish the basic principles of the Mendelian-chromosome theory of heredity, and the 1931 determination of the role of crossing-over and recombination. Many influential geneticists spurned the Society as being based on principles that were either scientifically outmoded or politically biased pseudoscience, and several also found its preconceptions antipathetic from the viewpoint of their Far Left political stance. Even so, Blacker endeavored to construct at least personal connections with figures such as J. B. S. Haldane (1892–1964), Lancelot Hogben (1895–1975), and Lionel Penrose (1898–1972). Penrose's work on the etiology of Down syndrome led to his 1934 publication of its relationship to maternal age rather than any obvious genetic factor. This underscored the geneticists' perception that even if factors making for "feeblemindedness" did lie in heredity, in most cases they were due to recessive genes that it would be impossible to identify and eradicate from the population at large through sterilization.[61]

The labor movement was also largely hostile to voluntary sterilization, seeing it as anti-working-class, although as Macnicol points out, organized working-class women were much more receptive, making "an intuitive but confused connection [with]...broader issues of maternity [and] birth control," as well as "the punishment of male sex offenders" (given beliefs that the operation curbed the male sex drive). However, while he plausibly suggests that this "reveals the dark and unhappy side of female working-class sexuality,"[62] a case might also be made for women's concerns over the deleterious impact upon family life of caring for "feeble-minded" members, and also of attitudes of the respectable self-improving working class toward the non-respectable and feckless.

While sterilization was aimed at curbing the multiplication of "undesirables," there was also some interest in aiding, via artificial reproduction, the multiplication of the "desirables." Its strongest advocate within the Society was the marginal figure of Herbert Brewer,[63] a left-wing post-office clerk, but other more influential members also considered it research-worthy. For perceived reasons of practicality, the focus was on artificial insemination by donor (AID), which fitted with the persisting tendency to locate eugenic value in the male and to perceive the woman in the equation as merely the vessel to incubate desirable seed. This led the Society into supporting various initiatives that were largely about assisting infertile couples to have children, and the "budding off" of an AID Investigation Council. As with birth control, those who benefited from the Society's interest in this area had rather different aims.[64]

AFTER WORLD WAR II

In light of the revelations in the late 1930s about the Nazi regime, it might be supposed that eugenics was no longer a subject that could be promoted and that the Society would at least rebrand itself into something less evocative of the horrors of racial hygiene. In fact, the backlash against eugenics was considerably delayed. The Society retained its name until 1989, despite some earlier internal discussions about changing it. Blacker himself was the person chosen to produce the scientific report on the "eugenic" experiments of the Nazis, and he commented, "rarely have I performed a more distasteful task." He argued that their policies had been "widely, though I think erroneously, connected with eugenics" and vigorously condemned their human experiments in sterilization as unnecessary, false science, and productive of no useful data.[65]

Eugenics continued to exert influence into the postwar years. Kevles has suggested that reform eugenists had pursued a policy of insinuating their ideas into the medical curriculum by offering lectures to medical students and by writing textbooks such as Blacker's own 1934 *Chances of Morbid Inheritance*.[66] The effect of this strategy was probably more long-term than immediate and thus may have influenced medical thinking in the 1940s and beyond. Pat Starkey has similarly drawn attention to the influence of interwar eugenic theories on social workers during and after the war, in particular in the development of the discourse of "problem families" within the Family Service Units. The latter emerged out of the Pacifist Service Units' casework with wartime families in difficulties. Although they were strongly based in a humanitarian service ethic, the influence of eugenist thinkers such as David Caradog Jones (1883–1974) in Liverpool had a significant impact on the terms in which they defined the "problem family." To some extent, ideas about the innate unfitness of certain elements of the community became even more acute once the postwar welfare state provided a safety net against the worst ravages of poverty. Starkey also notes implicit assumptions about innate intelligence underlying the newly minted three-tier educational system and selection criteria for secondary education.[67] While the Eugenics Society supported investigation into "problem families" in the immediate postwar era,[68] it also wanted to do something for "promising families," in particular, encouraging such families to have more children than they felt able to afford. The Society suggested that children could be identified as "promising" in primary school and their parents given incentives to have more, or even that "promising" mothers might be identifiable in antenatal clinics.[69]

By the 1970s, social, political and cultural changes had rendered these crypto-eugenic assumptions no longer respectable, as became apparent from the furor over Sir Keith Joseph's 1974 speech to Birmingham Conservatives invoking the dangers of the excessive fertility of the "least fitted mothers."[70] When, around the same period, scholars began investigating early-twentieth-century movements and individuals and encountered the prevalence of eugenics, the lens through which this was initially viewed was the racial politics of the Nazis. In 1999 a conference of what was now called The Galton Institute was disrupted by protesters for this reason.[71] However, it is arguable that with the rise of various biotechnological advances, decisions with a eugenic component relating to disorders with a genetic element are being made in the sphere of private reproductive choice. Thus, although explicit eugenic measures are currently unlikely to be enacted at a governmental level, the influence of eugenic thinking is still playing out in practice at an individual level.[72]

NOTES

1. Charles Darwin, *Descent of Man and Selection in Relation to Sex*, 2nd ed. (London: 1874; London: John Murray, 1922), 945.

2. Nancy Stepan, *The Idea of Race in Science: Great Britain, 1800–1960* (London: Macmillan, 1982), 113.

3. Charles Booth, *Labour and Life of People in London*, 17 vols. (London: Williams and Norgate, 1889–1903); B. Seebohm Rowntree, *Poverty: A Study of Town Life* (London: Macmillan, 1901).

4. Sir William Taylor, "An Address on the Medical Profession in Relation to the Army," *Lancet* 2 (October 18, 1902), 1088–1091.

5. Gareth Stedman Jones, *Outcast London* (London: Penguin, 1976).

6. R. A. Soloway, *Demography and Degeneration: Eugenics and the Declining Birthrate in Twentieth Century Britain* (Chapel Hill, NC: University of North Carolina Press, 1990), xviii.

7. Sidney Webb, *The Decline in the Birth Rate* (London: Fabian Society, 1907), 17.

8. Stepan, *The Idea of Race in Science*, xviii.

9. See Kenan Malik, *The Meaning of Race: Race, History and Culture in Western Society* (New York: New York University Press, 1996).

10. *Sociological Papers*, 3 vols., 1904–1906 (London: Macmillan, 1905–1907), 1–2.

11. Daniel J. Kevles, *In the Name of Eugenics* (Cambridge, MA: Harvard University Press, 1995), chap. 11.

12. Ibid. 104.

13. "Number of Members and Election to Membership, 1908–1953," Eugenics Society Papers, SA/EUG/A.85, Wellcome Library, London.

14. Lucy Bland, *Banishing the Beast: English Feminism and Sexual Morality, 1885–1914* (London: Penguin, 1995), chap. 6; Lesley Hall, "Women, Feminism and Eugenics," in *Essays in the History of Eugenics*, ed. Robert Peel (London: The Galton Institute, 1998); Angelique Richardson, *Love and Eugenics in the Late Nineteenth Century* (Oxford: Oxford University Press, 2003).

15. Elizabeth Sloan Chesser, *Perfect Health for Women and Children* (London: Cassell, 1914); Mary Scharlieb, *Womanhood and Race Regeneration* (London: Cassell, 1912); see Anna Davin, "Imperialism and Motherhood," *History Workshop* 5 (1978): 9–65.

16. Alice Vickery, "Response to Galton's Studies in National Eugenics," in *Sociological Papers*, vol. 2, 1905 (London: Macmillian, 1906), 22. See writings of Constance Gasquoine Hartley, *The Truth about Women* (London: Eveleigh Nash, 1913) and *Motherhood and the Relationships of the Sexes* (London: Eveleigh Nash, 1917).

17. "National Society for Women's Service," Eugenics Society Papers, SA/EUG/D.144; see E. Wilks, "The Eugenic Aspect of Conception Control," Medical Women's Federation archives, SA/MWF/B.4/4/3, Wellcome Library; "National Union of Societies for Equal Citizenship," Eugenics Society Papers, SA/EUG/D.147.

18. See Soloway, *Demography and Degeneration*, chap. 7.

19. C. P. Blacker to the Bishop of Derby, 25 June 1945, "Artificial Insemination," Eugenics Society Papers, SA/EUG/D.6.

20. Kevles, *In the Name of Eugenics* chap. 11; Soloway, *Demography and Degeneration*, chap. 9.

21. Michael Freeden, "Eugenics and Progressive Thought: A Study in Ideological Affinity," *The Historical Journal* 22, no. 3 (1979): 645–671.

22. Dan Stone, "Ludovici, Anthony Mario (1882–1971)," *Oxford Dictionary of National Biography*, Oxford University Press, 2004, www.oxforddnb.com/view/article/71825 (accessed

Dec 9, 2008); A. M. Ludovici, "The Psycho- and Physiological Objections to the Use of Contraceptives and an Alternative," lecture to the British Society for the Study of Sex Psychology, ca. 1925, British Sexological Society archives, Harry Ransom Humanities Research Center, University of Texas, Austin.

23. In a symposium held under the auspices of the British Society for the Study of Sex Psychology and published in the US journal *Medical Critic and Guide* 25/6 (June 1922): 210–220.

24. G. R. Searle, "Saleeby, Caleb Williams Elijah (1878–1940)," *Oxford Dictionary of National Biography,* Oxford University Press, 2004, www.oxforddnb.com/view/article/47854 (accessed 9 Dec 2008).

25. Marie C. Stopes, *Radiant Motherhood: A Book for Those Who Are Creating the Future* (London: G. P. Putnam's Sons, 1920), 177, 159.

26. Blacker to H. Brewer, April 18, 1932, Eugenics Society Papers, SA/EUG/C.42.

27. "Advice and Enquiries," Eugenics Society Papers, SA/EUG/D.3–4; "Reports on Lectures and Meetings," Eugenics Society Papers, SA/EUG/G.1–20.

28. Soloway, *Demography and Degeneration,* 145.

29. "Advice and Enquiries," Eugenics Society Papers, SA/EUG/D.3–4; "Pre-Marital Health Schedule," Eugenics Society Papers, SA/EUG/D.164–165.

30. Lesley A. Hall, "Marie Stopes and Her Correspondents: Personalising Population Decline in an Era of Demographic Change," in *Marie Stopes, Eugenics and the English Birth Control Movement,* ed. Robert Peel (London: The Galton Institute, 1997), 27–48.

31. "Notes of the Quarter," *Eugenics Review* 25 (April 1933–January 1934): 76–77, reprinted in *Sexology Uncensored: the Documents of Sexual Science,* eds. Lucy Bland and Laura Doan (Oxford: Polity, 1998), 183–184.

32. Julian Huxley to C. P. Blacker, May 29, 1933, Eugenics Society Papers, SA/EUG/C.209; letter, *The Lancet* 1 (1933): 1265–1266. See also Julian Huxley, A. C. Haddon, and A. M. Carr-Saunders, *We Europeans: A Survey of "Racial" Problems* (London: Jonathan Cape, 1935).

33. Soloway, *Demography and Degeneration,* 213–214.

34. Reprint of "Aims and Objects of the Eugenics Society" (1935) in Bland and Doan, *Sexology Uncensored,* 184–189.

35. Kevles, *In the Name of Eugenics,* 76. Barbara Bush suggests that British eugenics was "a strong element in inter-war racism." *Imperialism, Race and Resistance* (London and New York: Routledge, 1999), 28.

36. Galton, *Inquiries into Human Faculty,* 25 (our emphasis). See also Dan Stone, *Breeding Superman: Nietzsche, Race and Eugenics in Edwardian and Interwar Britain* (Liverpool: Liverpool University Press, 2002), 95.

37. "Eugenics and Imperial Development," *Eugenics Review* 11, no. 3 (1919): 126.

38. "Letter to the Premiers on the Occasion of Their Conference in London, 1923," *Eugenics Review* 15, no. 3 (January 1924): 647. See E. J. Lidbetter, "Eugenics and Imperial Development," *Eugenics Review* 11, no. 3 (1919): 132.

39. Mrs. Hodson to Prof. Fleure, September 8, 1924, Eugenics Society Papers, SA/EUG/D.179.

40. Donald MacKenzie, *Statistics in Britain, 1865–1930* (Edinburgh: Edinburgh University Press, 1981), 64.

41. Karl Pearson and Margaret Moul, "The Problem of Alien Immigration into Great Britain, Illustrated by an Examination of Russian and Polish Jewish Children," *Annals of Eugenics* 1 (1925–26): 5–127; 2 (1927): 111–244; 3 (1928): 1–70, 201–264.

42. Nikolas Rose, "The Psychological Complex: Mental Measurement and Social Administration," *Ideology & Consciousness* 5 (1979): 5–68.

43. See George W. Stocking, Jr., *Race, Culture and Evolution: Essays in the History of Anthropology*, 2nd ed. (Chicago, IL: Chicago University Press, 1982).

44. Elazar Barkan, *The Retreat of Scientific Racism* (Cambridge: Cambridge University Press, 1992), 65. See also Gavin Schaffer, "'Like a Baby with a Box of Matches': British Scientists and the Concept of 'Race' in the Inter-war Period," *British Journal for the History of Science* 38, no. 3 (2005): 307–324.

45. Mackenzie, *Statistics in Britain*, 126.

46. R. M. Fleming, "Anthropological Studies of Children," *Eugenics Review* 18, no. 4 (1927): 299.

47. "Mongolians" were generally seen as higher up the evolutionary scale than "negroes," with some anthropologists placing them as a sub-category of "Aryan." Malik, *The Meaning of Race*, 120.

48. Constance King and Harold King, *The Nation: The Life and Work of the Liverpool Settlement Movement* (London: University Press of Liverpool, 1938), 132.

49. Lucy Bland, "British Eugenics and 'Race Crossing': A Study of an Interwar Investigation," *New Formations* 60 (2007): 66–78.

50. R. M. Fleming, "Physical Heredity in Human Hybrids," *Annals of Eugenics* 9 (1939): 55–81.

51. "Notes of the Quarter," *Eugenics Review* 28, no. 2 (1936): 100; J. C. Trevor, "Some Anthropological Characteristics of Hybrid Populations," *Eugenics Review* 30, no. 1 (April 1938): 21–31.

52. "Immigrants, Research Information", 1954–1966, Eugenics Society Papers, SA/EUG/D.104.

53. "Advice and Enquiries," Eugenics Society Papers, SA/EUG/D.3–4.

54. Harvey Simmons, "Explaining Social Policy: The English Mental Deficiency Act 1913," *Journal of Social History* 11, no. 3 (1978): 395.

55. Nikolas Rose, *The Psychological Complex: Psychology, Politics and Society in England, 1869–1939* (London: Routledge, Kegan and Paul, 1985), 108.

56. Bland, *Banishing the Beast*, 239–242.

57. Stedman Jones, *Outcast London*, chap. 16.

58. John Macnicol, "Eugenics and the Campaign for Voluntary Sterilization in Britain between the Wars," *Social History of Medicine* 2, no. 2 (1989): 154.

59. Ibid., 157–159.

60. Lesley A. Hall, "No Sex, Please, We're Socialists: The Labour Party Prefers to Close its Eyes and Think of the Electorate," in *Socialist History*, 36 (2010): 11–12.

61. Kevles, *In the Name of Eugenics*, chap. 10.

62. John Macnicol, "The Voluntary Sterilization Campaign in Britain, 1918–1939," in *Forbidden History: The State, Society, and the Regulation of Sexuality in Modern Europe*, ed. John C. Fout (Chicago, IL: University of Chicago Press, 1992), 317–333.

63. See Herbert Brewer, "Eutelegenesis," *Eugenics Review* 27 (April 1935–January 1936), reprinted in Bland and Doan, *Sexology Uncensored*, 189–194.

64. "AID," ca. 1934–ca. 1961, Eugenics Society Papers, SA/EUG.D.6–7, and see also correspondence with Herbert Brewer, 1925–1963, Eugenics Society Papers, SA/EUG/C.42–44.

65. "'Eugenic' Experiments Conducted by the Nazis on Human Subjects," December 14, 1951, C. P. Blacker papers, PP/CPB/H.1/27, Wellcome Library; and his published article "Eugenic Experiments Conducted by the Nazis on Human Subjects," *Eugenics Review* 44, no. 1 (1952): 9–19.

66. Kevles, *In the Name of Eugenics*, 176–178.

67. Pat Starkey, *Families and Social Workers: The Work of Family Service Units, 1940–1985* (Liverpool: Liverpool University Press, 2000), chap. 2.

68. "Problem Families," 1940s–1950s, Eugenics Society Papers, SA/EUG/D.168–173.

69. "Promising Families," 1953–1959, Eugenics Society Papers, SA/EUG/D.174–175.

70. Soloway, *Demography and Degeneration*, 359–360.

71. Jay Griffiths, "Science Friction," *The Guardian*, September 22, 1999, www.guardian. co.uk/society/1999/sep/22/guardiansocietysupplement2.

72. *New Formations*, no. 60 (2007).

FURTHER READING

Barkan, Elazar. *The Retreat of Scientific Racism* (Cambridge: Cambridge University Press, 1992).

Bush, Barbara. *Imperialism, Race and Resistance* (London and New York: Routledge, 1999).

Farrall, Lyndsay. *The Origins and Growth of the English Eugenics Movement, 1865–1915* (New York and London: Garland Publishing, 1985).

Kevles, Daniel J. *In the Name of Eugenics* (Cambridge, MA: Harvard University Press, 1995).

Searle, G. R. *Eugenics and Politics in Britain, 1900–1914* (Leiden: Noordhoff International, 1976).

Schaffer, Gavin. *Racial Science and British Society, 1930–62* (Basingstoke: Palgrave, 2008).

Soloway, R. A. *Demography and Degeneration: Eugenics and the Declining Birthrate in Twentieth Century Britain* (Chapel Hill, NC: University of North Carolina Press, 1990).

Starkey, Pat. *Families and Social Workers: The Work of Family Service Units, 1940–1985* (Liverpool: Liverpool University Press, 2000).

Stone, Dan. *Breeding Superman: Nietzsche, Race and Eugenics in Edwardian and Interwar Britain* (Liverpool: Liverpool University Press, 2002).

CHAPTER 12

SOUTH ASIA'S EUGENIC PAST

SARAH HODGES

EUGENICS in colonial India, principally in the 1920s and 1930s, consisted initially of voluntary associations advocating birth control. As the possibility of formal political independence came more sharply into view in the late 1930s and 1940s, nationalist feminists became increasingly important in the eugenics movement. These women were able to put a maternalist eugenics, in particular a preoccupation with the strategic importance of women's reproductive health, centrally into the plan for postcolonial state strategies. By the 1950s, when independent South Asian governments began to implement these plans in earnest, however, maternalist eugenics became subsumed into the agenda of U.S.-led neo-Malthusian international population control policies. The strong continuities between colonial eugenics agendas and postcolonial population control efforts are striking elements in the history of eugenics in South Asia. Yet the different strands within colonial eugenics—particularly neo-Malthusianism—dominate, at different points in time and in the region's different postcolonial nations.

EUGENICS IN COLONIAL INDIA

In colonial India from the 1920s until formal political independence in 1947, most social and political debate was informed and energized by eugenic thinking. Instead of offering an explicit model for understanding heritability, eugenics in a poverty-stricken colonial context provided a powerful and enduring template for connecting reproductive behavior to the task of revitalizing the nation as a whole.

To these ends, Indians established many voluntary organizations to promote eugenics. The Indian Eugenics Society was established in Lahore in 1921, the Sholapur Eugenics Education Society in 1929, the Eugenic Society in Bombay in 1930, and the Society for the Study and Promotion of Family Hygiene there as well in 1935. Many associations were run from private homes and sometimes included small libraries or reading rooms. These societies held public meetings, published and distributed propaganda, and occasionally ran clinics.

Through these voluntary associations, eugenically minded Indians set out to introduce the benefits of eugenic education by holding public meetings at private clubs in cities and undertaking propaganda tours during their spare time. However, unlike their counterparts in Europe and the Americas, Indian eugenics societies did not act as pressure groups lobbying for legislation that would empower committees to adjudicate and then sterilize the eugenically "unfit." Neither did they found substantial research programs. Instead, Indian eugenic associations' most immediate contribution was the distribution of contraceptives and contraceptive information to their membership.[1]

Eugenics and Contraception

The history of eugenics in colonial India thus cannot be separated from the history of birth control advocacy. With the significant exception of the nationalist leader M. K. Gandhi (1869–1948), many prominent Indians favored birth control, and many eugenics associations were practically indistinguishable from birth control societies. Whereas in Britain contraceptive manufacturers and advertisers were constantly under threat of prosecution from obscenity laws, it was not unusual for mainstream Indian newspapers to advertise contraceptive products or birth control books prominently. From the 1920s, manufactured, mass-produced contraceptives were widely advertised and available to affluent, urban Indians.[2] Moreover, prominent Indian members of the colonial bureaucracy were often centrally involved in founding associations and promoting eugenic contraceptive use among their members. One such organization was the Madras Neo-Malthusian League, founded in 1928 by two of the most distinguished colonial public servants in the city.[3]

Why should the promotion of birth control have been, relatively speaking, so uncontroversial in India and so intimately a part of Indians' eugenics activities? Indian eugenicists linked India's poverty to its population dynamics. This was due in large part to the central role played by the decennial censuses published by the Government of India. These censuses constituted colonial "media events."[4] Indian commentators eagerly consumed their contents and weighed in on the state of the nation with highly critical commentaries which blamed colonial mismanagement—particularly its extractive economic policies and antidemocratic, poor governance—for India's enduring high rates of poverty, mortality and widespread ill health.

Thus middle-class colonial Indian eugenicists, although not necessarily outspoken critics of colonialism, connected a commonly held set of linked criticisms of poverty and colonial mis-rule with the technological possibilities presented by contraception. Eugenicists asserted that Indians could manage their own reproduction and in so doing breed a better India. Some connected individual reproductive self-governance to demonstrating fitness for formal political autonomy. Elected Indian officials in provincial ministries repeatedly called on the government to fund contraceptive advice as part of maternal and infant welfare initiatives.[5]

The colonial administration failed to grant these demands, however, and as a result of colonial administrative inaction, most birth control work was conducted by private associations often operating under the name of "eugenics." Yet, rather than preaching to the poor (as they demanded of government), middle-class Indian eugenicists most commonly preached to each other about the benefits of controlling their own fertility. Many eugenics societies took up the project of contraceptive distribution—not to the general public, but to their own membership. Other social reform movements—such as the Self Respect Movement in the Tamil-speaking south—advocated contraception as part of a broader radical agenda of self-emancipation.[6] In short, while not all contraceptive advocacy was necessarily eugenically inclined, the eugenics movement embraced contraception.

Imperial Connections

Eugenics and its promise of a simple and total system for the improvement of society captivated the imaginations of well-read, idealistic, and scientifically inclined Indians who were inspired to start societies of their own on an international model. Indeed, Indian eugenics societies had long-running and involved correspondence with organizations like the London-based Eugenics Society, the International Planned Parenthood Committee, and its predecessor, the Birth Control International Information Centre. The Eugenics Society provided Indian associations with reference works and general eugenics education materials. And in turn the Society journal, *Eugenics Review,* as well as *Birth Control News,* the London paper run by British birth control pioneer and eugenicist Marie Stopes, ran regular news items sent from eugenics workers in India and elsewhere across the globe.

Although Indian eugenicists used these international relationships to guide their own attempts at institution-building in India, they found themselves repeatedly rebuffed in their attempts to join the international eugenics community as *scientists* rather than as *specimens.* While the Eugenics Society provided Indian eugenic associations with books and periodicals, the distances between Indian and British eugenics went beyond the mere geographical. For example, C. P. Blacker (1895–1975) was general secretary of the Eugenics Society during his lengthy correspondence with A. P. Pillay (1890–1956), one of the central figures in the Indian eugenics movement in the 1930s and 1940s.[7] Blacker initially supported Pillay's organizations by sending requested materials. However, in the mid-1940s, when Pillay tried to elicit support for his journal, *Marriage Hygiene,* Blacker was cool to both the journal and its editor. Blacker complained to his British colleagues that Pillay should be content to participate in discussions of eugenics only insofar as he might be able to contribute to the international community's knowledge of unusual eugenic conditions prevalent in India.[8]

Popular Eugenics Publishing in India

In addition to the eugenics associations that held public meetings and advocated contraceptive use, publishing was the other major mode of eugenics activity in India. Vast numbers of tracts, pamphlets, and books written on eugenics (in English as well as in most Indian languages) circulated in India in the interwar years, many by authors who do not appear to have been active in associational eugenics. For example, Kartik Chandra Bose published *Sex Hygiene* in 1915, Pramatha N. Bose published *Survival of the Hindu Civilization Part II: Physical Degeneration—Its Causes and Remedies* in 1921, J. Krishnan published *Sex Education of Children in India* in 1930, S. Sundaresa Iyer published *How to Evolve a White Race* (Volume 1) in 1934, and M. V. Krishna Rao published *Hindu Ideals of Health and Eugenics* in 1942. These authors responded critically to India's status as a colony, but in terms quite different from those who unsuccessfully demanded the opening of birth control clinics as a remedy for national poverty. Instead, many of these authors invoked a widely held understanding of colonial rule as heralding a time of civilizational decay in India. The eugenics version of this story of civilizational decline under colonial rule focused on certain Hindu cultural practices such as caste endogamy and astrologically based arranged marriage. These authors argued that an inherently eugenical set of "laws" had governed pre-colonial Hindu family life and therefore, although currently colonized and poverty-stricken, Indians were not "behind" the West. Instead, these authors argued, Indians' ancient scriptures held the secrets to national regeneration that the West had only begun to discover. Thus, these authors went on to argue that Indians themselves held the key to their own national revitalization.[9]

India's Eugenic Categories: Religion, Caste, and Race

Unlike eugenicists elsewhere, eugenicists in India were unconcerned with understanding the specific workings of heredity. The relative insignificance of heredity to Indian eugenics must be understood in light of the conditions for the development of eugenic science in India. Like other scientists working under colonial conditions, Indian eugenicists were faced with severe limitations in terms of either carrying out research or instituting effective public education drives.[10] Thanks to the generosity of rich patrons, during the first decades of the twentieth century the Eugenics Society in London was busy carrying out a pedigree project, while the United States was home to a heavily endowed and growing Eugenics Record Office. In contrast, Indian eugenicists were dependent on their personal income and donations from abroad to fund their activities.

Further, "caste" posed a unique problem for understanding heredity in India. Caste refers to a hereditary Hindu system of occupation, endogamy, and social culture (that has largely overlapped with class and access to political power). Although caste technically exists only for Hindus (the religion of the majority of Indians), many converts to Christianity also observe caste practices and beliefs. From the eighteenth century, caste emerged in colonial bureaucracy as the defining marker for understanding India's social organization. Its centrality caused significant problems for conducting research into heredity in India.

Researchers failed to reach consensus regarding which groups should be singled out for eugenic study. While most experts in the early twentieth century agreed that "race" did not satisfactorily distinguish among Indians, there was no agreement regarding how caste might stand in for race as *the* taxonomy within which to undertake eugenic analysis. Caste was notionally transmitted though birth, but it was seldom regarded as a biological (rather than a social) category. Thus, even if caste was the unit of hereditary analysis, there were no explicit models developed (beyond that of arranged marriage) through which traits were believed to be passed from generation to generation.

Rather than through caste, eugenic-racial theories found their most popular application in Hindu diatribes against Muslims. These outbursts framed Hindus as India's supposed "originary" inhabitants, casting Muslims as an invading race.[11] In particular, Hindu sectarianism in the 1920s and 1930s was infused with anxieties about relative numbers of different religious groups across India. Sectarian authors regularly speculated as to the reproductive efficiency (or profligate dangers) of one or other religious community.[12] Contemporary historians have largely understood these arguments as both statistically unfounded and as fueled by Hindu religious prejudice against Muslims. For the purposes of this chapter, the example of Hindu sectarianism underscores how the possible categories for eugenics research remained contested. Specific eugenic research questions regarding mechanisms for understanding the heritability of various traits remained tangential to much eugenics work in colonial India.

Eugenics, Feminism, and Anti-colonial Nationalism in India

Although many Indians held broadly eugenic beliefs about the possibilities of effecting positive social engineering though monitoring and guiding individuals' reproductive behavior, nationalist feminists made some of the most enduring contributions to institutionalizing eugenics sensibilities in twentieth-century South Asia.[13] Indian women increasingly entered public life in the 1920s and 1930s as part of the struggle for political independence. Through their organizations like the All-India Women's Conference (AIWC), and India's premier nationalist party, the Indian National Congress (INC) women promoted a feminist message of maternalism. Indian nationalist feminists framed the provision of adequate resources for maternal and infant welfare as a duty no nation—colonized or independent—could afford to ignore. Laxmibai Rajwade (1887–1984), who would go on to serve as president of the AIWC as well as chair of the Women's Subcommittee of the National Planning Committee of the INC, explained the necessary relationships among national progress, women's health, and eugenics in India. She wrote:

> In addition to raising the marriageable age it is necessary to ensure that a person
> aged 25 years or more and unable to find employment or maintain a home should

not marry. An unemployed young man with a litter of children and perhaps an ailing wife is the greatest handicap to national efficiency and progress...Frequent child-birth emaciates the mother, makes her a victim to diseases while the children are invariably underfed and neglected. Rickety from childhood they develop into weaklings—a hindrance to the growth of a better race.[14]

In late colonial India, Indian feminists forged an important place within the nationalist movement. They argued that only healthy mothers could produce strong children, and that only a healthy race (a term they used interchangeably with "nation" or "national inhabitants") could hope to wrest from foreign rulers the right to self-government. Unlike earlier eugenics associations, these women were less concerned with contraceptive distribution (with the notable exception of a clinic they ran by a local affiliate group in Bombay) and more concerned with arguing for the centrality of women's and children's health to governance projects. In so doing, nationalist feminism effectively connected women's reproductive health to the possibility of national progress under an independent future government.

POPULATION CONTROL AND THE QUESTION OF EUGENICS IN POSTCOLONIAL SOUTH ASIA

As was the case across most of the globe from the 1950s, "eugenics" was not a term used by South Asians after independence to describe their associations or beliefs. Yet strong family resemblances endured between late colonial eugenicists' efforts to manage their own fertility and global post-independence attempts to manage the fertility of the poor. After the formal political independence of India and Pakistan in 1947 and Sri Lanka in 1948, family planning and population control programs were, by and large, delivered through a combination of voluntary associations (which, in some cases, were based on already existing late colonial institutional and individual arrangements) and the governments of these newly independent South Asian nations, often in conjunction with donor agencies based in the United States or Europe (particularly Sweden).

The dominant understanding of the relationship between colonial and post-Independence population control is quite straightforward. In the wake of Nazi eugenics atrocities during World War II, eugenics in South Asia, as elsewhere, simply started calling itself by a new name: "population control." Although somewhat simplistic, this "renaming" does capture the significant continuity in message and in leadership during the 1940s, 1950s, and in some cases, into the 1960s. During these decades, countless historical documents make it clear that Indian eugenics and population control shared a commitment to social engineering and improvement (principally the reduction of poverty) through intervening in individuals' reproductive behavior. Additionally, many Indians active in eugenics and birth control advocacy at the close of the colonial period took up the leadership of birth control, family planning, and/or population control efforts in independent South Asian nations. Similarly, the earlier connections forged among eugenics associations in Britain, the United States, and independent South Asian nations endured and, in some cases, intensified as voluntary family planning associations administered population control development aid on behalf of state agencies. Finally, South Asian censuses remained central to post-independence population control policy-makers. Within the global framing of population control, South Asian nations—and in particular their demographic data sets—emerged as important models for population control policy-making for much of the rest of the world.

The major qualification to the straightforward argument of "renaming," or continuity, is that, perhaps surprisingly, South Asian population control efforts were often far more "eugenic" than eugenics advocates in colonial India had ever been. Certainly some colonial Indians had been concerned about the possible dangers that an over-large population might pose for national progress. But their postcolonial descendents were uniformly convinced that without tackling population, national progress was una ttainable.[15] In the final decades of the twentieth century, South Asian population control policies principally targeted the poorer members of society and, in some cases, deployed coercive measures to effect policies of negative eugenics among the poor. Although this had always been an aspect of eugenics and birth control rhetoric in colonial India, its postcolonial dominance at both the rhetorical and practical policy level was new. While there is no consensus among historians as to the reasons for these changes, it is likely that it was due in large part to U.S. leadership in promoting population control as a condition for development aid (in combination with the American eugenics heritage of selective if strategic eugenic coercion, directed at vulnerable groups), alongside the existence of regimes in South Asia that sought to silence opposition to population control measures.[16]

Over the course of the twentieth century, eugenics across the globe meant different things to people in different locations. In colonial India and postcolonial South Asia, the continuities between colonial eugenics and postcolonial population control look far more complicated when one begins to examine which aspects dominated and which receded during a given set of historical circumstances. A commitment to undertaking strategic reproduction in order to build a strong India dominated colonial eugenics. While many colonial Indians who advocated eugenics were also concerned about the role played by the grinding, widespread, and enduring poverty in the region, this was a secondary concern to the immediate task of improving their communities' or families' eugenic health. In contrast, population controllers reversed the relative importance of these relationships in the postcolonial period. The neo-Malthusian imperative came to dominate; the drive to reduce poverty was eventually collapsed into a drive to reduce the potentially unruly poor. Historically, a geopolitical desire to contain or avert potential political disorder drove postwar and postcolonial population controllers' attempts to intervene in Indians' reproductive practices.[17]

South Asian Population Control: The Role of International Development Agencies

Within the realm of postwar expert knowledge—principally demographic and economic—South Asia (especially the major independent nations of the former British Empire in the region: India, Pakistan, Bangladesh, and Sri Lanka) came to assume prominence in global population control efforts. Particularly after the revolution in China in 1949, which closed the doors to international aid and the traffic in international experts central to the development and consolidation of postwar international aid regimes, South Asia emerged as a particularly attractive and convenient site of international development. Foreign experts were heartened by the so-called modernizing attitudes of the British-educated Indian political elites, including the first prime minister of independent India, Jawaharlal Nehru (1889–1964).[18] Within this context, population control was peddled by both foreign experts as well as South Asian modernizers as a tool of emancipation. In their view, population control followed naturally from, and reinforced, the emancipatory trajectory of formal political independence. According to development economists, who dominated neo-Malthusian policy thinking in the period, by adopting population control, South Asians would be able to breed themselves out of poverty.

One of the most important sites for the development of US-led population control policy was the Rockefeller-funded Office of Population Research (OPR) at Princeton University. Kingsley Davis (1908–1997), in his *The Population of India and Pakistan* (1951), relied on the extensive Indian census data collected decennially from 1871 to chart and evaluate long-term demographic trends and recent changes. His was the first major regional study to employ "demographic transition theory" as developed by his OPR colleague, Frank Notestein (1902–1983), as a predictive, rather than an explanatory, device. Demographic transition theory proponents, much like eugenicists before them, argued in terms of civilizational progress. Demographic regimes characterized by high fertility and high mortality were classed as "premodern" and thereby in need of modernization. South Asia's population was thus both a demographer's data set as well as a policy analyst's political opportunity.

The final sections of this chapter deal with South Asia's four major nations: India, Sri Lanka, Pakistan, and Bangladesh as a way of explicating the changing relationships between eugenics and population control in postcolonial contexts.

Independent India

Of Indian eugenics advocates, the career of A. P. Pillay sheds particular light on the interconnections between eugenicists and population controllers in the middle decades of the twentieth century. One of the few physicians involved with eugenics and early birth control advocacy in India, Pillay was the honorary medical director for the Sholapur Society in 1929, and in 1931 he opened a Eugenics Clinic in Bombay. In 1934, Pillay launched *Marriage Hygiene,* a journal devoted exclusively to eugenics; in 1935, along with other Bombay professionals, he formed the Society for the Study and Promotion of Family Hygiene. In 1938, this society held the first All-India Conference on Family Hygiene in Bombay in conjunction with the All-India Conference on Population. And in 1940 in Bombay, the society merged with the Bhangini Samaj who were running a family planning clinic run under the auspices of the AIWC, to become the Family Planning Society. In 1949 this society became the Family Planning Association of India (FPAI), founded by two women: Dhanvanthi Rama Rau (1893–1987) and Avabai Wadia (1913–2005) of the AIWC, with Pillay as the honorary medical advisor.

From 1952 the FPAI was allocated Indian government funds. Thus,, although family planning and population control were in the government of India's first Five Year Plan of 1952, it was a program pursued alongside substantial voluntary efforts. Also in 1952, the Indian government welcomed a population control pilot program of the World Health Organization (WHO), a project limited to the promotion of fertility control through the "rhythm method." Although there was debate within the WHO (as a United Nations agency) between population control's supporters and Roman Catholic nations opposed to the promotion of contraception, within independent India's planning debates, opposition to population control was largely a legacy of Gandhian opposition to contraception.

From 1955, with the aid of the Ford Foundation, the government extended official population control efforts beyond the rhythm method, with particular attention given to vasectomy. By the early 1960s, mobile camps were set up to sterilize men, but by the close of the decade, demographic data did not show that these efforts had any significant effect. By the 1970s, the government introduced financial incentives for vasectomies, and in 1975, Prime Minister Indira Gandhi (1917–1984) announced the suspension of constitutional democracy, a period known as the "Emergency."[19] During the Emergency, the government ran an intense sterilization campaign across the country.[20]

To what extent is it possible to understand the history of population control and family planning in independent India as part of a longer history of eugenics? Clearly, there were continuities in terms of leadership, the promotion of contraception, and the degree of international connections between Indians and like-minded population controllers across the globe. But the scope and neo-Malthusian tenor of population control efforts in the independent period far outstripped the imaginations of eugenicists in colonial India. Among elite advocates of eugenics in late colonial India, social and economic hierarchies worked not only in advocating contraception for the poor but also in denying it to them. For all the propaganda of many eugenicists, their most intensive work was within their own demographic cohort. The neo-Malthusianism that undergirded population control projects in newly independent India sought to eradicate poverty by intervening directly and robustly in the reproductive practices of all Indians. Population control efforts created a new common-sense in (a smaller) ideal family size that cut across most groups, rich or poor. But it was the poor whose bodies bore the brunt of the state's attempts to reduce the aggregate rates of population growth.

Pakistan

Despite the founding of the Indian Eugenics Society of Lahore in 1921, there was little substantial eugenics activity in Pakistan before the 1950s. Initially, family planning was promoted in Pakistan in the 1950s by voluntary organizations, particularly by the Family Planning Association of Pakistan (FPAP; founded in 1953), an affiliate of what became the International Planned Parenthood Federation. The Pakistani government allocated funds to FPAP (which operated out of a room in a patron's house), and in the 1950s FPAP provided the only family planning services available in Pakistan.[21] It is unclear whether or not there were any specific connections between Pakistani family planners and earlier eugenics advocates or advocacy. By 1970 the government provided the majority of clinical services, and voluntary organizations reoriented their activities toward research.[22] Under General Ayub Khan (1907–1974), who ruled Pakistan from 1958 to 1969, family planning efforts were incorporated into official state policy. As was the case in other independent South Asian nations, international donor agencies were also involved in promoting family planning in Pakistan, particularly after the country's economic crises in the 1950s.[23] The consistently cozy relationship with the United States during the Ayub Khan years facilitated the mobilization of international demographic expertise into Pakistan. Between 1960 and 1964, international donor agencies established training and research centers for population control, and one doctor who came to prominence as early as 1965, Nafis Sadik, went on to lead the global family planning efforts through her long-standing involvement with and ultimately directorship of the United Nations Population Fund. In this role Sadik also chaired the International Conference on Population and Development, held in Cairo in 1994.

Ayub Khan's status at home and internationally as a "military modernizer" put a strong stamp on the nature of family planning program design and implementation in 1960s Pakistan. However, because family planning became so closely associated with Ayub Khan, subsequent leaders sought to distance themselves from family planning regimes as part of their self-fashioning. Although there was a strong set of beliefs in the neo-Malthusian, or economic, value of population control and although the strategies of voluntarism administering the duties of the state and a rhetoric of maternalism characterize both periods, the discontinuities in terms of statecraft are perhaps more striking than any continuities. As one observer wryly noted after Ayub Khan was deposed: "The strength of Pakistan's family planning program [was] closely associated with the factors that have spelled disruption and breakdown for Pakistan's [demographic] political development."[24] In other words, Pakistani population control was autocratic rather than democratic.

Sri Lanka

Inspired in equal measures by eugenics and a concern for the welfare of mothers and infants, the Canadian-born Mary Rutnam (1873–1962) is credited with opening the first family planning clinic in the capital city of Colombo in 1937. However, as was the case in India, the clinic was unable to operate during World War II.[25] It was not until 1948, the year of Sri Lankan independence, that voluntary family planning efforts were reinstated in the island nation, culminating in the founding of the Family Planning Association of Sri Lanka (FPASL) in 1953. Sylvia Fernando (1904–1983) was the first president; like Rutnam before her, Fernando reportedly came to support family planning as a result of watching women come regularly to her father's medical practice. She concluded that only a reduction in women's overall number of pregnancies would improve the health of the poor and augment their prospects for wealth.[26] Sri Lankan voluntary efforts were funded by the Sri Lankan government soon after independence. After ten years of funding voluntary associations to promote family planning, in 1956 the government incorporated family planning into its official policy.[27]

Population control and family planning efforts were concentrated in the capital, Colombo, but also included a network of activities and clinics across the country. In addition to government funding, Sri Lankan family planning initiatives were funded by international donors, particularly from Sweden. Development economists dwelled upon correlations among low fertility, a welfarist legacy of high literacy, and low infant and maternal mortality. Sri Lanka's demographic profile was taken as evidence that a strong social welfare system would be more effective in controlling population growth than a broader international development policy that viewed population control as a rung on the ladder to economic growth.[28] In the context of increased and violent Tamil-Sinhala ethnic tensions from the mid-1950s, there was a wide (if unofficial) concern that family planning efforts might threaten the continued robust existence of the majority Sinhalese community. From the 1960s, the Sri Lankan government lowered the profile of its family planning program in order to avoid being seen by Sinhalese as attempting to reduce their relative numbers.[29] Subsequent research has pointed to Sri Lanka's low fertility rate less as an outcome of family planning policies and more (particularly coupled with a high rate of abortion) as an effect of women's historically later age at marriage.[30]

It is difficult to connect directly the post-independence history of family planning and population control in Sri Lanka to that of the history of eugenics and birth control in colonial Ceylon, for there was no prominent colonial eugenics association. Rather, Ceylon and Sri Lanka represent two aspects of the changing relationship between eugenics and population control in postcolonial South Asia. First, it is possible that the legacy of a eugenic preoccupation with infant and maternal welfare in the late colonial period contributed to the widespread awareness of the nation's low fertility after independence. However, far more historical research is needed to investigate this relationship. Second, the Sri Lankan story illustrates the complexities of postcolonial population politics. In this case, a newly independent state's desires to contain ethnic, or racial, tensions were more important than their desire to effect population control. It is possible that Sri Lanka's overall low fertility also served to make population control a less urgent issue than in neighboring India. Again, more research is needed to substantiate this claim. Finally, Sri Lanka serves as a problematic example of the way that women's reproductive health within eugenics and population control thinking has been understood both as a cause of economic growth as well as its result.

Bangladesh

In 1952 the voluntary Family Planning Association of Bangladesh was established, but the East Pakistan (now Bangladesh) administration did not incorporate family planning into state policy until the 1960s. Like other countries in South Asia, neo-Malthusian population control efforts in East Pakistan by the late 1960s focused primarily on the industrial working poor. Unlike the pattern of organization in India, Pakistan, and Sri Lanka, however, from the outset the Bangladesh government took a proactive stance toward the regulation of its citizens' fertility, rather than relying on voluntary organizations. Bangladesh declared independence from West Pakistan (now Pakistan) in 1971. The use of rape as a tool of war was widespread during the war of independence and independent Bangladesh incorporated raped women alongside male soldiers as "war heroes."[31] As a result, independent Bangladesh witnessed a large-scale, explicit institutionalization of abortion services in the early 1970s. Sheikh Mujibur Rahuman (1920–1975), prime minister and then president of the newly independent Bangladesh from 1971 to 1975, included population control (primarily female sterilization) alongside abortion services in the country's first Five Year Plan (1973–1978).[32] This early period also witnessed a consolidation of relationships between Bangladesh state fertility services and international family planning organizations such as the International Planned Parenthood Federation.[33]

Bangladesh has held a historically privileged place as a site of study for population control research. In 1974 the technique for female sterilization known as the "minilap" (transverse incision, local anesthesia, intravenous analgesia) was invented at one of the model clinics in Dhaka and then delivered, large-scale, to the countryside in Bangladesh and throughout the globe beginning in 1976.[34] Since 1966, extensive demographic data has been collected in and around Matlab as part of a project to understand the morbidity and mortality of diarrheal diseases. This extremely detailed data has made Matlab in particular and Bangladesh in general among international demographers' favorite sites for research and intervention. Matlab data became particularly important in the 1990s for its central role in debates regarding how changes in fertility might take place in the absence of corresponding social sector advances such as literacy or "empowerment."[35] These debates (as well as some research based on India's 1991 census reports) signaled a new era for connecting neo-liberal economic policies with neo-Malthusian population control policy and research.[36] Whereas neo-Malthusian policy a few decades earlier sought to curtail population growth in order to stimulate economic growth, the neo-Malthusianism of Matlab research sought to curtail population growth as a straightforward way to reduce the absolute number of poor people.

CONCLUSION

What are the connections between colonial eugenics and postcolonial population control politics over the course of the twentieth century in South Asia? Eugenics provided a way for South Asians to conceptualize the management of their population through linking broad systems of social classification—the poor and the rich, caste groups, Hindus and Muslims, Tamils and Sinhalese, Bangladeshi or Pakistani—with specific reproductive practices. In some national contexts (such as India), postcolonial population control efforts relied on earlier eugenic strategies and rhetoric in their direct attempts to manage fertility rates. In other national contexts (such as Sri Lanka), these classificatory systems worked against the state's direct management of fertility. It is striking that although neo-Malthusianism played itself out in different ways in different South Asian nations, postcolonial population control efforts all involved substantial collaboration with international development agencies. Seen this way, the eugenic legacy of South Asian postcolonial population control is as much a product of eugenics in countries such as Sweden and the United States as it is of eugenics in South Asia.

ACKNOWLEDGMENTS

Hearty thanks to Alison Bashford and Philippa Levine—for their clear vision for this volume and robust editorial engagement with this article.

NOTES

1. See Susanne Klausen and Alison Bashford, chap. 5, this volume.

2. Sarah Hodges, *Contraception, Colonialism and Commerce: Birth Control in South India, 1920–1940* (Aldershot: Ashgate, 2008), 105–138.

3. Ibid., 47–75.

4. David Arnold, "Official Attitudes to Population, Birth Control and Reproductive Health in India, 1921–1946," in *Reproductive Health in India: History, Politics, Controversies,* ed. Sarah Hodges (Delhi: Orient Longman, 2006), 22–50.

5. Hodges, *Contraception, Colonialism and Commerce,* 37–38.

6. Ibid., 77–104.

7. Pillay is often described in the recent historiography as a "Tamil Brahmin." This is incorrect. He was either a non-Brahmin Tamil Vellalar (a different caste group) or a Malayali.

8. Sarah Hodges, *Conjugality, Progeny and Progress: Family and Modernity in India* (PhD diss., University of Chicago, 1999), 137–139.

9. Sarah Hodges, "Indian Eugenics in an Age of Reform," in Hodges, *Reproductive Health in India*, 115–138.

10. On the restrictions on practicing science under colonial Indian conditions, see Deepak Kumar, *Science and the Raj, 1857–1905* (Delhi: Oxford University Press, 1995).

11. Pradip Kumar Datta, "Dying Hindus: Production of Hindu Communal Common Sense in Early Twentieth-Century Bengal," *Economic and Political Weekly*, (19 June 1993): 1305–1319.

12. Charu Gupta, *Sexuality, Obscenity, Community: Women, Muslims and the Hindu Public in Colonial North India* (Delhi: Permanent Black, 2001).

13. See Sanjam Ahluwalia, *Reproductive Restraints: Birth Control in India, 1877–1947* (Bloomington, IN: University of Indiana Press, 2008); Barbara Ramusack, "Embattled Advocates: The Debate over Birth Control in India, 1920–1940," *Journal of Women's History* 1, no. 2 (1989): 34–64.

14. Laxmibai Rajwade, "The Indian Mother and Her Problems," in *Our Cause: A Symposium By Indian Women*, ed. Shyam Kumari Nehru (Allahabad: Kitabistan, c. 1938), 84–85.

15. For a more elaborate version of this point, see Sarah Hodges, "Governmentality, Population and the Reproductive Family in Modern India," *Economic and Political Weekly* 39, no. 11 (2004): 1157–1163.

16. For more on the population control conditions of development aid, see Matthew Connelly, *Fatal Misconception: The Struggle to Control World Population* (Cambridge, MA: Harvard University Press, 2008).

17. Ibid., 4–5.

18. George Rosen, *Western Economists and Eastern Societies: Agents of Change in South Asia, 1950–1970* (Baltimore, MD: Johns Hopkins University Press, 1985).

19. Marika Vicziany, "Coercion in a Soft State: The Family Planning Program of India, Part I: The Myth of Voluntarism," *Pacific Affairs* 55, no. 3 (1982): 373–402.

20. Oscar Harkavy and Krishna Roy, "Emergence of the Indian National Family Planning Program," in *The Global Family Planning Revolution: Three Decades of Population Policies and Programs*, eds. Warren Robinson and John Ross (Washington, DC: World Bank, 2007), 304–305.

21. Rahnuma—Family Planning Association of Pakistan, www.fpapak.org (accessed 25 January 2008); A. Iqbal Begum, "The Voluntary Organization in a Family Planning Programme," in *Proceedings of the National Family Planning Conference, 1969* (Lahore: Pakistan Family Planning Association, 1970), 29–32.

22. Iqbal Begum, "The Voluntary Organization in a Family Planning Programme," 32. See also *Proceedings [of the] Second Conference of the Region for Europe, Near East and Africa, the Hague, 11–17 May, 1960: Psychological and Social Aspects of Family Planning* (Amsterdam; New York: Excerpta Medica Foundation, c. 1960), 139–149.

23. Much of the following discussion is drawn from Jason Finkle, "Politics, Development Strategy, and Family Planning Programs in India and Pakistan," *Journal of Comparative Administration* 3, no. 3 (1971): 261.

24. Ibid., 291.

25. Nicholas Wright, "Early Family Planning Efforts in Sri Lanka," in Robinson and Ross, eds., *The Global Family Planning Revolution*, 341–362.

26. Perdita Hudson, *Motherhood by Choice: Pioneers in Women's Health and Family Planning* (New York: International Planned Parenthood Association, 1994), 43–45.

27. Dallas F. S. Fernando, "Recent Fertility Decline in Ceylon," *Population Studies* 26, no. 3 (1972): 449.

28. Much of this social welfare versus economic growth argument for family planning successes in Sri Lanka is outlined in the three-volume series edited by Jean Dreze and Amartya Sen, *The Political Economy of Hunger*, 3 vols. (Oxford: Clarendon, 1990–91).

29. Wright, "Early Family Planning Efforts in Sri Lanka," 345, 359.

30. Ibid.

31. Nayanika Mookherjee, "Available Motherhood: Legal Technologies, 'State of Exception' and the Dekinning of 'War-Babies' in Bangladesh," *Childhood* 14 (2007): 339–354.

32. Kelley Lee and Gill Walt, "Linking National and Global Population Agendas: Case Studies from Eight Developing Countries," *Third World Quarterly* 16, no. 2 (1995): 265; Finkle, "Politics, Development Strategy, and Family Planning," 267.

33. For a critique of these relationships, see Betsy Hartmann, *Reproductive Rights and Wrongs: The Global Politics of Population Control and Contraceptive Choice* (New York: Harper and Row, 1987).

34. S. Begum, "Evolution of Female Sterilization Technique in Bangladesh," *Bangladesh Fertility Research Programme. Second Contributors' Conference on Fertility Regulation Techniques, Dacca, Bangladesh, November 18, 1977* (Dacca, Bangladesh: Bangladesh Fertility Research Programme, [1978]), 34–6.

35. See John Cleland, James E. Phillips, Sajeda Amin, G. M. Kamal, *The Determinants of Reproductive Change in Bangladesh: Success in a Challenging Environment* (Washington, DC: World Bank, 1994); in critical response, see John Caldwell, Barkat-e-Khuda, Bruce Caldwell, Indrani Pieris, and Pat Caldwell, "The Bangladesh Fertility Decline: An Interpretation," *Population and Development Review* 25, no. 1 (1999): 67–84.

36. For a review of the role of Tamil Nadu's fertility in these post-1991 debates, see Hodges, *Contraception, Colonialism and Commerce*, 139–152.

FURTHER READING

Ahluwalia, Sanjam. *Reproductive Restraints: Birth Control in India, 1877–1947* (Bloomington, IN: University of Indiana Press, 2008).

Connelly, Matthew. *Fatal Misconception: The Struggle to Control World Population* (Cambridge, MA: Harvard University Press, 2008).

Hodges, Sarah. *Contraception, Colonialism and Commerce: Birth Control in South India, 1920–1940* (Aldershot: Ashgate, 2008).

Hodges, Sarah, ed. *Reproductive Health in India: History, Politics, Controversies* (Delhi: Orient Longman, 2006).

Hartmann, Betsy. *Reproductive Rights and Wrongs: The Global Politics of Population Control and Contraceptive Choice* (New York: Harper and Row, 1987).

Rama Rau, Dhanvanthi. *An Inheritance: The Memoirs of Dhanvanthi Rama Rau* (London: Heinemann, 1987), chaps. 27–33.

Robinson, Warren, and John Ross, eds. *The Global Family Planning Revolution: Three Decades of Population Policies and Programs* (Washington, DC: World Bank, 2007).

....

CHAPTER 13

EUGENICS IN AUSTRALIA AND NEW ZEALAND: LABORATORIES OF RACIAL SCIENCE

....

STEPHEN GARTON

EUGENICS, in Australia and New Zealand, was everywhere, nowhere, and eventually somewhere. Everywhere because eugenics was much discussed: an influential discourse in colonial cultures saturated in anxieties about national fitness, racial decline, the threat of invasion, miscegenation, the fate of whiteness in the tropics, and the precariousness of European cultures perched so far from the metropolitan center. Australians and New Zealanders were active participants in international dialogues and movements seeking to promote the propagation of the fit and prevent the multiplication of the inferior. And yet eugenics was also, in a sense, nowhere: its conspicuous achievements in terms of legislation and policy pitifully few—no sterilization acts were ever proclaimed, and campaigns to segregate mental defectives faced considerable legislative obstacles. Even efforts to encourage "healthy" unions met with mixed success. Marriage and fertility clinics designed to ensure that prospective spouses were free of disease and informed in matters of appropriate sex behavior found a secure niche in the advice market but were never overwhelmed with applicants. Physical culture and other health movements to improve the quality of the race had passionate adherents and thrived for a time but never captured the imagination of the majority. State welfare efforts to improve infant and maternal hygiene may have had some impact on the steady decline in infant mortality, but improvements in water supply and sewerage were palpably more important. And procedures such as vasectomy, designed to curb the propagation of the "unfit," actually found enthusiasts largely among "the fit." Yet eugenics was also somewhere, making headway quietly, unobtrusively, behind the scenes in the interstices of government bureaucracies, such as prisons, lunacy, health, education, and child welfare, where innovation without legislative sanction was always possible.

The question for scholars of eugenics in Australia and New Zealand is not whether eugenics thrived as a currency for negotiating some of the great questions of the day—it did—but why it failed to have the influence its proponents hoped. Why did this seemingly influential movement, one commanding the support of so many significant and powerful citizens, fall short of achieving its ostensible aims? Why did Australia and New Zealand prove to be stony soil for a seed that many saw as essential for the survival of white civilization in these southern regions?

EUGENICS EVERYWHERE

The list of eugenicists in Australia and New Zealand is long and illustrious. In New Zealand, notable eugenicists included such politicians as the minister for health, St. Maui Pomare (d. 1930); prominent doctors like Frederick Truby King (1858–1938), William Triggs, W. A. Chapple (1864–1936), and health, education, and feminist reformers such as Doris Clifton Gordon (1890–1956), Elizabeth Gunn (1879–1963), and Ettie Rout (1877–1936).[1] Its political adherents in Australia were equally distinguished. Prime Minister Alfred Deakin (1856–1919) was certainly vexed by the problem of immigration and the future of the white race in the Southern lands, and his concerns about white civilization in the South were echoed by many on all sides of politics: from nationalist Richard Arthur (1865–1932), New South Wales (NSW) minister for health (1927–1930), to Labor politician John Eldridge (1872–1954), undersecretary for motherhood (1920–1921). Adherents also included doctors and academics, such as Harvey Sutton (1882–1963; professor of preventive medicine, University of Sydney), W. E. Agar (1882–1951; professor of zoology, University of Melbourne) and R. J. A. Berry (1867–1962; professor of anatomy, University of Melbourne), educationists, trade unionists, maternal welfare reformers, and birth control advocates like Lillie Goodisson (1860?–1947), and feminists such as Marion Piddington (1869–1950).[2] In short, eugenics was the preserve of the reforming classes—child welfare reformers, birth controllers, moral purity campaigners, temperance advocates, liberals, progressives, radicals, socialists, and feminists.

Late–nineteenth- and early-twentieth-century Australian and New Zealand believers in the importance of national vigor and racial improvement actively propagated eugenic theories. In journals such as the *Australasian Medical Gazette* and the *Medical Journal of Australia,* and at trans-Tasman meetings such as the Australasian Medical Congresses, doctors debated the importance of hereditary factors in patterns of disease, particularly mental disease, and the potential of mental hygiene to prevent the realization of hereditary flaws.[3] Many eugenicists, however, sought to reach a wider audience. If eugenics was to make headway, it was essential to press the case that threats to racial health were urgent and action essential. In New Zealand, W. A. Chapple's (1864–1936) *Fertility of the Unfit* (1904) was a widely read and influential text.[4] In Australia, similar authors sought a wide audience among politicians, opinion makers, and a middle-class readership, hoping to persuade them of the looming threats to civilization in the Southern Hemisphere and the urgent necessity for decisive measures to tackle the "population problem"—a constellation of anxieties arising from a falling birthrate, the belief that the "unfit" were increasing in number while the "fit" were decreasing, and the unique fear that vast unutilized lands and proximity to Asia made Australia and New Zealand particularly vulnerable to immigration, even invasion, from undesirable races to the immediate north. The answer was to populate the Antipodes with a vigorous race of white settlers. Numerous organizations published pamphlets to push the eugenic cause.[5] In New Zealand, the Women's Division of the Farmer's Union highlighted the importance of maternal health in ensuring racial vigor, and the Five Million Club eagerly promoted increasing the birthrate and outlawing contraception.[6] The Women's Christian Temperance Union, active on both sides of the Tasman, had a "Heredity Division" that highlighted the perils of inherited degeneracy.[7] In Australia, organizations as diverse as the Workers' Educational Association, the Women's Reform League, the Victorian Mother's Club, and the Free Kindergarten Union embraced eugenic discourses.[8]

Many reformers banded together to lobby for eugenic policies. In New Zealand a Eugenics Board was established by the Government in 1928, and various eugenic and racial improvement societies flourished in the 1930s. The history of eugenics organizations in Australia was more chequered. In 1911 a subcommittee on eugenics was established by the South Australian branch of the British Science Guild but only seems to have lasted a year or two. The following year Richard Arthur and John Eldridge helped establish the Eugenics Education Society of NSW, but it lost steam in the early 1920s and folded. Equally short-lived was the Eugenics Education Society of Melbourne, established in 1914. During the interwar years formal organization met with greater success. The Race Improvement Society in NSW, established in 1926, drew on a wide membership, including doctors, lawyers, social thinkers, clergy, and maternal welfare advocates. The Society—later the Racial Hygiene Association— held regular public forums, published numerous tracts on sex education and preparation for marriage, and sponsored radio programs, booklets, posters, documentary films, and even a play, *Just One Slip*. From 1933 to 1935 there was a short-lived Eugenics Society at the University of Western Australia.[9] And in 1936 prominent reformers established a new Eugenics Society of Victoria to advance the cause of "scientific education" and disseminate knowledge to prevent "race suicide."[10]

Australian and New Zealand reformers were also active on the international stage. At the first International Eugenics Conference in London in 1912, there were six official delegates from Australia and New Zealand.[11] Australian reformers were in active communication with leading overseas scholars. Commonwealth statistician

George Knibbs (1858–1929) corresponded with noted Norwegian eugenicist Jon Alfred Mjøen (1860–1939) and was vice president of the 1921 International Eugenics Congress in New York. Victor Wallace (1893–1977), founder of the Eugenics Education Society in Victoria, corresponded with Eugenics Education Society secretary C. P. Blacker (1895–1975). The intellectual traffic was not all one-way. Victorian politician and educationist Charles Pearson's (1830–1894) *National Life and Character* (1893) had a significant impact on American race theorist Lothrop Stoddard. And conversely, Charles Davenport (1866–1944) did some of his earliest empirical work on "race crossing" in New South Wales. Some also left to play important roles in movements overseas. Australian psychiatrist Ralph Noble (1892–1965) became a leading figure in the mental hygiene movement in the United States. Eugenicists in the Antipodes saw themselves as part of an international community of reformers concerned to advance scientific solutions to troubling social problems such as crime, poverty, insanity, sexual psychopathology, and poor educational performance.[12]

In general historians have seen eugenicists as falling into two broad camps—those who focused on the threat of mental defectiveness and the necessity of controlling their reproduction (through sterilization and permanent institutionalization); and those who stressed the importance of racial improvement through physical culture, mental hygiene, sex education, physical examination before marriage, maternal and infant welfare policies, child endowment, public health initiatives, and other mechanisms for improving the race. As many scholars have noted, eugenics often exhibited a complex, even contradictory, mix of Mendelian and Lamarckian assumptions, extreme hereditarian ideas, and an environmentalist faith in the capacity of the race to improve.[13] It is essential to see that these were not mutually exclusive positions: most eugenicists promoted both hereditarian and environmentalist ideas, although there were clear differences of opinion over where to draw the line between the irredeemable, whose condition was overwhelmingly hereditary, and the redeemable, whose deficiencies might be overcome because they were social, economic, or psychological in origin. Prominent members of the reforming classes in Australia and New Zealand clearly felt that eugenic ideas and policies were scientific, useful, and essential to the repertoire of policies that governments and reformers should pursue to promote social progress.

EUGENICS NOWHERE

In the Antipodes, however, legislative endorsement of eugenic ideas and practices was remarkably patchy. Despite all the research into mental defect and the numerous tracts, articles, alarmist stories in professional and popular media, pamphlets, public speeches, and lobbying of governments, legislation significantly extending the power of governments to control "defectives" and prevent their propagation was meager. In 1911 New Zealand did pass a Mental Defectives Act authorizing detention, and in 1924 the New Zealand government instituted a wide-ranging inquiry into mental defectiveness and sexual offenders, which recommended the establishment of a eugenics board to oversee the implementation of segregated colonies, forced sterilization, and marriage prohibition. Four years later such a board was instituted, although it lacked the power to authorize sterilization.

In Australia, eugenicists had to struggle state by state for legislative success. In 1913 South Australia enacted the first Mental Defectives Act, although it conferred no new powers to confine "defectives" than those usually contained in colonial lunacy legislation. In 1920 Tasmania passed a Mental Defectives Act and created a Mental Defectives Board, which operated a psychological clinic to test children for potential defectiveness, although persistent conflict between the Board and the Children of the State Department, which had jurisdiction over wayward and neglected children, effectively stymied the operation of the Board.[14] In 1929 a mental defectives bill authorizing compulsory sterilization made it to a second reading in Western Australia but lapsed on the resumption of Parliament. Victoria passed mental deficiency bills through the Legislative Assembly in 1926 and 1929 but these failed to achieve Legislative Council assent. In 1939 a third bill passed both Houses but was never proclaimed.[15] In the late 1930s a few states, notably New South Wales and Queensland, passed lunacy and mental defectives acts designed to give authorities powers to incarcerate sexual offenders for longer periods. This Australian legislation, however, fell well short of the success achieved in some American states and in Alberta, Canada.

Even New Zealand's relative success in establishing a board to oversee compulsory confinement of defectives was more apparent than real. Both countries had long had extensive powers through lunacy acts to confine mental defectives suffering serious hereditary and congenital disorders. For eugenicists, however, the most serious threat came from the feebleminded, those on the borderlands of deficiency who could hide their defectiveness, earn a living, and allegedly thrive in criminal and juvenile delinquent subcultures. This was the group that eugenicists believed represented the greater threat. The seeming normality of the feebleminded meant they could propagate, threatening the racial fitness of the entire population. This was the group, however, that largely remained outside the purview of all the mental defective and lunacy acts passed in the early twentieth century. The feebleminded, because of their relatively greater social integration, were harder to classify, diagnose, and hence to segregate.

The question remains, however, as to why eugenicists in Australia and New Zealand had little success enforcing even segregation, let alone sterilization legislation in comparison to parts of Europe, the United States, and Canada. Four reasons present themselves. First, eugenics in Australia and New Zealand did not go unopposed. There were powerful institutions, movements, and people who actively campaigned against eugenic legislation. In general, the labor movement, and trade unions in particular, feared that mental defectives legislation would adversely and unfairly target working-class children. Similarly, many of the churches, particularly the Catholic Church, with theological objections to any interference in "natural reproduction" and, in the Antipodes, a large Irish working-class flock, feared that a scientific solution would undermine their religious work.[16] Moreover, scientific opinion was never unanimous in its support of eugenic theories. Alternatives flourished. For instance, geographer Griffith Taylor (1880–1963) espoused theories of "racial hybridity," casting serious doubt on the race purity assumptions that framed eugenics.[17] Second, Australian and New Zealand legal cultures were committed to principles of habeas corpus. Compulsory incarceration, without extensive medical certification guidelines or unambiguous scientific evidence confirming defect, gave pause to critics inclined to stress the paramount importance of protecting citizens from arbitrary imprisonment.[18] Third, some medical practitioners feared the consequences of extensive sterilization powers, anxious that doctors would be vulnerable to legal challenge without the legal protection of informed consent. Others were concerned that sterilization might promote promiscuity and increase the incidence of venereal disease. Segregation was a safer alternative.[19]

Similar opposition and arguments, however, confronted eugenic movements in Britain, Europe, and North America. There was another factor, peculiar to Australia and New Zealand, which undermined the campaign for sterilization and tougher segregation laws. In 1922, George Arnold Wood (1865–1928), Challis Professor of History at Sydney University, published a groundbreaking reassessment of the convicts transported to Australia. Instead of being the dregs of Britain's criminal class, as long believed, Wood argued they were innocent victims of the Industrial Revolution, vigorous, enterprising laborers brought undone by a rapidly changing economy and forced to turn to crime to survive.[20] Throughout the nineteenth century, many Australians believed that the "hated convict stain" was responsible for higher rates of crime and insanity in colonial populations.[21] Wood drew on a different cultural tradition. By the late nineteenth century, colonial boosters were trumpeting Australasia as a region of the "coming man"—vigorous frontier types untainted by the baleful effects of urbanization, overcrowding, and sedentary, decadent lifestyles common in Britain and Europe. And the acclaimed gallantry of Australian and New Zealand soldiers during World War I seemed to Wood to confirm the "coming man" hypothesis.[22] Thus for Wood and many other Australians and New Zealanders, the people of the Antipodes were not inferior stock, but a race inherently more vigorous and less prone to degeneracy than other peoples.

If the white race in the Antipodes was indeed more vigorous, then the greatest threat to sustaining national efficiency was not so much mental defectiveness as "inferior" types seeking to enter Australia and New Zealand: race anxieties were more focused on external than internal threats. Australians and New Zealanders feared the import of degeneracy. The 1899 New Zealand Immigration Restriction Act imposed an English language test on all migrants. Australia followed suit in founding legislation of the Commonwealth of Australia, the 1901 Immigration Restriction Act (commonly known as the "white Australia policy").[23] Both countries also had extensive and effective quarantine legislation. Threats of all kind to the purity of the land and its people were to be policed at the national borders. Australian and New Zealand historians of eugenics have, with the notable exception of Alison Bashford, failed to recognize the significance of the *cordon sanitaire* for eugenics in the Antipodes.[24] It was the "essential safeguard" against the threat of "inferior types." In the last analysis, anxieties about proximity to Asia and fantasies about a fertile interior sustaining a substantial population outweighed fears that the propagation of the unfit would weaken civilization in the Antipodes.

EUGENICS SOMEWHERE

Immigration restriction may have been the conspicuous success story of eugenic public policy in Australia and New Zealand, but in the more conventional areas of eugenic concern—segregation, sterilization, marriage advice, maternal and infant welfare—the legislative record fell short of the hopes of many Australian and New Zealand eugenicists. Nonetheless, in particular areas—physical culture, mental hygiene, and marriage advice; the treatment and education of those deemed backward or wayward; and finally the transformation of incarceration practices— eugenics did have significant and lasting impact.

Voluntary movements for improving physical culture, promoting mental hygiene, and encouraging medical examination before marriage flourished in the early to mid-twentieth century. The range of organizations promoting healthy out- door activities to encourage city-bred children to escape the unhealthy cities was enormous—ranging from Boy Scouts to the Rights of Childhood League.[25] Other organizations promoted healthy outdoor lifestyles to ensure physical vigor—ranging from extreme naturalist movements to hiking and bush-walking clubs.[26] Under- pinning such movements was a pervasive fear of the city as a site of decadence, decrepitude, indolence, speed, nervous dissipation, and racial decline. Numerous medical practices thrived, catering to a market concerned about a supposed increase in nervous debility.[27] Another revealing "fad" was the cult of physical perfectibility. Strongmen, such as Eugene Sandow (1867–1925), flourished, catering to eager audi- ences fascinated with exploring the limits of human strength and endurance and thus repairing the degeneration caused by the horrors of war.[28] More prosaically numerous fitness and physical culture clubs, such as the Bjelke-Petersen Gymnasiums, encouraged children to foster strength, health, and flexibility through exercises, gymnastics, and physical regimen. Reformers promoted the virtues of playgrounds and sports. Many of these organizations relied on subscriptions to survive and thus catered to a middle-class clientele. But churches, charities, and other organizations (such as Police Citizen Boys' Clubs) spread the physical culture message to the urban working classes, offering free classes and excursions.[29]

Another significant area of voluntary activity was marriage and sex advice. Eugenicists hoped to promote healthy unions that would produce a more vigorous population, but venereal disease, particularly after revelations concerning the number of infected returning soldiers, and alcohol represented major threats to racial health. Legislation to force medical practitioners to notify health departments of patients with venereal diseases was enacted in various Australian states, and temperance groups flourished, supported by eugenicists, who saw abstinence as a means of eradicating a "racial poison" that destroyed health and weakened progeny. A number of prominent feminists in Australia and New Zealand, as elsewhere, were attracted to eugenics, arguing that women and children were the victims of men who brought drink and disease into the home, exacting a toll on future generations. These diverse reform groups were united around key campaigns to protect families and the "white race" through sex education, marriage advice, and physical and mental examination for those intending marriage. Through these means the "fit" could be encouraged to form unions and those who failed such tests dissuaded from marriage. Marriage guidance and family planning services were established, and leading eugenic organizations, such as the Racial Hygiene Association, created marriage, sex education, and family planning clinics. The weakness of such organizations was that they were voluntary, and, with on average 50,000 marriages a year in Australia, the clientele sustaining one or two clinics in most major cities was an infinitesimal proportion of the problem imagined by eugenicists.[30]

In the early twentieth century the declining birthrate and high rates of infant and maternal mortality encouraged many governments to introduce maternal and infant welfare policies and services. Baby health clinics, home visiting nurses, motherhood training (for example Tresillian nurses), pamphlets, and advice manuals proliferated, seeking to educate mothers in better nutrition and effective childcare techniques. Truby King was a highly influential advocate of new child-rearing techniques on both sides of the Tasman. King focused on sleep and swaddling techniques, feeding regimen for infants, and guidance on common infant diseases so that parents could seek timely medical advice. There were many doctors active in this flourishing market for medical and nursing services. Governments also supported families through new forms of welfare payment. In 1912 Australia introduced a maternity allowance (the "baby bonus") to give mothers the financial resources to meet the costs of giving birth and caring for infants in the first few weeks of life. Eugenicists and feminists were united in their campaign for child endowment policies to better enable families to support children.[31]

For many eugenicists, however, the urban criminal and delinquent underclass were the group of most concern. Many believed that hereditary deficiency, degeneracy, and mental defectiveness were the root causes of social alienation. Worse, in the early twentieth century, rates of crime, delinquency, and insanity appeared to be on the rise.[32] If the Anglo-Saxon race in the Antipodes was to be protected from the "tainted classes," then the key area for social intervention was to arrest the propagation of the depraved. For eugenicists the major flaw in the way societies dealt with such classes was an excessive commitment to the protection of individual rights. Eugenicists believed that such priorities had to be reversed. Instead of safeguarding the individual and fitting the punishment to the crime, the law needed to assess the nature of the individual and tailor treatment to avert damage to the wider society and future generations. Thus eugenicists favored early intervention, more careful assessment and classification systems (Bertillon measurements, finger printing, IQ tests, eventually psychological assessment) to uncover those with a real "criminal propensity." Once the hereditary criminal, delinquent, and psychologically malad-justed were identified, these groups needed to be streamed out of the ordinary sys-tems of criminal justice and child welfare and either sterilized or permanently segregated in institutions to prevent them from passing on their defectiveness. Governments, however, shied away from potentially controversial policies even when pressed by public servants. When Cecil Cook (1897–1985), Chief Protector of Aborigines in the Northern Territory, sought permission from the Commonwealth to sterilize "half-caste" girls he considered unmarriageable, he was refused.[33] As Eric Sinclair (1860–1925), Comptroller-General of the Insane in NSW, argued, "laws in the past have taken more care of the legal requirements than the medical and have laid such stress on the protection of the liberty of the subject."[34]

Legislation, however, was not essential to success. Reformers and bureaucrats could work around legal frameworks, utilizing procedural rules, departmental memoranda, or new institutions and policies within particular departments and bureaucracies to achieve their aims. And many doctors, psychiatrists, educationists, and child welfare reformers within government bureaucracies in Australia and New Zealand believed that the source of many of their problems—increasing num-bers of criminals, delinquents, and lunatics, rising rates of recidivism, the accumulation of chronic patients—required urgent address, even if Parliament was paralyzed. Concepts of mental defectiveness were immensely appealing as an expla-nation for the failure of traditional incarceration practices. Institutional decline became less the flaw of incarceration itself—poor discipline, a paucity of resources, or inadequate treatment and education—and more the inherent incapacity of "defectives" to reform. Thus segregation became an essential part of the institu-tional landscape of Australia and New Zealand. The challenge for administrators was to distinguish the redeemable from those whose hereditary deficiency required permanent sequestration. Critical were effective mechanisms for distinguishing between different categories of people—intelligence tests and increasingly more sophisticated psychological examinations were deployed in schools, reformatories, prisons, and child welfare institutions in an effort to make informed decisions about the best course of treatment for each inmate. Classification had significant conse-quences. Those considered curable, educable, and reformable were increasingly streamed out of institutions into alternative education and treatment facilities or back into the wider society supported by social workers—special schools, cottage homes, boarding out, agricultural farms, probation, first offenders early release pro-grams, and mental wards. Those whose deficiency was considered inherent entered institutions, usually for longer periods of time—habitual offender sentences, back wards of mental hospitals, asylums for mental defectives, child welfare homes, shel-tered workshops, and special education schools. There was, however, a gap in these institutional schemes. Child welfare and juvenile delinquent programs usually only covered inmates until they reached the age of eighteen years. Thereafter they had to be released, sometimes to the care of parents or charities. In the worst cases, however, juveniles were certified as insane on reaching maturity and then were admitted to a mental defectives asylum for life, thus ensuring permanent segregation through the operation of two institutional bureaucracies rather than one.[35]

Through these measures, eugenics made considerable headway in the day-to-day operation of government bureaucracies, significantly expanding the reach of governments into the regulation of social life and profoundly transforming the institutional landscape for those caught within the classification net.[36] Nonetheless, many were deeply concerned that the group considered the greatest threat—the feebleminded and borderline deficient—remained outside the complex network of policies and institutions that were deployed to ensnare them. Increasingly, however, further research began to complicate simple eugenic distinctions between fit and unfit. Criminologists and psychiatrists discovered a large number of serious delinquents with high intelligence but little moral sense of right and wrong. These "moral imbeciles" (or psychopaths) defied eugenic categorization. They were often exceptionally intelligent and at the same time resistant to many forms of social amelioration. These inmates seemed to suffer complex psychological maladjustments.[37] By the late 1930s, eugenics was increasingly seen as a crude and inadequate analysis of social problems, a discourse whose remedies failed to tackle the deeper underlying problems in the production of deficiency.

EUGENICS RECONSIDERED

Australian historian Rob Watts sees the first half of the twentieth century as "the age of eugenics."[38] In this context, Australian and New Zealand historians have been avid participants in international debates about the history of eugenics. Their primary aim has been to add these particular national stories into the larger narrative of eugenics in the West. A small but thriving historiography now exists, charting the diverse movements that sought to propagate eugenic ideas, the work of notable eugenicists, their influence, the effect of eugenic ideas in a number of spheres, the fate of efforts to pass eugenic legislation, and the ways that particular practices of classification and segregation were shaped by eugenic philosophies. We now have a much more complex and sophisticated understanding of the diverse contributions of eugenics to the development of early-twentieth-century social reform. Despite the effort of some historians to depict eugenics as narrow, pessimistic, and conservative, more recent work has ably demonstrated that eugenics was a powerful ideology that influenced many of the most significant progressive social reform movements in both countries.[39] These debates, however, raise important questions about what actually constituted eugenics and the extent to which it was distinct from other influential racial discourses in Australia and New Zealand.

Where should one draw the line between eugenics and other discourses on race and social progress? The majority of Australian and New Zealand historians have adopted the approach of overseas scholars, such as Daniel Kevles, widening the scope of eugenics to encompass a diverse range of reform programs. Diana Wyndham and Helen Smyth, for example, see eugenics as a broad church, encompassing hereditarian, environmentalist, neo-Malthusian, and many other approaches to race fitness and national efficiency. These historians have used concepts such as hard, mainstream, or classical eugenics (sterilization, compulsory segregation) and soft or reform eugenics (healthy lifestyles, sex education, encouraging marriage, and maternal welfare) to cover the diversity of movements for reform. Is this a fruitful approach? I don't believe so. It blurs fundamental differences crucial to understanding the operation of racial sciences in the Antipodes.

Australian and New Zealand reformers held a wide diversity of views on the great "race" questions of the day—was Western civilization in decline? What was the course of human evolution? Was the greatest threat to progress the propagation of the unfit? Could the white man survive in the tropics? Were indigenous peoples destined for extinction? Could we overcome inherent defects through rigorous physical and mental regimen? And in seeking solutions to these challenges, prominent reformers, doctors, feminists, public health advocates, and progressives often promoted both hereditarian and environmentalist ideas and policies (and the key issue is to explain how this was possible). Historians committed to broadening the ambit of eugenics want to sweep the contradictions away, homogenizing a complex field of discourses and practices. In doing so, they misrepresent the significance of eugenics.

This is evident when we examine particular policies in detail, and more importantly shift our focus from the discourses contesting to shape policy to the outcomes of those contests. For example, the 1903 NSW Birth Rate Royal Commission and the New Zealand Five Million Club have been seen as examples of the power and pervasiveness of eugenics.[40] Certainly eugenicists, like Octavius Beale (1850–1930), one of the Royal Commissioners, were vitally interested in the birthrate. Moreover, the birthrate debate could accommodate a variety of perspectives. Eugenicists and neo-Malthusians could agree that reducing the propagation of the "unfit" was essential, while eugenicists and pronatalists shared an enthusiasm for increasing the birthrate of productive and useful citizens. But which views held sway? The recommendations of the Commission and latter policies that flowed out of this population debate, such as maternity allowances and child endowment, did not distinguish between "fit" and "unfit" citizens. All, regardless of their capacity or incapacity, could access these benefits. Thus the pronatalist emphasis on "populate or perish" triumphed over eugenicist concerns to limit the reproduction of the unfit.[41] The fear of Asian invasion trumped anxieties about mental defectiveness.[42]

Similarly, the regulation of indigenous populations was an important arena where many racial sciences contended to shape policy, especially in Australia, where Aboriginal peoples were commonly seen as a "dying race." By the early years of the twentieth century, however, miscegenation and the consequent growth of a substantial "mixed population" raised important questions about how to deal with this "nowhere people."[43] The major policy response of Australian governments was not segregation or sterilization, as Cecil Cook discovered, but the forced removal of "half-caste" children from their families and their incarceration in welfare homes to be trained as domestics and apprentices—the now infamous "stolen generations." The philosophy underpinning this policy was "absorption" and "uplift," whereby Aborigines and Maoris were actually seen as "primitive Caucasians," held back by culture but with proper training and education capable of entering into normal society. Here the aim was to "breed out" rather than prevent propagation of a despised people. Absorption, of course, was a destructive form of biological management of reproduction, sharing much in common with eugenics, but as a philosophy and a policy it also differed significantly from traditional eugenic strategies. Absorption entailed the introduction of the biological potential of "half-castes" into the wider population. It was based on a belief that "half-castes" would be biologically improved through gradual assimilation. It was not grounded in a fear that they would exacerbate biological taints feeding the propagation of the unfit. Absorption trumped eugenics in the regulation of indigenous peoples.[44]

The Antipodes was a genuine laboratory for race theories and practices, where scholars, bureaucrats, philanthropists, churches, and politicians debated a range of ideas and approaches and deployed different policies and practices in quite pragmatic ways. In uncovering that past, historians need to step back and be clear about the range of competing ideas that jostled for space in the crowded market place of ideas. It is useful to distinguish between eugenics and other approaches to the questions of evolution, race, and the global color line in the Antipodes—pro-natalism, environmentalism, neo-Malthusianism, theosophy, spiritualism, quarantine, absorption, mental hygiene, naturalism, maternalism, and more. While many in the past adopted more than one of these approaches, it assists our understanding of the past if we see that these were often competing approaches to the challenges posed by evolution and race. Though eugenics was an important tributary that flowed into the larger river of racial sciences shaping the cultivation of whiteness and racial vigor in the Antipodes, it was but one tributary among many.

NOTES

1. See Helen Smyth, *Rocking the Cradle: Contraception, Sex, and Politics in New Zealand* (Wellington: Steele Roberts, 2000), 11–33.

2. For example, Diana Wyndham, *Eugenics in Australia: Striving for National Fitness* (London: Galton Institute, 2003); Michael Roe, *Nine Australian Progressives: Vitalism and Bourgeois Social Thought 1890–1960* (St. Lucia: University of Queensland Press, 1984); David McCallum, *The Social Production of Merit: Education, Psychology and Politics in Australia, 1900–1950* (London: Falmer Press, 1990); Martin Crotty, John Germov, and Grant Rodwell, eds., *"A Race for a Place:" Eugenics, Darwinism and Social Thought and Practice in Australia* (University of Newcastle, Proceedings of the History and Sociology of Eugenics Conference, 2000).

3. For example, W. A. Chapple, "The Fertility of the Unfit," *Transactions/Intercolonial Medical Congress* (1899): 472–482; Harvey Sutton, "The Feeble-minded: Their Classification and Importance," *Transactions/Australasian Medical Congress* (1911): 894–905; and Andrew Davidson, "Feeble-minded Children," *Australasian Medical Gazette* 30 (1911): 436–441.

4. W. A. Chapple, *The Fertility of the Unfit* (Melbourne: Witcombe and Tombs Ltd., 1904).

5. C. K. Mackellar and D. A. Welsh, *Mental Deficiency: A Medico-Sociological Study of Feeble-mindedness* (Sydney: Government Printer, 1917); W. E. Agar, *Eugenics and the Future of the Australian Population* (Melbourne: Eugenics Society of Victoria, 1939); and John Bostock and L. J. J. Nye, *Wither Away: A Study of Race Psychology and the Factors Leading to Australia's National Decline* (Sydney: Angus & Robertson, 1934).

6. See Smyth, *Rocking the Cradle*, 11–33.

7. Angela Wanhalla, "To 'Better the Breed of Men': Women and Eugenics in New Zealand, 1900–1935," *Women's History Review* 16, no. 2 (2007): 164–168.

8. See Ann Curthoys, "Eugenics, Feminism and Birth Control: The Case of Marion Piddington," *Hecate* 15, no. 1 (1989): 73–89.

9. See Wyndham, *Eugenics in Australia*, 53–102.

10. See Rob Watts, "Beyond Nature and Nurture: Eugenics in Twentieth Century Australian History," *Australian Journal of Politics and History* 40, no. 3 (1994): 318–334.

11. Eugenics Education Society, *Problems in Eugenics: Papers Communicated at the First International Eugenics Congress, University of London, 1912* (London: Eugenics Education Society, 1912), xi–xvii.

12. See G. H. Knibbs to Dr. Jon Alfred Mjøen, September 30, 1924, Commonwealth Institute of Science and Industry Papers, National Archives of Australia, Canberra, 175/4; V. H. Wallace, ed., *A World Population Policy as a Factor in Maintaining Peace* (Carlton: Melbourne University Press, 1957); Stephen Garton, "Sound Minds and Healthy Bodies: Reconsidering Eugenics in Australia 1914–1940," *Australian Historical Studies* 26, no. 103 (October 1994): 163–181; and Marilyn Lake and Henry Reynolds, *Drawing the Global Colour Line: White Men's Countries and the Question of Racial Equality* (Carlton: Melbourne University Publishing, 2008), 314.

13. See Smyth, *Rocking the Cradle*, 11–21, Carol Bacchi, "The Nature-Nurture Debate in Australia, 1900–1914," *Historical Studies* 19, no. 75 (1980): 199–212; Rob Watts, "Beyond Nature and Nurture," 318–334; and Stephen Garton, "Sir Charles Mackellar: Psychiatry, Eugenics and Child Welfare in New South Wales, 1890–1914," *Historical Studies* 22, no. 86 (1986): 21–34.

14. Caroline Evans and Naomi Parry, "Vessels of Progressivism? Tasmanian State Girls and Eugenics, 1900–1940," *Australian Historical Studies* 32, no. 117 (2001): 322–333.

15. Ross L. Jones, "The Master Potter and the Rejected Pots: Eugenic Legislation in Victoria, 1918–39," *Australian Historical Studies* 30, no. 113 (1999): 319–342. Jones considers the failure to proclaim the 1939 Bill "a mystery" but suggests that by then stories of what might be happening in Nazi Germany were causing alarm.

16. On the broader religious and labor responses and attitudes to eugenics see Wyndham, *Eugenics in Australia*, 7–54.

17. Carolyn Strange and Alison Bashford, *Griffith Taylor: Visionary, Environmentalist, Explorer* (Canberra: National Library of Australia Press, 2008), 88–113.

18. See Stephen Garton, "The 'Tyranny' of Doctors: The Citizen's Liberty League in NSW, 1920–39," *Australian Historical Studies* 24, no. 97 (1991): 340–358.

19. See Stephen Garton, *Medicine and Madness: A Social History of Insanity in NSW, 1880–1940* (Kensington: University of New South Wales Press, 1988), 76–92; and Jones, "The Master Potter and the Rejected Pots," 328–329.

20. George Arnold Wood, "Convicts," *Journal of the Royal Australian Historical Society* 8, no. 4 (1922): 177–208.

21. Henry Reynolds, "That Hated Stain: The Aftermath of Transportation in Tasmania," *Historical Studies* 14, no. 53 (1969): 19–31.

22. Richard White, *Inventing Australia: Images and Identity 1688–1980* (Sydney: Allen & Unwin, 1981), 77–85.

23. Lake and Reynolds, *Drawing the Global Colour Line*, 137–65. See also Myra Willard, *History of the White Australia Policy* (Carlton: Melbourne University Press, 1923); and A. T. Yarwood, *Asian Migration to Australia: The Background to Exclusion 1896–1923* (Carlton: Melbourne University Press, 1964).

24. Alison Bashford, *Imperial Hygiene: A Critical History of Colonialism, Nationalism, and Public Health* (Basingstoke: Palgrave, 2004), 164–185.

25. See Graeme Davison, "The City-bred Child and Urban Reform in Melbourne, 1900–1940" in *Social Process and the City*, ed. Peter Williams (Sydney: Allen & Unwin, 1983), 143–174; and Caroline Daley, *Leisure and Pleasure: Reshaping and Revealing the New Zealand Body 1900–1960* (Auckland: Auckland University Press, 2003), 193–225.

26. See Daley, *Leisure & Pleasure*, 161–193; Ana Carden-Coyne, "Classical Heroism and Modern Life: Bodybuilding and Masculinity in the Early Twentieth Century," *Journal of Australian Studies* 63 (1999): 138–149; and Melissa Harper, *The Ways of the Bushwalker: On Foot in Australia* (Kensington: University of New South Wales Press, 2007).

27. David Walker, "Modern Nerves, Nervous Moderns: A Note on Male Neurasthenia," in *Australian Cultural History*, eds. S. L. Goldberg and F. B. Smith (Cambridge and Melbourne: Cambridge University Press, 1988), 123–137.

28. Daley, *Leisure and Pleasure*, 13–82; and Carden-Coyne, "Classical Heroism and Modern Life," 138–149.

29. Daley, *Leisure and Pleasure*, 193–225; Richard Waterhouse, *Private Pleasures, Public Leisure: A History of Australian Popular Culture since 1788* (Melbourne: Longman, 1995), 165–173 and Carden-Coyne, "Classical Heroism and Modern Life," 138–149.

30. See Curthoys, "Eugenics, Feminism and Birth Control," 73–89; and Wyndham, *Eugenics in Australia*, 219–280.

31. See Philippa Mein-Smith, *A Concise History of New Zealand* (Cambridge and Melbourne: Cambridge University Press, 2005), 132–147; and Kerreen Reiger, *The Disenchantment of the Home: Modernising the Australian Family 1880–1940* (Oxford and Melbourne: Oxford University Press, 1985).

32. Stephen Garton, "Bad or Mad?: Developments in Incarceration in NSW 1880–1920" in *What Rough Beast? The State and Social Order in Australian History*, ed. Sydney Labour History Group (Sydney: Allen & Unwin, 1982), 89–110.

33. See Samia Hossain, "Norman Haire and Cecil Cook on Procedures of Sterilisation in the Inter-War Period," in *Historicising Whiteness: Transnational Perspectives on the Construction of an Identity*, eds. Leigh Boucher, Jane Carey, and Katherine Ellinghaus (Melbourne: RMIT Publishing, 2007), 454–463.

34. Eric Sinclair to W. A. Holman (Premier), May 13, 1914, "Papers re Proposed Amendments to the Lunacy Act 1902–37," Inspector-General of the Insane Special Bundle, State Records NSW, Kingswood, 12/1412.1.

35. Garton, *Medicine and Madness*, 76–92.

36. Watts, "Beyond Nature and Nurture," 319.

37. See Jill Levenberg, *Unequal Allies: Law, Psychiatry and the Administration of Criminal Justice in NSW, c1880–1960* (PhD diss., University of Sydney, 2003); and Garton, *Medicine and Madness*, 84–85.

38. Watts, "Beyond Nature and Nurture," 319.

39. For the narrow, pessimistic view, see Carol Bacchi, "The Nature-Nurture Debate in Australia, 1900–1914," *Historical Studies* 19, no. 75 (1980): 199–212. For opposing views see Watts, "Beyond Nature and Nurture," 318–334; Garton, "Sir Charles MacKellar," 21–34; and Roe, *Nine Australian Progressives*.

40. Wyndham, *Eugenics in Australia*, 168–218; and Smyth, *Rocking the Cradle*, 11–21.

41. Neville Hicks, *'This Sin and Scandal:' Australia's Population Debate, 1891–1911* (Canberra: Australian National University Press, 1978); and Judith Allen, *Sex and Secrets: Crimes Involving Australian Women Since 1880* (Oxford and Melbourne: Oxford University Press, 1990), 67–72.

42. For the deeper anxieties about Asia, see David Walker, *Anxious Nation: Australia and the Rise of Asia, 1850–1939* (St Lucia: University of Queensland Press, 1999).

43. See Henry Reynolds, *Nowhere People* (Camberwell: Penguin Books, 2005).

44. See Russell McGregor, *Imagined Destinies: Aboriginal Australians and the Doomed Race Theory, 1880–1939* (Carlton: Melbourne University Press, 1997); Reynolds, *Nowhere People*, 131–187; and Warwick Anderson, *The Cultivation of Whiteness: Science, Health and Racial Destiny in Australia* (Carlton: Melbourne University Press, 2002), 181–243.

FURTHER READING

Anderson, Warwick. *The Cultivation of Whiteness: Science, Health and Racial Destiny in Australia* (Carlton: Melbourne University Press, 2002).

Bacchi, Carol. "The Nature-Nurture Debate in Australia, 1900–1914," *Historical Studies* 19, no. 75 (1980): 199–212.

Bashford, Alison. *Imperial Hygiene: A Critical History of Colonialism, Nationalism, and Public Health* (Basingstoke: Palgrave, 2004).

Curthoys, Ann. "Eugenics, Feminism and Birth Control: The Case of Marion Piddington," *Hecate* 15, no. 1 (1989): 73–89.

Daley, Caroline. *Leisure and Pleasure: Reshaping and Revealing the New Zealand Body 1900–1960* (Auckland: Auckland University Press, 2003).

Garton, Stephen. "Sound Minds and Healthy Bodies: Reconsidering Eugenics in Australia 1914–1940," *Australian Historical Studies* 26, no. 103 (1994): 163–81.

Hossain, Samia. "Norman Haire and Cecil Cook on Procedures of Sterilisation in the Inter-War Period," in *Historicising Whiteness: Transnational Perspectives on the Construction of an Identity*, eds. Leigh Boucher, Jane Carey, and Katherine Ellinghaus (Melbourne: RMIT Publishing, 2007), 454–463.

Jones, Ross L. "The Master Potter and the Rejected Pots: Eugenic Legislation in Victoria, 1918–39," *Australian Historical Studies* 30, no. 113 (1999): 319–342.

Roe, Michael. *Nine Australian Progressives: Vitalism and Bourgeois Social Thought 1890–1960* (St. Lucia: University of Queensland Press, 1984).

Smyth, Helen. *Rocking the Cradle: Contraception, Sex, and Politics in New Zealand* (Wellington: Steele Roberts, 2000).

Wanhalla, Angela. "To 'Better the Breed of Men': Women and Eugenics in New Zealand, 1900–1935," *Women's History Review* 16, no. 2 (2007): 163–182.

Watts, Rob. "Beyond Nature and Nurture: Eugenics in Twentieth Century Australian History," *Australian Journal of Politics and History* 40, no. 3 (1994): 318–334.

Wyndham, Diana. *Eugenics in Australia: Striving for National Fitness* (London: Galton Institute, 2003).

CHAPTER 14

EUGENICS IN CHINA AND HONG KONG: NATIONALISM AND COLONIALISM, 1890s–1940s

YUEHTSEN JULIETTE CHUNG

From the 1890s, eugenics became an important element in Chinese political reforms allowing a critique of imperialist encroachment while offering a program for improving and strengthening the nation. The eugenics movement in China developed along paths rather different than those in the West. Becoming fit while remaining "Chinese" was a challenging dilemma—a parallel to the modernization dilemma of "how to become modern while not losing one's identity"—with which Chinese eugenicists wrestled. East Asian notions of racial improvement emerged first in Japan, where yellow-white intermarriage was sometimes promoted.[1] However, other than Kang Youwei, a Confucian scholar and reformer, few Chinese eugenicists advocated interbreeding. Thus eugenicists had to redefine a racial hierarchy, situate Chinese genetic traits, and determine their fit and unfit characteristics within the domain of the national body before they could put forward specific eugenic solutions.

In doing so, Chinese geneticists in the 1920s and 1930s were wary of using Mendelism, viewing it as appropriate only for animal and plant breeding. In Mendelian theory, newly acquired somatic modifications could not be transmitted to succeeding generations. Thus, if Mendelism were applied to human beings, racial improvement could be achieved only by preventing the procreation of the unfit. In this case, Chinese—inferior in the eyes of social Darwinists in the West—could become "fit" only by interbreeding for centuries with the supposedly superior white races. This, in turn, raised the question of what it would mean to talk of a distinct "Chinese" race. As a result, Lamarckian ideas played a more prominent role in the eugenics movements in China and Hong Kong. Lamarckism provided a foundation for the optimistic belief that evolution was necessarily progressive. The idea that somatic modifications acquired from an organism's development of particular habits would pass on to the offspring, under appropriate conditions, sustained the prospect of improving the human race through social reform and suggested that an improved environment would produce better people. Few of the critics and advocates I shall discuss here were Lamarckian biologists in a strict sense. Nonetheless, this chapter considers the appropriation of Lamarckism as a series of ideas emphasizing environmental factors, which could thus be used to develop social control projects based on the inheritance of acquired characteristics.

My consideration of Lamarckian appropriation is inspired by and grounded upon Stepan's studies of Lamarckism in eugenic projects in Latin America, especially Brazil. Stepan shows that whereas a Lamarckian-style genetics could accommodate the language of modern Mendelism and accept Mendelian laws of inheritance, it still left a space for the idea that social influences could permanently modify the germ plasm. Many Latin American doctors saw Lamarckian ideas such as *homiculture* and *puériculture* (the scientific cultivation of children involving knowledge of prenatal care, medicine, and obstetrics) as extending principles of public health into the special sphere of heredity in reproduction. "Eugenics thus became linked to obstetrics, population policies, infant welfare, and made common cause with campaigns against alcoholism, tuberculosis and venereal disease."[2] In early 1920s Brazil, eugenics was structurally and scientifically congruent with sanitation science and was perceived as simply a new branch of hygiene. Brazilian eugenicists furthermore insisted that "to sanitize is to eugenize."[3] Obviously, the meaning of eugenics in the Brazilian context was inseparable from public hygiene and other related environmental programs, and a similar merging of these two seemingly disparate ideas occurred in the Chinese and Hong Kong context.

Chinese eugenics developed when Pan Guangdan (1899–1967), who studied under Charles Davenport (1866–1944) at Columbia University, returned to China in the 1920s. Pan Guangdan set up the *Eugenics Monthly* (*Yousheng yuekan*) in 1931 to raise public awareness and involve the state in social reform programs. In 1936 the Eugenics League was formed in Hong Kong, focusing on birth control activities, changing its name to the Family Planning Association of Hong Kong in 1950 and becoming an official service of the government. This use of eugenics to promote birth control was in part supported as a practical solution to the unsolved problems of ongoing female child slavery—the *mui-tsai* system—and the customs of infanticide and abandonment of baby girls and disabled children.

EUGENICS AND THE DISCOURSE OF
CHINESE NATIONAL CHARACTER IN
HONG KONG AND CHINA

After its defeat in the Opium War in 1840, China was forced to cede the island of Hong Kong to Great Britain. Between 1840 and the first Sino-Japanese War in 1894–1895, China suffered a series of defeats in international military campaigns, and its sovereignty was threatened not only by the European imperialist powers but also by Japan. China was forced to sign unequal treaties, pay enormous indemnities for its defeats, lease out treaty ports as well as mining, railway, and waterway privileges, and even cede the island of Taiwan to Japan in 1895. The 1899–1900 Boxer uprising and the subsequent looting of Beijing in August 1900 by foreign troops from Japan, Russia, Britain, France, and the United States gave rise to a collective consciousness of crisis.

These national crises prompted campaigns for political reforms. In his 1898 proposal to Emperor Guangxu for constitutional reform, Kang Youwei (1858–1927) argued, "Given ferocious international competition, following the habitual rule of uniformity will lead to the demise of the system. If we do not boldly point out such sickness and announce it to raise awareness, China will subsequently perish."[4] In addition to the weakness of mind and intelligence that Kang articulated, China had to combat the national shame of bodily disability, highlighted most vividly in the discourse over women's bound feet. Previously concealed in petite golden-lotus shoes by women who hobbled around in secluded domestic spaces, bound feet were a hidden ethnic marker for Han Chinese resisting the Manchu's political dominance. They were also a cultural symbol of beauty, civility, and status among the Chinese upper class. From the time of the Taiping Rebellion (1850–1864), led by ethnic Hakkas, bound feet began to be viewed as a physical barrier preventing women from making a productive contribution to society. Bound feet changed from a symbol of high status to one of primitiveness: under Western influence, foot binding was increasingly medicalized and viewed as pathological.[5] Chinese scholars in Canton and Hong Kong felt that women's bound feet made a mockery of China among Westerners and pleaded for the practice to be penalized. On the grounds of hygiene, physical weakening, and racial degeneration, Kang Youwei and his disciple, Liang Qichao (1873–1929), launched anti–foot binding societies nationwide in 1897, convincing members to match their sons only with girls with natural feet. Kang and Liang also championed pre-natal care and women's primary education, sterilization of patients with mental illness or facial disfiguration, and racial interbreeding for human betterment. Their promotion of women's education, focused on training in prenatal care and virtuous motherhood, rendered Chinese women as breeders of the nation.

Foot binding was not the only cause of national shame. The rhetoric of sanitation—already an issue in Britain—became a focal point of discourse as Westerners traveled and lived in China. Europeans viewed the Chinese in Hong Kong as having no concept of public hygiene and urged sanitary improvements. Osbert Chadwick

(1844–1913), appointed medical officer in Hong Kong in 1882, wrote, "the dwellings of the Chinese working classes are inconvenient, filthy and unwholesome... Above all the water supply is miserable. It is unjust to condemn them as a hopelessly filthy race till they have been provided with reasonable means for cleanliness."[6] In Shanghai, similar images of Chinese sanitation and its relationship to Chinese national character were common. And to the puzzlement of Western commentators, there was no easy fit between filth and ill health. The English missionary physician William Lockhart (1811–1896) depicted Shanghai as a place where, despite no sewage systems and rubbish piling up over the ditches, the local population seemed adapted to filthy environments and survived them vigorously.[7] Such depictions provoked confrontations between Westerners and Chinese residents over public health and systems of disease control. Westerners viewed public hygiene as civilizational progress and modern necessity; the Chinese viewed the absence of hygiene as a humiliating reminder of national shame and Western superiority.[8] Regenerating a failed national character became a trope within Chinese scientific as well as literary and cultural discourses.

The problem of Chinese national character in the terrain of public health illuminated the symptomatic traits that eugenics advocates sought to transform. In the May Fourth era of the 1920s, depictions of national character resonated with critiques of cultural decadence and racial degeneration, evoked by leaders of Chinese vernacular literature reform such as Lu Xun (1881–1936) and Chen Duxiu (1879–1942).[9] Chen Duxiu, using the metaphor of new and old cells to represent youth and the elderly, claimed that in China the new and lively cells had been infected by the "virus" of the old and decaying ones. Lu Xun observed that "Chinese males and females tend to age ahead of their time; before they reach twenty, they are already senile."[10]

This degeneration discourse, found also throughout Europe in the late nineteenth century, created fertile ground in which eugenic ideas could become a source of inspiration for national salvation. Pan Guangdan saw the Chinese collectively as a sickly youth struggling to grow into a strong mature man. He thus gave the name *Huanian*, an abbreviation of a phrase meaning "helping the Chinese nation to reach maturity," to the eugenics journal he established in April 1932, immediately after his earlier *Yousheng Yuekan* (*Eugenics Monthly*) was discontinued. Conversely, Pan thought Chinese cultural creativity and scientific education inadequate, pointing to selfishness as an impediment to political solidarity. Pan's critique of the Chinese character and his presentation of eugenic proposals as an antidote wrestled with the clash between a social Darwinist identification of Chinese inferiority on the one hand, and national pride on the other. Pan had to overcome the agony of admitting national disability in order to promote eugenics as a tool to help China survive increasingly relentless global competition. As already discussed, none of the symptomatic traits of weakness identified by Chinese intellectuals and eugenicists were genetic, but were rather cultural. In this way intellectuals were able to resolve the potential impasse between national identity and inherent inferiority: reform the culture and the polity will follow.

REMEDIES IN CHINA: A CULTURAL SYNTHESIS OF EUGENICS VERSUS PUBLIC HYGIENE

Public health in China in the first half of the twentieth century was not well developed. The renowned anti-plague hero Dr. Wu Lien-teh (1879–1960) estimated in 1930 that half the children born in China died before they reached their first birthday.[11] Tuberculosis was widespread. According to the Chinese Mission to Lepers, China's most reliable source of the time, venereal diseases were also widespread in China: the rate of syphilis was 219.3 per thousand and more than 350 per thousand in Suzhou and Beijing, far higher than in European countries. Chinese hygienists, sociologists, cultural theorists, and educators promoted various diagnoses and remedies, radically different from the Western eugenicists' approach of strictly biological restraint.

Eugenic ideas were incorporated into social hygiene. From its establishment in 1915, the National Medical Association (later the Chinese Medical Association) and its journal, *National Medical Journal of China* (*NMJC*), promoted a synthesis. For example, in "Shehui weisheng lun" (Treatise on Social Hygiene, 1916), translated from the Japanese journal *Chuo koron* (without acknowledging the author and its source), Japanese public hygiene measures were recommended for China, including nutrition, home hygiene, public baths, procreation, motherhood, breast-feeding, school hygiene, and social welfare.

The relative merits of eugenic and public health measures were debated in the *NMJC* by Wu Lien-teh and Yu Fengbin (1844–1930), two of the journal's founding members. Wu expressed confidence in the future health of the Chinese nation and race. He thought that the adoption of preventive anti-epidemic plans, mass education in public hygiene, and an improvement in medical facilities would raise the health of the nation, allowing the state to become strong. For Wu, plagues, infectious diseases, famine, civil wars, and unsanitary infrastructure were at the core of national and racial weakness. In contrast, Yu promoted a more explicitly eugenic agenda focused on the causal relationship between marriage and family hygiene. He emphasized genetic defectiveness and the danger of reproducing a sickly family, and thereby an impoverished society and long-suffering nation. Yu praised the eugenic elements in American marriage laws and reminded his fellow countrymen of the importance of careful spousal selection. He evoked the ancient exhortation that inbreeding through kin marriage often produced handicapped offspring. He also warned against the practice of early marriage as violating the eugenic principle. People were never accidentally born of robust or ailing physique, he believed; therefore, it was important to investigate family genealogy before marriage. However, Yu also believed that syphilis, tuberculosis, alcoholism, and narcotics abuse poisoned the body cells and subsequently damaged the germ cells of the developing fetus. Yu implored people who cared about their family's prosperity and health to eradicate unhygienic habits and to select their spouse with the utmost care.[12]

The incorporation of eugenics into marriage and public hygiene was also advocated by Hu Xuanming (1887–1965; M.D., Johns Hopkins University), another *NMJC* founding member, whose work as the head of the municipal health department in Canton during the 1920s provided a model for other cities.[13] His article "Hunyin zhesixue" (Eugenics in Marriage) praised the eugenic marriage laws implemented in some American states for reducing the incidence of congenital venereal diseases. Hu recommended that women demand that men obtain a health certificate from a venereal disease clinic before proposing marriage.[14] He maintained that eugenic considerations in marriage should be a widespread, commonsense practice and that the state should preclude undesirable elements from marriage.[15]

The pattern of eugenic ideas favored by the hygienists was also followed by the German-trained physician, Hu Dingan (1898–?). In his medical commentaries, Hu blamed Chinese weakness on an overemphasis on mental activities to the detriment of military spirit and physical exercise. This historical tendency was worsened by the depraved customs of foot binding and opium addiction, ignorance of medical knowledge, the absence of national identity, and a national health policy administered by the state, something that would only emerge in 1928 after the nationalists came to power. Hu proposed the revitalization of national military training by pursuing national sports activities to reinvigorate physical strength and martial spirit. He recommended improved racial stock through better breeding to increase the average standard of intelligence, character, and morality. According to Hu, eugenics involved childbirth improvement, marriage counseling, and prevention of infectious and contagious diseases, mental illness, and narcotics abuse. He advocated a national health plan implemented alongside sports education from the primary level of the school system in order to safeguard the foundation of a healthy nation.[16]

This inclusive approach to social hygiene, incorporating elements of eugenics was also evident in the campaigns of the Young Men's Christian Association (established in China in 1895). From 1912, the Association organized a lecture bureau to propagate public health knowledge. In order to convey the importance of national health, the bureau employed visual aids such as cartoons, popular literature, slides, films, and exhibits to attract a large general audience, and mobilized student volunteers, doctors, and local elites to form an efficient community network in each city.[17] In addition to the social service and educational projects, the Association's student department attracted a new generation of educated urban youths who were earnestly searching for ways to strengthen China.[18] The YMCA in Shanghai also sponsored the eugenics journals established by Pan Guangdan.[19]

Such hygiene campaigns were regarded by mainstream eugenicists as providing merely temporary and cosmetic change.[20] Their fundamentally Mendelian position was different from that of the hygienists, cultural theorists, socialists, and educators, and provoked a series of debates. From these debates, which shaped the multilateral meaning of eugenics, we can gain a better grasp of the difference between the biological restraint and "social control" approaches, and their nuances in the Chinese context.

As an example of this difference of opinion, we might consider the debate between Pan Guangdan and Zhou Jianren (1888–1984; Lu Xun's younger brother and translator of Darwin's *On the Origin of Species* in 1947) in *Eastern Miscellaneous Magazine* in 1924–1925. Pan argued that survival and progress of a civilization relies upon the mechanism of cultural selection rather than natural selection. Before Westernization, the effects of poverty, diseases, natural disasters, famine, wars, and illiteracy meant that the law of natural selection largely governed the evolutionary process in China in a Malthusian fashion. With little cultural selection, the Chinese germ plasm must have been vigorous to survive centuries of natural selection. Given the high infant mortality rate in China, the survivors were generally the fittest. Pan affirmed conventional Chinese mechanisms of cultural selection, such as arranged marriage between those of equal social standing, the public service examination system, filial piety, and lineage systems. Zhou, however, felt that manmade selection based on conventional values did not conform to the interests of race or nation, but to those of individual family and lineage. Therefore, Zhou encouraged "free love" modeled after the natural courtship in the animal kingdom to meet the need of racial reproduction and national strengthening.[21] He suggested that in addition to wisdom and morality, the sexual characteristics of male robustness and female buxomness conformed not only to the standards of natural beauty but also to the needs of racial reproduction.

In 1929 Sun Benwen (1892–1979), who standardized Chinese sociological terminology denounced four fallacies in Pan Guangdan's eugenics: applying animal breeding as a model for human rearing; considering cultural influences as biological determinants; using the Intelligence Quotient test as a sufficient criterion to distinguish "superior" from "inferior"; and measuring a person's ability by their wealth and power.[22] Pan responded that eugenics was not an application of animal breeding to the human subject, because he followed the approach of Francis Galton's (1822–1911) genealogical studies on hereditary genius. Though his fourth fallacy is truly Galtonian, he argued there were biological components in cultural influences that even cultural sociologists could not deny. The issue for Pan was not whether IQ tests were plausible, but the ways in which one could ascertain the accuracy of measurement. Pan denied that eugenicists judged people's ability by wealth and power. In China, poverty was a chronic problem, and poor scholars were both common and highly respected.

In 1931, Ren Zhuoxuan (1896–1990; a Nationalist Party strategist pen-named Ru Song or Ye Qing) weighed in on these debates. Instead of rejecting eugenics, Ren recommended a revisionist environmentalist eugenics. He suggested, on the one hand, an improvement in social environment favorable to all classes, and on the other hand, research into hereditary diseases to clarify their congenital or acquired nature, as well as to investigate how society could provide the most congenial surroundings for gifted elements. Ren believed his reconciliation of the different approaches of Sun, Zhou, and Pan in a revisionist eugenic plan would avoid class privilege, racial prejudice, and social injustice.[23]

After Zhou, Sun, and Ren, other scholars proposed measures such as dietary improvement, physical education, geographical and meteorological analysis, bodily and public hygiene, and economic reform. In the 1930s this eugenic-inflected program gained ground. These initiatives were collected in a book entitled *Kexue de minzu fuxing* (Scientific National Revival), published by the Science Society of China in 1937.[24] Among these proposals, the most important were the New Life Movement initiated by Chiang Kai-shek (1887–1975),[25] and the subsequent campaigns of Cultural Construction (*wenhua jianshe*) directed by Chen Lifu (1900–2001); minister of education from 1934, in which the social debates arising out of eugenics and public hygiene since the 1920s finally spurred the state to action. The New Life movement aimed to eliminate narcotics use, to improve bodily and environmental hygiene, to promote women's education for war mobilization, and to reduce China's dependence on foreign imports.[26] This focus on moral and physical cleanliness linked four Confucian virtues, *li* (propriety), *yi* (justice), *lian* (integrity), and *chi* (shame, conscientiousness), with physical reforms such as gymnastic exercise, and the avoidance of spitting, smoking, prostitution, drinking, opium addiction, and bodily exposure. Together, these defined a bodily discipline and generated an awareness among citizens of being part of the nation. The definition and embodiment of citizenship as a whole distinguished the desirable from the undesirable. Alongside the formation of citizenship and a focal point for national identity, the state was granted full constitutional authority and hence was able to exercise power upon each individual body. People conformed actively and enthusiastically to the collective authority symbolized by the state.

However, individual bodies perished, and the results of moral and bodily disciplines vanished with them. Hence, Chen Lifu's Cultural Construction campaigns were aimed at the perpetuation of a cultural body from which each desirable individual body could be reproduced. In "Wholesale China-centered Cultural Construction" in 1935, Pan Guangdan came up with a eugenics proposal markedly different from the European and Japanese advocacy of eugenics laws.[27] He proposed instead environmental remedial actions: elevate people's living standard by reducing famine, preserve environmental resources, and improve the economy. He looked to control the speed of urbanization as a source of such problems as high mortality, sexually transmitted diseases, prostitution, high suicide rates, and narcotics abuse. He wanted to remold family values to foster eugenic ideas and education; to retain freedom of speech, thought, scholarship, and, most importantly, the examination system to select talented elements; and finally he wanted to encourage humanism and ethnic identity in education.[28] None of the elements proposed in Pan's eugenics plan fit the conventional understanding of the eugenics movement or eugenics legislation elsewhere in the world.

In 1936 the journal *Wenhua jianshe* (Cultural Construction) published a prospectus entitled *Yaxiya xueyuan jihua dagang* (Program for an Asian Academy), incorporating a school of racial improvement (*Renzhong gaizao xueyuan*) designed to foster ethno-racial studies of Japanese, Indians, and Chinese as a means of racial improvement.[29] In this way, the multilateral meaning of eugenics generated from these debates both synthesized different approaches between biological restraint and social control. Pan's eugenic measures emphasizing cultural mechanisms and environmental components entailed Lamarckian appropriation: conventional Chinese culture was perceived as a source of problems for survival and Lamarckian social control as an antidote. Hence, Lamarckism offered a solution to the dilemma of how to become fit while remaining "Chinese."

PROTECTION OF WOMEN AND THE HONG KONG EUGENICS LEAGUE'S BIRTH CONTROL CAMPAIGNS

The British acquired Hong Kong Island for berth and trade in 1841, and expanded to Kowloon in 1860 and the leased New Territory in 1898. Like most of the colonial world, medical services, hospitals, sanitation, and litter service were provided to serve the needs of officers and troops, just as colonial medicine existed "to make the tropics fit for the white man to inhabit."[30] In the early days of British rule in Hong Kong, infectious diseases were the primary cause of death; one-quarter of the English garrison and one-tenth of European traders died of malaria in 1843.[31] The majority of Hong Kong's population was Chinese immigrants, numbering 125,500 in 1865 and overwhelmingly (63 percent) male.[32] This imbalanced sex ratio made Hong Kong a recognized center for prostitution, with rates of venereal disease, especially syphilis, running high. The 1876 census and the police report in 1877 indicated that five-sixths of the almost 25,000 Chinese women in Hong Kong were prostitutes,[33] with a high rate of venereal disease infection. To control this state of affairs, the Colonial Office introduced a Contagious Diseases Ordinance to Hong Kong in 1857 authorizing the compulsory medical examination of women prostitutes and regulating the licensing of brothels by the registrar general, an office established by Governor John Bowring (1792–1872) in the 1850s. The ordinance punished prostitutes and brothel keepers in cases where women allegedly communicated venereal diseases to a client.[34] In practice, only prostitutes serving European soldiers and police were inspected and regulated. The colonial government's inability to eradicate VD helped perpetuate the system of *mui-tsai* (little sisters) to provide a source of "clean Chinese women" to a community of male immigrants. The *mui-tsai* system, which sold poor young girls into domestic servitude, was prevalent in Hong Kong until the 1940s, sustained by the colonial mindset of sexual exploitation and the skewed sex ratio in Hong Kong population.

One unintended outcome of *mui-tsai* and prostitution in Hong Kong was the emergence of a Eurasian community, problematic for both the Chinese and Europeans. The colonial government viewed white men's unions with native women as a colonial transgression likely to result in racial degeneration and moral and intellectual regression. Laws such as the Light and Pass Ordinance in 1857 and the Peak Reservation Ordinances in 1888 and 1904 had served to maintain the segregation of the two races. Traditional Chinese attitudes toward mixed marriage were equally forbidding. Even though the renowned reformer Kang Youwei once advocated racial intermarriage in the hope of whitening the Chinese people, racial mixing more often evoked impressions of degeneration, transgression, adulteration, impurity, regression, betrayal, and moral laxity in Chinese, as in British, circles.[35] The ambiguous identity as well as uncertain citizenship claims of Eurasians made them a subject of suspicion and dispute for both the colonial state and the Chinese population.

In 1920, C. G. Alabaster, a member of the Hong Kong Legislative Council and later attorney general, submitted an opinion piece titled "Some Observations on Race Mixture in Hong Kong" to London's *Eugenics Review*. Alabaster pressed the colonial government to impose "laws declaring marriage between certain races invalid or a punishable offence, or at least certain decisions as to the degree of blood making a particular person a member of one race or another."[36] He saw the emergence of Eurasians as a problem dating from 1911, because "before that year classification could be effected easily without too close an inquiry into a person's pedigree." Before 1911, there were three distinct groups of Eurasians: those descended from Portuguese with strong Roman Catholic ties and Portuguese names; the Chinese-identified, who kept Chinese names, clothes, a queue hairstyle, and who observed Chinese customs;[37] and the British-identified, with English names and clothes in the British community. The year 1911 changed China from an empire to a republic and blurred the differentiation between the English and the Chinese Eurasians, when the latter cut their hair queues and adopted European attire. Moreover, the establishment of the University of Hong Kong in 1911 helped advance Chinese bilingual capacities and enabled Chinese Eurasians to secure a controlling influence in the commercial community.[38] Of the fourteen Legislative Council members before 1922, four were Eurasians.[39] Alabaster's demand was bolstered by his fear that the postwar liquidation of German firms would result in the formation of new firms controlled by Eurasians who had profited from the war and were busily discarding their Chinese identities. War profit had helped the Chinese Eurasians attain a social elite status and challenged the dominance of the British race as "trustees and law-givers" of the "Asiatic and African people."[40] Alabaster's recommendations were never implemented, but his proposition nonetheless reflected "a deep-seated uneasiness about the shifting identities of the Eurasians on the part of the European communities, as well as a potential distrust of the Eurasians by the Chinese communities."[41]

Alabaster was involved not only in the debate over race-mixing but also in that circulating around female enslavement. In 1917 he defended a client charged with kidnapping, and the attention the case garnered led to concern, discussion, agitation, the formation of reform societies and finally, in 1923, an Ordinance in the Hong Kong Legislature to abolish the system.[42] Eugenics activists entered the debate on *mui-tsai,* arguing that the refusal of information about contraception to poor women resulted in "criminal abortion or in unwanted children who in Hong Kong and China are frequently given away, maintaining the system of Mui-Tsai."[43] In March 1936, American birth-control activist Margaret Sanger and British activist Edith How-Martyn (1875–1954) visited Hong Kong and generated considerable interest in a eugenic solution to the *mui-tsai* system. The initial plan of establishing a clinic to propagate knowledge of contraception was expanded to the formation of the Hong Kong Eugenics League in April that year.[44] Its supporters were well-placed in government and medical circles: professor of gynecology at Hong Kong University, W. C. W. Nixon

(1903–1966), served as the first president of the League, and P. S. Selwyn-Clark (1893–1976), director of medical services, oversaw it from 1938 to 1941.[45]

On June 26, 1936, Hong Kong's first birth control clinic opened. The majority of the patients came from the working classes. The clinic was used to help train midwives from the Tsan Yuk Hospital in administering contraception. Previously, personal hygiene and "mothercraft" were taught to women attending maternity centers, and domestic hygiene was taught by health nurses visiting homes. Adding the new channel of midwifery allowed knowledge of contraception and venereal disease prevention to penetrate to the poorest households. In 1939, clinic sessions were expanded to include infant welfare and maternity centers and maternity hospitals, the result largely of a sympathetic attitude on the part of the Hong Kong government. In 1937, the British Ministry of Health issued a circular to the Hong Kong government recommending postnatal contraception advice at the gynecological clinics.[46] Selwyn-Clark made clear the League's aim of relieving poverty by providing women with contraceptive advice and "the importance of the birth control sessions as an integral part of the pre-natal, post-natal and infant welfare work carried out through the Health Centers."[47]

Inevitably, the Hong Kong Eugenic League encountered criticism. Lord Fitzalan (1855–1947), president of the Catholic Union of Great Britain, complained to the Colonial Office in 1937 that the League's promotion of birth control violated Chinese law banning the sale of contraceptives and the public decency promoted by the New Life Movement. Fitzalan feared that the League's birth-control campaigns would impede the spread of Christianity in China. He also complained that R. D. Forrest, secretary for Chinese affairs in the Hong Kong government, served as the League's honorary treasurer. Fitzalan thought Forrest's position would allow him to circulate birth-control propaganda literature among the poor in Hong Kong.[48]

Government officials in Hong Kong informed the Colonial Office that Forrest was acting in a purely personal capacity as honorary treasurer to the League. They were unable to corroborate Fitzalan's allegation that the sale of contraceptives was illegal in South China. They confirmed that contraceptives were available in pharmacy stores in Canton and that its two leading hospitals, the Canton Hospital and the Hackett Memorial Hospital, had birth control clinics. Other such clinics were known to exist in Beijing and Shanghai.[49] Despite the government's sympathy for the birth control campaign, the subsequent correspondence between Hong Kong governor Geoffry Northcote (1881–1948) and the Colonial Office ensured that the Hong Kong Eugenics League was not officially linked to the Hong Kong government, and hence the advertisements of the League were subject to assiduous scrutiny.[50]

Such incidents did not deter the government from supporting the League's birth-control campaigns unofficially, since the League shared with the government the goal of limiting the number of unwanted births, especially among the poor. Moreover, the League had maintained contact with the parent body in Great Britain, the National Birth Control Association, to secure its support. The League had also experimented at the Tsan Yuk Clinic and produced a new contraceptive jelly at a price less than half of that made in Great Britain. Such jelly was perceived by the government to be suitable for contraceptive work in India.[51] Hence, the League only became inactive during the Japanese occupation between 1941–1945 and resumed as a governmental organ in 1950 with a new name of "Family Planning Association."

If in the 1950s birth control officially became "family planning," in the 1930s, birth control labeled "eugenics" was implicitly a response to the *mui-tsai* system and the social issues it created: child abandonment, infanticide, abortion, and mixed-race population. For example, documentation on the Eugenics League was officially archived under the case-heading of the "*mui-tasi* system of female child slavery," suggesting that for government, this was the major field under which birth control was to be addressed, and in which it functioned. For the official medical staff as well as the Chinese and Eurasian merchants who established the League, eugenics (primarily understood as "birth control") may well have been viewed as a key practical solution to the unsolved problems of the *mui-tsai* system.

CONCLUSION

Compared to Hong Kong, the birth-control movement in China was an urban middle-class phenomenon. Of the 99 women treated by the Peking Committee on Maternal Health in 1934, 96 came for contraception and 3 for sterilization, and all but one were from the middle and upper classes.[52] The birth-control campaigns did not penetrate into the peasantry and rural areas.[53] Chinese eugenicists such as Pan Guangdan considered birth control a double-edged sword likely to destabilize the class structure and in the long run extinguish the upper and middle classes, a view found also in Europe and in Japan. He suggested that birth control be selectively applied to those who could not afford a better upbringing, and among women who suffered from overreproduction and physical fragility.[54] Pan's suggestion seems more in line with the public interest of limiting unwanted births among the poor in Hong Kong.

At the time of Chinese wartime mobilization in 1941, Pan Guangdan and his colleagues were asked by the Nationalist government to participate in drafting guidelines for a National Population Policy. These guidelines incorporated the eugenic principle of preventing the proliferation of defective hereditary elements via sterilization and marriage prohibition. They prohibited abortion, infanticide, concubinage, abduction, and human trafficking and increased the frontier population through public health measures, as well as increasing educational facilities and industrialization and promoting environmental improvement. These measures were not concerned with women per se and did not benefit women only. Nevertheless, these campaigns provided women the legal protection and maternal health care that converged with an important goal in women's movements in China, and especially in the anti-*mui-tsai* campaigns in Hong Kong. Eugenics as an idea never disappeared because it spoke to a human desire for a better life, embraced by both the political Right and Left.

Most intriguingly, the wartime guidelines encouraged interracial and interethnic marriage as a means to strengthen national unity and provide human resources for military conscription.[55] In spite of his practical concern with ethnic minorities as a source for military conscription, Pan did not see the Han Chinese and minorities as necessarily inferior. He believed that superior and inferior lineage could be located within the same racial group, and within every racial group. Pan suggested that the Chinese state carefully "elevate the cultural standard of the minorities" without downgrading their vigorous genetic quality, which he thought the overly civilized Han Chinese were both lacking and seeking to supplement. Pan hoped that the Han Chinese and the frontier minorities could supplement one another in order to reproduce better Chinese offspring.[56] This particular feature of interethnic and interracial marriage encouragement among ethnic Chinese was in direct contrast to Alabaster's antimiscegenation position on the Chinese Eurasians in Hong Kong.

The discourse on national character in Hong Kong legitimated the British racial hierarchical view of Chinese, while in China it worked as a mechanism of self-criticism. The Chinese elite, less confident of their country's national status, depicted the Chinese as a hybrid, mobile population yet to be molded into the great people they hoped to become. In a nation formed of 56 ethnic groups (and although Han Chinese constituted 91 percent of the population), it was impossible to assert "one race, one nation." Thus theorists like Pan Guangdan supported the idea of an "ethnic nation" which included all ethnic nationalities and promoted intermarriage among them. Pan's view surpassed not only his contemporaries but also many Chinese today who are Han-Chinese-centered.

Acknowledgments

This article has been supported by the R. O. C. National Science Council in Taiwan, grant NSC 96–2411-H-007–007, and by National Tsing Hua University, grant #95N25E1. I would like to thank Matsubara Yoko, Sumiko Otsubo, Victoria F. Caplan, Philippa Levine, Alison Bashford, Matsubara Yōko, and my colleagues and students at Tsing Hua University for their help.

NOTES

1. Suzuki Zenji, "Geneticists and the Eugenics Movement in Japan," *Japanese Studies in the History of Science*, no. 14 (1975): 157–158.

2. Nancy Leys Stepan, *"The Hour of Eugenics:" Race, Gender, and Nation in Latin America* (Ithaca, NY: Cornell University Press, 1991), 81.

3. Nancy Leys Stepan, "Eugenics in Brazil: 1917–1940," in *The Wellborn Science: Eugenics in Germany, France, Brazil, and Russia*, ed. Mark B. Adams (Oxford: Oxford University Press, 1990), 121.

4. Sixth memorial of Kang Youwei to Emperor Guangxu, see *Wuxu bianfa* (Shanghai: Shanghai renmin, 2000), vol. 2: 198.

5. Dorothy Ko, *Cinderella's Sisters: A Revisionist History of Footbinding* (Berkeley, CA: University of California Press, 2005), chaps. 1–2.

6. Quoted in Susan Schoenbauer Thurin, *Victorian Travelers and the Opening of China, 1842–1907* (Athens, OH: Ohio University Press, 1999), 258.

7. William Lockhart, *The Medical Missionary in China: A Narrative of Twenty Years Experience* (London: Hurst and Blackett, 1861), 36–37. Cheng Hu has a more detailed account in his Chinese article, "The Image of the 'Unsanitary Chinese:' Different Narratives of Foreigners and Chinese—Observations Based on Hygiene in Shanghai, 1860–1911," *Bulletin of the Institute of Modern History Academia Sinica*, no. 56 (2007): 1–43.

8. Hu, "The Image of the 'Unsanitary Chinese,'" 27–33.

9. Chen was the founder of the *New Youth Magazine* in 1915 that launched the vernacular reform and the New Cultural Movement, and cofounder of the Chinese Communist Party in 1921. Lu was an independent literary thinker who began studying medicine and turned to literature.

10. See Lung-Kee Sun, "The Presence of the Fin-de-Siècle in the May Fourth Era," in *Remapping China: Fissures in Historical Terrain*, eds. Gail Hershatter, Emily Honig, Jonathan N. Lipman, and Randall Stross (Stanford, CA: Stanford University Press, 1996), 194–209.

11. Herbert D. Lamson, *Social Pathology in China: A Source Book for the Study of Problems of Livelihood, Health and the Family* (Shanghai: The Commercial Press, 1935), 272. Lamson used Wu's estimates. Social science research was underdeveloped at this time in China, and Lamson's work constitutes the most convincing data of the period. *Social Pathology* took Lamson six years to produce and became a standard textbook of sociology in China nationwide.

12. Wu's "Duiyu zhongyang yiyuan zhi ganyan" (Comments on the Establishment of the Central Hospital in Beijing) and Yu's "Hunyin yu jiating zhi guanxi" (On the Relationship of Marriage and Family Hygiene) are juxtaposed in the *National Medical Journal of China* 3, no. 4 (1917): 1–6.

13. Ka-che Yip, *Health and National Reconstruction in Nationalist China: The Development of Modern Health Services, 1928–1937* (Ann Arbor, MI: Association for Asian Studies, 1995), 47.

14. Even though Hu did not indicate the source of the original work, from the footnote in Pan Guangdan's article "Yousheng gailun," we know that Hu was translating Charles B. Davenport's *Heredity in Relation to Eugenics* (1911). See Pan's *Collected Works [Pan Guangdan wenji]*, 14 vols. (Beijing: Peking University Press, 1993–2002), 1: 263.

15. Hu Xuanming, "Hunyin zhesixue," in *Zhonghua yixue zazhi [National Medical Journal of China]* vol. 5, no. 3 (1919): 144–148 and vol. 5, no. 4 (1919): 216–224; vol. 6, no. 1 (1920): 50–57; no. 2: 121–132; no. 3: 174–187; no. 4: 256–268; vol. 7, no. 1 (1921): 60–71.

16. Hu Dingan, "Minzu de liliang zai guomin jiankang [The strength of a nation relies upon the health of the people]," in his collection of medical commentaries *Hu Dingan yishi yanlunji* (Shanghi: Shangwu, 1935), 63–70. Chinese pursuit of national sports has been recently examined by Andrew Morris in *Marrow of the Nation: A History of Sport and Physical Culture in Republican China* (Stanford, CA: Stanford University Press, 2004).

17. Shirley S. Garrett, *Social Reformers in Urban China: The Chinese Y.M.C.A., 1895–1926* (Cambridge, MA: Harvard University Press, 1970), 140–148.

18. Kimberly A. Risedorph, *Reformers, Athletes, and Students: The YMCA in China, 1895–1935* (PhD diss., Washington University, 1994).

19. Pan's affiliation with the YMCA has not appeared in any studies on the YMCA. When I interviewed Pan's daughter, Pan Naimu, she said Pan was a Christian initially but later rejected Christianity.

20. On this fundamental issue, Pan Guangdan stood on the side of the geneticists.

21. For a detailed account of the debate, see Yuehtsen Juliette Chung, *Struggle for National Survival: Eugenics in Sino-Japanese Contexts, 1896–1945* (London and New York: Routledge, 2002), chap. 3. And for Zhou Jianren's discussion on sexuality, see Frank Dikötter, *Sex, Culture and Modernity in China* (Honolulu, HI: University of Hawaii Press, 1995), 38–9, 110–111.

22. Sun's article "Wenhua yu youshengxue [Culture and eugenics]," and Pan's response "Yousheng yu wenhua [Eugenics and culture]," and Sun's response to Pan's response "Zailun wenhua yu youshengxue," were all published in *Shehui xuekan* 1, no. 2 (1929): 1–45.

23. See Ren's article, "Ping Youshengxue yu huanjinglun de lunzheng," *Ershi shiji* 1, no. 1 (1931): 57–124.

24. In addition, there was Zhang Junjun's *Minzu suzhi zhi gaizao* (Chongqing: The Commercial Press, 1944), which focused on Chinese dietary improvement and physical education.

25. As a newly baptized Christian, Chiang Kai-shek initiated the New Life Movement to synthesize Christian and Confucian values of bodily discipline.

26. Arif Dirlik, "The Ideological Foundations of the New Life Movement: A Study in Counterrevolution," *Journal of Asian Studies* 34, no. 4 (1975): 945–980.

27. For Japanese eugenics, see Chung, *Struggle for National Survival*, and Sumiko Otsubo, *Eugenics in Imperial Japan: Some Ironies of Modernity, 1883–1945* (PhD diss., Ohio State University, 1998).

28. Pan Guangdan, *Minzu texing yu minzuweisheng*, in Pan's *Collected Works*, vol. 3, 31–39.

29. This prospectus was drafted by Fu Youren in *Wenhua jianshe* 2, no. 5 (1936): 26–28.

30. John Farley, "Bilharzia: A Problem of 'Native Health,' 1900–1950," in *Imperial Medicine and Indigenous Societies*, ed. David Arnold (Manchester and New York: Manchester University Press, 1988), 189.

31. S. Griffiths, "One Country, Two Systems: Public Health in China," *Public Health* 122, no. 8 (2008): 754–761.

32. Jung-fang Tsai, *Hong Kong in Chinese History: Community and Social Unrest in the British Colony, 1842–1913* (New York: Columbia University Press, 1993), 47.

33. John M. Carroll, *A Concise History of Hong Kong* (Hong Kong: Hong Kong University Press, 2007), 56.

34. Philippa Levine, "Modernity, Medicine, and Colonialism: The Contagious Diseases Ordinances in Hong Kong and the Straits Settlements," *positions* 6, no. 3 (1998): 675–705.

35. Vicky Lee, *Being Eurasian: Memories across Racial Divides* (Hong Kong: Hong Kong University Press, 2004), 4.

36. C. G. Alabaster, "Some Observations on Race Mixture in Hong Kong," *Eugenics Review* 11 (1919–1920): 247–248, and Lee, *Being Eurasian*, 22–25.

37. The Qing Chinese shaved their front heads and braided their back hair into a queue.

38. Alabaster, "Some Observations on Race Mixture," 247–248.

39. Chan, *The Making of Hong Kong Society*, 116.

40. Alabaster, "Some Observations on Race Mixture," 248.

41. Lee, *Being Eurasian*, 24.

42. Carl T. Smith, "The Chinese Church, Labour and Elites and the Mui Tsai Question in the 1920s," *Journal of the Hong Kong Branch of the Royal Asiatic Society* 21 (1981): 91–113.

43. *Hong Kong Eugenics League Annual Report 1937–38*, Eugenics Society Papers, Wellcome Library, London, SA/EUG/E.20.

44. Ibid.

45. Victoria F. Caplan, *Maternity and Modernity in Hong Kong* (MPhil diss., University of Hong Kong, 2005), 37–38.

46. See "Maternity and Child Welfare," in *Report of the Medical Department for the Year 1937*, 41–42.

47. "Hong Kong Eugenics League, Annual Report 1939–1940," *Report of the Medical Department for the year 1939*, appendix 3, 112–116.

48. Lord Fitzalan to Ormsby-Gore, July 16, 1937, The National Archives, London [TNA], CO 129/565/2: 42–44.

49. Northcote to Ormsby-Gore, August 9, 1937, TNA, CO 129/565/2: 37–39.

50. Northcote to H. R. Cowell, July 8, 1938, TNA, CO 129/571/19: 14–23.

51. "Hong Kong Eugenics League, Annual Report 1939–1940."

52. See *The Chinese Medical Journal* 48, no. 7 (1934): 786–791. The reasons for the three sterilization cases were unknown.

53. See Su's *Birth-control in China* (MA diss., University of Chicago, 1946), chap. 5 and the conclusion.

54. "Shengyu xianzhi yu yousheng xue" (Birth-control and eugenics), which appeared in the *Lady's Journal* in June 1925, was included in Pan's *Collected Works* [*Pan Guangdan wenji*], vol. 1, 349–359.

55. Long Guanghai, *Zhongguo renkou* (Taipei: Zhonghua shuju, 1955), appendix, 1–7 and Pan Guangdan, *Yousheng yu kangzhan* (Chongqing: Shanwu shuju, 1944), 35–46.

56. Ibid.

FURTHER READING

Caplan, Victoria F. *Maternity and Modernity in Hong Kong* (MPhil diss., University of Hong Kong, 2005).

Chung, Yuehtsen Juliette. *Struggle for National Survival: Eugenics in Sino-Japanese Contexts, 1896–1945* (London and New York: Routledge, 2002).

Chung, Yuehtsen Juliette. "Struggle for National Survival: Eugenics in the Second Sino-Japanese War and Population Policies," in *Trans-Pacific Relations: America, Europe and Asia in the Twentieth Century*, ed. Richard Jensen, Jon Davidann, and Yoneyuki Sugita (Westport, CT: Praeger, 2003).

Dikötter, Frank. *The Discourse of Race in Modern China* (Hong Kong: Hong Kong University Press, 1992).

Dikötter, Frank. *Sex, Culture and Modernity in China* (Honolulu, HI: University of Hawaii Press, 1995).

Dikötter, Frank. *Imperfect Conceptions: Medical Knowledge, Birth Defects, and Eugenics in China* (New York: Columbia University Press, 1998).

Lee, Gerald H. J. *Pan Guangdan and the Concept of Minzu* (MPhil diss., Cambridge University, 1996).

Lee, Vicky. *Being Eurasian: Memories Across Racial Divides* (Hong Kong: Hong Kong University Press, 2004).

Levine, Philippa. "Modernity, Medicine, and Colonialism: The Contagious Diseases Ordinances in Hong Kong and the Straits Settlements," *positions* 6, no. 3 (1998): 675–705.

Otsubo, Sumiko. *Eugenics in Imperial Japan: Some Ironies of Modernity, 1883–1945* (PhD diss., Ohio State University, 1998).

....

CHAPTER 15

SOUTH AFRICA: PARADOXES IN THE PLACE OF RACE

....

SAUL DUBOW

THAT twentieth-century South Africa was fundamentally constituted by ideas of race may seem a statement of the obvious: it is difficult to think of any society elsewhere in the world (including the American South) in which color-based discrimination was more overt or deeply entrenched in law. Racial categories and ascriptions determined all aspects of South Africans' lives from birth to death, and they intruded as much on private as public life. One might therefore expect that eugenics and related scientific ideas played a major role in validating the systems of apartheid (1948–1994) and its predecessor, racial segregation (ca. 1902–1948). This proposition, though substantially true, needs to be qualified in several respects. South African eugenics was inescapably linked to race, but racial discrimination was by no means dependent on eugenic ideas.

So thoroughly were racial hierarchies internalized and enforced by the apartheid regime that eugenic ideas were never of primary importance within the framework of white supremacy. One hundred and fifty years of slavery and many more of servitude imprinted paternalism and deference in the lived relations between whites and blacks. By the time a comprehensive scheme of racial segregation was elaborated as a national program in the first decades of the twentieth century, finely calibrated distinctions between different races and ethnic groups were thoroughly assimilated in the habits of mind and social behavior of South Africans. Racial divisions were thus, to a considerable extent, naturalized. When eugenic ideas were most freely in circulation—in the first half of the twentieth century—they were as often mobilized in the context of intra-white conflict (that is, in the battle for ethnic

ascendancy between English and Afrikaans-speakers) than in the struggle to maintain overall white supremacy over blacks. Indeed, until the 1930s, the problem of
race tended to refer to battles between "Boer and Brit" within white society; the
"color" question was conventionally regarded as something else entirely. From the
1940s, when apartheid was theorized and implemented, there was often reluctance
to deploy eugenic arguments as a justification of white supremacy and race. Although
of utility to apartheid theory, eugenics sat uneasily with Afrikaner theology and
posed uncomfortable questions about the origins and persistence of white poverty.

BACKGROUND

While there are good grounds for tracing racial consciousness to the very beginnings of European settlement at the Cape in the mid-seventeenth century, careful
account needs to be taken of changes in the patterns of racial awareness and
discrimination: for example, the shift from social hierarchies based on status
(Christian or non-Christian, slave or manumitted) in the period of Dutch colonization, to those founded on race typology in the course of the nineteenth century.
    Systematic debate about the equality or otherwise of South Africa's complex
array of peoples and cultures began when British rule began to modernize the
country and its institutions in the early nineteenth century.[1] Paradoxically, it required
a conception of the unity of humankind to provoke theorized assertions of intrinsic
racial difference. Thus, racial awareness was prompted, variously, by the presence at
the Cape of a vocal and well-connected emancipationist and humanitarian lobby,
which urged equality in law for all indigenous peoples; by the eastward extension of
the Colony's settler frontier to include lands belonging to Xhosa-speaking Africans;
and by the emergence of a purposive and increasingly interventionist colonial state.[2]
Settler insistence on ineradicable differences between blacks and whites were in part
a response to missionary and emancipationist beliefs that all God's children were
potentially equal (although the cultural superiority of Christianity and the necessity
of material and moral progress went almost unquestioned).
    There is substantial evidence that questions of race were being discussed in the
language of science by the mid-nineteenth century, and even earlier. Robert Knox
(1791–1862), the controversial Edinburgh anatomist who worked as an army surgeon on the hotly contested eastern Cape frontier between 1817 and 1820, helped to
frame such views in the British world, and Knox's landmark text *The Races of Men*
(1850) owed much to his experience at the Cape. Yet it was only in the mid-1870s
that this racial discourse became more thoroughgoing in South Africa. Several
processes converged to hasten the crystallization of racial ideology: the development
of the "new" imperialism focused European attentions on the subcontinent; the discovery of diamonds (1867) and then gold (1886) sparked a rapid process of industrialization in the South African interior which created a huge demand for a ready

supply of cheap African labor; the need to control a vast African proletariat persuaded opinion-formers to disavow liberal hopes of gradually assimilating individual Africans within colonial society; Darwinian (or Spencerian) theories of natural selection framed discussions about the Africans' innate capacity to progress up the scale of civilization.

It was as a result of this explosive coalescence of geopolitical, economic, and ideological factors, along with the desire to bring an unruly, confused, and disparate region under firm cognitive and administrative control, that the study of southern African societies was encouraged, especially from the final quarter of the nineteenth century. Investigations conducted by a growing corpus of colonial-based intellectuals in fields as diverse as geology, paleontology, and philology prompted new theories about the age of the subcontinent and the relationship of different races to one another. The defining characteristics of so-called Bushmen, Hottentots, and Bantu were described and detailed with reference to their language, culture, historical origins, and relative position in the hierarchy of humankind. Sequences of population movements (prior to and including colonial occupation) became closely associated with underlying racial competence.[3]

Speculation about the continuing strength of African societies abounded. While it was generally agreed that the aboriginal bushmen were a "dying race" who no longer posed a threat to colonial society, this diagnosis differed in respect to Nguni-speaking Africans who were portrayed as virile and racially "vigorous." Some thought "tribal" Africans were natural eugenists because they did not artificially protect their weaker brethren and were disposed to internecine warfare. Most settlers therefore regarded Africans' prolific fertility as a political threat—while coveting their labor as an untapped economic resource. This mixture of fear and greed led the imperial and colonial powers during the 1870s and 1880s to conquer the still powerful African kingdoms and polities of the Xhosa, Sotho, Tswana, and Zulu.

It was not only blacks who came under racial scrutiny at this time. As British attention became focused on the future of the independent South African Republic, wherein the vast goldfields of the Witwatersrand were located, stereotypes of indolent and retrogressive Boer farmers acquired new force. Alfred Milner (1845–1925), the British high commissioner, increased pressure on President Paul Kruger to modernize the economic and social structures of his "feudal" South African Republic and to grant political rights to Britons living within its borders. Milner, who styled himself a "British race patriot" and absorbed many of the social Darwinist nostrums of the day, was convinced by 1898 that Kruger's "mediaeval race oligarchy" would have to be swept aside.[4] The Anglo-Boer or South African War erupted a year later.

Not all British imperialists subscribed to the Milnerite view of primitive, retrograde Boers. A counternarrative, articulated by writers like the British historian J. A. Froude (1818–1894) in the 1870s, portrayed Boers rather more positively as simple and devout Protestant farmers who were ideally suited to African conditions. Arthur Conan Doyle (1859–1930) characterized Boers as a rugged and unconquerable Teutonic race, while Olive Schreiner (1855–1920) looked forward to co-mingling between two nationalities whose blood and character were essentially compatible.

During the period of reconstruction that followed the South African War, culminating in the creation of the Union of South Africa (1910), a great deal of ideological and political labor was expended on assuaging Afrikaner resentment so as to build a common white South African identity. Milner's successor as high commissioner, Lord Selborne (1859–1942), drafted a *Memorandum* in 1907 which spoke of the need for the two principal Teutonic "races" of South Africa—British and Dutch—to overcome their historic differences. Selborne inverted standard eugenic tropes in order to portray racial mixture between them advantageous to the making of a new nation.[5] The obverse of this eugenic inclusiveness regarding those of European descent was a growing emphasis on incommensurable differences between blacks and whites.

It was in the period of political reconstruction after 1902 that racial segregation was devised as a systematic policy. English-speaking intellectuals, some liberal-minded, others with strong imperial links, played a central role in its formulation.[6] Segregationist ideologues were quick to absorb eugenic thinking and drew readily on lessons from the post-bellum American South as well as Britain and its African empire. Central tenets of the developing body of race thinking in South Africa included the view that Africans should be protected from the corrosive effects of modern industrial society (except where they were to be used as migrant labor); that they were naturally suited to a pastoral existence; and that they were mentally ill-equipped to benefit from Western education. Comparative anatomists measured skulls in order to determine brain size and to define the racial types that comprised the subcontinent's peoples. In prehistory and physical anthropology (fields of scholarship that brought national distinction to South Africa), the search for the missing link in hominid evolution was overlaid with racial typing and taxonomy and was further elaborated by reference to racially based theories of cultural diffusionism and population movements.[7]

During the first three decades of the twentieth century, then, eugenic and related forms of scientific racial thought developed in tandem with policies of racial segregation. Growing interest among educationists and psychologists in the technology of mental testing promised to settle the question of the "educability" of Africans. Variants of psychometric tests were devised for use in schools and in the mining industry. Government experts based in the National Bureau of Educational and Social Research (established in 1929 with substantial funding from the Carnegie Corporation of New York), as well as academics in the rapidly expanding university sector, developed large-scale IQ testing programs. Considerable efforts were directed to the study of white schools and industrial institutes, where the underperformance of Afrikaans relative to English-speakers was a source of concern.[8] Such work highlighted social and ethnic fissures within the white community, as well as indicating eugenic weaknesses within the white race as a whole.

Enthusiasm for psychometric testing was linked to the professionalization of knowledge in schools, universities, and state organizations. Eugenics was enthusiastically endorsed by individual members of the medical profession and also by psychiatrists and physicians attached to mental institutions. J. T. Dunston (1875–1937), physician superintendent of the Pretoria Mental Hospital, was an enthusiastic eugenist who played a significant role in framing the 1916 Mental Disorders Act. This measure represented the first overarching effort to provide a typology of "defective" persons within official discourse.[9] The annual reports supplied by Dunston to the government, in his capacity as commissioner of mentally disordered and defective persons, stressed the dangers to society, as well as the burden to the state, posed by the feebleminded.[10]

Dunston's anxieties, and indeed the bulk of mental testing activities, were focused on differential intelligence in the white community. Yet, psychometric tests were also utilized in order to prove the apparent inherent mental inferiority of Africans—and hence their unsuitability for the privileges of common citizenship. Such studies overlapped with anthropologically oriented work addressing the nature of "native mentality." Culturally oriented (and qualitative rather than quantitative by orientation) questions generated by this approach considered whether Africans were capable of original thought, whether they were organically disposed to believe in magic and superstition, and whether Africans' cognitive development was "arrested" at the point of adolescence. The answers provided tended to reinforce the view that white experts and employers should "know the native mind"—a common phrase that neatly conflates an objectified scientific view of African mentality with established folk-wisdom shaped by long-standing relations of agrarian paternalism.

Eugenic ideas also informed popular fears about African sexuality. Intermittent moral panics and waves of hysteria about the putative sexual threat posed to white women by black men highlighted the social dangers posed by "detribalized" unmarried men and women living in uncontrolled conditions in urban areas.[11] Laws were introduced so as to restrict the right of blacks to live in "white" urban areas and to assuage fears of moral corruption and social disorder. The 1929 "black peril" election, won by J. B. M. Hertzog's (1866–1942) National Party, was a harbinger of the 1948 election in which the dangers of white South Africa being "swamped" by a wave of urban Africans were ruthlessly exploited by the incoming apartheid government. The 1950 Immorality Act, forbidding sexual relations across the color line, was rigorously enforced by the new apartheid regime. Although justified principally on social, political, and moral grounds, its impulse and justification may also be seen as eugenic insofar as the maintenance of racial purity was a primary objective.

Like so much apartheid legislation, the 1950 Immorality Act built upon measures passed in the segregation era, in this case a measure passed in 1927 prohibiting "carnal intercourse between Europeans and Natives and other acts in relation thereto." It was also a response to fears that miscegenation threatened the "prestige" of the white race. As such, it drew readily on available stereotypes of black male sexual rapacity. Anxieties about "blood intermixture" focused especially on the creole "colored" population whose ambiguous racial status was seen as destabilizing.[12] The prospect of Mendelian "throwbacks" being born in families generally considered to be white was another concern. Coloreds were often said to be susceptible to diseases such as tuberculosis and alcoholism. In the 1920s, two of South Africa's most dedicated eugenists, the Wits University zoologist H. B. Fantham (1876–1937) and his wife, Annie Porter (1880–1963), a parasitologist, compiled case-based evidence that purported to show that racial mixture resulted in physical and organic abnormalities.[13]

Consensus on the social undesirability of sexual intermixture was almost universal among whites. This view was also supported by socially conservative African leaders, even by those who otherwise rejected political segregation. Gender-based concerns about the degradation of women frequently crossed lines of color—though it should be noted that African patriarchs were more likely to see white men as the peril, and with good reason. Curiously, eugenic research was ambiguous on the question of racial decline caused by racial crossing in respect to non-whites. Eugen Fischer (1874–1967), who was to become a leading academic figure in the Nazi race hygiene movement, published research in 1913 based on his doctoral work on the Baster community in South West Africa (Namibia) which aimed to study the operation of Mendelian principles in a mixed-race "bastard" community. Fischer conceded that miscegenation could result in "hybrid vigor," a view reiterated by the London university biologist and eugenist Reginald Ruggles Gates (1882–1962), who visited South Africa in 1929.[14] But the theory of hybrid vigor did not mean that men like Gates or Fischer approved of intermixture with whites—on the contrary, it was assumed that whites were always diminished by such contact.

INSTITUTIONS

Although widely pervasive, eugenics did not have a strong institutional footing in South Africa and, while a Eugenics Society was briefly in existence under Fantham's leadership, it has left no trace. The influence of eugenics was instead borne indirectly through the agency of opinion-forming individuals based in university and government departments. Explicit discussions took place within the medical profession: in 1926, and again in 1928 eugenics formed the subject of presidential addresses delivered to the South African Medical Association. Proponents like doctors E. G. Dru Drury (1872–1947) and P. W. Laidler (1885–1945) enjoyed some success in alerting their colleagues to the dangers of race degeneration and reminding them of their responsibilities to ensure the improvement of the biological stock.

The failure to focus eugenic interests in a single organization was not necessarily a constraint on the promotion of eugenic awareness. In countries like Britain or the United States there were intense political wranglings within and between institutions committed to eugenics, but in societies like South Africa, where the critical mass of intellectuals was far less concentrated, eugenic ideas were disseminated in more dilute, albeit no less insidious, ways. Eugenic enthusiasts enjoyed some success in introducing their ideas to scientific, professional, and official bodies, using their own status as intellectual collateral. Part of the appeal lay in the fact that, as well as being radical and dangerous, eugenics was modern, scientific, and spoke compellingly to issues of contemporary concern. It also offered scope for the expansion of research in new fields of education, social policy, penal science, and anthropological study. These areas in turn provided a recruiting base for new adherents.

The Race Welfare Society, established in 1930 in Johannesburg, was probably the clearest instance of a public organization deliberately geared to the advancement of eugenics. It illustrates well the reciprocal process whereby eugenics fed on, but also stimulated, policies of social intervention. The original purpose of the Race Welfare Society was to tackle, in a practical fashion, the "evils" of hereditary disease, "poor white-ism," and race degeneration. Its creation was a signal success for H. B. Fantham, who also managed to introduce eugenics into the research remit of the South African Association for the Advancement of Science. But Fantham's efforts to foster a "eugenic conscience" in the public at large (for example, by forming study circles or persuading schools in the Transvaal to include eugenics in the science syllabus) proved less successful, principally because of its implications for intra-white ethnic relations.

The Race Welfare Society pursued its program of practical eugenics through a network of birth control clinics that spread through South Africa in the 1930s. Its activities were supported by public health reformers within the state, like E. H. Cluver, whose official positions constrained them from advocating birth control measures. The strong presence of doctors and other professionals within the Race Welfare Society, coupled with its autonomous status, facilitated the spread of advice on birth-spacing to mainly working-class women. In this manner the Society allowed committed eugenists like Fantham to pursue "race improvement," while simultaneously providing a protective umbrella for those, frequently female, practitioners who were primarily concerned with the welfare of women. Klausen has amply demonstrated how birth control clinics, operating under the aegis of the Race Welfare Society, soon came under the influence of liberal social reformers whose main concern was with maternal health and the problems faced by the urban poor rather than with race degeneration as such.[15] The convergence of gender, color, class, and ethnic debates within the Society says much about the plasticity of eugenics in South Africa, as well as indicating how a coalition of professionals and self-appointed experts, with divergent political interests, could work together with some success.

Another aim of eugenists was sterilization of the mentally unfit, a measure strongly urged by Fantham and Dunston in the 1920s as well as by doctors like the Union Medical Officer of Health, Dr. Mitchell, and R. A. Forster, physician superintendent of the Alexandra Institute for the Feebleminded. Conversely, warnings of dire consequences for the white race and costs to the taxpayer were strongly refuted by members of the church as well as by doctors like H. Egerton Brown, superintendent of the Maritzburg Mental Hospital, who cited evidence from overseas, Britain in particular, indicating that opinion was swinging away from eugenic sterilization.[16]

Among those who cautioned against sterilization was Lancelot Hogben (1895–1975), then professor of zoology at the University of Cape Town. In 1931 the noted Afrikaans doctor and literary figure, C. Louis Leipoldt (1880–1947), retracted his earlier support, observing that the practice of sterilization was "fraught with grave dangers to the community."[17] The *Cape Times* began an editorial on "Frenzied Eugenics" in 1933 with the statement "Eugenics is not a science" and went on to warn about insidious developments in Nazi Germany.[18] A government interdepartmental committee into mental deficiency (focusing solely on feeblemindedness among whites) refrained from recommending compulsory sterilization when it reported in 1930. Debates about sterilization persisted into the mid-1930s, but the majority of public opinion was not in favor. In 1933 Department of Justice legal advisers concluded that in the absence of specific legislation, sterilization without consent would be legally tantamount to the infliction of serious bodily harm.

The vogue for sterilization in South Africa declined from the early 1930s, as it did in Britain which, as the ex-colonial power, continued to serve as an exemplar.[19] But there were reasons specific to South African conditions that made the prospect of eugenic sterilization controversial. Most important was the phenomenon of "poor white-ism," which came to the fore in the 1920s and 1930s as a social and economic problem requiring urgent attention. The great majority of these poor whites were Afrikaans-speakers. Afrikaner nationalist politicians were sensitive to any suggestion that white poverty was a result of innate "weakness," since this might imply that "their" people were unworthy of social support.[20] Instead, great emphasis was placed on the need to incorporate poor Afrikaners within the "volk" so as to build an ethnically based coalition capable of resisting imperial (and Jewish) economic power. Ideologues within the Afrikaner nationalist movement, as well as some English-speaking white labor leaders, insisted that unfair economic competition with blacks was the main reason for white poverty in the urban areas.

From 1924 to 1933 Hertzog's Afrikaner National Party governed in coalition with Labour. Extensive measures to protect "civilized" (white) workers from black competition in the workplace were introduced during this decade. Advocates of laissez-faire economics were wholly opposed to such protectionist policies and often argued that artificial support of inefficient whites was economically—as well as eugenically—counterproductive. For racial theorists like Fantham, white supremacy could only be maintained by ensuring that the quality of the white race, and its moral "prestige", would be maintained by means of eugenic policies and practices.

An alternative eugenic view was developed by the Rhodes University zoologist and ostrich-breeding expert, James E. Duerden (1865–1937), who thought white supremacy could be maintained by means of social reform rather than sterilization of the unfit. Duerden was sanguine about the possibility of achieving solidarity between the white "races." Since both ultimately derived from Dutch and British stock, "two of the most virile nations of Europe," they might together achieve "a new South African nationalism" compatible with membership of the emergent white commonwealth. Elaborating this theme to a scientific audience in an address on genetics and eugenics in 1925, Duerden criticized Fantham's hard biological determinism (he also rejected Weismann's views on the insoluble power of the "germ plasm") by pointing out that heredity was a process whose outcome involved complex interaction between genes as well as with environmental influences. For Duerden the prognosis for the reclamation of indigent whites was good if suitable investment in training and education was made available.[21]

AFRIKANER NATIONALISM AND APARTHEID

The effects of the 1929 world economic depression greatly intensified awareness of white poverty. But many Afrikaner nationalists were reluctant to mobilize publicly around an issue that could be a source of communal embarrassment. In 1929 the Afrikaans press had been vociferous in its criticism of E. G. Malherbe (1896–1983), a leading Afrikaans-speaking investigator on the Carnegie Commission, for pronouncing that white poverty was a "skeleton" in the Afrikaner cupboard and that a psychological "inferiority complex" caused by unconscious feelings of vulnerability had mistakenly led Afrikaners to blame "poor white-ism" on black competition in the labor market.[22] One Afrikaner intellectual who appreciated the severity of white poverty and saw how it could be utilized to pursue wider political objectives was Hendrik Verwoerd (1901–1966), the Stellenbosch University social psychologist who subsequently rose to international prominence as the principal architect of high apartheid in the 1950s and 1960s. In 1934 Verwoerd played a leading role in organizing a "Volkskongres" on the poor white question, insisting that the Afrikaner nation could save itself through a combination of state intervention and communal activity. Verwoerd had no qualms about dealing with black labor competition through discriminatory measures, yet it is worth noting that neither in his political nor in his academic career did he base the case of white supremacy on grounds of innate superiority.[23]

Afrikaner Nationalist unease with eugenics was intensified by religious sensibilities: it could not be overlooked that eugenics and allied forms of social Darwinism depended on a view of evolution that challenged scriptural orthodoxy. Such concerns were intensely felt by Christian-Nationalists, whose hold on radical Afrikaner politics strengthened from the 1930s.[24] Yet, nationalist intellectuals did not altogether disavow eugenic ideas. In the late 1930s, practitioners of psychometric testing, like M. L. Fick and J. A. J. van Rensburg, conducted tests that purported to demonstrate the intellectual inferiority of blacks. Their findings were eagerly adopted by Gerrie Eloff, a geneticist and member of the militant fascist Ossewabrandwag movement, who sought to reconcile eugenic ideas with Christian-National conceptions of the divine destiny of the Afrikaners. Eloff laid much store on what he saw as the Afrikaners' inherent aversion to racial intermixture. But he also believed that the Afrikaners' racial constitution, based on their unique genetic inheritance (Nordic and Alpine), was ideally suited to life in the African continent.

Eloff's ideas were enthusiastically picked up by Geoffrey Cronjé (1907–1992), a Pretoria university criminologist, who wrote a series of highly influential books in the 1940s elaborating the need for full-scale apartheid. Cronjé evinced a visceral brand of racism, assuring his audiences that biological research had proved that racial intermixture produced inferior human material (though he was also concerned that whites with the lowest mental capacities might not be able to compete with more able blacks). In Cronjé's view, only a policy of total apartheid could provide a solution to the racial question.[25]

The coincidence of extreme nationalism and scientific racism in the work of Eloff and Cronjé reached a peak in the early to mid-1940s, when fascist and Nazi ideas gained rapid ground within the Afrikaner nationalist leadership. Yet the appeal of fascism was offset by concerns that totalitarian ideologies venerating the state or a charismatic leader might displace the authority of the Church. Support for Hitler began to wane as Afrikaner political leaders realized that the Axis powers were losing the war, and the deeply divided Afrikaner nationalist movement gradually reunited around the political faction committed to pursuing the parliamentary road to apartheid. This was achieved in 1948 with the electoral triumph of the National Party.

Apartheid's victory occurred just as international opinion began to take stock of the horrors of the holocaust. The United Nations Declaration of Human Rights was signed in 1948, and it was at this time that UNESCO began work on a series of statements on race in an effort to engineer scientific consensus around the view that race was less a biological than a cultural and social phenomenon. The postwar era also witnessed the rise of mass nationalism and the beginnings of decolonization in Africa. Such developments all placed pressure on the new and still insecure Afrikaner regime to disclaim biological supremacy as a fundamental justification of apartheid. While there were always some who were ready to make the case, apartheid's ideologues in fact had no need to over-invest in concepts of biological race.[26] Appeals to the more flexible language of cultural difference and ethnic nationalism were in many ways better suited to nationalist needs: they fitted in well with romantic Christian-National beliefs in the divine calling of the Afrikaner *volk*; they facilitated the claim that South Africa was founded on the just principle of "unity in diversity"; and they permitted apartheid's apologists to reject accusations of racism by maintaining that the country's policies were based around a positive recognition of human difference, which took into account historical and social realities.

A new, specialized field of *volkekunde* (*volks* anthropology) emerged from the 1930s to dignify these claims and helped considerably to pave the path for the balkanization of the country through the creation of officially defined tribal/ethnic units or Bantu homelands from the 1960s. Clothed heavily in the precepts of ethnos theory, *volkekunde* reiterated the divinely ordained imperative for ethnically defined groups to express their inner nationalism by living in separate, bounded communities. To be sure, culturalist or ethnic-nationalist thinking did not dispense with race; rather, it amounted to an alternative form of essentialist discourse that gestured to, without depending on, biological determinism.

Eugenic ideas may have played no more than an ancillary role in the elaboration of apartheid theory, but they were always available for use, and they were sufficiently familiar to be referred to indirectly or inferentially. Along with appeals to tradition, culture, and the values of western Christian civilization, eugenic subtones were unavoidably present in the obsessive preoccupation with purity of blood and descent, in ever more absurd taxonomies of difference, and in the quest for an ordered, bounded, and regular society cleansed of polluting racial elements. Demographic anxieties evoked constant fears of *oorstrooming,* or inundation. Taken together, one might refer to this as a manifestation of popular or demotic eugenics. Liberal critics frequently argued that apartheid marked an atavistic return to pre-modern ways of thought, and that apartheid represented the victory of unscientific religious values over the mores of a sophisticated industrial society. This view overlooks the reality that apartheid's determined and remorseless imposition of racial constructs depended on a sophisticated, modern society with a developed state bureaucracy, legal system, and economy. Keith Breckenridge, who refers suggestively to South Africa as a "biometric state," has traced the use of systematic fingerprinting in the South African mines and in police records back to the beginnings of formalized segregation in 1902 (drawing a suggestive link to Francis Galton's views on the utility of fingerprints in colonial governance). The notorious pass law (or *dompas*) system, which was extended to all Africans in the 1950s, depended heavily on an ambitious (and ultimately chaotic) system of universal fingerprinting whose scope was, in its time, unprecedented in the world.[27]

Verwoerd's biometric project was predicated on the 1950 Population Registration Act that assigned a preset racial category to every individual in the country. Apartheid's social engineers devised sophisticated techniques of enumeration in the pursuit of what Deborah Posel calls a "high-modernist fantasy"[28]—a modern eugenic dystopia, one might add. Yet, it is well to remember that racial classification was not overreliant on scientific-based typologies: rough and ready techniques, including pencils inserted into hair to judge the springiness of curls, proved more than adequate to the task. Social convention, bureaucratic logic, legality, and the authority of lived experience, remained the key arbiters of racial belonging. Thus, while apartheid fully expressed the biopolitics of racial rule, it was sustained by wider social structures and popular racist fears that continued to be embedded in white society over the twentieth century.

FRONTIER LABORATORIES: SOUTHERN AFRICA

The recent tendency to see eugenics as a trans-national phenomenon fits well with reevaluations of the spread of scientific knowledge that eschew mechanistic models of the transmission of ideas from "core" to "periphery." Although intellectuals in colonial societies like South Africa looked to metropolitan science to validate their ideas and social standing, the ideologies they developed were seldom merely derivative. New contexts required fresh adaptations, and the confluence of different variants of racial thinking could mean that eugenics acquired a degree of hybrid vigor. The influence of eugenic ideas may have been particularly potent when they were introduced into societies where intellectual elites were relatively small, where there was fresh scope for social experimentation, and where scientific access to decision-makers was more immediate than may have been the case in mature European societies.

Scholars of empire have shown that practitioners of applied science, in fields ranging from medicine and veterinary science to agriculture and forestry, frequently exerted disproportionate influence in the colonial context. The permeable "periphery" could itself be a "frontier" for testing out new ideas. This was one reason why so many scientists, eugenists among them, traveled to the colonies to establish their reputations. Indeed, several key figures in international racial science—among them Francis Galton, Robert Knox, Eugen Fischer, as well as that articulate critic of eugenics, Lancelot Hogben—were shaped by their formative experiences in South Africa.

Strictly speaking, the term "southern Africa" may be more apt because, in the case of Galton and Fischer, their research activity actually took place in present-day Namibia. A German colony until South Africa took control of the territory during World War I, it was in Namibia that Hereros were systematically massacred in the 1904–1907 war—an event that in recent years has increasingly come to be seen as a prototypical act of racial genocide.[29] Southern Rhodesia (Zimbabwe) was also closely linked to South Africa until it cut itself off from formal association with the Union by electing to become a self-governing colony from 1923; the workings of the Rhodesian native affairs department and the pattern of its segregationist legislation bear ready comparison with that of South Africa, and Rhodesian missionaries and anthropologists developed similar discussions about the nature of the "native mind."

As in South Africa, eugenics was widely discussed by opinion-formers in the context of discussions about segregation and degeneration.[30] A Rhodesian magistrate, Peter Nielsen, wrote a trenchant anti-racist tract in 1922, affirming that the characteristics and capacities of whites and blacks were fundamentally the same. The title of his book, *The Black Man's Place in South Africa*, suggests that he was thinking of the region as a whole. Yet, there are significant differences: Southern Rhodesian settler society was far smaller than in South Africa, political divisions between Afrikaans- and English-speakers were much less marked, and it was industrialized to a far lesser degree than its neighbor to the south. To this extent, the intellectual culture of Rhodesia seems to bear closer comparison with colonial Kenya, where eugenics was narrowly concentrated around a relatively few individuals.[31]

South African society was sufficiently complex—as well as economically advanced and institutionally developed—to sustain more than a single core of intellectuals and politicians with an interest in eugenics. The study of eugenics formed part of a wider effort to modernize racial rule in the country. It offered new justifications of innate difference, allowed its adherents and experts to make claims for resources, and played an important role in promoting South Africa as a field for international scientific discovery. Indeed, in the interwar years politician-statesmen like Jan Hofmeyr (1894–1948) and Jan Smuts (1870–1950) went out of their way to represent the country's potential as an international "laboratory" for the study of racial problems.

Eugenics took on its own local coloring in South Africa because it featured as part of an ideological amalgam that supported segregationist as well as apartheid thinking. The capacity of segregationist and apartheid logic speak to different constituencies and to draw on multiple sources of authority—even if these were internally inconsistent or contradictory—helps to explain the persistence of racial rule in South Africa through the twentieth century. Eugenics was an important resource, but it was never relied upon as the sole form of authority. The problematic status of poor whites in the segregationist era and the rapidly changing international climate of opinion on racial difference during the apartheid period meant that eugenics had only limited utility.

We have seen that eugenic ideas were sometimes expressed in conventional terms and contexts, most obviously in the intelligence testing movement, in psychiatry, and in attempts to introduce birth control and sterilization. More often it registered its presence within other concerns. It aroused the greatest degree of popular concern around the fear of miscegenation and bodily pollution, but in most cases such fears were confirmed by an awareness of eugenics rather than aroused by it. Eugenic ideas were also evident in wider intellectual treatments of race—for instance, in the claims of physical anthropology, in historical accounts of the peopling of the subcontinent, and also in explorations of "whiteness." Under apartheid, an undeclared form of state eugenics was practiced through the process of ordering, enumerating, and controlling black South Africans. Racial Malthusianism was also prominent in apartheid demography.

As in other contexts, South African eugenics operated both intra- and interracially. Whether experts were grounded in the views of Mendel and Weismann, on the one hand, or of Lamarck on the other, was relatively unimportant—it was perfectly possible to be a Mendelian in theory but a Lamarckian in practice. Similarly, in accounts of racial difference, cultural essentialism merged with biological determinism. Such inconsistencies could be an ideological strength, since advocates of racial superiority were often more concerned to lay claim to scientific authority and apt to make selective use of racial theories than they were with abiding by the internal logic of an argument. Thus, eugenics provided a discursive resource that was seized upon by intellectuals and politicians seeking authority for their actions and ideas—albeit with little concern for argumentative rigor or formal coherence. As a result, it might be useful to see eugenics as a scavenger science, or perhaps even a virus, feeding on whatever was available, utilized by political hosts, and adapting itself in the process.

ACKNOWLEDGMENTS

Thanks to Susanne Klausen for her comments.

NOTES

1. Zine Magubane, *Bringing the Empire Home: Race, Class, and Gender in Britain and Colonial South Africa* (Chicago, IL: University of Chicago Press, 2004).

2. Alan Lester, *Imperial Networks: Creating Identities in Nineteenth-century South Africa and Britain* (London and New York: Routledge, 2001).

3. See for example, George W. Stow, *The Native Races of South Africa* (London: S. Sonnenschein, 1905); Sir Harry H. Johnston, *A History of the Colonization of Africa by Alien Races* (Cambridge: Cambridge University Press, 1899); George McCall Theal, *The Yellow and Dark-Skinned People of South Africa South of the Zambesi* (London: Swan Sonnenschein, 1910).

4. C. Headlam (ed.) *The Milner Papers. South Africa, 1897–1899*, 2 vols. (London: Cassell and Co., 1931), 1: 234, Milner to Selborne, 9 May 1898.

5. "A Review of the Present Mutual Relations of the British South African Colonies. Memorandum Prepared by the Earl of Selborne at the Request of the Government of Cape Colony, 1 January, 1907," in *Select Documents Relating to the Unification of South Africa*, ed. Arthur Percival Newton, 2 vols. (London: Frank Cass, 1968), 2: 54–5. Compare, with the Colonial Office memorandum drafted by Selborne in 1896 which reflected on "racial rivalries" in the following terms: "Dutch and English; English and Dutch. Most curiously though sprung from the same stock, the two races do not amalgamate. It shows what a lot of Celtic and Norman blood must be infused in us." Cited in R. Robinson and John Gallagher, *Africa and the Victorians* (London: Macmillan, 1961), 435.

6. Paul Rich, "Race, Science, and the Legitimization of White Supremacy in South Africa, 1902–1940," *The International Journal of African Historical Studies* 23, no. 4 (1990): 665–686.

7. Saul Dubow, *Scientific Racism in Modern South Africa* (Cambridge: Cambridge University Press, 1995); Dubow, *A Commonwealth of Knowledge: Science, Sensibility and White South Africa, 1820–2000* (Oxford and New York: Oxford University Press, 2006).

8. Rich, "Race, Science," 679–680.

9. Don Foster, "Historical and Legal Traces 1800–1990," in *Perspectives on Mental Handicap in South Africa*, eds. Susan Lea and Don Foster (Durban: Butterworths, 1990).

10. Dubow, *Scientific Racism*, 147–149.

11. See for example, Timothy Keegan, "Gender, Degeneration and Sexual Danger: Imagining Race and Class in South Africa, ca. 1912," *Journal of Southern African Studies (JSAS)* 27, no. 3 (2001): 459–477.

12. Mohamed Adhikari, *Not White Enough, Not Black Enough. Racial Identity in the South African Coloured Community* (Athens, OH: Ohio University Press, 2005), 24–25.

13. See for example, H. B. Fantham, "Some Factors in Eugenics, together with Notes on Some South African Cases," *South African Journal of Science (SAJS)* 22 (1925): 400–424; H. B. Fantham and Annie Porter, "Notes on Some Cases of Racial Admixture in South Africa," *SAJS* 24 (1927): 476–485.

14. Reginald Ruggles Gates, *Heredity in Man* (London: Constable, 1929), 329, 332, 333.

15. Susanne M. Klausen, "The Race Welfare Society: Eugenics and Birth Control in Johannesburg, 1930–40," in *Science and Society in Southern Africa*, ed. Saul Dubow(Manchester: Manchester University Press, 2000).

16. H. Egerton Brown, "The Sterilisation of the Mentally Defective," *South African Medical Journal* 6, no. 4 (1932): 107–111.

17. *Cape Times*, 15 June 1928; *Cape Times*, September 18, 1931.

18. "Frenzied Eugenics," *Cape Times*, August 5, 1933.

19. Desmond King and Randall Hansen, "Experts at Work: State Autonomy, Social Learning and Eugenic Sterilisation in 1930s Britain," *British Journal of Political Science* 29, no. 1 (1999): 77–107.

20. Saul Dubow, "Scientism, Social Research and the Limits of South Africanism: The Case of E. G. Malherbe," *South African Historical Journal* 44 (2001): 99–142.

21. J. E. Duerden, "Social Anthropology in South Africa: Problems of Race and Nationality," *SAJS* 18 (1921): 1–31; Duerden, "Genetics and Eugenics in South Africa: Heredity and Environment," *SAJS* 22 (1925): 59–72; Duerden, "Genesis and Reclamation of the Poor White in South Africa," *The Eugenics Review* XIV (1922–1923).

22. Dubow, "Scientism."

23. Roberta Balstad Miller, "Science and Society in the Early Career of H.F. Verwoerd," *JSAS* 19, no. 4 (1993): 634–661.

24. Saul Dubow, "Afrikaner Nationalism, Apartheid and the Conceptualisation of 'Race,'" *Journal of African History* 33, no. 2 (1992): 209–237.

25. Dr. G. Cronjé, *'n Tuiste vir die Nageslag* (Johannesburg: Publicité Handelsreklamediens, 1945); Cronjé, *Voogdyskap en Apartheid* (Pretoria: Van Schaik, 1948).

26. Hermann Giliomee, *The Afrikaners, Biography of a People* (London: Hurst, 2003), 470.

27. Keith Breckenridge, "Verwoerd's Bureau of Proof: Total Information in the Making of Apartheid," *History Workshop Journal* 59, no. 1 (2005): 83–108.

28. Deborah Posel, "Race as Common Sense: Racial Classification in Twentieth-Century South Africa," *African Studies Review* 44, no. 2 (2001), 100.

29. See, for example, Tilman Dedering, "The German-Herero War of 1904: Revisionism of Genocide or Imaginary Historiography?" *JSAS* 19, no. 1 (1993): 80–88.

30. Diana Jeater, *Law, Language, and Science. The Invention of the "Native Mind" in Southern Rhodesia, 1890–1930* (Portsmouth: Heinemann, 2007).

31. Chloe Campbell, *Race and Empire: Eugenics in Colonial Kenya* (Manchester: Manchester University Press, 2007).

FURTHER READING

Appel, Stephen W. " 'Outstanding Individuals Do Not Arise from Ancestrally Poor Stock': Racial Science and the Education of Black South Africans," *The Journal of Negro Education* 58, no. 4 (1989): 544–557.

Bank, Andrew. "Of 'Native Skulls' and 'Noble Caucasians': Phrenology in Colonial South Africa," *Journal of Southern African Studies* 22, no. 3 (1996): 387–403.

Coetzee, J. M. *White Writing: On the Culture of Letters in South Africa* (New Haven, CT: Yale University Press, 1989).

Distiller, Natasha and Steyn, Melissa (eds.). *Under Construction: 'Race' and Identity in South Africa Today* (Sandton: Heinemann, 2004).

Klausen, Susanne M. *Race, Maternity and the Politics of Birth Control in South Africa, 1910–1939* (Basingstoke: Palgrave, 2004).

MacDonald, Michael. *Why Race Matters in South Africa* (Cambridge, MA: Harvard University Press, 2006).

Thompson, Leonard. *The Political Mythology of Apartheid* (New Haven, CT: Yale University Press, 1985).

CHAPTER 16

EUGENICS IN COLONIAL KENYA

CHLOE CAMPBELL

IN the British East African colony of Kenya, a small but vociferous eugenics movement emerged in the 1930s. This chapter will provide an overview of how eugenic thought manifested in Kenya and will explain why the Kenyan movement failed to make the impact its members had hoped to achieve, both locally and within the British establishment. While the flurry of eugenic activity that emanated from Nairobi in the 1930s was at one level a minor sideshow in the colony's broader history, it nonetheless constitutes a telling chapter in the history of the relationship between eugenics and colonial culture, showing us how British mainline eugenics could be applied to colonial debates on racial affairs.

Kenya's eugenicists came from the colony's small British population, which numbered some 16,800 in 1931. Both the official community, which worked as a part of the colonial administration, and the non-official settler population, which had been establishing itself in gradually increasing numbers since the late nineteenth century, took an interest in eugenics. The Kenya Society for the Study of Race Improvement (KSSRI) was formed in Nairobi in 1933. These "Race Improvers" were interested in eugenics and social hygiene in their broader forms, but more specifically they became connected with contentious research on race and intelligence, which gave Kenyan eugenics a particular notoriety and vehemence. The Kenyan eugenicists' work became controversial when they sought to acquire funds from the British government to establish a program of research into the differences in brain structure and mental development among East Africans and Europeans. Central to the Kenyan eugenicists' claims about the importance of promoting a colonial eugenic research center was their apparent finding that the mental development reached by the average East African adult was that of the average European boy of about eight.[1]

THE KENYAN EUGENICIST DOCTORS

The application of eugenics to a new environment raises questions about the individuals who served as conduits for these ideas. In Britain, the Eugenics Society tended to attract experts in related, specialized fields, such as genetics. In contrast, the main sources of information on eugenics in Kenya were British medical doctors, who either worked in general practice as colonial medical officers or whose field of practice was unrelated to genetic science. For example, Henry Laing Gordon (1865–1947) was a psychiatrist and James Sequeira (1865–1948) a dermatologist, and though neither was expert in genetics or evolutionary biology, they enjoyed high professional repute in Kenya. Their audience, while consisting of doctors and those who formed the educated, "literary" section of the settler community, was not in a position to make alternative assertions about the processes of human heredity. Hence local knowledge of eugenics was largely enforced by the expertise and interests of Henry Gordon, in particular.

Gordon had settled in Kenya in 1925, having acquired land under a scheme to provide greater access to medical facilities for settlers. He became increasingly interested in mental health and set up a private practice in Nairobi, in 1929 becoming a private consultant for European cases at Mathari Mental Hospital, the only mental health facility in the colony at the time. In 1931 Gordon's role expanded to that of visiting physician, responsible for the psychiatric treatment of all races at Mathari. Gordon was a key early figure in an East African school of psychiatry that achieved "a degree of intellectual autonomy and authority within the colonies as representative of baseline psychological research conducted from the field."[2] By the 1930s, toward the end of his career, much of his thinking was informed by an increasingly dated brand of "mainline" eugenics that was being contested by critics both within and outside the Eugenics Society in Britain. Mainline eugenics in Britain was characterized by an often politically conservative bent that accommodated simplistic generalizations about race and gender hierarchies; it was, as Kevles has argued, superseded, in the 1930s, by the more nuanced and scientifically informed "reform" eugenics.[3] Kenyan eugenics in the 1930s showed no sign of this development from mainline to reform thinking. Of special significance in the translation of eugenics to Kenya was that when examining race, an area for which British eugenics had not prescribed a methodology, the Kenyan doctors used biological measurements of brain capacity and cell structure rather than the pedigrees, statistics, and population surveys that were applied at that time in Britain to the measurement of social class and intelligence.

In the 1930s eugenics became a serious preoccupation within the medical profession in Kenya; Kenyan eugenicist doctors made their agenda central to debates about African welfare and development and related medico-legal questions. Missionary doctors, however, were conspicuously absent in supporting eugenic research. The Dean of Nairobi Cathedral, Reverend Wright, was a high-profile supporter of the KSSRI, but, as one missionary pointed out in the correspondence pages of the *East African Standard (EAS)*, the KSSRI had no official approval of any Church authority.[4] The incompatibility of missions and eugenics had various underlying causes. Eugenics was almost never accepted by the Roman Catholic Church. Protestant missionaries, although not doctrinally opposed to eugenics as were Catholics, were likely to be suspicious of eugenics because of the long-standing association of atheism and the Darwinian roots of eugenics.

The division between these traditions was compounded in Kenya by the question of native interests; the education and development being encouraged by missionaries were contrary to Kenyan eugenic fears that meliorative practices were unsuitable and even dangerous when applied to Africans. In a letter to the British Eugenics Society, Gordon himself wrote that he was viewed with suspicion by the missionary organizations in Kenya, which saw him as hostile to their work in African education and development.[5]

However, senior members of the Colonial Medical Administration were actively supportive of eugenics. Two directors of Medical and Sanitary Services in Kenya, Dr. John Gilks (1881–1971) and Dr. Albert Paterson (1885–1959), two directors of Medical Services in Uganda, Dr. William Kauntze (1887–1947) and Dr. Hugh Trowell (1904–1989), and the long-serving editor of the *East African Medical Journal (EAMJ)*, James Sequeira, were involved. Eugenic thinking was therefore more than peripheral among Kenyan doctors; it was expounded by some of the most powerful people within the profession. John Gilks, for example, was director of Medical and Sanitary Services until his retirement in 1933, when he returned to England and was elected a member of the Council of the British Medical Association (BMA). In 1934 Gilks joined the Council of the British Eugenics Society and in 1936 he became deputy chairman of the Dominions Committee of the BMA. Gilks became an important figure in Gordon's campaign because of his seniority and because he provided a well-connected base in Britain; he was also well-known for the work that he undertook on public health and nutrition in Kenya.[6]

One of the reasons why the theories of the Kenyan eugenicists about African mental capacity were considered so compelling by this milieu was because they were applied to the concept of colonial trusteeship: the idea that colonial rule involved an obligation to protect the interests of the native population. In Kenya in the interwar period, this also implied the protection of African interests in the face of the vexed political issues arising from the competing demands of both the European and Indian communities. The eugenicist doctors argued that a modern notion of trusteeship should involve a program of "scientific colonization" and that the colonial project presented an unprecedented opportunity to build new societies on modern, eugenic principles.

The Kenyan eugenicists were particularly vocal in the areas of juvenile delinquency, education, and the diagnosis and treatment of the criminally insane. This in itself flags one of the apparent paradoxes of Kenyan eugenics, but one that builds on a theme commonly found in eugenic thought in many different contexts: Kenya's white eugenicists, whether they came from the colonial administration or the wider settler community, were not exclusively drawn from the most racially hostile members of the European community. Indeed, Kenyan eugenicists were often concerned with native development and welfare, issues that were dismissed by more politically extreme settlers for whom African welfare was a waste of resources. Some of those who supported establishing a center for research on race and intelligence in Nairobi were colonial officials regarded by other Europeans within the colony as dangerously "pro-native." William Kauntze (1912–1945) is a good example. Director of the Colonial Medical Service in Uganda from 1933, an editorial committee member of the *EAMJ*, and later chief medical adviser to the Colonial Office in London, Kauntze was "a doctor of strong humanitarian principles" and actively encouraged the training of African laboratory assistants.[7] He was certainly not a man who followed the vein of violent race hostility that characterized a strong strand of colonial settler culture. Kauntze was, however, frequently cited as a high-profile supporter of the campaign to promote research on race and intelligence. Race was such a preoccupation in colonial Kenya, and the use of biological language when discussing race so rooted, that eugenic attitudes appear pervasive, even among people who would not necessarily have described themselves as eugenicists. This slippage was intensified by the fact that eugenic thinking was so flexible, accommodating quite different motivations and levels of commitment. In Kenya, there was considerable shared ground between "mainline" or traditional eugenicists and those who were prepared to involve themselves in the scientific problematizing of racial difference.

The case of Albert Paterson (1885–1959) provides another example of the difficulty in defining how an interest in eugenics and support for research on mental development in Africa, did not imply necessary collusion with the more typical Kenyan eugenicist stance on race and intelligence. Paterson was deputy director of Medical and Sanitary Services in Kenya from 1920 to 1933, when he succeeded Gilks as director, a post he held until his retirement in 1943. Paterson was on the committee of the KSSRI,[8] and became embroiled in the campaign for the funding of a research project on the East African brain. Much of Paterson's writing tended toward environmentalism.[9] Although this largely precluded a belief in biologically innate mental difference, for Paterson the function of education in Kenya and the purpose of the research lay in aiding the project of African modernization and development.[10] His approach fell into the social hygiene category which encompassed both environmentalist and eugenic approaches in the pursuit of a biologically improved society. Paterson's case underscores the lack of homogeneity in eugenic thinking; his outlook was quite different from Gordon's; yet, as director of Medical Services, he won the support of the Kenyan government for research funding. He also attempted, less successfully, to acquire the support of the British Government. The involvement of these liberal colonial medical officials with a meliorist agenda demonstrates that the theories propounded by the Kenyan eugenicists were not exclusively the scientific expression of belligerent settler racism, although their ideas were associated with that perspective. Eugenics and its application to race and intelligence took root in the Kenyan medical profession because it promised biological solutions to perceived social problems, in particular African "backwardness" and the shape of future African development.

The first piece of research that Gordon undertook on African intelligence was his 1930 study of mental deficiency at Kabete Reformatory for juvenile offenders.[11] Gordon's work was significant partly because the results were produced at a time when a serious review of the reformatory and the management of juvenile offenders in Kenya was beginning, and although the study was not published, it was widely read among officials and gave Gordon credibility.[12] As director of Medical Services, Gilks circulated the report widely.[13] Gordon's experiment at the Reformatory used a range of methods to come to the extraordinary conclusion that of the 219 inmates he measured, not one attained the European standard of normal intelligence. This led him to conclude that the normative standard of African intelligence was different and that the level of this difference had to be established. In the course of his inquiry, Gordon made over 40 visits to the Reformatory and used a combination of measurements and tests: "Anthropological measurements, of physiological tests, of clinical examination more particularly of the nervous system and to detect abnormalities attributable to defects of germ plasm (so-called stigmata), and of psychological or mental tests."[14] Gordon borrowed this combination of methods from the eminent English anatomist and eugenicist Professor Richard Berry (1867–1962).

In 1930 Gordon published an article in the *Kenya and East African Medical Journal* (renamed the *East African Medical Journal* in 1931), which built on his report on Kabete and lay the basis for much of the Kenyan eugenic argument about the innate mental capacity of the native and the implications for social policy. The theory was that among "raw natives"—those untouched by Western culture—the cultural level was so low that high-grade "aments" could flourish:[15]

> ...free breeding of high grade aments under primitive conditions may be a hidden eugenic factor in racial retardation in Africa, just as it may be (and is believed to be) a grave threat of racial degeneration in Europe. It is conceivable that absence of economic pressure and of industrial competition, coupled with advantages of tribal life in Reserves, leaves unrestricted the fecundity of high grade aments.[16]

The problems of amentia were most acute when the native was no longer on the reserve but urbanized, and in European employment or education. Native amentia was thus linked to development. The incidence of amentia was so high that it became the normative level within the African population. The numbers were too great to enable the application of traditional eugenic policies of segregation and sterilization: the possibility of sterilization does not seem to have been an option proposed by the Kenyan eugenicists. The Kenyan response to the possibility of the segregation of the mentally unfit was to establish different standards for the entire African population that in effect meant segregation at a profound intellectual as well as practical level.

Following Gordon's work,[17] the government pathologist F. W. Vint published several articles on the subject of race and intelligence that were felt, both by the eugenicist doctors and also by officials, to add empirical weight to Gordon's theories.

His first major statement, "A Preliminary Note on the Cell Content of the Prefrontal Cortex of the East African Native" was published in the *EAMJ* in 1932.[18] A further article was published in the prestigious British *Journal of Anatomy* in 1934, entitled "The Brain of the Kenya Native."[19] Vint reported post-mortem analyses of adult male brains he had obtained from the native hospitals of Nairobi. By this stage Vint had performed macroscopic and microscopic examinations on 100 brains. He reported that his research indicated that the brain of the East African was smaller than that of the European and, even more significantly, that both the cortex and the cells in the cortex were smaller.[20] Vint's research was particularly potent because he was far less overtly political than Gordon and the other Race Improvers of Nairobi, and he was viewed as having serious scientific credentials.[21] The combination of Vint's apparent authoritative empiricism and Gordon and Gilks's vocal, high-profile connections with the British Eugenics Society seemed to create a potent basis for a campaign for funding to establish a full program of research on racial differences.

NAIROBI'S "RACE IMPROVERS"

Beyond Kenyan medical circles, public interest in eugenics was strong enough to justify the formation of the KSSRI in 1933. Early in 1933 a public lecture Gordon gave on eugenics was so successful that a repeat was requested to accommodate a larger audience. Held in March 1933, the lecture led to the formation of the Race Improvement Society.[22] An impression of the content of Kenyan eugenic discourse can be made from a pamphlet entitled "Eugenics and the Truth about Ourselves in Kenya."[23] Based on one of Gordon's public lectures, it was a dramatic and urgent exposition of eugenics and its importance in the colonial environment. The pamphlet explained the tenets of eugenics, emphasizing that "Eugenics aims to raise the average ability of the race at birth, by greater attention to nature." Gordon warned that currently "daily, hourly, too few normals, too many subnormals, are added to the population. *If this is allowed to go on we cannot avoid the sinking to a level beyond rescue*."[24] Gordon proceeded to apply the principles of mainline British eugenics to the racial circumstances of Kenya: the African population replaced the British urban working classes as the genetically inferior stock, threatening to swamp the country. The damaging effect of the presence of poor whites was felt to add additional urgency to the eugenic situation in Kenya:

> We are developing a *poor white group, a submerged Asiatic group,* and a *huge African group* of alarming potentialities. The reason is most evident in the case of the native. TRUSTEESHIP is being interpreted as *nurture* only. We are trying to create a new civilisation by repeating the old problem of neglecting nature.[25]

Gordon urged that in the face of these dangers, it was essential that only fertile, high-quality British stock be admitted to the colony: "not retired breeders from Anglo-India or elsewhere." Race improvement, in this context, was addressed to the white population as much as the native population.

On forming the KSSRI, Gordon wrote to the Eugenics Society in Britain, asking for support.[26] He was met with enthusiasm and the offer of a supply of eugenic literature, as well as interest from the National Council of Mental Hygiene and the Child Guidance Council. Also circulating among Kenyan eugenicists was South African literature on the problem of poor whites.[27] Gordon and his colleagues saw eugenics as an imperial movement with international implications. Emphasis was also placed on the high status of its Kenyan members, as "great leaders" in the areas of "Church, Medicine, Law and Science."[28] The rules for the KSSRI stated that membership was open only to Europeans. Members of the Indian community attended the public lectures but were not permitted membership. As Gordon put it: "Possibly 10 per cent [of the audience] would be Indian, equally intelligent [as the European population] but recklessly prolific in procreation."[29]

The membership of the KSSRI in 1933 was about 60.[30] Seemingly small, but given that the KSSRI only permitted European members, in fact it attracted a greater number in relation to overall population than the British Eugenics Society (768 in 1932). Membership numbers, moreover, do not tell the whole story. As Geoffrey Searle has argued in relation to Britain, eugenics advocates were more interested in attracting influential and academically esteemed members than in mass recruitment.[31] Gordon described those interested in his lectures as "mostly British of the intelligent middle-upper class, including civil servants."[32] The *EAS* reported that the inaugural meeting, held at Nairobi's New Stanley Hotel, was attended by "leading professional and businessmen."[33] Members of the KSSRI tended to move in the circles of Kenya's social and administrative elite, for example Daphne Moore, who was on the committee of the KSSRI; her husband, Sir Henry Monck-Mason Moore (1887–1964) was colonial secretary in the early 1930s and acting governor for five months in 1933. The chairman of the society was R. F. Mayer, an influential figure in the European settler community owing to his control of the *East African Standard*. Another influential member on the KSSRI committee was the Reverend R. V. Wright, Dean of Nairobi Cathedral. Grant described him as "the next best man to Gordon... He is terrifically eugenic minded."[34]

Judging by the descriptions of public meetings, which permitted non-members, there was also significant general interest in eugenics among European settlers. One Race Improver, Eleanor Grant (1885–1977), spoke of there being "100s of people" at the first meeting of the KSSRI, and later wrote of people "flocking in to the RI [Race Improvement] Society."[35] There was enough interest in "Race Improvement" to lead to the foundation of another branch of the KSSRI at Nakuru in November 1933.[36] The letters written by Eleanor Grant to her daughter, the writer Elspeth Huxley (1907–1997), provide a useful account of the social composition and attitudes that characterized the eugenics movement in Kenya. Grant was of the settler social elite; of British aristocratic background, her values, in particular her devotion to the creation of a rural, agricultural idyll in the colony, reflected the anti-urban inclinations of settler society. Along with this conservatism, Grant also displayed a modern interest and faith in the progressive nature of science, particularly biology; her letters convey a typically eugenic espousal of a materialist, biological pragmatism that she placed in opposition to Victorian squeamishness and sentimentalism.

The KSSRI was active for just a few years in the 1930s; it petered out as it lost some of its key members. Many of its leaders—Gordon, Gilks, Sequeira—were heavily focused on the objective of obtaining high-profile support in Britain for their cause, and they did not have strong institutional or localized policy ambitions within the colony.[37] As Kenya's leading eugenicists became increasingly involved in the campaign in Britain, it seems they were less interested in the day-to-day running of a local society and Kenya's settler population did not generate the local personnel to sustain an organization such as the KSSRI independently.

METROPOLITAN RESPONSES

In order to understand the demise of the Kenyan eugenics movement, it is necessary to investigate its reception in Britain. In the 1930s the Kenyan eugenicists became involved in a campaign to obtain funding from the British government to establish a large research program in Nairobi dedicated to investigating the causes of African mental backwardness. The Kenyan colonial administration was unable to fund such a program, so it was essential to obtain intellectual legitimacy from British experts and to convince the British government that this was a project worth supporting. The reception of the Kenyan work in Britain was mixed. It garnered great initial interest, but the controversial nature of the research also raised considerable concern at a time when the question of race in science was being contested. Ultimately, these concerns, coupled with the suspicions of the British government about the racial agenda for which Kenyan settler politics had become notorious, meant that official backing was rejected.

Connections between the British and Kenyan eugenicists seem to have been initially forged in 1930, when Gordon sent a copy of his report on Kabete Reformatory to the British Eugenics Society.[38] The paper went over very well, described as being "of great interest and value."[39] Gordon continued a cordial correspondence with Carlos Blacker (1895–1975), general secretary of the Eugenics Society from 1931 to 1952, and the Eugenics Society gave its support and promised to do its "utmost to assist" the newly formed KSSRI.[40] The links between the Kenyan eugenicist doctors and the British Eugenics Society intensified in 1933, when Gordon was given special leave by the Kenyan medical department to visit London to publicize his theories and to pursue funding. During his stay Gordon addressed a meeting of the Eugenics Society with the paper "Amentia in the East African," which was published in the *Eugenics Review* the following year.[41]

In November 1933 the British Eugenics Society publicized the Kenyan research in letters to *The Times,* the Colonial Office, and the Economic Advisory Council (EAC),[42] hoping to spark a debate about the Kenyan research on race and intelligence.

The letters called for Gordon and Vint's research to be given more serious consideration, and pointed to the need for a more extended inquiry, arguing that: "successful native policy can only be laid down on a sure foundation of ascertained fact, and a correct evaluation of the capacity of the peoples concerned."[43] The signatories included high-profile figures from the British Eugenics Society, such as Sir Humphrey Rolleston (1862–1944), president of the Eugenics Society; Frank Crew (1886–1973), professor of Genetics at the Animal Breeding Research Institute at Edinburgh University; and Julian Huxley (1887–1975).[44] Interestingly, Frank Crew was one of the reform geneticists who warned of the danger of underestimating the role of environment in human behavior and development. Similarly, Huxley was a key figure in the emergence of reform eugenics and can be seen as a kind of hinge character in questioning the formulation of race in science. Elazar Barkan describes a "duality" in Huxley's ideas about race in the early 1930s: "At this stage Huxley was non-racist in his descriptions and analyses, but continued to take a racist stand when it came to conjectures."[45]

The Kenyan research was immediately recognized as controversial in Britain. The physical anthropologist Louis Leakey (1903–1972), who had grown up in Kenya with his missionary parents, was among the first to react, with a wide-ranging critique of the methodology and assumptions of the research.[46] Further notable criticism came from the eminent left-wing geneticist J. B. S. Haldane (1892–1964).[47] Staff at the Colonial Office in London followed this debate about African intelligence with growing distaste, particularly after *The Times* published follow-up letters by Gilks and Gordon, which did nothing to allay official concerns about the extremity of the Kenyan position.[48] The Colonial Office had initially been tolerant of the Kenyan eugenicists, receiving their requests for funding and support with either genuine engagement or, more often, polite but fundamentally unimpressed interest. In 1934 the governor, Joseph Byrne (1874–1942), wrote to the Colonial Office supporting the work of the Kenyan doctors.[49] Eventually the prime minister, Ramsay MacDonald (1866–1937), referred the request to Sir Malcolm Hailey (1872–1969), who was embarking on his famous review of African conditions, *An African Survey*.[50] MacDonald was particularly anxious that government involvement might have political ramifications in South Africa. Political concerns, along with the sense that investment in this type of research was not the business of government, constituted a firm basis for vetoing official involvement with the project.

Malcolm Hailey and his colleagues on *An African Survey* were skeptical about the Kenyan research, regarding it as "amateurish and inadequate."[51] As early as 1933, concerns had been raised about the suspiciously immaculate nature of Gordon's findings by those involved in the African Research Survey in Oxford. Hilda Matheson (1888–1940), the secretary of the Survey, wrote of Gordon's results, "they are too perfect to convince anyone, and...no scientist ever gets results where everything appears to fit your theory so completely and nothing occurs to be placed on the other side."[52]

These doubts bring us to a wider point about Gordon's research, which apparently tested an enormous subject group of 3,444 individuals and involved a large and time-consuming range of tests.[53] It is not clear how or when Gordon was able to undertake this extensive program of research, with neither financial assistance nor expert research personnel.[54] The claims of the Kenyan eugenicists to have science on their side looked increasingly weak when examined by British experts. The final blow to the Kenyan eugenics campaign came with the publication of *An African Survey* in 1938, which dismissed the possibility of an inquiry into mental capacity of the African brain as incapable of producing results of any social and political value, and further questioning the objectivity of the Kenyan work.[55]

The Kenyan eugenics movement was supported, to different degrees, by successive governors, directors of education and health, the acting chief native commissioner, as well as district commissioners. The dean of Nairobi Cathedral, both the managing director and editor of the main daily newspaper of the colony, as well as many socially influential settlers were involved in the movement. By the late 1930s, although there had been no radical change in settler attitudes toward race and no upheaval in the policy or personnel of the colonial administration, the enthusiasm for eugenics in Kenya faded, at least in public discourse. Without British support, Kenyan eugenics could not be sustained: the Kenyan European community lacked a critical mass of individuals with the intellectual and scientific interests and authority to establish a lasting, self-sufficient organization. The significance of the Kenyan eugenics movement lies largely in its revelations of the complexities of racial thinking in the colonial environment; how eugenic ideas enabled notions of race to creep into liberal colonial thinking, as well as serving the more obvious settler supremacist agenda of a colonial society so brutally shaped by racial division.

NOTES

1. F. W. Vint, "A Preliminary Note on the Cell Content of the Prefrontal Cortex of the East African Native," *East African Medical Journal (EAMJ)* 9, no. 32 (1932): 36.

2. Sloan Mahone, "East African Psychiatry and the Practical Problems of Empire," in *Psychiatry and Empire,* eds. Sloan Mahone and Megan Vaughan (Basingstoke: Macmillan, 2007), 41–66; see also Jock McCulloch, *Colonial Psychiatry and "the African Mind"* (Cambridge and New York: Cambridge University Press, 1995).

3. See Daniel J. Kevles, *In the Name of Eugenics: Genetics and the Uses of Human Heredity* (Cambridge, MA: Harvard University Press, 1995).

4. "Inquirer," to *East African Standard (EAS),* July 8, 1933, 35.

5. Gordon to Blacker, October 5, 1930, Eugenics Society Papers, SA/EUG/C.129, Wellcome Library, London. Permission to cite these papers has been kindly given by the Galton Institute, London.

6. J. L. Gilks and J. B. Orr, "The Nutritional Condition of the East African Native," *EAMJ* 4, no. 3 (1927): 85–90.

7. J. Iliffe, *East African Doctors* (Cambridge: Cambridge University Press, 1998), 47.

8. Enclosed notice with letter from Shaw to Blacker, July 4, 1933, Eugenics Society Papers, SA/EUG/C.129.

9. A. R. Paterson, "The Education of Backward Peoples," *EAMJ* 8, no. 11 (1932): 302.

10. Paterson, "The Education of Backward Peoples," 302.

11. H. L. Gordon, "Report of a Survey of the Inmates of Kabete Reformatory for the Purpose of Detecting the Presence of Amentia (Mental Deficiency)," Eugenics Society Papers, SA/EUG/C.129.

12. A fuller discussion of the role of eugenics in the discourse on juvenile delinquency can be found in Chloe Campbell, "Juvenile Delinquency in Colonial Kenya, 1900–1939," *Historical Journal* 45, no. 1 (2002): 129–151.

13. Gilks to Colonial Secretary, March 3, 1931, AP/1/699, Kenya National Archives (hereafter KNA), Nairobi; Minutes of the Meeting of the Committee of Visitors, December 3, 1930, AP/1/700, KNA.

14. Gordon, "Report of a Survey of the Inmates of Kabete Reformatory," 8.

15. "Amentia" was a term for mental deficiency; high-grade amentia was considered the least severe form of mental deficiency.

16. H. L. Gordon, "A Note on the Diagnosis of Amentia," *Kenya and East African Medical Journal* 7, no. 8 (1930): 210.

17. See H. L. Gordon, "Correspondence. The Educable Capacity of the African," *EAMJ* 9, no. 7 (1932): 210–212; H. L. Gordon, "Amentia in The East African," *Eugenics Review* 25, no. 4 (1934): 223–235; H. L. Gordon, "The Intentional Improvement of Backward Tribes," *EAMJ* 11, no. 5 (1934): 143–156.

18. F. W. Vint, "A Preliminary Note on the Cell Content."

19. F. W. Vint, "The Brain of the Kenya Native," *Journal of Anatomy* 68, no. 2 (1934): 216–223.

20. Ibid., 216.

21. Comment by Flood, May 17, 1937, CO 822/78/19, The National Archives of the UK (hereafter TNA), London.

22. "The Improvement of the Race," *EAS*, March 25, 1933.

23. H. L. Gordon, "Eugenics and the Truth about Ourselves in Kenya," CO 822/55/1, TNA.

24. Ibid., 2 [original italics].

25. Ibid., 3 [original italics].

26. Gordon to Moore, March 25, 1933, Eugenics Society Papers, SA/EUG/C.129.

27. "To Study Improvement of the Race," *EAS*, June 3, 1933.

28. Ibid.

29. Grant to Mrs Collyer, September 26, 1938, Eugenics Society Papers, SA/EUG/D.69.

30. Grant to Huxley, July 12, 1933, MSS Afr. s. 2154/1/1, Bodleian Library, University of Oxford.

31. G. R. Searle, "Eugenics and Politics in Britain in the 1930s," *Annals of Science* 36, no. 2 (1979): 160.

32. Gordon to Mrs. Collyer, September 26, 1938, Eugenics Society Papers, SA/EUG/D.69.

33. "To Study Improvement of the Race," *EAS*, June 3, 1933.

34. Grant to Huxley, July 12, 1933, MSS Afr. s. 2154/1/1, Bodleian Library.

35. Grant to Huxley, July 12, 1933; September 28, 1933, MSS Afr. s. 2154/1/1, Bodleian Library.

36. Grant to Huxley, November 9, 1933, MSS Afr. s. 2154/1/1, Bodleian Library.

37. Grant to Huxley, July 12, 1933, MSS Afr. s. 2154/1/1, Bodleian Library.

38. H. L. Gordon, "Report of a Survey of the Inmates of Kabete Reformatory," Eugenics Society Papers, SA/EUG/C.129.

39. Secretary to Gordon, January 21, 1931, Eugenics Society Papers, SA/EUG/C.129.

40. Blacker To Gordon, March 27, 1933, Eugenics Society Papers, SA/EUG/C.129.

41. Gordon, "Amentia in the East African," 223–235.

42. The EAC was set up in 1930 by Ramsay MacDonald. Its purpose was to establish a group of economic experts to advise the government on issues relating to economic policy.

43. Dawson of Penn, Lord Horder, H. Rolleston, A. Keith and E. Smith to *The Times,* November 25, 1933.

44. Huxley was only used as a signatory to the letters to the EAC and the Colonial Office.

45. Elazar Barkan, *The Retreat of Scientific Racism* (Cambridge: Cambridge University Press, 1992), 241–242.

46. Leakey to *The Times,* December 13, 1933.

47. Haldane to *The Times,* December 19, 1933.

48. Gilks to *The Times,* December 30, 1933; Gordon to *The Times,* January 22, 1934.

49. Dispatch from Governor Byrne to Cunliffe-Lister, July 5, 1934, CO 822/61/14, TNA.

50. Hemming to Freeston, November 16, 1934, CO 822/61/14, TNA.

51. Coupland to Hailey, March 13, 1936, MSS Afr. s. 1829/1/3, Bodleian Library.

52. Matheson to Oldham, December 14, 1933, MSS Afr. s. 1829/1/3, Bodleian Library.

53. Gordon, "Amentia in the East African," 223–235.

54. For more on this, see Chloe Campbell, *Race and Empire: Eugenics in Colonial Kenya* (Manchester: Manchester University Press, 2007), 58–59.

55. Lord Hailey, *An African Survey: A Study of Problems Arising in Africa South of the Sahara* (London: Oxford University Press, 1938), 38.

FURTHER READING

Anderson, David. *Histories of the Hanged: Britain's Dirty War in Kenya and the End of Empire* (London: Weidenfeld & Nicolson, 2005).

Barkan, Elazar. *The Retreat of Scientific Racism: Changing Concepts of Race in Britain and the United States between the World Wars* (Cambridge: Cambridge University Press, 1992).

Campbell, Chloe. *Race and Empire: Eugenics in Colonial Kenya* (Manchester: Manchester University Press, 2007).

Dubow, Saul. *Scientific Racism in Modern South Africa* (Cambridge: Cambridge University Press, 1995).

Dubow, Saul, ed. *Science and Society in Southern Africa* (Manchester: Manchester University Press, 2000).

Elkins, Caroline. *Britain's Gulag: The Brutal End of Empire in Kenya* (London: Jonathan Cape, 2005).

Kennedy, Dane. *Islands of White: Settler Society and Culture in Kenya and Southern Rhodesia, 1890–1939* (Durham. NC: Duke University Press, 1987).

Lewis, Joanna. *Empire State-Building: War and Welfare in Kenya, 1925–52* (Oxford: James Currey, 2000).

Mahone, Sloan, and Megan Vaughan, eds. *Psychiatry and Empire* (Basingstoke: Palgrave, 2007).

McCulloch, Jock. *Colonial Psychiatry and "the African Mind"* (Cambridge: Cambridge University Press, 1995).

Semmel, Bernard. *Imperialism and Social Reform: English Social-Imperial Thought 1895–1914* (London: George Allen & Unwin, 1960).

Vaughan, Megan. *Curing Their Ills: Colonial Power and African Illness* (Stanford, CA: Stanford University Press, 1991).

CHAPTER 17

EUGENICS IN POSTCOLONIAL SOUTHEAST ASIA

SUNIL S. AMRITH

SOUTHEAST Asia has not featured prominently in the historiography of global eugenics. For their part, histories of social and political thought in Southeast Asia pay little attention to eugenics.[1] To situate eugenics in modern Southeast Asian history, the rich vein of writing on race and racial thought in the region provides an essential point of entry. Focusing on the experience of postcolonial Malaysia and Singapore, this chapter suggests that traces of eugenic thought and practice have played a role in shaping strategies of state-directed development from the 1950s. The "science of racial improvement" exerted a powerful influence on the political elite of both countries, providing a rationale and a model for many attempts to understand, differentiate, and "improve" the population. In modern Malaysia and Singapore, eugenics has formed part of a long-term political project to govern diversity, in a region shaped by an extended history of migration.

The biological determinism of the colonial period has had a lasting effect across Southeast Asia, well beyond Malaysia and Singapore, in the internalization and popularization of particular notions of inherited "racial" traits. In the postcolonial era, confidence in the developmental project loosened, but never overcame, the notion that these traits were immutable. Throughout the region, the results of this ambivalent but pervasive eugenic imagination ranged from a raft of intrusive (if sometimes "effective") state interventions to brutal violence.

There is no clear narrative of the "rise and fall" of eugenics in post-colonial Southeast Asia; first because its "rise" was muted and its effects often indirect; and second because when eugenics *did* have an explicit influence on policy, it was in the

1970s and 1980s, by which point eugenic thought and practice had passed its global heyday and had lost much of its legitimacy elsewhere.

The Colonial Inheritance

Eugenics in its late-Victorian variant underwent an inevitable process of translation and transformation in colonial Southeast Asia. The language of modern eugenics in Southeast Asia informed and drew upon much older colonial debates about race and place. To the extent that naming and categorizing "others" was an integral part of the colonial enterprise, this proved particularly fraught in Southeast Asia, where Europeans encountered a region with a deep history of migration and mobility. Early discussions of race and space in colonial Southeast Asia were often shaped by environmental considerations. As in many other regions of the "tropics," fears for the health of Europeans, of degeneration in hot climes, were widespread.

More lastingly, the colonial discourse on race in Southeast Asia focused upon characterizing and differentiating between migrant groups. For instance, John Crawfurd (1783–1868), a Scottish administrator and amateur ethnographer, observed in the 1850s that "numerous vessels" from southeastern India "bring annually, with the setting in of the westerly monsoon, shoals of these people, literally to seek their fortunes in a country richer by nature than their own...in their character these adventurers are shrewd, supple, unwarlike, mendacious and avaricious," he declared.[2] The Chinese, on another view, were "the most successful traders and most patient toilers in the East," whose "love of combinations, of the guilds and unions in which all Chinamen delight, tempts them too far."[3] Colonial observers in Malaya commented on the ambiguous and sometimes murky origins of the individuals and communities they tried to place; an official report concluded in 1856 that "although this Asiatic population is classed under three heads, Chinese, Mahometan and Hindoo, no correct opinion can be formed of its composition from these distinctive appellations."[4] In this context, the Dutch administration in the East Indies went furthest in marking the Chinese out as both homogenous and different, requiring them to carry passes, and imposing restrictions on their movements and their places of residence.[5]

From the outset, race—and, in particular, racial diversity—dominated European visions of Asian society in Southeast Asia. However, environmental factors (climate, above all) and systems of law and administration were held to explain these traits and to naturalize the economic division of labor: the Chinese were industrious but fractious; Tamils were docile, good for hard labor. The first explicit discussions of heredity took place in connection with the myriad of Southeast Asia's creolized or hybrid communities, which emerged as a source of anxiety for the colonial state. The "Jawi Peranakan"—a community that emerged from intermarriage between south Indian Muslim men and Malay women—was the object of special condemnation. Of the Jawi Peranakan, Crawfurd wrote: "The motley race formed by these unions is a compound character of no very amiable description, partaking of the vices of both parent stocks." Peranakan Chinese families, too, represented "a race inferior in energy and spirit to the original settler, but speaking the language, wearing the garb, professing the religion, and affecting the manners of the parent country."[6] This way of characterizing creole communities was not immutable. Culture still mattered: many colonial officials viewed the highly educated, Anglophone (and often Christian) Straits Chinese elite as loyal and effective collaborators.

The late nineteenth century was a time when anxieties about racial mixing reached new levels of intensity. As Ann Laura Stoler has shown in detail, the arrival of increasing numbers of European women in colonial Southeast Asia provoked new anxieties about the boundaries of "whiteness" and new efforts to police that boundary with vigor.[7] The "Eurasian problem" came to the fore, most particularly in the Dutch East Indies and French Indochina, where unions between European men and local women had been widespread. Within creole communities, too, tensions began to emerge. Influenced by Chinese nationalism and Chinese ideas about racial purity, leaders of the Indonesian Chinese community condemned the "laughable combination or mixing" that occurred as young Peranakan children were "engulfed in native practices and customs...firmly and fanatically" through the influence of their Javanese mothers.[8] Yet here, too, the emphasis remained on acquired traits and habits ("culture") rather than heredity.

The desire to erect firm boundaries around race was one rationale for the introduction of the census in Southeast Asia; Malaya's first census took place in 1871. As Charles Hirschman has shown, the advent of the census was accompanied by a changing conception of race on the part of the colonial elite, "founded on the idea that peoples were different not only in appearance and culture, but also in inherent capacities."[9] By 1891, the census listed the various "races" and "tribes" under the major headings that continue to shape official conceptions of race in Singapore and Malaysia to this day: Chinese, Malays, Indians, and "Others." By the turn of the twentieth century, the most significant creole communities no longer appeared in the census: Straits Chinese were merely "Chinese," and from 1911 the Jawi Peranakan were listed as "Malay."

Nevertheless, the hardening of racial categories left a significant residue of ambiguity. The census commissioner of 1931, C. Vlieland (1890?–1974), made this quite clear:

> It is impossible to define the sense in which the term "race" is used for census purposes: it is, in reality, a judicious blend, for practical ends, of the ideas of geographic and ethnographic origin, political allegiance and racial and social affinities and sympathies.[10]

In particular, colonial census-takers found it difficult to disentangle the threads of "racial," ethnic, and religious affiliations, and to map these upon fixed "origins." Vlieland lamented that:

> The difficulty of achieving anything like a scientific or logically consistent classification is enhanced by the fact that most Oriental peoples themselves have no clear conception of race, and commonly regard religion as the most important, if not the determinant, element.[11]

What, then, did eugenics—the "science of racial improvement"—mean in the context of colonial Southeast Asia? The modern state in Southeast Asia held to a conception of multiple, discrete populations rather than a homogenous national body. As a result, rather than seeking to improve *the* population—after the fashion of eugenics in Europe, or indeed in China or India—the colonial state in Southeast Asia devised carefully targeted interventions to improve particular populations in all their diversity.

Given the high death rates on the plantations, medical services were directed entirely toward ensuring the productivity and the reproduction of Indian labor; in the case of the Chinese in Malaya, the colonial state sought to work through Chinese intermediaries and to harness Chinese voluntary associations as a tool of government. By the early twentieth century, however, the population that the colonial state most sought to improve was the "indigenous" Malay population—the "myth of the lazy native," as Syed Hussen Alatas called it, took deep roots in the early twentieth century.[12] If eugenic policies can be identified in colonial Southeast Asia, they were almost entirely framed in terms of policies to restrict immigration and settlement, to "reserve" land and employment for the natives.

The eugenic impetus can be traced to the origins of a discourse on indigeneity, on the responsibility of colonial power to "protect" vulnerable Malays or Burmese from the threat posed by more "energetic" immigrant groups. Initially, explanations for indigenous backwardness tended to be historicist, cultural, and environmental in nature, rather than explicitly racial. The problem was increasingly framed in terms of the ostensibly superior genetic-cultural inheritance of the Chinese immigrants, disposing them to be hardworking, devious, cunning, and more economically successful than the "natives." The introduction by the colonial state of Malay Reservations in 1913—preventing the transfer of land into non-Malay hands within prescribed areas—was a portent of things to come. By the 1930s, and in the aftermath of violence directed against "immigrant" Indians, Burma too introduced legislation to limit landholding and commercial activity by peoples not deemed indigenous.[13] Throughout colonial Southeast Asia, the economic depression of the 1930s led to the rise of immigration restriction, almost invariably justified in terms of improving the lot of the native populations, ill-equipped to compete with "immigrant races" better endowed by nature and by culture.

The coming of limited colonial democracy in the 1930s, in the form of representative councils, deepened the eugenic imagination of Southeast Asia's nascent nationalists. In Malaya, as in Burma, local nationalists turned their hostility against so-called immigrants—the Chinese and the Indians—long before they targeted the colonial state. It is in this context that the problem of balancing racial numbers became absolutely central to the problem of government on the Malay peninsula, which had a larger "immigrant" population than anywhere else in the region. Writing in the flourishing Malay-language press of the 1930s a Malay intellectual declared that:

> the government can inform these foreigners that the "protection" of the Malays
> isn't like the protection of the deer in the forest by the game warden, who sees to

it that the deer isn't killed by hunters but allows it to be preyed upon by other enemies such as the tiger and other carnivorous animals living in the same forest.[14]

This indicates the complex mixture of crude social Darwinism ("the survival of the fittest;" the "laws of the jungle") and the close connection between debates on race and racial aptitudes, and the politics of immigration control and colonial "reservations." From the outset, eugenic policies in Southeast Asia focused on using state power to rebalance the "plural society," and "racial improvement" began to signify the identification and exclusion of particular peoples.

MALAYSIA: RACE AND POSTCOLONIAL DEVELOPMENT

In Malaysia since independence, politics has been organized almost entirely along the lines of race. This phenomenon has deep roots, as the earlier part of this chapter tried to show. The Japanese occupation of Southeast Asia produced new kinds of distinction between different populations—new definitions of loyal and disloyal, martial and effete peoples and "races." The most immediate cause of the racialization of Malaysia's politics, however, was the need to build a conservative ruling coalition against the Communist insurgency that erupted in 1948.[15] For a number of reasons—to do with the division of labor, patterns of settlement, and Japanese policy during the war—the Malayan Communist Party (MCP) had a primarily Chinese support base, though it never considered itself an ethnically based party. The colonial state, however, used the threat of a Chinese insurgency to rally support among Malay conservatives and to restore the authority of the Chinese business elite, which the war had undermined.

The language of biological racism suffused the colonial counterinsurgency—all Chinese were suspect, "infected" with a "secret society complex"—and the resettlement of over 500,000 Chinese in heavily fortified New Villages marked both a "positive" and a "negative" attempt to manage race: the New Villages isolated the Chinese peasantry and urban poor from the MCP, while attempting to "rehabilitate" them with education, public health facilities, and organized social welfare. Among the other aims of the counterinsurgency were the "improvement" of the Chinese population of Malaya; not genetically, but culturally and politically.

At the core of the Alliance, which won the elections of 1955 and took power at independence in 1957, was an entrenchment of political representation along racial lines. The political settlement at independence recognized that the "sons of the soil"—the Malay population—would have preferential access to political power, as a way of lifting them from their historical "backwardness" as well as recognizing them as indigenous (where Chinese and Indians remained outsiders, however many generations had passed since their settlement in Malaya). After a traumatic episode of interethnic violence in May 1969, government policy shifted toward a more concerted attempt at "racial uplift." The New Economic Policy, inaugurated in 1971, aimed at a fundamental redistribution of wealth by "eradicating poverty" and "restructuring society," to create a class of Malay capitalists. The effect was to consolidate the economic power of the Malay ruling class, facilitating the growth of a number of business conglomerates with close links to the ruling party.[16] Clearly, the New Economic Policy was rooted in a quest to consolidate political and economic power in the hands of the Malay elite, though the egalitarian motivations behind it, the desire to reduce Malay poverty, must not be discounted.

For the purposes of this volume, however, what is most striking is the way in which the language of eugenics made a strong impression on public discourse around this time, as a rationale for and justification of the redistribution of wealth and power in Malaysia. In *The Malay Dilemma*—which was initially banned upon publication as "inflammatory"—the ultra-nationalist doctor Mahathir Mohamad (b. 1925), who would become Malaysia's longest-serving prime minister, invoked explicitly eugenic concerns in the aftermath of the 1969 "racial riots."

As race constituted the essence of entitlement in post-colonial Malaysia, the impetus to purify and mold the "Malay race" emerged strongly. Eugenics, in this case, was an amalgam of state policies of affirmative action, targeted birth control, the promotion of more "rational" marriage practices, the reform of personal laws, and the education of Malay mothers. The counterpart to this in the economic sphere would be the creation of a class of Malay capitalists, to lead by example.

In *The Malay Dilemma*, Mahathir Mohamad reframed the commonsense colonial vision of the "plural society" in the language of eugenics. "That hereditary factors play an important part in the development of a race is an accepted fact," he argued, suggesting a sense of certainty about race that was at odds with the prevailing scientific consensus.[17] Mahathir's vision of the Malay race was shaped by both genetic and environmental factors. The narrative underpinning Mahathir's conception of the "Malay dilemma" is worth quoting at length:

> The effect of Chinese immigration on the Malays was conflict between two contrasting racial groups which resulted from two entirely different sets of hereditary and environmental influences.... For the Chinese people life was one continuous struggle for survival. In the process the weak in mind and body lost out to the strong and the resourceful. For generation after generation, through four thousand years or more, this weeding out of the unfit went on.... But, as if this was not enough to produce a hardy race, Chinese custom decreed that marriage should not be within the same clan. This resulted in more cross-breeding than in-breeding, in direct contrast to the Malay partiality towards in-breeding.[18]

Indicating the complex mix of cultural, environmental, and genetic explanations for current socioeconomic arrangements, Mahathir invoked a familiar discourse on early marriage as an explanation for the decreasing "quality" of the Malay population. "Malays abhor the state of celibacy," he declared, so the poor and the disabled "survive, reproduce and propagate their species. The cumulative effect of this can be left to the imagination."[19]

What is distinctive about this particular vision of eugenics, however, is its confidence that political power could bring about a transformation in the relative "qualities" of Malaysia's different racial groups. In Mahathir's view, the evolutionary shock that awakened the Malay race and transformed its character came in the form of World War II and the struggle for control of the state: "Under the stress of this rapid destruction of their hopes, the Malay character underwent a metamorphosis. Seeing their salvation in politics, the previously docile Malays, with remarkable rapidity and initiative, organized themselves." This was not without ambivalence. He invoked the possibility that gaining political power "will not be good for the Malays," by making them "softer and less able to overcome difficulties on their own." Conversely he argued, harking back to the discourse of early Malay nationalism in the 1930s, that "removal of all protection would subject the Malays to the primitive laws that enable only the fittest to survive."[20]

Mahathir's polemic is perhaps the most sustained, certainly the most widely known, eugenicist text in modern Southeast Asia. It was written with specific political objectives in mind, and it was an intervention in debates within the ruling United Malays National Organization (UMNO) party as much as it was aimed at a wide audience. Yet the policies that resulted from the shift in political alignment in the 1970s—and which Mahathir developed under his reign—cannot be identified as explicitly eugenic. They consisted of providing differential access—on grounds of "race"—to political power, educational and social facilities; strategies of state-linked capital accumulation by a Malay business elite; and broader policies of social welfare, including a wide-reaching public health program and efforts to reduce population growth.[21] The political interventions of the 1970s and 1980s aimed either to erase or to naturalize divisions within the Malay community as much as between Malays and others.

In this context, the significance of eugenics in shaping policy lay in its ability to lend the support of scientific language as a rationale for policies that had complex, sometimes contradictory motivations. The deepest effect may well lie in the way in which the language of hereditary traits seeped into the everyday language of racial difference in modern Malaysia. Racial characteristics, on this view, were immutable and immediately recognizable. Mahathir put it quite starkly, but he was not alone in thinking this way:

> The Jews for example are not merely hook-nosed, but understand money instinctively. The Europeans are not only fair-skinned, but have an insatiable curiosity. The Malays are not merely brown, but are also easy-going and tolerant. And the Chinese are not just almond-eyed people, but are also inherently good businessmen....It can be seen that these characteristics determine the relationship between races when they come in contact with each other.[22]

Yet in recent years it has become clear that an issue which the colonial census-takers of the early twentieth century encountered remains fraught in contemporary Malaysia, and that is the question of where to draw the line between inherited identities and self-identification, particularly where the intersection between religion and "race" is concerned. While modern Malaysians undoubtedly have "clear conceptions of race," nevertheless—as Vlieland pointed out back in 1931—many still "commonly regard religion as the most important, if not the determinant, element."[23]

Singapore: Eugenics and "National Survival"

Eugenic policies came closer to realization in postcolonial Singapore, which developed, in many ways, as a political inversion of Malaysia. In Singapore, too, the eugenic imperative after independence came from the political elite, and built upon commonsense notions of race and diversity inherited from the colonial era. Singapore remained a British colony after the Federation of Malaya became independent, but joined the Federation in 1963. To simplify a complex story, Singapore's inclusion in Malaysia, with its large Chinese working-class population and its tradition of left-wing politics, threatened Malaysia's conservative racial accommodation. Upon its ejection from the Federation in 1965, Singapore has founded itself upon a narrative of struggle, as a "Chinese island in a Malay sea." In contrast to Malaysia, Singapore has held to an ideology of multiracial meritocracy, which served to obscure deep fractures and inequalities.

From the time of its "accidental" independence, the Singapore state became obsessed with molding and disciplining a multiracial citizenry. Engineering the "quality" and the "quantity" of population, the state put into place an extensive population control program and expanded the disciplinary apparatus of the state—most significantly, instituting compulsory military service—to stop the population from "going soft" and succumbing to the lassitude of the tropics. The key was to produce a "new man": self-subjecting, efficient, with a merciless work ethic, allowing Singapore to achieve its strategy of development through the attraction of foreign capital. Natural metaphors pervaded public discourse in the 1960s: Singapore would be drowned in a Malay sea; its vitality sapped by the tropical environment, "infected" with communism or lassitude.[24]

As the ruling People's Action Party in Singapore swept away (or imprisoned) its opponents, eugenic arguments emerged with force to justify the political order of things. Prime Minister Lee Kuan Yew (b. 1923)—a member of the Straits Chinese elite and a Cambridge-educated lawyer—made these arguments quite explicit. He declared in 1967 that "no more than five percent" of any population were "more than ordinarily endowed physically and mentally," and it was this "five percent" who should rule in the interests of all.[25] This conception of society had an effect upon Singapore's family planning program, aggressively pursued by the government after 1965.

An elite movement in support of family planning dates back to the years after World War II. The Family Planning Association of Singapore emerged in 1949 and was one of the founding members of the International Planned Parenthood Federation (1953). By the time of Singapore's independence, the new political elite was acutely concerned with the specter of overpopulation on a small island. Of particular concern, however, was the "quality" of the population. Supporting a new "abortion and voluntary sterilization bill" in parliament in 1969, Lee lamented that "free education and subsidised housing lead to a situation where the less economically productive people in the community are reproducing themselves at rates higher than the rest." The rationale for his government's family planning policy was to

> devise a system of disincentives, so that the irresponsible, the social delinquents, do not believe that all they have to do is to produce their children…One of the crucial yardsticks by which we shall have to judge the results of the new abortion law combined with the voluntary sterilization law will be whether it tends to raise or lower the total quality of our population…we will regret the time lost if we do not now take the first tentative steps towards correcting a trend which can leave our society with a large number of the physically, intellectually and culturally anaemic.[26]

The "take up rate" of oral contraceptives was rapid; but the state's hope that the "disincentives" would change the class composition of the population proved frustrating. Thus, by the early 1980s, the Singapore state made a further attempt to formulate "eugenic" population policies, this time by providing special benefits (tax breaks and other incentives) to highly educated women in order to encourage them to have *more* children.

Concerned, by 1980, that the population control program had been too successful (the birthrate among educated women was falling much faster than among the less educated), Lee lamented its consequence:

> If we continue to reproduce ourselves in this lop-sided way, we will be unable to maintain our present standards. Levels of competence will decline. Our economy will falter; administration will suffer; and society will decline.[27]

The Graduate Mothers Scheme of 1984, which introduced selective benefits for educated women who had more children, encountered unexpected and unwonted opposition in Singapore, leading to the formation of the Association of Women for Action and Research (AWARE), which became the leading women's nongovernmental organization (NGO) in Singapore.[28] Indeed, this was precisely the kind of elite feminist mobilization that may, in an earlier era, have supported eugenics. Public opposition led to the withdrawal of the Graduate Mothers Scheme. What remained was a "selectively pro-natal" policy, the eugenic implications of which were somewhat muted: "have three or more, if you can afford it" was the slogan of the late 1980s.[29] At the same time, the government's Social Development Unit organized romantic cruises and retreats for carefully selected elite graduates, trying to create the "right" sorts of marriages.

Eugenics in independent Singapore shaped every aspect of government inter-vention in society, and its imagination of "society" itself. Even if the more overt attempts to impose eugenic policies failed, eugenic ideas played a central role in maintaining Singapore's self-image as Malaysia's or Indonesia's antithesis: modern, Chinese, prosperous, well-governed, fit, and efficient.

The influence of eugenics may have faded in the last decade, but it is still pre-sent, and now shapes the discourse on immigration. In recent decades, the Singapore state has evinced extreme concern about relationships between working-class Singaporeans and outsiders—Filipina domestic workers; construction workers from India, Bangladesh, Burma, and Thailand. This has led to draconian laws requiring special permission for marriages between migrant workers and Singaporeans, and providing for the deportation of female migrant workers who become pregnant. The legislation specifically prohibits foreign workers from "breaking up Singaporean families."[30] At the same time, the state has actively encour-aged, since the 1980s, migration from China, seen as a "racially" preferable alternative to migration from neighboring Southeast Asia or from South Asia.

Singapore's "eugenic" immigration policy consists of differentiating sharply between different kinds of immigrants. On the one hand, highly skilled profes-sionals ("foreign talent," in local parlance) are actively sought and are encouraged to settle to add to the quality of Singapore's population. On the other hand, an army of low-skilled, low paid "foreign workers" bear the costs of Singapore's development, kept under constant surveillance and discipline, and barred from incorporation into the national population.[31]

CONCLUSION: WIDER COMPARISONS

Singapore and Malaysia are distinctive in the region in being overtly wedded to an ideology of multiracialism. It was in the context of balancing and managing diver-sity that eugenics had its greatest impact on government in Malaysia and Singapore. Other parts of the region share similar histories of migration, and a similar development of categories of minorities and majorities. In a region where diversity is a constant, Southeast Asian nations that did not embrace a negotiated form of multicultural government swung between attempts to erase cultural, linguistic, or "racial" differences ("assimilation"), and more or less violent attempts to eliminate them.

In terms of practical application, it was most often through the massive population control programs of the postcolonial era that eugenic assumptions about population quality, as well as quantity, surfaced. To the extent that the global project of population control was shaped by the legacy of eugenics, then its lasting effects can be seen in the Philippines, Indonesia, and Thailand, three of the most enthusiastic participants in that global enterprise. In each case, population-control policies were imbued with a number of assumptions about social class and about minorities.[32] Repeated attempts to "assimilate" indigenous or "tribal" minorities across the region have had strong eugenic overtones and have tended to emphasize the hereditary incapacity of indigenous peoples.

The other major measure through which almost all Southeast Asian states have attempted to "balance" the population is migration policy: for example, the state-directed mass migration of Christian Filipinos to Mindanao after World War II was an attempt to dilute the "Muslim" character of the south.[33] The massive *transmigrasi* program in Indonesia, started in colonial times, aimed to recalibrate the balance of population between Java and the outer islands, creating national cohesion in the process.[34] In each of these cases, it is difficult to isolate the influence of eugenics from broader concerns with governability, with majorities and minorities, and with the quest for political power and representation.

Perhaps the most lasting and damaging legacy of biologically based racial determinism is that markers of ethnic and cultural difference, translated into the apparently immutable language of "race," could never truly be erased. The language of heredity has surfaced time and again in modern Southeast Asia in pursuit of the "enemies within" modern nation-states.

Few communities in Southeast Asia have encountered this more concertedly than Southeast Asia's Chinese. As Ariel Heryanto has written of Indonesia under Suharto's New Order, "the stigma of being Chinese and hence ideologically 'unclean,' or that of being Chinese and hence having been 'involved in the 1965 coup' were declared contagious and hereditary." Under Suharto's "assimilation program," Chinese Indonesians were urged to assume "native" names and modes of dress, and intermarriage was ostensibly encouraged. Yet "Chinese identities are never totally to be wiped out. They are carefully and continually reproduced, but always under erasure. In fact, the negation is a necessary element of the making of this ethnic Other." Most pervasive is the fact that as a result of popular characterizations of the Chinese, their "work ethic, industriousness, thrift or perseverance," the "Chinese have been literally stuck with a very narrow range of human characteristics, making it difficult to both imagine and image them in any other way."[35] Even in Thailand, where the Chinese population was most clearly "assimilated" into the middle and upper class, a sense of distinctiveness remained, but arguably this was voluntary as much as it was imposed and had to do with "culture" as much as "race."[36] It would not be difficult to see the furthest and most perverse extension of colonial/postcolonial racial thinking in Southeast Asia in the definition of racial and class enemies for extermination—the fate that befell "Vietnamese" residents and intellectuals in Cambodia under the Khmer Rouge, possessed of a particularly murderous conception of inherent racial difference.[37]

The language of heredity was always, of course, open to subversion. The prominent Indonesian novelist and writer Pramoedya Ananta Toer (1925–2006) was imprisoned in part because of his strident defense of Indonesia's Chinese in the early 1960s, in a series of newspaper articles in which he posed the most provocative question to the Indonesian nationalist persecutors of the Chinese: "There is not a single Indonesian or Chinese who can prove they are of such pure blood. Is there not one drop or cell of blood of another people flowing in their veins?" Indonesian history made such certainty unlikely, if not absurd.[38]

On the whole, the legacy of eugenics in modern Southeast Asia lies in the quotidian production and government of difference and diversity. Its expression as policy has more often than not been through the all-encompassing quest for "development." In the third quarter of the twentieth century, when developmental interventions in Southeast Asia were at their most ambitious, this tended to revolve around the two poles of population control policy and mass education. Both of these approaches have been lauded in accounts of the Southeast Asian "model" of development; this chapter has shown that more complex, and sometimes darker, eugenic motivations shaped a number of these interventions.

The particular moment of eugenics' impact on Southeast Asia—coincident with the global Cold War—has added another distinctive element to its manifestations in the region. In modern Southeast Asia, the language of eugenics has often been used to characterize or even to predict *political* affiliations, in terms of particular "racial" susceptibilities to communism, separatism (or, lately, terrorism). The language of heredity is used in a sense that is partly metaphorical and partly literal, to define the enemies of the state—or, in the case of the poor or indigenous peoples, enemies of progress.

Conversely, however, nation-builders in Southeast Asia have often shied away from truly embracing the language of blood and origins, for—as Pramoedya Ananta Toer suggested—to pursue that line of thinking too far could produce some discomfiting results, challenging notions of racial purity, of insiders and outsiders, in a region characterized, above all, by histories of mobility.

NOTES

1. There is, to the best of my knowledge, no single volume on the history of eugenics in Southeast Asia, or even in any single Southeast Asian country; even the specialized journal literature is very limited.

2. John Crawfurd, *History of the Indian Archipelago: Containing an Account of the Manners, Arts, Languages, Religions, Institutions and Commerce of Its Inhabitants*, 3 vols. (Edinburgh: Archibald Constable, 1820), 1: 133–134.

3. John Thomson, *The Straits of Malacca, Indo-China and China, or, Ten Years' Travels, Adventures and Residence Abroad* (London: Sampson Low, Marston, Low & Searle, 1875), 12–14.

4. *Report on the Administration of the Straits Settlements, during the Year 1855–56*, (Singapore, 1857), 20.

5. Benedict Anderson, *Spectre of Comparisons: Nationalism, Southeast Asia, the World* (London: Verso, 1998), chap. 15.

6. Crawfurd, *Indian Archipelago*, 133–134.

7. Ann Laura Stoler, *Race and the Education of Desire: Foucault's History of Sexuality and the Colonial Order of Things* (Durham, NC: Duke University Press, 1995); Stoler,

"Rethinking Colonial Categories: European Communities and the Boundaries of Rule," *Comparative Studies in Society and History* 31, no. 1 (1989): 134–161.

8. Kwee Tek Hoay, *The Origins of the Modern Chinese Movement in Indonesia* [trans. of "Atsal Moelahnja Tomboel Pergerakan Tonghoa jang Modern di Indonesia," *Moestika romans*, nos. 73–84, 1936–1939] ed. and trans. Lea E. Williams (Ithaca, NY: Modern Indonesia Project, Southeast Asia Program, Cornell University, 1969).

9. Charles Hirschman, "The Meaning and Measurement of Ethnicity in Malaya: An Analysis of Census Classifications," *Journal of Asian Studies* 46, no. 3 (1987): 568.

10. C. Vlieland, *British Malaya. A Report on the 1931 Census and Certain Problems of Vital Statistics* (London: Crown Agents for the Colonies, 1932), 74–75.

11. Ibid.

12. Syed Hussein Alatas, *The Myth of the Lazy Native* (London: Frank Cass, 1977).

13. The debate on indigeneity, of course, opened up divisions between the Burmese majority and other indigenous minorities, including the Karen, the Kachin, and the Shan.

14. Cited in William Roff, *The Origins of Malay Nationalism* (New Haven, CT: Yale University Press, 1967).

15. T. N. Harper, *The End of Empire and the Making of Malaya* (Cambridge: Cambridge University Press, 1999).

16. Edmund Terence Gomez and K. S. Jomo, *Malaysia's Political Economy: Politics, Patronage and Profits* (Cambridge: Cambridge University Press, 1997), chap. 3.

17. Mahathir Bin Mohamad, *The Malay Dilemma* [1970] (Singapore: Times Books, 1992), 17, 19.

18. Ibid., 24.

19. Ibid., 27.

20. Ibid., 27.

21. Kai Hong Phua and Mary Lai Lin Wong, "From Colonial Economy to Social Equity: History of Public Health in Malaysia," in *Public Health in Asia and the Pacific Historical and Comparative Perspectives*, eds. Milton J. Lewis and Kerrie L. Macpherson (London and New York: Routledge, 2007), 170–187.

22. Mahathir, *Malay Dilemma*, 84–85.

23. Vlieland, *British Malaya*, 74–75.

24. Carl A. Trocki, *Singapore: Wealth, Power and the Culture of Control* (London and New York: Routledge, 2006).

25. Christopher Tremewan, *The Political Economy of Social Control in Singapore* (New York: St Martin's Press, 1994), 100.

26. Ibid., 103.

27. Trocki, *Singapore*.

28. Lenore Lyons, *A State of Ambivalence: The Women's Movement in Singapore* (Leiden: Brill, 2004).

29. Mui Teng Yap, "Singapore's 'Three or More' Policy: The First Five Years," *Asia Pacific Population Journal* 10, no. 4 (1995): 39–52.

30. Singapore, Ministry of Manpower, *Employment of Foreign Manpower Act*, July 2007 (chapter 91A); see especially the provisions 9–11 under the Fourth Schedule of the Act.

31. Pheng Cheah, *Inhuman Conditions: On Cosmopolitanism and Human Rights* (Cambridge, MA: Harvard University Press, 2007).

32. For the global context, see Matthew Connelly, *Fatal Misconception: The Struggle to Control World Population* (Cambridge, MA: Harvard University Press, 2008).

33. Thomas Mckenna, *Muslim Rulers and Rebels: Everyday Politics and Armed Separatism in the Southern Philippines* (Berkeley, CA: University of California Press, 1998).

34. J. M. Hardjono, *Transmigration in Indonesia* (Kuala Lumpur: Oxford University Press, 1997).

35. Ariel Heryanto, "Ethnic Identities and Erasure: Chinese Indonesians in Public Culture," in *Southeast Asian Identities: Culture and the Politics of Representation in Indonesia, Malaysia, Singapore and Thailand*, ed. Joel S. Kahn (Singapore: ISEAS, 1998), 99, 103–104.

36. Craig J. Reynolds, "Globalization and Cultural Nationalism in Modern Thailand," in Kahn, *Southeast Asian Identities*, 115–145.

37. See Ben Kiernan, *The Pol Pot Regime: Race, Power and Genocide in Cambodia Under the Khmer Rouge, 1975–79*, 2nd edition (New Haven, CT: Yale University Press, 2002).

38. Pramoedya Ananta Toer, *The Chinese in Indonesia: An English translation of Hoakiau di Indonesia* [1960], trans. Max Lane (Singapore: Select Books, 2008), 76.

FURTHER READING

Alatas, Syed Hussein. *The Myth of the Lazy Native: A Study of the Image of the Malays, Filipinos and Javanese from the 16th to the 20th Century and Its Function in the Ideology of Colonial Capitalism* (London: Frank Cass, 1977).

Anderson, Benedict. *Imagined Communities: Reflections on the Origins and Spread of Nationalism*, 2nd ed. (London: Verso, 1991).

Anderson, Benedict. *The Spectre of Comparisons: Nationalism, Southeast Asia, and the World* (London: Verso, 1998).

Connelly, Matthew. *Fatal Misconception: The Struggle to Control World Population* (Cambridge, MA: Harvard University Press, 2008).

Harper, T. N. *The End of Empire and the Making of Malaya* (Cambridge: Cambridge University Press, 1999).

Hirschman, Charles. "The Meaning and Measurement of Ethnicity in Malaya: An Analysis of Census Classifications," *Journal of Asian Studies* 46, no. 3 (1987): 555–582.

Kahn, Joel S., ed. *Southeast Asian Identities: Culture and the Politics of Representation in Indonesia, Malaysia, Singapore and Thailand* (Singapore: ISEAS, 1998).

Mahathir Bin Mohamad. *The Malay Dilemma* [1970] (Singapore: Times Books, 1992).

Toer, Pramoedya Ananta. *The Chinese in Indonesia: An English translation of Hoakiau di Indonesia* [1960], trans. Max Lane (Singapore: Select Books, 2008).

Stoler, Ann Laura. *Race and the Education of Desire: Foucault's History of Sexuality and the Colonial Order of Things* (Durham, NC: Duke University Press, 1995).

Trocki, Carl A. *Singapore: Wealth, Power and the Culture of Control* (London and New York: Routledge, 2006).

CHAPTER 18

GERMAN EUGENICS AND THE WIDER WORLD: BEYOND THE RACIAL STATE

PAUL WEINDLING

GERMAN eugenics—or, as it was often called, "racial hygiene"—incorporated two strands, one racial and the other welfare oriented. Both targeted the reproduction of future generations in a period of rapid industrialization and two world wars. Eugenics in Germany was also characterized by its intention to reach out to a wider world of German colonies and German ethnic groups beyond the frontiers of the state. Austria, German-Swiss cantons, and German settlements in eastern Europe and the Baltics all had eugenic advocates and groupings. German eugenicists desired to influence the development of eugenics internationally, notably in Nordic Scandinavia and in the United States, which had a large German immigrant population.

In 1905 the world's first eugenic organization, the *Gesellschaft für Rassenhygiene* (Racial Hygiene Society), was founded in Berlin, with the core message that fitness was a duty to the race. The periodical, *Archiv für Rassen- und Gesellschaftsbiologie,* which Alfred Ploetz (1860–1940) launched in 1904, a year before he founded the Racial Hygiene Society, took particular interest in the inheritance of diseases and physical traits, as well as the declining birthrate among supposedly elite population groups, notably the educated middle class. The task of fitness involved not only the pursuit of racial purity, but also the promotion of healthy families and the prevention of inherited diseases. Alcohol, tobacco, sexually transmitted diseases, and tuberculosis were condemned as "racial poisons," damaging the health not just of the individual but of the population and future generations, and indeed of the race. The German eugenics movement saw these problems as an outgrowth of modernity, and thus addressed key issues such as rapid industrialization and urban growth and associated changes in morbidity, family size and structure, and sexuality. Both Imperial Germany and Austria-Hungary at the end of the nineteenth century had rapidly expanding cities, declining birthrates, high rates of children born outside marriage, and were host to a range of infectious, chronic degenerative, and psychiatric diseases. Eugenicists therefore addressed the symptoms of rapid modernization and social dislocation through the interpretive lens of degeneration.

After World War I, the loss of territories and German colonies prompted eugenicists to join demands for an expansion of German "living space" (*Lebensraum*), especially in eastern Europe. The simultaneous development of welfare systems encouraged eugenicists to envision how they might contribute to schemes of social regeneration. Race and welfare were fused in 1933 when Hitler took office. Once racial hygiene was *gleichgeschaltet* (coordinated) with offices of racial health, there was a rapid nazification of the German welfare state, with Nazi planners appropriating and incorporating eugenics as they implemented racial policy and genocide.

RACIAL HYGIENE

In 1891 the German psychiatrist Wilhelm Schallmayer (1857–1919) had outlined a system of public health in which eugenically trained physicians served the race and nation rather than merely the sick individual. Schallmayer developed a scheme of corporate national racial service (*Rassedienst*), and the improvement of the hereditary elements in the population (*Volkseugenik*) by means of health passports.[1] This model for eugenic public health opened the way for physicians to stigmatize not just racial otherness but also a range of medical conditions, behaviors, and identities, as a pathological threat to the body politic. Biology and medicine were permeated by the language of the state as an organism, as well as of the social and national body, or *Volkskörper*. Professionals in fields like medicine and social work sought control over a range of social phenomena and offered "solutions" to those perceived as social problems.[2]

Austrian interests were developing along similar lines,[3] and Austrian scientists were prominent in the Berlin nucleus around Ploetz's new Racial Hygiene Society. The anthropologist Felix von Luschan (1854–1924), born in Hollabrunn bei Wien, joined the society early in 1907. The Austrian ethnologist Richard Thurnwald (1869–1954) collaborated with Ploetz in Berlin, and the Viennese anthropologist Rudolf Pöch (1870–1921) came to know Ploetz, first when they were both medical students in Zürich and then through the international anti-alcohol movement.[4] Ploetz moved to Munich, where a new local chapter of the Society was founded, supported by Austrians like the Munich professor of hygiene Max von Gruber (1853–1927) and the Lamarckian Ignaz Kaup (1870–1944), a follower of the Austrian anti-Semite Georg von Schönerer (1842–1921). The Society, then, was broadly "greater German," or *Grossdeutsch,* in orientation, in that they wished to separate "German Austria" politically from the rest of the largely Slav and Magyar Habsburg Empire.

In Austria itself, the social reformer Rudolf Goldscheid (1870–1931), the left-leaning zoologist Paul Kammerer (1880–1926), and the anatomist Julius Tandler (1869–1936) established what amounted to a eugenics society in 1912, the section for "Social Biology and Eugenics" of the Sociological Society of Vienna. Ploetz, meanwhile, was in touch with Swiss psychiatrists, notably August Forel (1848–1931) and Ernst Rüdin (1874–1952). Zürich and Basel continued to be centers of eugenic activity, evident in the anti-alcohol campaigns, and in a eugenic approach to psychiatry. Likewise, eugenic ideals attracted people in areas of German settlement in eastern, northeastern, and southeastern Europe, such as the Siebenbürgen Saxons of Transylvania, the Sudeten Germans in what would become interwar Czechoslovakia, the Baltic Germans, and the Volga Germans.[5] By the 1920s a eugenics society had been established in Saratov in the Volga German Republic of the Soviet Union, with an ethnic German component.

The Racial Hygiene Society was proclaimed the International Society for Racial Hygiene in 1907, and by March 1910 a national German umbrella organization was instituted. The Society rapidly expanded, forming branches in Berlin, Munich, and Freiburg. By 1913 it had a membership of 425, composed of physicians, university academics, and other professionals. Numbers climbed to 1,085 in 1931. The German Racial Hygiene Society only sought mass recruitment in the Nazi period after 1933;[6] in the earlier period, it was more exclusive. Members had to submit to a medical examination to assess their reproductive health, for example, and Ploetz proclaimed the *Gesellschaft für Rassenhygiene* as itself an elite breeding group, encouraging the admission of wives and children, and of students.

The term "racial hygiene"—originally coined by Ploetz in 1895—was, as Marius Turda discusses in this volume, an academic hybrid, a cross between the biological concept of race (variously defined as a breeding community, or population group, or even the human race in general), and the science of hygiene, involving bacteriology and sanitary approaches to public health. But the term "racial hygiene" was ambivalent, as it could also imply the purification of the Germanic race along with a racial "cleansing" of supposedly polluting elements. Ploetz played opportunistically on the ambivalence of the terms "race" (defined demographically as a breeding group) and "hygiene," as a medical specialism. His main goal was the acceptance of *Rassenhygiene* as a science, understanding it as a branch of public health that stressed hereditary factors in a population. At the same time, he pursued a cultural agenda, seeking to recover "primitive" racial vigor as an antidote to degenerative modernism.[7] Ploetz cultivated connections with German groups in North America (he lived in Springfield, Massachusetts, and then Meriden, Connecticut, from 1890–1892), and later he sustained links with American as well as Argentinian eugenicists. His associate Thurnwald was frequently in the United States, writing on such issues as racial segregation.

The biologist Ernst Haeckel (1834–1919), an honorary member of the Racial Hygiene Society, postulated an evolutionary tree from "ape men," splitting to a

primitive branch on the one side of "Negroes," "Kaffirs," "Hottentots," and "Papuas,"
and to the "higher" races (Magyars, Finns, Japanese, Chinese, Caucasians and—
highest of all—the Indo-Germanic races). Haeckel classified in all 12 human types
and 36 races.[8] The Indo-Germanic branch divided into Slavs, Balts, and—at the
most evolved level—Anglo-Saxons, and High Germans. According to Haeckel, Jews
had common descent with Arabs from a semitic branch.[9]

While most anthropology was based on measuring physique, Haeckel opened
the way to a biological approach to human variation and culture that developed,
after 1900, on the basis of Mendelian genetics. Eugen Fischer (1874–1967), an anatomist and anthropologist at Freiburg, studied interbreeding of "mixed-race" whites
and natives in the colonial territory of German South West Africa (Namibia). Fischer
saw this "bastard" (or hybrid) race as potentially healthy, strong, and fertile, ideally
adapted for military service and labor. Scientifically, Fischer's work was innovative
in its use of the Mendelian laws of heredity.[10] The grim reality, however, was that
between 1904 and 1908, German troops were engaged in a genocidal campaign to
suppress an indigenous Herero and Nama (called at the time Hottentot) rebellion
against their rule in the region. The German commander, Lothar von Trotha (1848–
1920), set out to exterminate the Herero by killing or by forcing them into a death
march across the parched Kalahari desert (see Dubow in this volume). By 1908,
German policy was to establish concentration or labor camps, and Fischer's
"solution"—a human cross-breed suited to colonial conditions—should be seen in
this context.

Racially minded doctors in the German colonies of Cameroon and Togo similarly supported racial hygiene research. Ludwig Kuelz (1875–1938) argued that to
prevent malaria, black and white peoples needed to be separated.[11] He accompanied
a medical and demographic expedition to German New Guinea, instigated by the
Reich Colonial Office in 1913–1914. The doctor, anthropologist, and racial hygienist
Rudolf Pöch similarly conducted expeditions to New Guinea in 1901–1906 and to
South Africa in 1907–1909 to study "primitive" races.[12] Racial hygienists aimed both
to find evidence of "primitive" peoples and to improve conditions of settlement of
the Germanic races.

JEWISHNESS AND RACIAL HYGIENE

While Jews were of interest to early eugenicists, eugenics was not fixated on the
"Jewish problem" until the Nazi takeover in 1933. The public health-oriented psychiatrist Wilhelm Schallmayer, who disseminated pioneering eugenic tracts, insisted
that nations were conglomerates of races. His writings show no clear hierarchy between European and Asiatic races, and he paid no special attention to the Jews.[13]
Ploetz, by contrast, deemed Jews a "civilized race" (*Kulturrasse*) on a par with the
other races that composed Germany. Indeed, in 1895 Ploetz prophesied that

democracy and science would sweep away anti-Semitism. He steered the *Deutsche Gesellschaft für Rassenhygiene* away from such populist racist groupings as the *Gobineau-Vereinigung* (Gobineau Association), *Mittgart-Bund* (Mittgart League), and *Alldeutscher Verband* (Pan German League), deemed to have given Hitler his ideas of Aryan superiority.

In its early years, it appeared immaterial whether a member of the Racial Hygiene Society was Jewish. Jewish members were, for the most part, expert in the prevention of chronic degenerative diseases, for example the dermatologist Alfred Blaschko (1858–1922), epidemiologist Adolf Gottstein (1857–1921), or ophthalmologist Arthur C(r)zellitzer[14] (1871–1942), who worked on problems of myopia and founded the Jewish Society for Family Research in 1924. Another Jewish physician, Max Hirsch (1877–1948), was the pioneer of "social gynecology," concerned with the reproductive risks to women of such hazardous situations as hard manual labor. The "half Jewish" medical and biological statistician, Wilhelm Weinberg (1862–1937), who chaired the Stuttgart Racial Hygiene Society, dealt with statistics of maternal mortality, tuberculosis, and hemophilia, as well as genetic ratios (contributing to the Hardy-Weinberg law). The geneticists Richard Goldschmidt (1878–1958) and Hermann Poll (1877–1937), both of whom were assimilated Jews and secular in their outlook, were advocates of eugenics. Poll and the Vienna anatomist Julius Tandler (1869–1936) argued for the determining role of the inherited "constitution" of the body, both as regards susceptibility to infection and chronic degenerative diseases. But there were latent tensions in the 1920s with the rightward move of some eugenicists and biological anthropologists. One manifestation of this tension was the split of the welfare-oriented *Deutscher Bund für Volksaufartung* (League for Regeneration) from the Racial Hygiene Society in 1925, as a body more hospitable to Jewish and socialist members.[15]

Notwithstanding Jewish involvement in eugenics, anti-Semitism was increasing from the 1880s (the term dates from 1882) and gaining a biologically articulated form. At a fundamental level, and despite his pronouncements about Jewish culture, Ploetz was an anti-Semite. Initially, this manifested as a debate on the anthropological characteristics of Jewish and Semitic races. Ploetz subsequently began noting who among recruits to the nascent racial hygiene movement was Jewish, and he sought allies to curb putative Jewish influence. A valued new recruit was the *völkisch* publisher Julius Lehmann (1864–1935), who was eager to cement alliances among the racial ultra-right in the 1920s, while drawing in right-wing advocates of racial hygiene. Lehmann supported the development of racial hygiene as a science of preventive medicine, in 1911 publishing the catalogue of the section on racial hygiene at the International Hygiene Exhibition, held in Dresden.[16] Ploetz sustained this double identity of the Racial Hygiene Society, appealing to the ultra-right and the center-left. On the one hand, a range of liberal and left-wing advocates of social medicine were involved, with his encouragement. On the other, he founded a Nordic body culture organization, *Der Bogen,* in May 1912 (the bow was a symbol of Nordic vitality) as a secret inner core within the Racial Hygiene Society. It continued after World War I as the *Widar-Bund* (Widar was the Nordic god of light), or the Widar League.

THE WEIMAR WELFARE STATE

After the cataclysmic defeat of Germany in World War I, German eugenicists feared that the German race would be exterminated by hunger and territorial loss. Prior to 1914, racial hygiene needs to be understood within the context of German imperialism, but the postwar loss of colonies, of territories to the new Polish state, and of Alsace-Lorraine to France created a shift of focus within the new welfare state. Racially minded critics of new republics in Germany and Austria demanded a Greater German state with revised borders including all German-speaking populations. The loss of colonies prompted a new stress on *Lebensraum* and racial health.

Eugenicists pursued the aim of regenerating Germany and recovering the primitive racial vigor said to exist among the Teutons or Aryans. Much effort went into rekindling this lost racial energy as an antidote to the degenerative effects of modernity. Here, eugenics can be seen as a blueprint for ideas of cultural rebirth and rejuvenation of social institutions. These ideas attracted support from a broad political spectrum. Ploetz was initially a socialist, and with other socialists like August Bebel (1840–1913) and Karl Kautsky (1854–1938) appreciated the relevance of biology and evolution to a modern outlook.

The rise of nationalist fervor increased the links between eugenics and the *völkisch* (the ultra-Germanic and nationalist) movement, shifting racial hygiene rightward from the later 1920s. Lehmann took a leading role in racializing eugenics by sponsoring Hans F. K. Günther (1891–1968) to write the *Rassenkunde des deutschen Volkes* (1922; Racial Study of the German Peoples) and works that later found favor among the Nazis.[17] Although Günther's work earned praise from Fritz Lenz (1887–1976), a human geneticist and leading eugenicist, and Eugen Fischer, other racial hygienists were skeptical about the scientific accuracy of his anthropology. Lehmann also published the journal *Volk und Rasse* from the mid-1920s, which subsequently infused the racial ideology of the extreme Nazi police and paramilitary organization, the SS (*Schutzstaffel*), as it extended its power under Heinrich Himmler (1900–1945).

In contrast to this strident racialization of eugenics, non-racist forms of eugenics emerged strongly in the Weimar welfare state. Positive welfare-oriented measures such as improved housing and education were implemented, and there were proposals to limit the spread of the so-called racial poisons, notably tuberculosis, sexually transmitted diseases, and alcoholism. It was the social hygienist Alfred Grotjahn (1869–1931) who suggested institutionalizing the degenerate as a means of preventing their reproduction, a policy that would later be extended to their sterilization. In the Depression, sterilization of the institutionalized was considered as a cost-saving measure.

Eugenicists were unrepentantly meritocratic. The various German eugenics movements were generally led by professional elites, often public health officers or demographers, but also administrators, lawyers, and priests. They shared common concerns about countering physical and psychological degeneration on the basis of redirecting the welfare state away from universalist to selective social measures, offering schemes like national hereditary biological surveys (*erbbiologischen Bestandsaufnahmen*), hereditary databanks, and mechanisms to segregate deviants and undesirables from the general population.

In 1927 the Jesuit biologist Hermann Muckermann (1877–1962) took a key role in founding a national eugenics institute in Berlin, the *Kaiser-Wilhelm-Institut für Anthropologie* (Kaiser Wilhelm Institute for Anthropology). Researchers there studied the fertility of elite population groups, such as army officers and the police. Deriving financial support from industrialists and state and municipal organizations, the idea was to establish norms for a healthy family life and for selective welfare benefits. The German Psychiatric Institute (*Deutsche Forschungsanstalt für Psychiatrie*) in Munich had a similar role, and this was where Ernst Rüdin established a genealogical-demographic department for research into such topics as criminal biology, the inheritance of schizophrenia, and other "deviant" traits, as well as positive traits such as the inheritance of genius. Biological quality was to be a basis for differential welfare entitlement, while deviancy could be curtailed by institutionalization and sterilization to prevent reproduction, about which the Prussian welfare authorities convened a meeting to prepare legislation in 1932. In this way, eugenics was a major element shaping the Weimar welfare state and social policy, driving means to assess the biological criteria of fitness, and measures for the social segregation of the "unfit."

The rise of eugenics was nonetheless met by critical refutations, particularly of racial hygiene. A long-standing critic was the Austrian social scientist Friedrich Hertz (1878–1964) who published *Moderne Rassentheorien* (Modern Race Theory) in 1904, and *Rasse und Kultur* in 1925. The latter appeared in translation in London and New York as *Race and Civilization* in 1928.[18] Hertz accepted the idea that races existed as physical types, although rarely pure, but could not accept the view that race and psychology were inextricably linked. He similarly rejected claims that intelligence and mental abilities were wholly due to inheritance, and noted how minor coincidences were posited as elaborate statistical proof.[19] He was scathing of the Nordic racism of Baur, Fischer, Lenz, and their popular ally, the Nordic propagandist Hans Günther (1891–1968).[20] Hertz presciently realized the ominous links between racial eugenics and the political Right.

Nazi Eugenics

The Nazi takeover marked a shift from an inclusive biological approach to welfare to one based on race, coercion, and violence against those deemed undesirable for biological and racial reasons. The expectation of race hygienists like Lenz (who had already advised the SS on fitness and reproductive health guidelines) that Hitler would assist eugenics was confirmed in July 1933, when the Nazis passed a sterilization law. The psychiatric geneticist, Rüdin, took a leading role in drawing up the law, which was targeted at a range of clinical conditions, notably schizophrenia, muscular dystrophy, Huntington's chorea, epilepsy, severe mental defect, inherited deafness, and chronic alcoholism. Sexual and mental abnormalities attracted particular interest as indications for sterilization. The law drew on a range of foreign models, including the Californian and Danish sterilization laws, but German eugenic experts provided the essential local impetus.[21] At least 375,000 individuals were sterilized by the German authorities (including some 6,000 in annexed Austria), and there were an estimated 5,000 deaths from complications.[22] There were also racially justified sterilizations, though these lacked a legal basis, since mixed race was not made a criterion for sterilization under the July 1933 law. Nonetheless, 385 African-German mixed-race children were forcibly sterilized in 1937, when a concerted roundup was held by the Nazi authorities and anthropologists. Subjected to extensive psychological, anthropological, and genetic evaluation, the sterilized children, aged between 13 and 16, were fathered by black French troops who occupied the Rhineland after World War I.[23]

The Nazi regime instituted new laws to pursue racial segregation. In September 1935, the Reich Citizenship Law (*Reichsbürgergesetz*) effectively limited citizenship to those of "German and related blood who through their behavior make it evident that they are willing and able faithfully to serve the German people and nation."[24] Jews and other non-Germans were reclassified as aliens and denied German citizenship. The Blood Protection Law (*Gesetz zum Schutz des deutschen Blutes und der deutschen Ehre*), proclaimed on the same day, forbade all sexual relations between Germans and non-Germans, based on citizenship, effectively forbidding marriages and sexual relations between Germans, Jews, and non-whites alike. These were the so-called *Nürnberger Gesetze* (Nuremberg Laws), based on the misconception that blood could be infected by sexual relations with someone of another race. The marital health law of 1935 (*Ehegesundheitsgesetz*), decreed at the same time as the Nuremberg (*Nürnberg*) Laws for racial separation, demanded hereditary health examinations prior to marriage. This was oriented to eugenic ends, but was not specifically racial in its wording, since it was directed to Germans themselves. Marriage certificates involved tests for sexually transmitted disease and genetic disease, and this augmented Nazi health policy that generally stressed preventive medicine.

Soon after these legal initiatives, policies of exclusion from the rights of citizenship and social life were launched against racial "undesirables." The Roma were targeted, along with Jews, for vicious persecution, indicating how the Nazi measures were not purely anti-Semitic but motivated by a general antipathy to supposedly inferior races. In June 1936, a Central Office to "Combat the Gypsy Nuisance" opened in Munich, the headquarters of a national data bank on so-called Gypsies. Robert Ritter (1901–1951), a medical anthropologist at the Reich Health Office, concluded that 90 percent of "Gypsies" native to Germany were "of mixed blood." He described them as "the products of matings with the German criminal asocial subproletariat," and as "primitive" people "incapable of real social adaptation."[25] Through the impositions of such ideas of racial order, long-standing and often well-integrated German citizens were excluded from civil society.

"Euthanasia"

The rationales and procedures for sterilization were radicalized in the Nazi killing of persons with mental illness, the so-called feebleminded and delinquent, and persons with physical disabilities. The system of registrations of people with disabilities for compulsory sterilization was a preliminary basis for "euthanasia," bureaucratically and institutionally isolating those deemed unworthy of life, and who were considered a financial and social burden on the state. Economic, eugenic, and racial policies were fused. The killings were ordered on the basis of medical records sent to the clandestine panel of adjudicating psychiatrists in Berlin.

Hitler did not mention killing the mentally ill and disabled in his book, *Mein Kampf.* But he did so at a Party rally in 1929, and once in power, a medical lobby around Hitler pressed for the introduction of the killing of the malformed and incurable from 1935. A law to legalize "euthanasia" killings was proposed and drafted but never implemented, and the practice was not introduced until 1939. The numbers killed in the initial phase of "euthanasia," code-named "T4" (after the administrative office at *Tiergartenstrasse* 4), according to one set of records amount to 70,273 persons.[26]

The links between eugenics and Nazi "euthanasia" measures (often, just cold-blooded killing) need to be analyzed critically. It was possible to be a eugenicist, advocate coercive sterilization, and yet not condone the killing of patients. Some eugenicists later distanced themselves from these practices. Fritz Lenz, for example, advocated "euthanasia", but from 1941 kept increasingly aloof from its implementation and from the deportations and killings of Jews. Others, however, were fully involved. The psychiatrist Paul Nitsche (1876–1948), an early member of the German Racial Hygiene Society, was involved in administering the "T4" killings. Rüdin and the psychiatrist Carl Schneider (1891–1946) were involved with murderous research on children in a psychiatric hospital at Heidelberg. These killings represent important continuities between sterilization, "euthanasia," and murderous human experiments by various eugenic, genetic, and medical individuals. However, since "euthanasia" was concealed by a special set of nominally secret killing institutions and authorities, the nature and extent of the continuities still requires documentation.

After the Allied liberation of Germany in 1945, doctors, biologists, and public health officials denied the links between eugenics and the killing of psychiatric patients. One of Hitler's medical followers, the surgeon Karl Brandt (1904–1947), said that the decision to implement euthanasia was a demand of the people. The father of a deformed baby wrote to the Führer asking that the child be put out of its misery. We know there was such a baby and that Brandt visited the family, but this likely happened after the decision had already been made among Hitler's close circle to impose euthanasia. At the outbreak of the war, Hitler backdated a secret order for "euthanasia" to Brandt and Philipp Bouhler (1899–1945), the head of his Chancellery.[27]

In 1941 strong condemnation from the Roman Catholic bishop of Münster, Clemens Galen (1878–1946), and some public opposition, particularly from distressed relatives, resulted in an official halt to the killings. "Euthanasia" personnel, including physicians and technicians, were transferred to the *Aktion Reinhardt*, which built and ran the extermination camps of Bełżec, Sobibór, and Treblinka: the use of carbon monoxide gas to kill inmates was a direct link between the killing centers for the psychiatric patients and the Holocaust. "Euthanasia"—selection of the infirm and disabled for killing in the gas chambers of the psychiatric hospitals—continued unabated in the wartime concentration camps. In so-called "special children's wards," children (we do not know the exact numbers, but one estimate by a postwar Frankfurt prosecutor puts the total at 5,000) were killed by injections and starvation. Physicians, assisted by nurses, killed victims by starvation and by administering deadly drugs. The groups killed included newborn babies, children with physical and mental disabilities, the mentally disturbed, and the infirm. Sometimes victims were killed merely for challenging the staff in institutions.[28]

GENETICS AND RACIAL RESEARCH

The number of victims killed for racial and hereditary biological research remains unknown. Yet many German medical researchers took advantage of the large number of killings in clinics, prisons, and concentration camps to pursue their scientific agendas in human genetics, reproductive physiology, and the genetic basis of immunity to infections. The professor of psychiatry Carl Schneider was not only an adjudicator for "euthanasia," but he also saw an opportunity for histo-pathological research, seeking to determine the difference between inherited and acquired mental deficiency. Fifty-two children were examined, each for six weeks. Twenty-one of them were killed deliberately, so as to compare the diagnosis made when they were alive with the post-mortem pathological evidence.[29]

Josef Mengele (1911–1979) was camp doctor at Auschwitz from 1943, where he combined sanitary responsibilities—supervising the "Gypsy Camp," protecting the camp staff from infection—with his duties to racially select newly arrived inmates. In this role, he identified twins and other persons of interest (notably, persons with growth anomalies) and pursued scientific research essentially as an informal, spare time activity. He had worked as assistant to Otmar Freiherr von Verschuer (1896–1969), an expert on the genetics of twins, and at Auschwitz he joined the medical anthropologist Siegfried Liebau (b. 1911), who also was associated with von Verschuer. Mengele exemplifies the scientific drive to produce new data. About 900 children endured Mengele's twin camp, and he scoured transports for growth deformities in the young and old. Most but not all were twins, children who often announced they were twins in the hope of surviving. They came from throughout eastern Europe: Romania, Hungary, Czechoslovakia, and Poland. Most were Jewish, although some were Sinti and Roma, who were killed when the Auschwitz "Gypsy Camp" was liquidated.[30]

From April 1943, Mengele built up his own research installation with a staff of prisoner pathologists, and Verschuer obtained a grant from the German Research Fund for research on hereditary pathology, focusing on blood proteins. Mengele injected his patients with infective agents to compare their effects, and cross-injected spinal fluid, sometimes ordering the killing of a victim so that internal organs could be analyzed. He also assisted in obtaining blood and body parts for Berlin colleagues. Under this project, Mengele assisted in supplying the heterochromic eyes of a Sinto family, studies which show the network of connected eugenic-genetic-race scientists associated with the camps. The eyes were sent to the geneticist—and Nazi activist—Karin Magnussen (d. 1997) at the Kaiser Wilhelm Institute for Anthropology in Berlin, who was carrying out serial research on iris structure of schoolchildren. When anomalies in the iris of the family of Otto Mechau from Oldenburg came to light, she examined them in August 1943 before their deportation to Auschwitz. She then assisted the SS anthropologist Liebau in Auschwitz and contacted Mengele to secure the victims' eyes.[31]

EUGENICS AND NAZI RACIAL PLANNING

The production and application of racial, eugenic, and hygienic knowledge provided a basis for Nazi racial planning and for genocide. Courses that had been organized at the Kaiser Wilhelm Institute for Anthropology in 1935–1936 for SS anthropologists were crucial in bridging scientific research with its eventual genocidal implementation. The training courses in genetics were for SS doctors, involved in supervising the hereditary health of SS recruits and in racial policy. Hans-Helmut Poppendick (1902–1994), for example, acquired expertise in human genetics, and then in the SS Race and Settlement Office worked closely with the eugenicist Fritz Lenz, who, in turn, advised the SS about criteria of selection of SS officers.[32] But Nazi racial categories were always subject to wide interpretation. Racial expertise remained contested and competitive without a single agency ever resolving the incommensurable issues in diverse theories of Aryan, Nordic, and Teutonic racial identity. The same was true of Slav identity. Roma, on the other hand, suffered because of a relatively well coordinated integration of anthropologists with police authorities based on notions of hereditary criminality.

Race scientists took a key role in administering and categorizing populations in the conquered territories, and in providing a planning framework for a gargantuan scheme to murder and to transplant population groups. In the occupied areas, the policies of identifying *Volksdeutsche,* and of displacements and forced labor, became intricately involved with the imposition of racial policy. Administratively the situation became ever more complex as the racial officers were required to categorize people as half and quarter Jew, as "Zigeuner," or "gypsies." Racial biology motivated and drove the persecution and genocide of the Sinti and Roma people. The Reich Health Office imposed severe measures against the Roma, and Robert Ritter (1901–1950) directed their registration and psychological evaluation, supported by a team of psychologists and racial anthropologists, notably Eva Justin (1909–1966).[33] Their observations were followed by incarceration of Roma in concentration camps, notably Auschwitz. After being studied by eugenically minded psychologists, the Roma were deported and later killed.[34]

In the effort to identify people racially, a dense network of local population and racial studies, notably anthropometric and serological researches, was appropriated and implemented for genocidal ends by the Nazi racial experts of the *Rassepolitisches Amt* (Racial Political Office), *SS Ahnenerbe* (Ancestral Inheritance), and the *SS Rasse-und Siedlungshauptamt* (Race and Settlement Office).[35] What can be demonstrated from atrocities like the Jewish skeleton collection at Strassburg is that networks of racial experts were involved in selecting and screening victims for transfer from concentration camps to the sites of atrocity. SS anthropologist Bruno Beger (1911–2009) at Auschwitz selected victims from all over Europe for transfer for killing and dissection in Strassburg.[36]

Nazi demographers were assisted by census techniques, and collected medical, health, and welfare data. Data on diseases and crime were analyzed, and states organized central registries. Hamburg had a Central Health Passport Archive, and Thuringia had an Office for Racial Welfare under the eugenicist Karl Astel (1898–1945) to centralize and analyze the statistics: the new technology of Hollerith punch cards, using an IBM patent, was used. These techniques assisted in calculating the numbers of Jews, how many had emigrated, and the location of those remaining. They calculated how many full, half, and quarter Jews still lived in the Reich. The SS demographer Richard Korherr's (b. 1903) calculations on numbers of Jews in the occupied territories assisted Adolf Eichmann (1906–1962) with the implementation of the Final Solution. In 1943 Korherr calculated for Himmler and Hitler how many Jews had been killed, country by country. Similar techniques were applied to identify social deviants and for the genocidal measures against the Roma. In the occupied territories, notably The Netherlands, census techniques were used in the deportation of Jews to the concentration and death camps of the east.

CONCLUDING PERSPECTIVES

The legacy of Nazism was immense. Medical and scientific elites in the postwar Federal Republic were tainted by the connection, although eugenicists continued to argue that sterilization, in particular, was justifiable. Nothing was offered by the Federal authorities in the way of medical care for the victims, apart from a belated and bureaucratic compensation program restricted to victims of human experiments rather than all racial health policies, and there was no publicly funded program to reverse sterilization. Despite limited compensation for victims of German biomedical research, full acknowledgement of the injustice has not been made.[37]

Eugenics was prominent at the Nuremberg trials, notably in the Medical Trial (Case One of the Nuremberg Military Tribunal) in 1946–1947, but this prominence neither stemmed eugenic practice in other countries nor always resulted in successful prosecution. The Allied attempt to prosecute perpetrators of sterilization proved difficult (with the exception of X-ray sterilization), in part because of the legal basis of the procedure prior to war in 1939. Moreover, much was made of the similarity between U.S. and German eugenics by the defense, who argued that German eugenics differed little from that practiced in the United States.[38] The case against Poppendick of the SS Race and Settlement Office also raised the involvement in Nazi practice of eugenicists at the Kaiser Wilhelm Institute for Anthropology in Berlin. Though Poppendick was condemned, after his release he gained a doctorate under von Verschuer (changing his name slightly to Poppendiek to conceal his conviction).[39] Other eugenicists or racial anthropologists were dismissed after 1945. Yet, though Rüdin was deprived of his Swiss nationality, sterilizations for schizophrenia or "moral idiocy" continued in Zürich until 1970.[40]

The German Racial Hygiene Society ceased to exist after the war, and its papers, alas, have never been located. Racial hygiene was rebranded "human genetics," with a focus on genetic malformations and premarital screening. Switzerland continued eugenic policies into the 1950s, with such measures as forced adoptions from Roma families (see Mottier in this volume). Aspects of Nazi ideology were ongoing in the conservative family policy of the Federal Republic. German conservative social policy, shielded by the Cold War, allowed former racial experts to continue their scientific careers in the Federal Republic. The issue of radiation fallout, for example, provided a new sphere for eugenically trained researchers in the 1950s, continuing previous studies in radiation genetics and in the study of malformations. Eugenicists like Lenz, the geneticist Hans Nachtsheim (1890–1979), the demographer Hans Harmsen (1899–1989), and Verschuer went on to have influential careers in human genetics and public health in the Federal Republic. Verschuer moved to an institute for Human Genetics at Muenster from 1951. Other racial experts remained among Austrian medical elites into the 1950s and 1960s. Indeed, the Viennese brain pathologist Heinrich Gross (1915–2005) continued research on the brains of child "euthanasia" victims.[41]

The student protests of 1968 initiated a break with the old elites, however, leading to such critical publications as those of geneticist Benno Müller-Hill and psychiatrist Klaus Doerner.[42] A new phase of concern about medicine and National Socialism served to liberalize repressive Federal German policies concerning birth control and abortion. By the 1980s, the new social history of medicine and the legacy of civil rights generated interest in eugenics as a scientized form of coercive power. Issues included abuses against the disabled and the mentally ill that culminated in Nazi medical killing, eugenic schemes of birth control and abortion, as well as racial atrocities against ethnic minorities. What is interesting is that marginal figures—left-wing doctors (often former activists in the 1960s protests), feminists, disability rights advocates, and others with human rights concerns— appreciated that eugenics represented a specifically medicalized form of power, while historians generally overlooked this. The standard interpretation in main-stream history was that anti-Semitic, right-wing racist groups laid the founda-tions for Nazi racial ideology and the Holocaust, and that racial atrocities were more the outcome of populist and anti-intellectual Nazi propaganda, than of medically imposed schemes of population and racial welfare planning. That eugenics and racial hygiene had a quite specific history, linked to the emerging welfare state and a range of populations construed as "social problem groups," was not appreciated.

New interest in the social history of medicine from the 1980s generated an examination of the links between eugenics and public health, and associated issues in population policy. In the Federal Republic of Germany, critical historians saw how elites and academic and medical power structures were linked from the 1960s back through the Nazi era to Weimar eugenics. For example, public health physician Hans Harmsen was analyzed through his association with the birth control organi-zation, Pro Familia, and the Protestant welfare group, the Innere Mission.[43] Historical work on eugenics in the German Democratic Republic from 1983 interpreted eugenics as a warning against authoritarian misuse of science and medicine.[44] Radical social history began to shape studies of the records of the persecuted and marginalized, either as life histories or through the records of sterilization courts and "euthanasia" killings.[45] A grassroots wave of interest in critical historical research identified collections of documents in the cellars of hospitals and held by academic and medical institutions reluctant to allow continuities with the Nazi era to be scrutinized.[46]

The cumulative effect of this new body of work in fringe journals and radical books and brochures was a sea change in German history, rendering central ques-tions of population and expertise on heredity and health in a range of disciplines, associations, and institutions. New interpretations of German eugenics by Proctor (stressing continuities) and Weindling (stressing discontinuities) argued for the specificity of eugenically oriented medicine and the need to examine social processes as professionalization.[47]

The idea of a "racial state" advanced by Michael Burleigh and Wolfgang Wipperman and an interpretative essay on modernity by Detlev Peukert provided a new synthetic historical framework for the study of eugenics.[48] Race became a central issue in German history, as opposed to the former concern with state repres-sion of liberal freedoms, and class tensions and inequalities. This contribution has developed a balanced approach, integrating different interpretative angles, and raising problematic and still not wholly resolved issues. While much remains to be researched regarding the politics of eugenics and health in German history, we can see a seismic shift since the late 1980s, bringing a hitherto marginalized terrain into the epicenter of German history.

NOTES

....

1. Wilhelm Schallmayer, *Über die drohende körperliche Entartung der Kulturmenschheit und die Verstaatlichung des ärztlichen Standes* (Berlin: Heuser, 1891).

2. Some historians, eager to emphasize continuities between eugenics and Nazism, have spoken of eugenics as presenting "the final solution of the social problem." Christian Pross and Götz Aly, eds., *Der Wert des Menschen: Medizin in Deutschland 1918–1945* (Berlin: Edition Hentrich, 1989).

3. Paul Weindling, *Health, Race and German Politics between National Unification and Nazism* (Cambridge: Cambridge University Press, 1989), 116.

4. Paul Weindling, "A City Regenerated: Eugenics, Race and Welfare in Interwar Vienna," in *Interwar Vienna: Culture between Tradition and Modernity*, eds. Deborah Holmes and Lisa Silverman (Rochester, NY: Camden House, 2009), 89–113; *Eugenik in Österreich. Biopolitische Strukturen von 1900 bis 1945*, eds. Gerhard Baader, Veronika Hofer, Thomas Mayer (Vienna: Czernin Verlag, 2007).

5. Tudor Georgescu, "In Pursuit of a Purged Eugenic Fortress: Alfred Csallner and the Transylvanian Saxon Eugenic Discourse in Interwar Romania," in *Hygiene, Health and Eugenics in Southeast Europe to 1945*, eds. Marius Turda, Sevasti Trubeta, and Christian Promitzer (Budapest: Central European University Press, forthcoming, 2010).

6. Weindling, *Health, Race, and German Politics*, 145–146.

7. Ibid.

8. Ernst Haeckel, *Natürliche Schöpfungsgeschichte* (Berlin: Reimer, 1909), 11th ed., vol. 2, 742–743.

9. Ibid., 764–765.

10. Eugen Fischer, *Die Rehobother Bastards und das Bastardisierungsproblem beim Menschen* (Jena: Gustav Fischer, 1911).

11. *Tropenarzt im Afrikanischen Busch* (Berlin: Wilhelm Süsserott Verlag, 1943), 3.

12. Rudolf Pöch, "Reisen ins Innere Südafrikas zum Studium der Buschmänner in den Jahren 1907 bis 1909," *Zeitschrift für Ethnologie* 42, no. 1 (1910): 357–362; Pöch, "Einige bemerkenswerte Ethnologika aus Neu-Guinea," *Mitteilungen der Anthropologischen Gesellschaft in Wien* 37 (1907): 57–71.

13. Wilhelm Schallmayer, *Vererbung und Auslese*, 4th ed. (Jena: Gustav Fischer, 1920).

14. Crzellizter/Czellitzer appears in two variant spellings.

15. Weindling, *Health, Race, and German Politics*, 408–409.

16. Paul Weindling, "The Medical Publisher J.F. Lehmann and Racial Hygiene," in *Die Geschichte des Julius-Friedrich-Lehmanns-Verlages 1890–1979*, ed. Sigrid Stoeckel (Munich: Lehmanns, 2002).

17. Hitler's library contained several of Günther's works. See Phillip Gassert and D. W. Mattern, *The Hitler Library: A Bibliography* (Santa Barbara, CA: Greenwood Press, 2001).

18. Friedrich Hertz, *Moderne Rassentheorien* (Vienna: C.W. Stern, 1904), 2nd ed. (Leipzig: Alfred Kröner Verlag, 1915); *Rasse und Kultur: Eine kritische Untersuchung der Rassentheorien* (Leipzig: Alfred Kröner Verlag, 1925).

19. Hertz, *Rasse und Kultur*, see chap. 3, "Rasse und Seelenleben."

20. The edition bearing Lehmann's dedication to Hitler is in the Library of Congress, Washington, DC. Erwin Baur, Eugen Fischer, and Fritz Lenz, *Grundriss der menschlichen Erblichkeitslehre und Rassenhygiene*, 2 vols. (München: Lehmanns Verlag, 1923).

21. Stefan Kühl, *The Nazi Connection: Eugenics, American Racism, and German National Socialism* (Oxford and New York: Oxford University Press, 1994).

22. Gisela Bock, *Zwangssterilisation im Nationalsozialismus* (Opladen: Westdeutscher Verlag, 1986); Claudia Andrea Spring, *Zwischen Krieg und Euthanasie: Zwangssterilisation in Wien 1940–1945* (Vienna: Böhlau, 2009).

23. Reiner Pommerin, *Sterilisierung der Rheinlandbastarde. d. Schicksal einer farbigen deutschen Minderheit 1918–1937* (Düsseldorf: Droste, 1979).

24. Robert Proctor, *Racial Hygiene: Medicine under the Nazis* (Cambridge, MA: Harvard University Press, 1988), 131.

25. Joachim S. Hohmann, *Robert Ritter und die Erben der Kriminalbiologie: "Zigeunerforschung im Nationalsozialismus und in Westdeutschland im Zeichen des Rassismus"* (Frankfurt a. M.: Peter Land, 1991).

26. Henry Friedlander, *The Origins of Nazi Genocide* (Chapel Hill, NC: University of North Carolina Press, 1995).

27. Udo Benzenhöfer, *Der Fall Leipzig (alias Fall "Kind Knauer") und die Planung der NS-"Kindereuthanasie"* (Münster: Klemm & Oelschläger, 2008).

28. Friedlander, *The Origins of Nazi Genocide*.

29. Christoph Mundt, Gerrit Hohendorf, and Maika Rotzell, eds., *Psychiatrische Forschung und NS Euthanasie. Beiträge zu einer Gedenkveranstaltung an der Psychiatrischen Universitätsklinik Heidelberg* (Heidelberg: Wunderhorn, 2001).

30. *Sinti and Roma: Victims of the Nazi Era, 1933–1945* (Washington, DC: United States Holocaust Memorial Museum, 2002).

31. Hans Hesse, *Augen aus Auschwitz* (Essen: Klartext, 2001).

32. Weindling, *Nazi Medicine and the Nuremberg Trials*.

33. Eva Justin, *Lebensschicksale artfremd erzogener Zigeunerkinder und ihrer Nachkommen,' Veröffentlichungen auf dem Gebiet des Volksgesundheitsdienstes* (MD diss. Berlin, 1944).

34. Michael Zimmermann, *Rassenutopie und Genozid: Die nationalsozialistische "Lösung der Zigeunerfrage* (Hamburg: Christians, 1996).

35. Michael Kater, *Das Ahnenerbe der SS 1935–1945: Ein Beitrag zur Kulturpolitik des Dritten Reiches* (München: R Oldenbourg, 1997); Isabel Heinemann, *"Rasse, Siedlung, deutsches Blut," Das Rasse- und Siedlungshauptamt der SS und die rassenpolitische Neuordnung Europas* (Göttingen: Wallstein Verlag, 2003).

36. Hans-Joachim Lang, *Die Namen der Nummern* (Hamburg: Hofmann und Campe, 2004).

37. Paul Weindling, "The Nazi Medical Experiments," in *The Oxford Textbook of Clinical Research Ethics,* ed. Ezekiel J. Emanuel et al. (Oxford and New York: Oxford University Press, 2008), 18–30.

38. Weindling, *Nazi Medicine and the Nuremberg Trials*.

39. Ibid.

40. Marietta Meier, Brigitta Bernet, and Roswitha Dubach, *Urs Germann, Zwang zur Ordnung: Psychiatrie im Kanton Zürich, 1870–1970* (Zürich: Chronos Verlag, 2007).

41. Weindling, *Health, Race, and German Politics,* 566–570; Matthias Diehl, "Endstation Spiegelgrund. Die Tötung behinderter Kinder während des Nationalsozialismus am Beispiel der Kinderfachabteilung in Wien," (Med. Diss. Göttingen 1996).

42. Benno Müller-Hill, *Murderous Science: Elimination by Scientific Selection of Jews, Gypsies, and Others in Germany, 1933–1945* (Cold Spring Harbor, NY: Cold Spring Harbor Laboratory Press, 1998). First edition as Benno Müller-Hill, *Tödliche Wissenschaft: Die Aussonderung von Juden, Zigeunern und Geisteskranken, 1933–45* (Reinbek: Rowohlt, 1984).

43. Hans Harmsen, *Bevölkerungsprobleme Frankreichs, unter besonderer Berücksichtigung des Geburtenrückganges* (Berlin: Vowinckel, 1927).

44. Achim Thom and Horst Spaar, eds., *Medizin im Faschismus* (Berlin: Akademie für ärztliche Fortbildung, 1983).

45. Bock, *Zwangssterilisation im Nationalsozialismus*; Klaus Doerner, "Nationalsozialismus und Lebensvernichtung," *Vierteljahreshefte fuer Zeitgeschichte*, 15 (1968): 121ff.

46. A difficulty in recovering the history of victims is the often blanket imposition of data-protection by German bureaucrats, a measure effectively protecting perpetrators, in covering up the life histories of victims.

47. Proctor, *Racial Hygiene*; Weindling, *Health, Race and German Politics*.

48. Michael Burleigh and Wolfgang Wipperman, *The Racial State: Germany 1933–1945* (Cambridge: Cambridge University Press, 1991); Detlev Peukert, "The Genesis of the 'Final Solution' from the Spirit of Science," in *Reevaluating the Third Reich*, eds. Thomas Childers and Jane Caplan (New York: Holmes & Meier, 1994), 234–252.

FURTHER READING

Burleigh, Michael and Wolfgang Wipperman. *The Racial State: Germany 1933–1945* (Cambridge: Cambridge University Press, 1991).

Friedlander, Henry. *The Origins of Nazi Genocide* (Chapel Hill, NC: University of North Carolina Press, 1995).

Müller-Hill, Benno. *Murderous Science: Science: Elimination by Scientific Selection of Jews, Gypsies, and Others in Germany, 1933–1945* (Cold Spring Harbor, NY: Cold Spring Harbor Laboratory Press, 1998).

Peukert, Detlev. "The Genesis of the 'Final Solution' from the Spirit of Science," *Reevaluating the Third Reich*, eds. Thomas Childers and Jane Caplan (New York: Holmes & Meier, 1994).

Proctor, Robert. *Racial Hygiene: Medicine under the Nazis* (Cambridge, MA: Harvard University Press, 1988).

Weindling, Paul. "A City Regenerated: Eugenics, Race and Welfare in Interwar Vienna," in *Vienna: The Forgotten City between the Wars*, eds. Deborah Holmes and Lisa Silverman (Rochester, NY: Camden House, 2009).

Weindling, Paul. *Health, Race and German Politics from National Unification to Nazism 1870–1945* (Cambridge: Cambridge University Press, 1989).

Weindling, Paul. *Nazi Medicine and the Nuremberg Trials* (Basingstoke: Palgrave, 2004).

Weiss, Sheila F. *Race Hygiene and National Efficiency: The Eugenics of Wilhelm Schallmayer* (Berkeley, CA: University of California Press, 1987).

CHAPTER 19

EUGENICS IN FRANCE AND THE COLONIES

RICHARD S. FOGARTY AND
MICHAEL A. OSBORNE

EUGENICS IN FRANCE *AVANT LA LETTRE:*
ENLIGHTENMENT ROOTS

The pre-history of French eugenics resides in early modern and Enlightenment ideas on human perfectibility, theories of generation and inheritance, and considerations of demography and national strength. Among French elites, the Marquis de Condorcet (1743–1794) and later the utopian Comte de Saint-Simon (1760–1825) and sociologist Auguste Comte (1798–1857) promoted versions of social and political progress. These general notions of progress and the nineteenth century's serial studies of poverty, ill health, and criminality informed social engineering projects of urban environments and their inhabitants. France's rather distinctive intellectual heritage framed modern discourse on population, eugenics, and hygiene. Eugenics and republican rights applied mostly to metropolitan citizens, as the French generally viewed colonized peoples as less perfectible than themselves.[1]

Condorcet's anti-clerical *Esquisse d'un tableau historique des progrès de l'esprit humain* (1795) argued that science, language, and other intellectual technologies promised betterment of the human condition. His optimistic, cumulative, progressive, and distinctly French views elicited pessimistic reaction from Thomas Robert Malthus (1766–1834), whose *Essay on Population* (1798) looms over subsequent discussions of population. In the nineteenth century, Comte's social physiology of the historical stages of civilization completed the general background for eugenic thought. Comtean progress also subordinated the needs of the individual to those of society, a theme prefiguring mature eugenic reasoning.

Natural history, biology, and medicine also framed thinking about human nature and the possibility of improvement. The Enlightenment naturalist Georges Louis Leclerc Comte de Buffon (1707–1788) and his ideas on the historical malleability of animal types, refined and radicalized by the biologist Jean Baptiste Pierre Antoine de Monet de Lamarck (1744–1829) and others, conceptualized nature and humanity as changing. For Buffon this change was a degeneration from a previous type and was premised on the idea of epigenetic embryological development. The bolder Lamarck arranged organisms from simple to complex and envisioned the former progressing to ever-greater complexity according to inner physiological drives and the whim of environmental circumstances.

THE STUDY OF POPULATION

By the 1630s, commercial interests in colonial Martinique prompted the collection of demographic information. Later, King Louis XIV's minister Jean-Baptiste Colbert (1619–1683) assembled information on French citizens, foreigners, creoles, and indigenous peoples throughout French North America, the Antilles, Cayenne, and the most important of all French colonies, Saint-Domingue. These surveys enumerated attributes of colonial populations, including age, place of birth, numbers of slaves, health information, number of men fit to bear arms, number of widows, and so on. Although France surrendered most of its colonial holdings to Britain in 1763, it conducted more than 250 additional surveys in the eighteenth century. The metropolitan population, which grew less robustly than France's continental neighbors prior to the Revolution, received less study, possibly because of the vast scale of the enterprise.[2]

Several eighteenth-century texts address human heredity and breeding, and by the 1770s the term "regeneration" had gained use in scientific and political lexicons.[3] For example, Benoît de Maillet (1656–1738), a French counsel to Egypt and author of *Telliamed* (1748), chronicled imagined conversations between a French missionary and Indian philosopher who considered race mixing to strengthen humanity and attain perfection. "Could we not say that there are certain races of men, like species of trees," observed one, "which must be grafted on to others in order to improve them?"[4] The grafting image appears frequently in subsequent French narratives of eugenics and colonialism. Also published near mid-century was the Parisian physician Charles Augustin Vandermonde's (1727–1762) *Essai sur la manière de perfectionner l'espèce humaine* (1796), which reasoned that Buffonian degeneration could be mitigated through proper procreative conduct and rational approaches to mate selection, child rearing, and education. René Antoine Ferchault de Réaumur's (1683–1757) breeding experiments on domestic fowl likely influenced Vandermonde, who argued that physicians like himself could sculpt and perfect humans by altering environmental factors and promoting rational conjugal hygiene.[5]

Marital and racial issues pervade French scientific discourse. A host of *philosophes* attacked the indissolubility of marriage as an anti-populationist measure trapping fertile individuals in childless unions. Denis Diderot's (1713–1784) *Supplément au voyage de Bougainville* (composed 1772, published 1796) dealt explicitly with biological regeneration and also asserted miscegenation's transformative power. Diderot's mythical Tahitian chief, Orou, actually promotes sexual contact between Frenchmen and Tahitian women to regenerate the intelligence of Tahitian peoples, spur population growth, and strengthen the nation.[6] Other Enlightenment observers argued against miscegenation, especially between black men and white women. For example, Guillaume Poncet de la Grave (1725–1803) campaigned against interracial marriage, claiming it exposed French blood to corruption and produced disfigured children. His efforts resulted in a seldom-enforced ban on interracial marriage instituted on April 5, 1778.[7] Later, the Napoleonic Code Civil of 1804 desacralized marriage and rendered it more open to surveillance by physicians and the state.

Nineteenth-century physicians and government administrators retained these proto-eugenic concerns: colonial and metropolitan demography, marriage, reproduction, degeneration, national strength, and miscegenation. The sphere of state action expanded to include child-rearing and later financial incentives for large families. Populationist, pronatalist, and hygienist concerns comingled with studies of poverty and criminality, and attempts to control them. For example, the German physician Johann Peter Frank (1745–1821) identified poverty as a root of illness, national weakness, and diminished procreative potential. His multivolume *System of Complete Medical Police* (1791–1794) urged legislation to stimulate population growth, protections for unwed mothers, adherence to proper conjugal hygiene, and the regulation of midwifery. A nascent French hygienic movement soon embraced his ideas.

From the Nineteenth Century to 1914: The Lamarckian Heritage and the Colonial Context

Once the science of eugenics emerged formally in the latter half of the nineteenth century, the French eugenics movement generally avoided "negative" measures to prevent the "unfit" from reproducing and stressed "positive" actions directed at environmental conditions to enhance the quality of the French population while simultaneously increasing the quantity.[8] Long lasting neo-Lamarckian views of heredity, notably the heritability of acquired characteristics, set French eugenics apart from other European eugenics movements.[9] Darwin's competing theories had received a rocky reception in France from the beginning, when Clémence Royer (1830–1902) translated *The Origin of Species* into French in 1862. As Yvette Conry has demonstrated, Darwinism was never really "introduced" in France as an operable scientific theory during the nineteenth century, or even during a good part of the twentieth.[10] French scientists attacked Darwinism for its non-quantitative, non-experimental, and admittedly speculative nature. Those French scientists who opted for a transformist philosophy generally supported varieties of neo-Lamarckianism rather than Darwin's thesis of natural selection.

In 1700, France was Europe's most populous nation. By the end of the nineteenth century, the birthrate had fallen, provoking acute fears of absolute and relative decline.[11] Accordingly, French eugenicists veered away from "negative" restrictions on procreation but sought increase in the reproductive activity of the more fit classes. Neo-Lamarckian views on heredity pointed to "positive" eugenic measures ameliorating the environment in which all French people procreated. If parents could pass on characteristics acquired during their lifetime to their children, then the imperative was not to restrict procreation and lower birthrates further, but to enhance the health of potential parents.

Such a positive approach allied French eugenics closely with the pronatalist and social hygiene movements, and French eugenicists embraced efforts that their counterparts in other countries regarded as futile. The German biologist August Weismann's (1834–1914) theory of the continuity of the "germ plasm" and the later rediscovery of Mendelian factors failed to alter the ideas of most French eugenicists. Both theories seemingly undercut attempts to improve the national stock by improving the general health of the population, but the social and political urgency of the "quantity" half of the eugenic equation in France shaped eugenicists' views. An announcement signaling the formation in 1912 of the French Eugenics Society noted the "urgency of stimulating the increase of the population in quantity, if one wants to obtain the quality."[12] Thus quantity was seen as a determinant of quality.

Colonial issues did not loom large in the formalized discussions of metropolitan eugenicists, who focused mainly on metropolitan citizens. Nonetheless, colonial authorities were concerned to optimize their populations. Colonial activities also informed thinking about race, health, and labor and had clear implications for anyone considering those issues within France itself. Colonies were supposed to benefit the metropole, so promoting colonial health and reproduction may have been seen as fulfilling economic promises. During the labor shortages of the interwar years, political figures like Albert Sarraut (1872–1962), a former governor-general of Indochina, minister of the colonies, and twice prime minister, reacted against American "negative" eugenics programs, preferring instead to "manage" the flow of colonial workers to France through environmental and social solutions.[13] Simultaneously, Jules Carde (1874–1949), governor-general of French West Africa, called for France to "*faire du noir*" in an effort to slow depopulation and optimize the reproductive capabilities of African populations to produce workers for French enterprises. Techniques for this effort included medical assistance and attention to demographic issues such as fecundity, infant mortality, and population size.[14]

With the rise of anthropology, anatomy and physiology became more central to conceptions of race. By World War I, the notion of interracial mixing to secure the empire had few adherents. In the colonies, segregation might preserve European seed from the dangers of miscegenation, disease, and the worst aspects of physical and moral degeneration. In the 1920s, France used Rockefeller monies to found a National Office of Social Hygiene and later added a division called the Colonial Social Hygiene Service, which was concerned with preserving health, the race, and with controlling infectious diseases such as tuberculosis. Both agencies maintained elements of eugenic programs. By 1930, however, they were only marginally concerned with population quantity and quality, and were beyond control by eugenicists.[15]

FEARS OF DEGENERATION AND THE FORMATION OF THE FRENCH EUGENICS SOCIETY

A morbid obsession with "degeneration" and national decline also sustained a peculiarly French style of eugenics.[16] France felt acutely the Europe-wide discourse on degeneration, possibly because of the loss of territory after the Franco-Prussian War of 1870–1871 and perceptions of economic decline relative to a united Germany and to Great Britain. Originally formulated as an individual psychiatric diagnosis by Bénédict-Auguste Morel (1809–1873) at mid-century, *dégénérescence* soon came to refer to the progressive devolution of the human species, and many with class-based fears used the theory of *dégénérescence* to define both the problem and its solution scientifically.[17]

The origins of the modern French eugenics movement lie in multifaceted movements for "regeneration" through various social hygiene and pronatalist organizations.[18] Regeneration activities included the promotion of sports and physical fitness and a quest by French doctors for a medical "social prophylaxis" that would address crime and afflictions that might be hereditary, including alcoholism, tuberculosis, and syphilis.[19] Even French psychiatry seemed obsessed with degeneration and addressed its causes and symptoms medically and eugenically via "mental prophylaxis."[20] Also conspicuous was a campaign for healthier babies led by the neo-Malthusian Paul Robin (1837–1912) and his *Ligue de la régénération humaine.*[21] Robin sought support from physicians and eugenicists and echoed the eugenicists' two main concerns, though he prioritized them differently, arguing "the preoccupation with *quality* should always precede that of *quantity.*"[22] But this Malthusian commitment to limiting births marginalized his efforts.[23]

Far more influential over the later course of French eugenics was Aldolphe Pinard's (1844–1934) pre- and post-natal health movement of the 1890s. This science of healthy babies, or *puériculture,* accorded prime importance to parents, since they would pass on healthy traits acquired from their environment to the child, not only during pregnancy but also at the moment of conception. Pinard and others promoted the good health of the reproductive population in order to preserve and improve the species, and while Robin and other neo-Malthusians claimed to share *puériculture*'s goals, their methods were quite different: Robin urged quality before quantity, while Pinard addressed both imperatives simultaneously.[24]

Enthusiasm brought back by the French delegation to the First International Eugenics Congress in London in 1912 led to the founding of the French Eugenics Society at the end of that year.[25] Pinard was a founding member and vice president, and Edmond Perrier (1844–1921), a prominent neo-Lamarckian zoologist and director of the Paris Muséum d'Histoire Naturelle, became the first president. Until the outbreak of war in 1914 (when formal activities were suspended until 1920), the Society met regularly to hear talks like Perrier's on "Eugenics and Biology" and faithfully published a slender monthly journal, *Eugénique.* Physicians constituted more than half the group's founding members.[26] The Society's agenda included government action to manage sexual activity, marriage, and birth and life expectancies via *puériculture,* social hygiene, and eugenics—clear examples of what Michel Foucault would later call "biopower."[27]

1914–1945: A Movement in Flux

During the 1920s and 1930s, the French Eugenics Society's enthusiastic activity and coherence gave way to organizational atrophy and marginalization. Simultaneously, advocacy of negative eugenic measures became more prominent and came to at least partial fruition after 1940, when Marshal Philippe Pétain's (1856–1951) National Revolution opened the way to more interventionist and restrictive eugenic measures.

Suspension of activities during World War I slowed the group's momentum and caused it to lose membership. The 1924 creation of the National Office of Social Hygiene incorporated some of the Society's agenda, and in 1926 *Eugénique* ceased publication. The Society met irregularly and faltered until 1941, when it merged with a branch of the International Institute of Anthropology. Yet the Great War's appalling demographic impact inspired French eugenicists to reemphasize social hygiene and positive eugenics to rejuvenate a French population facing greater and more specific threats than a vague, generalized "degeneration." Now, more than ever, the production of more and healthier children was critically urgent, and if the Society was organizationally weak, other institutions and actors were now more open to eugenic ideas.

Public discussions of eugenics proceeded, even if they did not rejuvenate the Society. In 1926 Pinard, now a member of the Chamber of Deputies, proposed legislation to require all French males to submit to a premarital medical examination. But years of debate over the scope of the examination, the state's responsibilities to its citizens, and the role of doctors in the process held up the bill's progress. Nonetheless, the 1930s witnessed increasing interest in eugenics, and even negative eugenic proposals unthinkable in earlier periods dominated by fears of depopulation.

Those fears had not entirely disappeared, of course. The mid-1930s were "Hollow Years," when the demographic losses of 1914–1918 meant that fewer young men achieved reproductive (and military) age.[28] But the push for premarital examinations signaled a shift toward the "quality" side of the eugenics equation, with "quantity" relegated to lesser priority. As immigration gained in importance, Eugène Apert (1868–1940), a Society founder and its president beginning in 1934, identified immigration as a priority for eugenic action. The physician René Martial (1852–1955), veteran of three years in Morocco and concerned over the diseases of colonial immigrants, argued that immigration endangered national efficiency and should be restricted to preserve the health of the French nation. In addition, prominent physicians like Just Sicard de Plauzoles (1872–1968) feared high rates of natality among France's poor and advocated birth control. These and other negative eugenics measures surfaced amidst the social pessimism and economic anxieties provoked in part by the Depression.[29] Religious Catholics, stimulated in part by papal condemnation of eugenics, opposed birth control and other negative eugenic measures, as did pronatalist groups who were still concerned about falling birthrates, and members of the political Left who preferred the positive eugenics approach of public hygiene.[30]

Resistance to negative eugenics is also evident in the cool reception given to the ideas of Charles Richet (1850–1935) and Alexis Carrel (1873–1944), the era's two most famous eugenicists. The accomplished physician and biologist Richet served as the president of the Society immediately after the war. His *Sélection humaine* (1919) accepted Lamarckian-style environmental factors as having powerful long term effects on species, but also counseled shorter term restrictive measures to improve the "race" based on the iron laws of heredity. Proposals included removal and quarantine of the sick, prohibitions on interracial marriage, "the elimination of the mentally deficient" (through neglect, not euthanasia), and prohibition of marriage for the "abnormal."[31] Yet, despite Richet's prestige and visibility in the French eugenics movement, few of his colleagues subscribed to what they regarded as his extreme views.

However, no figure better symbolizes the marginality of negative eugenics in France than the most internationally famous of French eugenicists, Alexis Carrel, who won the Nobel Prize for Physiology or Medicine for 1912 but remained largely outside French scientific and eugenics communities for most of his life.[32] The bulk of his career was spent in the United States at the Rockefeller Institute for Medical Research. In the 1930s, he and the aviator Charles Lindberg (1902–1974) worked on a perfusion pump for the *in vitro* cultivation of animal hearts, kidneys, ovaries, and other organs. The experiments sparked sensationalized rumors of Carrel's Frankensteinesque attempts to create an artificial human. Both men were interested in human engineering, biological regeneration, and the problems of civilization.

Carrel also had social and professional interactions with many American eugenicists, including Henry Fairfield Osborn (1857–1935), Charles Davenport (1866–1944), and John Harvey Kellogg (1852–1943), but few contacts with eugenicists in France. His most famous statement on eugenics, the astoundingly successful and popular book *Man, the Unknown,* appeared in French and American editions in 1935 and was also abridged by the *Reader's Digest.*

William Schneider portrays Carrel as promoting an idiosyncratic style of Franco-American eugenics linked to an organization for scientific study, modeled after the freedom of scientific investigation enjoyed at the Rockefeller Institute and Institut Pasteur. There, disinterested biopolitical researchers would improve society and enjoy occupational security for life.[33] Carrel's views ranged widely over biological holism and degeneration, mysticism and Roman Catholicism, telepathy and anti-materialism, and how the unfit burdened civilization. *Man, the Unknown* contained positive and negative eugenic ideas. Carrel's reputation as a proto-Nazi eugenicist who envisioned the Final Solution rests primarily on one passage of this wide-ranging book that suggested "humanely and economically" disposing of criminals and the criminally insane, "in small euthanasic institutions supplied with proper gases."[34] After Paris fell to the Germans, Carrel met with the head of the collaborationist government, Marshal Pétain, and agreed to head a new *Fondation Française pour l'étude des problèmes humaines,* founded in November 1941.

APOTHEOSIS: THE VICHY YEARS

Carrel's return to head a Vichy institution is indicative of newfound opportunities for eugenicists during the war years. Yet the history of France between 1940 and 1944 displays continuities with earlier trends, as well as new departures.[35] In the previous decades, some French eugenicists had considered negative measures and embraced Mendelian genetics, and in 1930 Georges Schreiber, a pediatrician and Society vice president, had written approvingly of therapeutic sterilization.[36] René Martial's calls to restrict immigration were firmly rooted in the rigid biological determinism of blood types and the dangers of careless "interracial grafting."[37] Yet, for all this intellectual activity, concrete restrictive measures were conspicuously absent. The only major proposed legislation directly related to eugenics, the premarital exam first proposed by Pinard in 1926 continued to languish in parliament. In the end, it would take the defeat of 1940, German occupation, and the installation of Pétain's Vichy government for eugenics to develop more fully in new directions. Even then, however, continuity would be in some ways as conspicuous as novelty.

In the occupied portion of France, the German authorities provided the impetus for indigenous French racism and anti-Semitism to be expressed in eugenic terms. The notorious *Commissariat général aux questions juives* (CGQJ), a center for racist and anti-Semitic propaganda, was instigated in 1941 by Germans, but created, mostly funded, and staffed by Frenchmen. The primary concern in this period, of course, was anti-Semitism, and eugenic justifications thereof, to which important strands of French medicine and Martial's ideas contributed.[38] To be sure, the anti-Semitism of the period cannot be reduced to eugenics, but eugenics often provided support and a vocabulary to buttress even the wildest anti-Jewish propaganda and the most sinister anti-Jewish measures. A particularly good example of this was CGQJ leader Louis Darquier de Pellepoix's (1897–1980) defense of the infamous 1942 Vel' d'Hiv roundup, and eventual deportation, of Parisian Jews as a "public hygiene" measure.[39] Vichy's most enduring eugenic legacy, the 1942 law instituting a premarital exam, remains in force to this day. Its sponsors correctly recognized it as "the first time [that] a eugenic measure appears in French legislation."[40]

Anne Carol presents the 1942 law as the culmination of the eugenics movement in France, particularly since this primarily medical measure emerged out of a movement that had always been largely defined by physicians, and because the law was consistent with the longer history of French eugenics. The requirement for a premarital exam—for both parties, within one month of marriage—was contained in a larger law "Relative to the Protection of Maternity and Newborns," designed to promote the health of mothers and infants by stipulating requirements for pre-natal, post-natal, maternal, and infant health care. Thus, the law was consistent with one of the most important precursors (or perhaps more accurately, adjuncts) to eugenics, *puériculture*, which had always focused on health from the preconception to the post-natal stages. So the 1942 law was "certainly the heir of a French tradition."[41] It was both symbolic and fitting that the most significant piece of eugenic legislation ever passed in France was embedded in a series of other measures promoting social hygiene and maternal health.

The premarital examination also reflects the peculiar context of its emergence. The exam was mandatory, but placed no restrictions on the right to marry, nor did it require the parties to divulge the results, even if they revealed a serious infectious disease. It was in this sense merely informative, and sought, in the words of the law's authors, "only to confront the future couple with their conscience and their responsibility."[42] The law was consistent with the cautious approach of French "liberal medicine" and earlier laissez-faire notions of state action. Thus, under Vichy France, eugenics avoided the "totalitarian ambitions" of extreme negative eugenics, even as that vision triumphed on the other side of the Rhine and spread its malign influence throughout much of Europe.[43]

Nonetheless, the Vichy regime did provide institutional support for eugenics in one additional way, by inviting Alexis Carrel to return to France and establish his *Fondation pour l'étude des problèmes humaines.*[44] The projects undertaken by the Foundation in its four years of existence show the influence of French eugenics, especially the older concerns of population quality and quantity, and a focus on children, the family, and health. The most important legacy of Carrel's foundation would be its contribution to the postwar study of demography, since the prestigious *Institut national d'études démographiques* (INED) would be formed in 1945 from elements of Carrel's foundation and with some of its personnel.[45]

In the end, World War II and the Vichy regime marked the high point of French eugenics activity. Yet France continued to define its own idiosyncratic vision of eugenics, and the Vichy regime itself, whose National Revolution called for a return to traditional Catholicism and sought to encourage large families and population growth rather than restrict them, failed to enact extreme negative eugenic measures such as sterilization, abortion, or euthanasia. Vichy legislation outlawing abortion was particularly forceful, so the fact that the 1942 law on premarital examinations was comparatively mild and that this was the high point of French eugenics are probably more significant than the circumstance of the legislation being enacted under Vichy.[46]

1945–PRESENT: THE END OF FRENCH EUGENICS OR AN "ETERNAL RETURN"?

French eugenics and biology became less idiosyncratic after World War II. Just as the more purely scientific mainstream biological science of inheritance traveled a path from national distinctiveness, even peculiarity, before 1940 to closer unity with international norms by the 1960s, so too French eugenic concerns have merged with international discussions of prenatal diagnosis, abortion, fertility treatment, genetic manipulation, and so-called "designer babies."[47] Still, eugenic ideas persist and the term "eugenics" provokes strong emotions, prompting some scholars to write of the topic's "eternal return."[48]

In the immediate postwar period, the population geneticist Jean Sutter (1910–1970), at INED, continued to promote eugenic solutions to traditional French problems associated with public health and population.[49] But eventually, the notoriety of Nazi-style eugenics and the merging of French genetics with international norms led advocates of social hygiene who would in the past have embraced a discourse of eugenics to define their efforts as "euthenics," an alternative to "the eugenics of exclusion," which stressed ameliorating the environment, outside of considerations of heredity.[50] The term euthenics was not new as American eugenicists had employed it as early as 1913. By the 1960s, one could find little trace of the former overt avowal of eugenics among French researchers, despite the continuities between the research agendas of earlier eugenicists and contemporary researchers in institutions like INED.

In recent years the term "eugenics" has been applied less to demographic reform than to individual manipulations of human life and "eugenic" decisions considered within the doctor and patient relationship. As Anne Carol has described it, the state has disappeared from the older eugenic trinity of family, state, and doctor.[51] French biologist and popular science writer Jean Rostand (1894–1977), a proponent of eugenics both before World War II and after, articulated this transformation of eugenic considerations as early as 1953, noting that if the issues developed out of scientific investigation, the role of the scientist would now be more focused on providing citizens information on which they could then act individually.[52] So today, given the enormous and growing power of modern medicine over human life, parents and doctors face problems many commentators do not hesitate to describe as "eugenic."[53]

As one recent observer has put it, "Formerly eugenics was focused on the selection of procreators; its modern forms are concerned more and more with the choice of gametes."[54] Thus, state or elite efforts to wield biopower are not where the controversies and debates focus, and in fact, when the state or the wider social body enters into these issues, it is in terms of law and jurisprudence.[55] This was particularly evident in the Nicholas Perruche affair, in which Nicholas and his parents sued the doctor and laboratory who had conducted a prenatal diagnostic test but failed to detect the rubella he had contracted *in utero* that left him severely handicapped. A court ruled that a person born handicapped could sue the administrators of a faulty prenatal diagnostic test if the results failed to provide a mother with the opportunity to abort the pregnancy. However, in 2002 the French National Assembly overturned this ruling with new legislation stipulating that the mere fact of being born could not constitute grounds for damages. The ensuing controversy has again raised the specter of eugenics, but on the level of individual decisions and actions by parents and doctors. Still, it is possible that state intervention in the matter, representing the putative rights of the unborn, places restrictions on reproductive freedoms.[56]

Eugenic concepts still shadow contemporary discussions of biotechnology and medical ethics. Scholars like Pierre-André Taguieff argue that contemporary debates about genetics and eugenics have freed themselves from the taint of racism that marked them in the past, and are purely scientific discussions about the best way to cure or prevent hereditary disorders.[57] Others fear new scientific knowledge and medical technology will be applied to "better the race" one birth at a time. The intention may be "philanthropic," as advocates have always claimed such efforts to be. Nonetheless, its implications remain sinister.[58] What is still at issue, then, is the core problematic that led scientists, doctors, and others to think in terms of race betterment and eugenics, that is, the "temptation," as many observers put it, to consider human life "as a material" and to arrange people hierarchically "according to the functional value attributed to their organism."[59]

Conclusion

French eugenics remains subtly imbricated with ideas of race, a circumstance heightened by the legacy of the nation's vast colonial empire. Connections between eugenics, race, and empire have not entirely faded from public memory. Indeed, these links reemerge in surprising ways. In December 2006, the government of

Niger declared that it intended to pursue a legal case in French courts against the author and television news presenter Pascal Sevran for racist statements. His *Le Privilège de Jonquilles* (2005) argued that Niger's high birthrate and extreme poverty constituted a crime, and that the perpetrators "sign their crime by copulating." In a later interview, he declared that poverty, hunger, and suffering meant that "it is necessary to sterilize half the planet!" The Niger government's response characterized Sevran's ideas as "fascist" and asserted, "They could not be more racist and they praise eugenics, in which Mr. Sevran is a thorough believer."[60]

That an African government would invoke eugenics to describe the Malthusian musings of a writer in the former French metropole is perhaps not too surprising, given the enduring legacies of imperialism, racism, and eugenics. In previous decades, Sevran's invocation of sterilization would have put him on the margins of a French eugenics movement that more often stressed positive eugenic measures, but his linkage of procreation, population, health, and race partook of a long tradition. Thus, in France and beyond, if anything guarantees an eternal return of eugenics, it is the rhetorical uses to which the term can still be put.

NOTES

1. Alice L. Conklin, *A Mission to Civilize: The Republican Idea of Empire in France and West Africa, 1895–1930* (Stanford, CA: Stanford University Press, 1997).

2. Jacques Dupâquier and Eric Vilquin, "Le pouvoir royal et la stastique demographique," in *Pour une histoire de la statistique*, 2 vols. (Paris: Institut National de la Statistique et des Études Économiques, 1976–1977), 1: 83–104.

3. Michael Winston, "Medicine, Marriage, and Human Degeneration in the French Enlightenment," *Eighteenth-Century Studies* 38, no. 2 (2005): 263–281; Winston, *From Perfectibility to Perversion: Meliorism in Eighteenth-Century France* (New York: Peter Lang, 2005); Kathleen Wellman, "Physicians and Philosophes: Physiology and Sexual Morality in the French Enlightenment," *Eighteenth-Century Studies* 35, no. 2 (2002): 267–277.

4. Quoted in Pamela Cheek, *Sexual Antipodes: Enlightenment Globalization and the Placing of Sex* (Stanford, CA: Stanford University Press, 2003), 174.

5. Anne C. Vila, *Enlightenment and Pathology: Sensibility in the Literature and Medicine of Eighteenth-Century France* (Baltimore, MD: Johns Hopkins University Press, 1998).

6. Cheek, *Sexual Antipodes*, 164–193.

7. Sue Peabody, *"There Are No Slaves in France": The Political Culture of Race and Slavery in the Ancien Régime* (Oxford and New York: Oxford University Press, 1996), 128–133.

8. See William H. Schneider's seminal and comprehensive work on eugenics in France, *Quality and Quantity: The Quest for Biological Regeneration in Twentieth-Century France* (Cambridge: Cambridge University Press, 1990).

9. Schneider, *Quality and Quantity*; Anne Carol, *Histoire de l'eugénisme en France: Les médecins et la procréation, XIXe-XXe siècle* (Paris: Seuil, 1995); Jacques Léonard, "Les origines et les conséquences de l'eugénique en France," *Annales de Démographie Historique* (1985): 203–214; Pierre-André Taguieff, "Eugénisme ou décadence? L'exception française," *Ethnologie française* 29 (1994): 81–103.

10. Yvette Conry, *L'introduction du Darwinisme en France au XIXe siècle* (Paris: Vrin, 1974). See also Schneider, *Quality and Quantity*, 55–58; Jacques Léonard, "Eugénisme et Darwinisme: Espoirs et perplexités chez des médecins français du XIXe siècle et du début du XXe siècle," in *De Darwin au Darwinisme: science et idéologie*, ed. Yvette Conry (Paris: Vrin, 1983): 187–207.

11. Joseph Spengler, *France Faces Depopulation* (New York: Greenwood Press, rpt. 1968); Joshua H. Cole, *The Power of Large Numbers: Population, Politics, and Gender in Nineteenth-Century France* (Ithaca, NY: Cornell University Press, 2000), 180–211.

12. *Chronique médicale*, February 1 (1913): 47.

13. Clifford Rosenberg, "Albert Sarraut and Republican Radical Thought," *French Politics, Culture and Society* 20, no. 3 (2002): 97–114.

14. Raymond R. Gervais and Issiaka Mandé, "Comment compter les sujets de l'Empire? Les étapes d'une démographie impériale de AOF avant 1946," *Vingtième siècle, revue d'histoire* 95 (2007): 63–74.

15. Schneider, *Quality and Quantity*, 134–145.

16. Schneider, "Puericulture and the Style of French Eugenics," *History and Philosophy of the Life Sciences* 8 (1986): 265–277.

17. Daniel Pick, *Faces of Degeneration: A European Disorder, c. 1848–c. 1918* (Cambridge and New York: Cambridge University Press, 1989); Jacques Hochmann, "La théorie de la dégénérescence de B.-A. Morel, ses origines et son évolution," in *Darwinisme et société*, ed. Patrick Tort (Paris: Presses Universitaires de France, 1992), 401–412; Robert A. Nye, *Crime, Madness, and Politics in Modern France: The Medical Concept of National Decline* (Princeton, NJ: Princeton University Press, 1984).

18. Alain Drouard, *L'eugénisme en questions: l'exemple de l'eugénisme* (Paris: Ellipses, 1999), 81–86.

19. Laurent Mucchielli, "Criminologie, hygénisme et eugénisme en France (1870–1914): débats médicaux sur l'élimination des criminels réputés <<incorrigibles>>," *Revue d'histoire des sciences humaines* 2, no. 3 (2000): 57–89.

20. Anne-Laure Simonnot, *Hygiénisme et eugénisme au XXe siècle à travers la psychiatrie française* (Paris: Seli Arslan, 1999).

21. Drouard, *Eugénisme en questions*, 103–109.

22. Paul Robin, *Dégénérescence de l'espèce humaine, causes et remèdes*, Nouvelle édition populaire (Paris: Librairie de "Régénération," 1905 [orig. 1896]), inside leaf, "Déclaration de la ligue de la Régénération humaine." Emphasis in original.

23. Alain Drouard, "Aux origines de l'eugénisme en France: l néo-malthusienisme (1896–1914)," *Population* 47, no. 2 (Mar–Apr 1992): 435–460; Schneider, *Quality and Quantity*, 33–37.

24. Schneider, *Quality and Quantity*, 63–83: Schneider, "Puericulture and the Style of French Eugenics," 265–277; Nadine Lefaucher, "La puériculture d'Adolphe Pinard," in Tort, *Darwinisme et société*.

25. Jacques Léonard, "Le premier Congrès international d'eugénique (Londres, 1912) et ses conséquences françaises," *Histoire des sciences médicales* 17, no. 2 (1983): 141–146; Schneider, *Quality and Quantity*, 84–94.

26. Schneider, *Quality and Quantity*, 92–94.

27. Michel Foucault, *The History of Sexuality, Volume I: An Introduction* (New York: Vintage, 1990).

28. Eugen Weber, *The Hollow Years: France in the 1930s* (New York: Norton, 1994).

29. Schneider, *Quality and Quantity*, 181.

30. William H. Schneider, "The Eugenics Movement in France, 1880–1940," in *The Wellborn Science: Eugenics in Germany, France, Brazil, and Russia*, ed. Mark B. Adams (New York: Oxford University Press, 1990), 79–84.

31. Schneider, *Quality and Quantity*, 110–113.

32. Andrés H. Reggiani, *God's Eugenicist: Alexis Carrel and the Sociology of Decline* (New York: Berghahn Books, 2007).

33. Schneider, *Quality and Quantity*, 256–282.

34. Alexis Carrel, *Man, the Unknown* (New York: Harper, 1935), 318–319, quoted in Schneider, *Quality and Quantity*, 276–277.

35. Robert O. Paxton, *Vichy France: Old Guard and New Order, 1940–1944* (New York: Knopf, 1972).

36. Schneider, *Quality and Quantity*, 186–190.

37. René Martial, *Traité de l'immigration et de la greffe inter-raciale* (Paris: Larose, 1931); Schneider, *Quality and Quantity*, 231–255.

38. See Henri Nahum, *La médecine française et les juifs, 1930–1945* (Paris: Harmattan, 2006).

39. Schneider, *Quality and Quantity*, 262.

40. Carol, *Histoire de l'eugénisme en France*, 331.

41. Ibid., 331.

42. Quoted in Ibid., 332.

43. Ibid., 312.

44. Alain Drouard *Une inconnue des sciences sociales: la Fondation Alexis Carrel, 1941–1945* (Paris: La Maison des Sciences de l'Homme, 1992).

45. Andrés Horacio Reggiani, "Alexis Carrel, the Unknown: Eugenics and Population Research under Vichy," *French Historical Studies* 25, no. 2 (2002): 331–356; Alain Drouard, "A propos de l'interface médecine-sciences sociales: la Fondation Française pour l'Étude des Problèmes Humains dite Fondation Carrel," *Histoire des sciences médicales* 28, no. 1 (1994): 49–56.

46. See Miranda Pollard, *Reign of Virtue: Mobilizing Gender in Vichy France* (Chicago, IL: University of Chicago Press, 1998).

47. Richard M. Burian and Jean Gayon, "The French School of Genetics: From Physiological and Population Genetics to Regulatory Molecular Genetics," *Annual Review of Genetics* 33 (1999): 313–349.

48. Jean Gayon and Daniel Jacobi, eds., *L'éternel retour de l'eugénisme* (Paris: Presses Universitaires de France, 2006). See also André Pichot, *L'eugénisme, ou les généticiens saisis par la philanthropie* (Paris: Hatier, 1995), 58–80.

49. Schneider, *Quality and Quantity*, 291.

50. Carol, *Histoire de l'eugénisme en France*, 351.

51. Ibid., 354.

52. Drouard, *Eugénisme en questions*, 122.

53. Danielle Moyse, "Le diagnostic prénatal, quelle sécurité? L'échographie ne peut devenir l'instrument d'un eugénisme déguisé," *Projet* 293 (2006): 24–27, and *Bien naître, bien être, bien mourir: propos sur l'eugénisme et l'euthanasie* (Paris: Érès, 2001); Jacques Milliez, *L'euthanasie de foetus: médecine ou eugénisme?* (Paris: Odile Jacob, 1999).

54. Zeynep Kivileim-Forsman, "Eugénisme et ses diverses formes," *Revue trimestrielle des droits de l'homme* 54, no. 14 (2003): 527.

55. Jean-Noël Missa and Charles Susanne, eds., *De l'eugénisme d'État à l'eugénisme privé* (Brussels: De Broeck & Larcier, 1999); Catherine Bachelard-Jobard, *L'eugénisme, la science et le droit* (Paris: Presses Universitaires de France, 2001).

56. Kivileim-Forsman, "Eugénisme et ses diverses formes," 531.

57. Pierre-André Taguieff, "Sur l'eugénisme: du fantasme au débat," *Pouvoirs* 56 (1991): 23–64, and "Retour sur l'eugénisme. Questions de définition," *Esprit* 200 (1994): 198–215.

For a full discussion of this contemporary debate, see Jean-Paul Thomas, *Les fondaments de l'eugénisme* (Paris: Presses Universitaires de France, 1995), 85–121.

58. Pichot, *L'eugénisme*.

59. Jacques Testart, *Le désir du gène* (Paris: Flammarion, 1994), 270.

60. Abdoulaye Massalatchi, "Niger Brings Racism Case against French Writer," *Reuters AlertNet*, December 16, 2006, www.alertnet.org/thenews/newsdesk/L16886757.htm.

FURTHER READING

Carol, Anne. *Histoire de l'eugénisme en France: Les médecins et la procréation, XIXe–XXe siècle* (Paris: Seuil, 1995).

Drouard, Alain. *Une inconnue des sciences sociales: la Fondation Alexis Carrel, 1941–1945* (Paris: La Maison des Sciences de l'Homme, 1992).

Drouard, Alain. *L'eugénisme en questions: l'exemple de l'eugénisme* (Paris: Ellipses, 1999).

La Haye Jousselin, Henri de. *L'idée eugénique en France: essai de bibliographie* (Paris: H. de La Haye Jousselin, 1989).

Léonard, Jacques. "Eugénisme et Darwinisme: espoirs et perplexités chez des médecins français du XIXe siècle et du début du XXe siècle," in *De Darwin au Darwinisme: science et idéologie*, ed. Yvette Conry (Paris: Vrin, 1983), 187–207.

Nye, Robert A. *Crime, Madness, and Politics in Modern France: The Medical Concept of National Decline* (Princeton, NJ: Princeton University Press, 1984).

Pick, Daniel. *Faces of Degeneration: A European Disorder, c. 1848–c. 1918* (Cambridge and New York: Cambridge University Press, 1989).

Reggiani, Andrés Horacio. *God's Eugenicist: Alexis Carrel and the Sociobiology of Decline* (New York: Berghahn, 2007).

Schneider, William H. *Quality and Quantity: The Quest for Biological Regeneration in Twentieth-Century France* (Cambridge: Cambridge University Press, 1990).

Taguieff, Pierre-André. "Eugénisme ou décadence? L'exception française," *Ethnologie française* 29 (1994): 81–103.

Thomas, Jean-Paul. *Les fondaments de l'eugénisme* (Paris: Presses Universitaires de France, 1995).

UNESCO. *Cloning, Gene Therapy, Human Behaviour, Eugenics... Six Lectures* (Paris: UNESCO, 2005).

Vila, Anne C. *Enlightenment and Pathology: Sensibility in the Literature and Medicine of Eighteenth-Century France* (Baltimore, MD: Johns Hopkins University Press, 1998).

Wellman, Kathleen. "Physicians and Philosophes: Physiology and Sexual Morality in the French Enlightenment," *Eighteenth-Century Studies* 35, no. 2 (2002): 267–277.

Winston, Michael. *From Perfectibility to Perversion: Meliorism in Eighteenth-Century France* (New York: Peter Lang, 2005).

....

CHAPTER 20

EUGENICS IN THE NETHERLANDS AND THE DUTCH EAST INDIES

....

HANS POLS

EUGENICS has never held broad appeal in the Netherlands. It was advocated by a small group of intellectuals but never captured the interest of elite scientists, the medical profession, leading advocates of the movement for social and hygienic reform, or the general public. From the 1880s, evolutionary theory, the ideas of Thomas Malthus (1766–1834), and, to a lesser extent, eugenics, were aired mostly by small groups of Dutch intellectuals. Eugenic ideas were mainly discussed by proponents of the public health movement, which encompassed a variety of initiatives that promised to increase the quality of the Dutch population through hygienic measures, increased educational opportunities, and moral reawakening. The first Dutch organization exclusively devoted to promote research in eugenics and the dissemination of eugenic ideas was founded in 1930, two decades after other countries. Even the most enthusiastic Dutch eugenicists were cautious and tentative about eugenics; they almost always emphasized the need for further research and rarely proposed practical applications. The only eugenic measure ever discussed in the Dutch parliament was the compulsory medical examination before marriage; it did not pass. German ideas on racial purity hardly registered in Dutch eugenic circles; when they arose, they were generally dismissed as unscientific.

In contrast, eugenics was taken up far more enthusiastically in the Dutch East Indies. An organization to promote eugenics was founded in Batavia in 1927. Unlike their counterparts in the Netherlands, advocates of eugenics in the Dutch East Indies explicitly discussed the importance of race. Eugenicists aimed to investigate the characteristics of the racial and ethnic groups that inhabited the Indonesian archipelago, acclimatization (the physiological and metabolic changes in individuals of European descent who lived in tropical regions), the consequences of crossbreeding, and the effects of rapid modernization on what they considered the primitive indigenous population. Theories on racial difference had been present in biological, anthropological, and medical thought from the start of the twentieth century. In the twentieth century, racial boundaries were drawn much more explicitly and policed more extensively in colonial public life. The colonial eugenics society achieved modest support, mainly among physicians, biologists, agricultural scientists, and higher civil servants. It was, for a period of five years, the most active and influential eugenics group in the Dutch empire.

EUGENICS IN THE NETHERLANDS BEFORE 1940

From the early twentieth century, a variety of social reformers, public health activists, physicians, progressive politicians, and concerned citizens began expressing deep concern about threats to the quality of the Dutch population. These social critics were concerned about a variety of social ills, including a (perceived) rise in alcoholism, prostitution, vagrancy, asocial activities, petty thievery, criminality, and other behaviors that attracted both moral reproach and medical concern. Their concerns were motivated by a more general "civilizing offensive" that was taking place at the time; the problematic behaviors were generally transgressions of middle-class moral codes.[1] Various interventions were proposed to promote the further advance of civilization and to stem tendencies leading to degeneration, which critics believed would lead to a general state of social decline characterized by moral and material squalor. Proposed interventions included sanitation, the provision of fresh drinking water, compulsory education, legal limits to the length of the work week, restrictions on the sale and consumption of alcohol, and the establishment of parks and playgrounds.

Physicians and public health activists were particularly concerned about three diseases which, according to them, constituted the greatest threat to the population of the Netherlands: tuberculosis, alcoholism, and venereal diseases. These diseases not only adversely affected public health and labor productivity, but threatened the health of future generations as well. The fear that they would be transmitted congenitally was based on a broad conception of reproduction rather than a specific understanding of the nature and quality of genetic inheritance, which only became dominant in the 1930s. The apprehension about the future of the germ plasm provided a rhetorical tool which connected a wide variety of vices with medical concerns; not surprisingly, proposals for highly moralistic health crusades followed. In the debates about the future of the Dutch population, public health and moral concerns became increasingly intertwined. Initially, eugenics was characterized by sociological and medical critiques on the state of the Netherlands as a modern country; its advocates expressed uneasiness about the low quality of identifiable sectors of the population. Because of the influence of the public health and social hygiene movements, in addition to the relative absence of interest in social Darwinism (ideas about the nature of society were generally phrased in moral and religious terms instead of in biological or economic ones), eugenic initiatives in the Netherlands initially focused on the hygiene of procreation and the health of future generations, rather than on genetics and inheritance of specific traits.[2] By the 1920s, however, there was a growing interest in genetic inheritance and the inherent inequality of human beings.

The plant breeder, botanist, and later professor of genetics M. J. Sirks (1889–1966) was central to the organizational efforts of the eugenics movement. His manual on the science of heredity (translated into English in 1956 as *General Genetics*) became a standard textbook in the Netherlands.[3] Sirks also edited three genetic journals for over forty years: *Genetica, Bibliographia Genetica,* and *Resumptio Genetica.* Other leading researchers in genetics, such as Hugo de Vries (1848–1935), J. P. Lotsy (1867–1931, and Tine Tammes (1871–1947), were less interested in eugenics, although they viewed human beings as inherently unequal. They doubted that simple eugenic measures would improve the genetic quality of the population, and they emphasized the need for further research, disavowing the overly simplistic approaches advocated by eugenicists.

Dutch social scientists, as opposed to biologists and geneticists, showed a greater interest in social Darwinism; some came to advocate eugenics explicitly. The ethnologist, sociologist, and social geographer S. R. Steinmetz (1862–1940), one of the founding fathers of the social sciences in the Netherlands, was strongly influenced by Herbert Spencer's (1820–1903) sociology. Steinmetz was one of the first individuals in the Netherlands to formulate a comprehensive eugenics program: he was convinced that there were significant differences between human beings, which were based on the qualities they had inherited. He lamented the higher fertility of the undesirable in comparison to the gifted classes, a phenomenon that, according to him, inevitably led to "race suicide." He proposed a variety of measures to stimulate the better social classes to procreate more to counter this trend. Steinmetz opposed measures aiding the feeble and the weak because they robbed Dutch society of the natural mechanisms for "weeding out the unfit." Only the ethnologist and, later, sociologist J. H. F. Kohlbrugge (1865–1941), who had spent two decades in the Dutch East Indies as a physician, embraced even more radical right-wing eugenic views.[4]

During the 1920s, Dutch eugenicists were pessimistic about the effects of the public health movement; they doubted whether environmental change, hygienic reform, and compulsory education would result in enduring improvements. They focused on promoting positive measures to stimulate "desirable" individuals to procreate; the most radical negative measure they advocated was a compulsory medical examination before marriage. Sterilization was hardly ever discussed. For the few individuals in the Netherlands who were interested in eugenics, it provided a discourse to critique modernity rather than a practical program for racial improvement. They emphasized the need for more extensive research that might, in a distant future, lead to practical initiatives.

In the 1930s, debates among public health activists interested in eugenics were mainly about ways to manage groups of "socially inferior" individuals. The concern about the rise in the prevalence of mental retardation and mental illness provided added impetus to these debates. Dutch psychiatrists had always been interested in eugenics; throughout the interwar years, the number of psychiatrists participating in discussions on eugenics increased. They were inspired by the international mental hygiene movement, which emphasized prevention.[5] Professor of psychiatry K. H. Bouman (1874–1947) had advocated eugenic measures since the 1910s. In 1924, hoping to establish a Dutch Society for Mental Hygiene, he expressed alarm about the increase in the number of asocial, maladjusted, and mentally disabled and disturbed individuals; despite his eloquence, the society only became active in the 1930s. Physician Gerrit Pieter Frets (1879–1958), who was associated with the psychiatric hospital Maasoord, near Rotterdam, was active in eugenic associations as well. He was known for his socialist leanings and his interest in finding pragmatic and scientific solutions for social problems. Frets had visited California to study the legal aspects of sterilization. He had also investigated families with Huntington's chorea who were living near (and in) Maasoord and often referred to this hereditary condition in his writings.[6] The psychiatrist and Protestant theologian J. van der Spek (1886–1982), who experimented with somatic treatments such as ECT and insulin treatment, also advocated the wider application of eugenics.[7] Psychiatrists interested in eugenics emphasized the importance of preventing mental inferiority. Even though they expressed concern about the increase in the number of mentally inferior individuals, they were reluctant to formulate measures that would control these individuals or decrease their progeny.

One of the most important advocates for eugenics in the Netherlands was the biologist Marie Anne van Herwerden (1874–1934). After distinguishing herself in plant cytology research, she was appointed research associate in biology at the University of Utrecht. After she was passed over for a professorship, she received a stipend to visit the United States. There she met the French eugenicist Alexis Carrel (1873–1944), the geneticists Edmund Wilson (1856–1939) and Thomas Hunt Morgan (1866–1945), as well as the eugenicist Charles B. Davenport (1866–1944). On her return home, van Herwerden became the most active promoter of eugenics in the Netherlands, held key positions in the few eugenic organizations there, and represented the Netherlands at the International Federation of Eugenics Organizations. Her *Human Heredity and Eugenics* became the standard manual of eugenics in the Netherlands.[8]

Eugenicists in the Netherlands were inspired by American initiatives and ideas and, to a lesser extent, by British ones. Despite the proximity of the Netherlands to Germany and the dominance of German medical thought before 1940, Dutch eugenicists were highly ambivalent about German ideas and activities. They admired the scholarship of leading German advocates of eugenics and envied their social prestige. Nevertheless, they had strong misgivings about their ideas on race, and about the eugenic measures they were proposing. These misgivings only increased after the Nazis took power in 1933 and such measures were implemented. Most Dutch eugenicists considered concerns about racial purity to be unscientific; consequently, racial issues were hardly ever discussed in the Dutch eugenic literature. In addition, they were generally not in favor of forced sterilization. At the 1934 conference of the International Federation of Eugenics Organizations in Zurich, Frets attacked the scientific justification for forced sterilization, which led to an angry altercation with Ernst Rüdin (1874–1952), the designer of the German sterilization laws.[9] He repeated his critique two years later, when the Federation met in Scheveningen, the Netherlands, where he was a rare voice of protest among eugenicists against German initiatives.[10] Although more individuals present might have had their misgivings, Frets was the only one who voiced them.

MEASURES

The public health discussions in which eugenicists participated focused on the quality of the future population of the Netherlands. In these debates, eugenicists advocated making medical examination before marriage compulsory and engaged in extensive discussions on the desirability, nature, and timing of this examination. The medical examination of future spouses would reveal the presence of venereal diseases, alcoholism, and tuberculosis; in addition, it would identify genetic vulnerabilities. Proposals to make medical examination before marriage compulsory were raised in parliament twice: in 1924 and again in 1953. At both times, it was discussed only briefly and dismissed as an excessive intrusion into the private affairs of citizens. Opponents claimed that this measure would be counterproductive by promoting extramarital relationships between individuals who were unlikely to pass, which in turn would lead to an increase in illegitimate births.[11] The fact that birth control, which was at the time highly controversial, in particular in denominational circles, would be one of the measures that could be taken if genetic defects were detected only made the situation more complicated. (The physician most responsible for the dissemination of information on birth control in the Netherlands, Jan Rutgers (1850–1924), was partly inspired by eugenic ideas.) Generally, advocates of the medical examination before marriage concluded that it should take place on a voluntary basis. It never became very popular; the few clinics that provided advice on birth control measures enjoyed much greater patronage.

In general, Dutch eugenicists were hesitant to propose eugenic measures, partly because they were convinced that this was premature, since the science of human heredity was only in its infancy, and partly because they did not want to advocate measures that had little chance of gaining popular and political acceptance. After compulsory sterilization laws had been passed in Germany, ethical misgivings strengthened this skeptical attitude. As biologist A. L. Hagedoorn (1880–1953) commented in 1938:

As long as the eugenics movement...limited itself to talking and to passing resolutions on congresses, it was possible for us scientists interested in heredity to ignore it all, although we preferred to be uninvolved in these spheres. However, now that very close in our neighborhood, in the middle of Europe, suddenly legal measures are pushed through in which science is completely set aside, we notice that we have been playing a dangerous game.[12]

EUGENICS ORGANIZATIONS IN THE NETHERLANDS

The Netherlands was not represented at the first International Congress of Eugenics in London in 1912. Dutch participation at the second Congress, held in 1921 in New York, was minimal. The first organization that aimed to promote eugenics in the Netherlands was founded in 1924 as the Central Committee of Collaborating Societies Promoting Research in Human Heredity (in 1930, the name was changed to the Dutch Eugenics Federation). This Committee represented five organizations with an interest in eugenics, groups interested in genetics, anthropology, a systematic study of the Dutch population, and compulsory medical examination. Later, the Eugenic Society of the Dutch East Indies and a group interested in the problems of population joined as well.[13] The range of organizations represented in the Central Committee might give the impression that widespread activity was taking place. This impression is misleading, however, since a small number of eugenicists played key roles in all these organizations. In addition, the Central Committee did not undertake any activities of its own.

The first Dutch periodical exclusively devoted to eugenics was *Ons Nageslacht* (Our Progeny), which started publishing in 1928 in Batavia, the capital of the Dutch East Indies. When Johan Christiaan van Schouwenburg (1873–1946), who had organized the Eugenics Society in the Dutch East Indies and was its motivating force, migrated to the Netherlands in 1933, he continued to promote eugenics activities there. Realizing that there was no similar periodical in the Netherlands, he founded *Erfelijkheid bij den Mensch* (Human Heredity), which first appeared in 1935 (the title changed into *Afkomst en Toekomst* [Descent and Future] in 1937). At its high point, this journal had about 300 subscribers. The journal ceased publication in 1941.

During the 1930s, eugenics in the Netherlands was at its peak in influence and public visibility. In 1933, plans were made to found an institute for the study of human heredity and racial biology, which was to be located in the Hague, with Sirks as chair. However, attempts to raise funds were unsuccessful. Despite the relative influence of eugenic ideas in the 1930s, Dutch eugenicists faced a number of challenges. Eugenic ideas were discussed by liberals and socialists, while denominational circles were disinterested and, at times, openly hostile. Membership in eugenics organizations decreased (partly as a consequence of economic conditions). Eugenic measures were criticized by biologists and geneticists because they were not backed by scientific research (even though most of these scientists were sympathetic to the aims of the eugenics movement). At the same time, Dutch eugenicists attempted to distance themselves from the initiatives that were undertaken in Germany, in particular the emphasis on racial purity and the institutionalization of forced sterilization laws.

EUGENICS IN THE DUTCH EAST INDIES

Eugenics, as already noted, enjoyed far more attention in the Dutch colonial world than in the Netherlands, in part because race was central in the social organization of the Dutch East Indies.[14] The European colonial group, which held a tight grip on power and controlled virtually all natural, economic, and military resources, attempted to maintain a strict social and spatial separation from the indigenous inhabitants of the colonies. The Dutch East Indies had three parallel legal codes: different sets of laws pertained to Europeans, the indigenous population, and "foreign Orientals" (which included those of Arab and Chinese descent, but not the Japanese, who were, after a trade agreement in 1898, included as Europeans). During the seventeenth and eighteenth centuries, under the rule of the United [Dutch] East Indies Company (VOC), most European visitors to the colonies were male; if they settled, they married indigenous women. Their offspring, Indo-Europeans, became the mainstay of the European inhabitants of the Indies.[15] From early in the twentieth century, an increasing number of European families settled in the Dutch East Indies.[16] Consequently, racial and ethnic boundaries were policed increasingly stringently. Nevertheless, in 1920, up to 13 percent of European men in the Indonesian archipelago married indigenous women, and up to 90 percent of the European population could be designated as Indo-European.[17]

During the first two decades of the twentieth century, the so-called "ethical policy" held sway in the Dutch East Indies, according to which the profits made by the Dutch in the Indies had to be reinvested locally to benefit the indigenous population. Educational opportunities for Indonesians were significantly expanded, irrigation works initiated, and a viable infrastructure established. In 1918, a parliament (the *Volksraad*) was established in Batavia in which the indigenous population enjoyed political representation for the first time. After 1920, social tensions in the Dutch East Indies increased markedly, with an ever more vocal nationalist movement demanding political rights and, later, independence. These demands were countered by an increasingly repressive colonial government. Indo-European individuals became more and more discontented with their social position because they felt marginalized by the increased number of Europeans in the colonies. At the same time, they were competing with an increasing number of educated indigenous individuals, who started to occupy positions in the lower ranks of the colonial administration that previously had been reserved for Indo-Europeans. The

Indo-European Association (IEV), founded in 1919, advocated special privileges for the group it represented and, until the mid-1930s, embraced the most conservative political ideology. The agitation from this group, in addition to the poverty of many Indo-Europeans, led many social commentators to write on the "Indo problem."[18]

Tensions between racial and ethnic groups provided the main context for a growing interest in eugenics in the Dutch East Indies. In contrast to the Netherlands, eugenics in the Dutch East Indies was primarily and almost exclusively concerned with issues of race and racial difference. Colonial advocates of eugenics presented the new science of human heredity as a tool that could potentially alleviate racial tensions by increasing mutual understanding based on scientific insights regarding the characteristics of the different ethnic and racial groups of the colonies. Like their counterparts in the Netherlands, eugenicists in the Dutch East Indies argued that vast amounts of research needed to be conducted because the science of human heredity was still in its infancy. They argued that the archipelago, which was home to more than 100 different ethnic groups speaking over 250 languages, could be transformed into a vast eugenic laboratory.[19] They were interested in investigating three issues: acclimatization (or the challenges Europeans faced when they attempted to live in tropical regions); cross-breeding; and the effects of rapid modernization on primitive races. Research leading to reliable information in these areas would, it was hoped, substantially aid colonial governance.

The research of C. D. de Langen (1887–1967), professor of internal medicine at the Batavia Medical Faculty from 1914 to 1935, focused on acclimatization. He investigated the physiological and metabolic effects of migration to the tropics on individuals of European descent.[20] Around the same time, colonial psychiatrists, among them F. H. van Loon (1886–1971) and P. H. M. Travaglino (1877–1950), had expressed views on the nature of the indigenous mind, which they characterized as childish, emotional, infantile, and unreliable. In a speech to a conservative political association, Travaglino built upon this analysis, arguing that an extensive study of the psychological characteristics of the different ethnic and racial groups should inform colonial rule.[21] Less subtle were the offensive statements of the Association of [European] Physicians, written by two members of its executive, J. J. van Lonkhuyzen (1877–1965) and O. Deggeller (1872–1941), who derided the depraved moral state, laziness, and unimpressive intellectual abilities of the indigenous population. Although their statements were widely criticized in the European and the indigenous press, both men nonetheless came to occupy influential positions in the Public Health Service.[22]

Eugenics Organizations in the Dutch East Indies

The *Eugenetische Vereeniging in Nederlansch-Indië* (Eugenics Society of the Dutch East Indies) was the outcome of a collaboration between a German medical researcher with a strong interest in the biology of race mixing (Ernst Rodenwaldt, 1878–1965), a retired forest manager and active member of the Indo-European Association (J. C. van Schouwenburg), and a leading civil servant working at the

archives of the colonial government, who had a long-standing interest in genealogical research, in particular of Java's Indo-European families (Paul Constant Bloys
van Treslong Prins, 1873–1940). The initiative to found an organization to promote
eugenics was taken by van Schouwenburg. In 1927, he published an article in the
progressive journal *Koloniale Studiën* (Colonial Studies), providing a eugenic perspective on the role of the Dutch colonial government in the Indies. He argued that
eugenics could alleviate social tensions in a society torn by racial antagonism. If the
characteristics of the different racial and ethnic groups in the Indies were unknown,
he argued, colonial administrators were essentially working blind.[23] He squarely
placed then-current discussions about the future direction of colonial policy,
including political participation by the indigenous population, within a eugenic
framework, asserting that it would be impossible to continue ruling the Dutch East
Indies without adequate scientific insights into the nature of its population. Eugenics
promised to realize a more harmonious colonial society. Aiming to stimulate interest
and research, van Schouwenburg emphasized that reliable scientific insights on
human heredity were barely available.

In late 1927, the *Eugenetische Vereeniging in Nederlansch-Indië* was founded. In
the early 1930s, when the society was at its peak, it was just short of 600 members.
In 1928, it started a journal, *Ons Nageslacht* (Our Progeny), which aimed to increase
public awareness of eugenics while disavowing any political implications.[24] The
Eugenics Society attracted higher-level civil servants, physicians, biologists, and
agricultural researchers; most of them had enjoyed higher education (in particular
in medicine, agriculture, and biology). A very small number of Javanese nobility
also joined. Deggeler, by then an inspector in the Public Health Service, was elected
first president, while Rodenwaldt became one of its most active members.[25]
Rodenwaldt knew van Schouwenburg well and provided the theoretical underpin-
nings of the work of the *Eugenetische Vereeniging*, as well as conducting several
research projects it funded. Bloys van Treslong Prins, who had access to data on the
births, deaths, and marriages of Europeans in the Dutch East Indies, provided
necessary information for Rodenwaldt's research. In the later volumes of *Ons
Nageslacht*, he published extensive genealogies of prominent Dutch East Indies
families.

Rodenwaldt, a specialist in tropical medicine, had migrated to the Dutch East
Indies in 1921, after Germany lost most of its empire during World War I. After
leading a number of successful malaria campaigns, he was appointed director of the
Eijkman Institute, Batavia's premier medical laboratory. From his student days,
Rodenwaldt had maintained a strong interest in studying race mixing, inspired by
his former teacher Eugen Fischer (1874–1967), who had studied the Rehoboth, the
descendants of the Boers and the Hottentots in South West Africa. His involvement
in malaria campaigns required Rodenwaldt to travel extensively throughout the
archipelago. During one of these trips, he visited the small island of Kisar, just east
of Timor, where a small number of soldiers of the United Dutch East Indies
Company had settled in the late seventeenth century.[26] They had married local
women, but their offspring had only married within their small group (which

entitled the men to enlist in the colonial armed forces). Consequently, this tribe of mestizos had been left undisturbed for the next century and a half, providing, in Rodenwaldt's words, an excellent natural experiment in race crossing.[27]

Rodenwaldt collected an enormous amount of physical data, including skin and eye color; hair color and texture; skull size and shape; limb length and shape; and the form of the nose. On the basis of extant information and extensive interviews, he reconstructed their family trees (greatly aided by Bloys van Treslong Prins). He also provided a fascinating account of the way this small group had survived on an isolated and mostly infertile island. On the basis of his research, Rodenwaldt concluded that earlier eugenic fears about the deleterious effects of interbreeding were mostly unfounded (a view that would not be popular among the European inhabitants of the Dutch East Indies, who generally feared interbreeding and contamination with the indigenous inhabitants of the Indies). He explained the success of some of the descendants of the Kisarese by the strength of their European inheritance. Rodenwaldt advocated more research, which in his view was essential for the future of the Dutch East Indies. At the same time, he cautioned against premature applications. Rodenwaldt's research gained international recognition in eugenic circles; he was invited to become a member of the Committee on Race Crossing of the International Federation of Eugenics Organizations.

Rodenwaldt hoped to interest Indo-Europeans in his research projects, both because he needed them as research material and because he was convinced that this group could benefit most from eugenic research. He was already collaborating with van Schouwenburg, who had been the president of the Berbek chapter of the Indo-European Association (IEV) and who was the editor of its periodical, *Onze Stem* (Our Voice). According to Rodenwaldt, Indo-Europeans, by combining features from two different races, were unusually well adapted to life in the tropics.[28] The Eugenics Society received funding from the IEV in 1930; nevertheless, it did not succeed in building an enduring alliance with this organization. Over the next few years, Rodenwaldt conducted several research projects through the Eugenics Society. He collected information on family pedigrees, using charts he had received from Davenport.[29] Through the use of questionnaires, he aimed to study the genital function of European and Indo-European women in the tropics with the aim of correcting the widespread opinion that white women became infertile and to ascertain the effects of cross-breeding on fertility. He concluded—despite the low number of questionnaires returned—that the tropical climate did not adversely influence fertility, libido, and menstrual pains in European women and that there were minimal differences in fertility between European and Indo-European women.[30] Rodenwaldt's questionnaire was widely criticized as being in bad taste; only a fraction was returned. Several newspapers objected to the immoral nature of the questions posed. Many Indo-Europeans felt uncomfortable answering questions about descent, which, in the 1920s and 1930s, could undermine their social position (which was partly based on suppressing and minimizing their indigenous descent).

In 1934, Rodenwaldt returned to Germany to teach Hygiene at the University of Kiel. A year later, he took up a professorship at the Medical Faculty at the University of Heidelberg, which by then had become notorious for its support of Nazi policies.[31] Rodenwaldt himself became a forceful apologist for Nazi eugenic measures (at one point, Ernst Rüdin warmly recommended him for a position at the Kaiser Wilhelm Institute for Genealogy in Munich as an excellent "Führer, teacher and organizer," while Alfred Ploetz (1860–1940), an influential German eugenicist and advocate of racial biology, praised his long association with Nazism).[32] In the meantime, his opinions about the effects of cross-breeding had changed dramatically. While he had previously reassured readers that the misgivings against crossbreeding were unfounded, his opinions had turned decidedly negative:

> He [the mixed-blood individual] never sleeps, interfering in all human
> relationships, undermining trust, even within his own family, when one of the
> partners is of pure blood. [...] Miscegenation is a risk for every human
> community. Since no one can estimate its consequences, the mixing of races is
> irresponsible. A people interbreeding without restraint with a people racially
> removed will see its numbers of self-assured leader personalities dwindle.[33]

Rodenwaldt now used sociological and psychological instead of biological and genetic arguments, which reflected the racial anxieties and preoccupations of the Nazis much better. He expressed strong doubts whether individuals of mixed descent had a constitution that was suitable to embody and transmit advanced Western European culture.[34]

EUGENICS IN THE NETHERLANDS DURING AND AFTER WORLD WAR II

The Dutch Eugenics Federation and the organizations associated with it ceased their activities in 1941, probably to prevent being co-opted by the German occupying forces. Physicians who were members of the NSB (National-Socialist Association) organized the Medical Front, which started publishing *Rashygiënische Mededeelingen* (Racial Hygiene Announcements) in February 1944. The biologist W. F. H. Ströer (1907–1979), who had received advanced training in Germany, was the only individual active in this organization who had also been involved in the Dutch eugenics movement before 1940. The Nazis hoped that he would be instrumental in implementing their racial policies in the Netherlands. The language of eugenics during the German occupation was more forceful and more intent on practical application than that utilized by its pre-war advocates. Authors in *Rashygiënische Mededeelingen* often disparaged earlier Dutch efforts as weak and merely academic.

After the war, Dutch eugenicists were afraid that links with Nazi policies had tainted eugenics as a whole. This, however, did not impede their activities, but the revival of the Dutch eugenics movement after the war proved to be short-lived. Public health activists and social reformers who had been active before the war reunited and proclaimed the urgency of measures to remake the Dutch population as a means to undo the damage of the occupation years.[35] Eugenicists explicitly distanced themselves from the German measures implemented during World War II, because they knew that this association would discredit their initiatives. Most of the ideas they had presented before the war reappeared during the late 1940s and early 1950s.

The Federation of Eugenics Societies was not revived after the war. Instead, in 1949, the Nederlandse Anthropogenetische Vereniging (Dutch Anthropogenetic Society) was founded, which aimed to coordinate anthropogenic research, stimulate educational initiatives, and raise funds to open an institute for the collection of data on the Dutch population. Nevertheless, the ideas and ideals of the pre-war era had vanished. Discussions among members of the Anthropogenetic Society focused on the desirability of preventing hereditary diseases on an individual basis. As a consequence, the medical examination before marriage was once more proposed as a beneficial measure. It was again brought up in parliament, and, yet again, dismissed.

SUCCESS AND INFLUENCE OF EUGENICS IN THE NETHERLANDS

In 1927, when the International Federation of Eugenics Societies met in Amsterdam with Leonard Darwin (1850–1943) as chairman, van Herwerden bemoaned the fact that the Dutch eugenicists could only offer hospitality, since they had very little else to show for themselves: Dutch initiatives had been feeble and hesitant from the beginning, she thought.[36] Other countries, most notably the United Kingdom, the United States, Germany, and Sweden had displayed much more initiative. Eugenics societies had been established there shortly after the turn of the century, and some of these countries had even opened institutions to conduct research in eugenics. Van Herwerden also observed that, in the Netherlands, eugenics was debated only in intellectual circles and never held popular appeal.[37]

The main reason for the lack of success of the rather moderate eugenics movement in the Netherlands is related to the so-called pillarization of Dutch society. Before 1960, the Netherlands was divided into three segments or pillars. Two of them were denominational in nature: Catholic and Protestant (although the latter segment can be divided further between the Dutch Reformed Church and stricter Calvinist denominations). The third segment was non-denominational and consisted of liberals, socialists, progressives, and others. Civil society was divided between these segments: the educational system, sports clubs, radio broadcasting companies, newspapers, social associations, and political parties were organized within each of them. Political compromise made governing a pillarized society possible: the government provided the basic structure of social life, while the pillars were responsible for all matters involving morality and theological concerns. Because the medical examination before marriage impinged on moral concerns and was considered excessively intrusive, the Dutch government viewed it as an initiative it could not support. In particular, the Catholic Church objected to a state-sanctioned medical intrusion into marriage, which it felt ought to be ruled by theological concerns.

The pillarization of Dutch society also explains the lack of popularity of social Darwinist ideas in the Netherlands. Theologians dismissed such ideas as vulgar and materialistic; according to them, human beings were motivated (or ought to be motivated) by ethical concerns rather than egoism, greed, or competition with their fellow human beings. Thus, the social organization of the Netherlands before 1960 made a public discussion of eugenic ideas very difficult, as it did not fit with the dominant moral discourse in the denominational pillars. Eugenics ideas were only discussed by socialists and liberals in the non-denominational pillar. In addition, the political compromise that pillarization entailed made it virtually impossible for eugenicists to propose measures to be implemented by the state. In addition, the eugenics movement in the Netherlands experienced its highest visibility and influence only in the early 1930s, a time when most geneticists had lost interest in it. For these reasons, eugenics failed to attain both popular and intellectual appeal; it remained limited to talking and to passing resolutions on congresses. The only way it could exert a limited influence was by participating in organizations that promoted public health and mental hygiene.

In the Dutch East Indies, religious denominations were much less influential. Social and political life was built on ethnic and racial distinctions, which were drawn and policed more stringently during the twentieth century. In this context of increasing racial and ethnic tension, eugenics, portrayed as the scientific study of racial and ethnic differences, was received much more favorably because it responded to widespread social concerns in colonial circles, among them the fear of contamination with indigenous society and the increased political antagonism (often perceived as racial antagonism) of the 1920s and 1930s. Eugenicists participated in debates on the nature of colonial society and proposed measures to bolster colonial governance. This would provide biologists and physicians with a politically significant role, which must have been enticing to them. For these reasons, eugenics held both popular and professional appeal in the Dutch East Indies. As a consequence, eugenics was more popular in the Dutch colonial periphery than in the metropolis.

NOTES

1. On the civilizing offensive in the Netherlands, see Piet de Rooy, *Werklozenzorg en Werkloosheidsbestrijding 1917–1940: Landelijk en Amsterdams Beleid* (Amsterdam: van Gennep, 1978); and Adriana Dercksen and Louise H. Verplanke, *Geschiedenis van de Onmaatschappelijkheidsbestrijding in Nederland, 1914–1970* (Meppel: Boom, 1987).

2. This is the main conclusion of the standard work on the history of eugenics in the Netherlands: Jan Noordman, *Om de Kwaliteit van het Nageslacht: Eugenetica in Nederland, 1900–1950* (Nijmegen: SUN, 1989).

3. Marius Jacob Sirks, *General Genetics*, trans. Jan Weijer and D. Weijer-Tolmie (The Hague: Martinus Nijhoff, 1956). The first (Dutch) edition of this manual appeared in 1922.

4. Hiskia G. Coumou, "Jacob Kohlbrugge: Sociaal pedagoog *malgré lui*," in *Sociale Pedagogiek in Nederland, 1900–1950* (Leiden: DSWO Press, 1998), 93–130.

5. For a history of the mental hygiene movement in the Netherlands, see Leonie de Goei, *De Psychohygiënisten: Psychiatrie, Cultuurkritiek en de Beweging voor Geestelijke Volksgezondheid in Nederland, 1924–1970* (Nijmegen: SUN, 2001). For an overview of the interest of Dutch psychiatrists in mental hygiene and eugenics, see Harry Oosterhuis and Marijke Gijswijt-Hofstra, *Verward van Geest en Ander Ongerief: Psychiatrie en Geestelijke Gezondheidszorg in Nederland (1870–2005)*, 3 vols. (Houten: Bohn Stafleu van Loghum, 2008)1: 384–391.

6. G. P. Frets, *Sterilisatie*, vol. 7, *Verslagen van het Psychiatrisch-Juridisch Gezelschap* (Amsterdam: Van Rossum, 1933); G. P. Frets, "De Erfelijkheid bij 15 Lijders aan Chronische, Progressieve Chorea (Huntington), die in de Jaren 1914–1941 in de Psychiatrische Inrichting *Maasoord* Verpleegd Zijn," *Genetica* 23, no. 1 (1943): 465–528. See also Ria van Hes, *Dansen aan Zee: De Ziekte van Huntington in Katwijk en Omstreken* (2006), available at www.dansenaanzee.web-log.nl/dansenaanzee/ (accessed October 14, 2008).

7. Goei, *De Psychohygiënisten;* Noordman, *Om de Kwaliteit van het Nageslacht,* 104–106.

8. M. A. van Herwerden, *Erfelijkheid bij den Mensch en Eugenetiek* [Human Heredity and Eugenics] (Amsterdam: Nederlandsche Bibliotheek, 1926). A second edition appeared in 1929; a third edition, edited by G. P. Frets, appeared in 1954.

9. Noordman, *Om de Kwaliteit van het Nageslacht,* 131. See also Stefan Kühl, *The Nazi Connection: Eugenics, American Racism, and German National Socialism* (Oxford and New York: Oxford University Press, 1994), 30.

10. Kühl, *Nazi Connection,* 30.

11. Noordman, *Om de Kwaliteit van het Nageslacht,* 150–169.

12. Quoted in ibid., 111.

13. For an overview of these organizations. see ibid., 93–145.

14. Ann L. Stoler, "Making Empire Respectable: The Politics of Race and Sexual Morality in 20th-Century Colonial Cultures," *American Ethnologist* 16, no. 4 (1989): 634–660.

15. At the founding meeting of the Indo-European Association in 1919, the definition of "Indo-European" was debated extensively; no consensus ensued. Naturally, any definition, then and now, is inherently contestable. Apart from individuals who had at least one Indonesian forebear, individuals with European parents who had been born in the Indies were included as well. The extent to which individuals identified themselves as Indo-European depended on a variety of social, cultural, and political factors. See J. Th. Koks, *De Indo* (Amsterdam: H. J. Paris, 1931) [Koks identified himself as Indo-European].

16. For the consequences of these changes in the colonies for individuals of mixed descent (initially called mestizos but later referred to as Indo-European individuals or "Indos"), see Jean Gelman Taylor, *The Social World of Batavia: European and Eurasian in Dutch Asia* (Madison, WI: University of Wisconsin Press, 1983); Ulbe Bosma and Remco Raben, *Being "Dutch" in the Indies: A History of Creolisation and Empire, 1500–1920,* trans. Wendie Shaffer (Singapore: National University of Singapore Press, 2008); Julia Clancy-Smith and Frances Gouda eds., *Domesticating the Empire: Race, Gender, and Family Life in French and Dutch Colonialism* (Charlottesville, VA: University of Virginia Press, 1998).

17. See Kleian, *Burgelijke Stand: Aanhangesel Behoorende bij het Adresboek van geheel Ned.-Indië* (Weltevreden: Landsdrukkerij, 1920).

18. Hans Meijer, *In Indië Geworteld: De Twintigste Eeuw* [Rooted in the Indies: The Twentieth Century] (Amsterdam: Bert Bakker, 2004); Bosma and Raben, *Being "Dutch" In the Indies*. See also Paul W. van der Veur, "The Eurasians of Indonesia: Castaways of Colonialism," *Pacific Affairs* 27, no. 2 (1954): 124–137; van der Veur, "Cultural Aspects of the Eurasian Community in Indonesian Colonial Society," *Indonesia* 6 (1968): 38–53; and Ann L. Stoler, "Sexual Affronts and Racial Frontiers: European Identities and the Cultural Politics of Exclusion in Colonial Southeast Asia," *Comparative Studies in Society and History* 34, no. 3 (1992): 514–551.

19. Anthropological research had already provided an overview of the many ethnic groups in the Dutch East Indies; see J. P. Kleiweg de Zwaan, *De Rassen van den Indischen Archipel* [The Races of the Indies Archipelago] (Amsterdam: Meulenhoff, 1925).

20. See, for example, C. D. de Langen and H. Schut, "Over Acclimatisatie [About Acclimatization]," *Mededeelingen van den Burgerlijken Geneeskundigen Dienst in Nederlandsch-Indië* 7, no. 3 (1918): 26–42.

21. Hans Pols, "Psychological Knowledge in a Colonial Context: Theories on the Nature of the 'Native' Mind in the Former Dutch East Indies," *History of Psychology* 10, no. 2 (2007): 111–131.

22. [O. Deggeler and J.J. van Lonkhuyzen], "Het Indisch Ontwerp 1913 [The Indies Proposal 1913]," *Bond van Geneesheeren in N.-I.,* no. 52–53 (1912): 25–29.

23. J. Ch. van Schouwenburg, "Hollands Taak in Indië: Beschouwd van een Eugenetisch Standpunt [The Task of the Netherlands in the Indies: Considered from a Eugenic Perspective]," *Koloniale Studiën* part 1 (1927): 45–56.

24. [J.Ch. van Schouwenburg], "Ter Inleiding van "Ons Nageslacht" bij zijn Lezers [Introduction of "Our Progeny" to its Readers]," *Ons Nageslacht* 1, no. 1 (1928): 1–6.

25. My thanks to Warwick Anderson for bringing Rodenwaldt to my attention. Anderson is investigating Rodenwaldt's research in the context of an ARC-funded research project on the Twentieth-Century Sciences of Human Hybridity.

26. The results were published as Ernst Rodenwaldt, *De Mestiezen op Kisar,* 2 vols. (Batavia: Mededeelingen van den Dienst der Volksgezondheid in Nederlandsch-Indië, 1925) [in Dutch] and Ernst Rodenwaldt, *Die Mestizen auf Kisar,* 2 vols. (Batavia: Mededeelingen van den Dienst der Volksgezondheid in Nederlandsch-Indië, 1928) [in German]. An overview of this research project also appeared in the first issue of *Ons Nageslacht:* J. C. van Schouwenburg, "Eugenetische Beschouwingen van Prof. Dr. Rodenwaldt [Eugenic Considerations by Prof. Dr. Rodenwaldt]," *Ons Nageslacht* 1, no. 1 (1928): 6–11.

27. Ernst Rodenwaldt, "De Mestiezen van Kisar [The Mestizos of Kisar]," in *Handelingen van het Vijfde Nederlandsch-Indisch Natuurwetenschappelijk Congres* (Batavia: Kolff, 1928), 141–142.

28. Ernst Rodenwaldt, "Eugenetische Problemen in Ned. Indië."

29. M. A. van Herwerden and H. H. Laughlin, "Een Stamlijst voor Internationaal Gebruik [A Chart for Family Research for International Use]," *Ons Nageslacht* 4 (1931): 77. The chart was provided by the Eugenics Record Office, Cold Spring Harbor, New York.

30. Ernst Rodenwaldt, "Invloed van de Tropen op het Geslachtsleven van de Vrouw: Voorloopige Mededeelingen omtrent de Resultaten der Enquete Boerma-Rodenwaldt [The Influence of the Tropics on the Sexuality of Women: Initial Announcements on the Results of the Survey Boerma-Rodenwaldt]," *Ons Nageslacht* 4 (1931): 6–11.

31. Steven P. Remy, *The Heidelberg Myth: The Nazification and Denazification of a German University* (Cambridge, MA: Harvard University Press, 2002).

32. Paul Weindling, *Health, Race and German Politics between National Unification and Nazism, 1870–1945* (Cambridge: Cambridge University Press, 1989), 510. Ploetz was also Rodenwaldt's father-in-law.

33. Ernst Rodenwaldt, "Vom Seelenkonflikt des Mischlings [The Mental Conflicts of Mixed-Race Individuals]," *Zeitschrift für Morphologie und Anthropologie,* special issue: "Festschrift für Eugen Fischer," 34 (1934): 364–375, quoted by Annegret Ehman, "From Colonial Racism to Nazi Population Policy: The Role of the So-Called *Mischlinge*," in *The Holocaust and History: The Known, the Unknown, the Disputed, and the Reexamined,* ed. Michael Berenbaum and Abraham Peck (Bloomington, IN: Indiana University Press, 1998), 120.

34. Wolfgang U. Eckhardt, *Medizin und Kolonialimperialismus: Deutschland 1884–1945* (Paderborn: Ferdinand Schöningh, 1997), 518–521. See also Eckhardt, "Generalarzt Ernst Rodenwaldt," in *Hitlers Militärische Elite,* vol. 1, *Von den Anfängen des Regimes bis Kriegsbegin,* ed. Gerd R. Ueberschär (Darmstadt: Primus Verlag, 1998), 210–222. In his postwar autobiography, Rodenwaldt mentions that the Nazi government had sought his advice about a sterilization program targeting Indo-Europeans living in occupied Netherlands. He stated that he could not recommend their sterilization because of the important contribution of German blood to this group—a conclusion Bloys van Treslong Prins would have seconded. See P. C. Bloys van Treslong Prins, *Die Deutschen in Niederländisch-Indien: Vortrag, Gehalten in der Ortsgruppe Batavia Am 30. Sept. 1935* (Tokyo: Deutsche Gesellschaft für Natur- und Völkerkunde Ostasiens, 1937).

35. Hansje Galesloot and Margreet Schrevel, *In Fatsoen Hersteld: Zedelijkheid en Wederopbouw na de Oorlog* (Amsterdam: SUA, 1989).

36. M. A. van Herwerden, *Erfelijkheid bij den Mensch en Eugenetiek* [Human Heredity and Eugenics], 2nd ed. (Amsterdam: Nederlandsche Bibliotheek, 1929), 377.

37. Maria Anna van Herwerden, "Eugenics Abroad, VI: Holland," *Eugenics Review* 24, no. 2 (1932): 131.

FURTHER READING

de Rooy, Piet, Ann Stoler, and Wim F. Wertheim, eds. *Imperial Monkey Business: Racial Supremacy in Social Darwinist Theory and Colonial Practice* (Amsterdam: Free University Press, 1990).

Noordman, Jan. *Om de Kwaliteit van het Nageslacht: Eugenetica in Nederland, 1900–1950* (Nijmegen: SUN, 1989).

Schellekens, Huub, and Rob Visser. *De Genetische Manipulatie* (Amsterdam: Meulenhoff, 1987).

Stoler, Ann L. *Carnal Knowledge and Imperial Power: Race and the Intimate in Colonial Rule* (Berkeley, CA: University of California Press, 2002).

Stoler, Ann L. "Making Empire Respectable: The Politics of Race and Sexual Morality in 20th-Century Colonial Cultures," *American Ethnologist* 16, no. 4 (1989): 634–660.

Stoler, Ann L. "Sexual Affronts and Racial Frontiers: European Identities and the Cultural Politics of Exclusion in Colonial Southeast Asia," *Comparative Studies in Society and History* 34, no. 3 (1992): 514–551.

CHAPTER 21

THE SCANDINAVIAN STATES: REFORMED EUGENICS APPLIED

MATTIAS TYDÉN

THE end of the twentieth century saw an urgent need to confront historical injustices. There were many different reasons to examine the apparent success stories of Western democracies: exploitation and suppression of indigenous peoples; neglect of the Jewish suffering by Allied and neutral countries during the Holocaust; mistreatment behind the walls of asylums, workhouses, and charitable institutions. Another contentious issue was abuses made in the name of eugenics, especially in Scandinavia. The revelation in 1997 that widespread eugenic sterilization had taken place in Sweden and its neighboring countries generated worldwide attention. The international press, quick to make radical comparisons, reported "a 40-year Nazi-style campaign of forced sterilization" and Swedish laws that "could have come out of a Nazi text book."[1] Eventually, the story of the Swedish sterilization program became one of the restitution cases in which history in various countries was put on trial. In the Swedish case, a government commission was established, and in the end financial compensation was paid out to some 1,600 individuals sterilized against their will or under questionable circumstances.

There were two reasons for the turmoil in the 1990s about Scandinavian eugenics. Not only did this topic put important questions on the agenda about morality and history, guilt and rehabilitation, but it also challenged the conventional conception of Scandinavian contemporary history. According to the standard narrative Denmark, Norway, and Sweden constituted peaceful and egalitarian democracies. In all three countries, Social Democratic parties came to power in the interwar years and successively established stable welfare regimes. Their mix of state planning and market economy, as well as their schemes of universally distributed social rights, came to be known as "the Scandinavian model."

The exposure of Scandinavian eugenics changed that account. And all the more so since the development of eugenics seemed to have evolved within the very welfare system that sought to protect and assist the poor and marginalized. This, however, might not come as a surprise for scholars familiar with the history of eugenics. A number of studies have shown the links between eugenics and progressive social thought. Due to its plasticity, eugenics could serve different political purposes and could be incorporated into different ideological contexts. The Scandinavian case, then, is the story of how eugenic polices were established within a democratic framework.

Historical research on Scandinavian eugenics is quite recent, probably due to the widespread and long-standing tendency to regard eugenics as something that "happened elsewhere." Early works include essays on Norwegian eugenics by Nils Roll-Hansen and studies of the eugenics movement in Sweden (Gunnar Broberg and Mattias Tydén) and Denmark (Lene Koch).[2] *Eugenics and the Welfare State: Sterilization Policy in Denmark, Sweden, Norway, and Finland,* edited by Broberg and Roll-Hansen and published in 1996, constitutes the first comparative study on Scandinavian eugenics including Finland. This book focused on the somewhat paradoxical fact that the democratic Nordic states were among the few nations that actually introduced sterilization laws in the 1930s. On the other hand, as Roll-Hansen put it, "a liberal democratic tradition [in Scandinavia] with emphasis on the rights on the individual provided for a moderate law and practice."[3]

Far more critical conclusions were put forward in the wake of the media coverage of Scandinavian eugenics in 1997. In a special issue of *Scandinavian Journal of History* (1999), Peter Weingart stressed the similarities between Nazi German and Swedish sterilizations, as well as the reluctance in Scandinavia to abandon eugenic practices after World War II: "it took more than a generation to disturb the peace of mind of public consciousness and to uncover their own involvement in the aberrations of a dark era."[4] Dorothy Porter and Paul Weindling took a somewhat more cautious position, sketching the broader international network in which Scandinavian eugenics was a receiving as well as a contributing element.[5]

A strong interest has remained regarding the case of eugenic sterilization in the Scandinavian countries. This is no doubt partly due to the political implications of this issue: how eugenics corresponded with the Scandinavian welfare model has continued to be a highly disputed topic. Another reason is the existence of abundant and detailed sources, especially in Sweden. As a result of centralized administration from the very start, the files of more than 60,000 persons sterilized from 1935 to 1975 are still available at the archives of the Swedish National Board of Health. This has made a detailed investigation of the rise and fall of the Swedish sterilization program possible.[6] Similarly comprehensive studies have been made concerning Denmark and Norway.[7]

EARLY SCANDINAVIAN EUGENICS

The three Scandinavian countries—Denmark, Norway, and Sweden[8]—share experiences that were important for the development of eugenic ideas and policies. During the late nineteenth and early twentieth centuries they went through a rapid stage of modernization with growing industries, urbanization, and political democratization. Class tensions, poverty, and urban slums were increasing causes of concern. Lower birthrates and extensive emigration added to the image of population decline. These social and demographic transformations provided a breeding ground for racial thought and eugenics with a conservative and patriotic touch. Moreover, Nordic nationalism around 1900 fueled such ethnocentric myths as the notion of a "pure Nordic race."

Eugenic ideas were introduced in the decades around 1900, mainly mirroring a transmission to Scandinavia from German, British, and American sources. Gradually alliances were formed around more specific eugenic programs, and pressure groups were established. As early as 1904 an "anthropological committee" (*Den antropologiske Komite*) was set up in Denmark, and in time it developed into a private eugenic society. A loosely organized "committee for racial hygiene" emerged in Norway in 1908, while Swedish academics in 1909 formed *Svenska sällskapet för rashygien* (the Swedish Society for Racial Hygiene), organizing public lectures and publishing popular books and booklets. More important from a scientific point of view was the founding of the Swedish *Mendelska sällskapet* (the Mendelian Society, 1910) and *Norsk forening for arvelighetsforskning* (the Norwegian Genetics Society, 1919). Primarily a platform for creating a network of Swedish geneticists, the Mendelian society also became important in spreading Scandinavian genetics internationally through its English-language journal *Hereditas* (1920–).[9] While the Mendelian Society—and the journal—focused on basic genetic research the connection between science and wider social issues was also upheld. The leaders of the Society stated in 1918 that "more directly than most other sciences genetics is to the advantage of practical life. Plant breeding and animal breeding as well as applied race biology find their basic principles therein. Race biology has a fundamental importance for the many social undertakings that will be topical in the near future, and for which a critical, strictly scientific perspective is necessary."[10]

Genetics and geneticists were only one of many sources for the growing interest in eugenics in late-nineteenth and early-twentieth-century Scandinavia. The theme of degeneration was dealt with in fiction by novelists such as Herman Bang (1875–1912) in Denmark and August Strindberg (1849–1912) in Sweden. The menace of degeneration—and salvation through eugenics—was also apparent in physical anthropology, a discipline attracting archaeologists and anatomists as well as geneticists, and with a strong position in Scandinavia since the pioneering work by the Swede Anders Retzius (1796–1860), who invented the cephalic index in the mid-1800s. Mental health professionals made up another important pressure group. In Denmark the practice of eugenic sterilization was developed in close connection with the institutional treatment of the "feebleminded." In Sweden the efforts to run a sterili-zation law through parliament were initiated by psychiatrist Alfred Petrén (1867–1964), a leader in the organization of the Swedish care of the mentally disabled.[11]

In the 1910s and 1920s, liberals and Social Democrats, as well as feminists, came to perceive eugenics as one of many paths to societal change and social reform. An early and possibly influential call for eugenics was made by Swedish feminist writer Ellen Key (1849–1926) in books such as *Barnets århundrade* (The Century of the Child, 1900), later published in Germany as well as in Great Britain, and *Livslinjer* (Lines of Life, 1903–1906). While Key stressed the importance of education and of dedicated and loving upbringing of children, at the same time she left the door open for state-controlled reproduction and even euthanasia.[12] Key's focus on free love and motherhood points forward to what Atina Grossmann has called the "motherhood-eugenics consensus" in the sexual reform movement.[13] In Scandinavia, too, sexual reformers, such as Norwegian-Swedish Elise Ottesen-Jensen (1886–1973), came to support the introduction of sterilization laws, partly in accordance with their eugenic aims, partly as a tool enabling women to control their reproduction.[14]

In sum eugenics—regarded as a social movement—became a platform for alli-ances where different aims could meet. This was by no means a phenomenon unique to Scandinavia.[15] But the achievements of early-twentieth-century Scandinavian eugenics must be attributed to "the special character of the social and cultural con-ditions that existed in the Nordic countries in this period:"[16] these were small, struc-turally centralized, and consensus-oriented societies where politics and science interacted in the development of social policies. Furthermore, and in contrast to countries with Catholic lobby groups, eugenics met no opposition from the Lutheran churches, which accepted reproductive control as long as it was for the purpose of the common good.[17]

EUGENICISTS DIVIDED

The development of Mendelism and a growing understanding of the complexity of heredity made for different views about the potential of racial hygiene and for tensions within the community of eugenicists. In the 1910s the leading geneticist in Denmark, Wilhelm Johannsen (1857–1927), founder of concepts such as "gene," "genotype," and "phenotype," strongly dissociated himself from the "dreamers and fanatics" of the contemporary eugenics movement.[18] In Norway a sharp dividing line developed from the mid-1910s between the alarmist and hard-core version of eugenics, quite successively propagated by the pharmacist Jon Alfred Mjøen (1860–1939) and his supporters on one hand, and the "moderate" or out-right critical position taken by medical and biological scientists such as Ragnar Vogt (1870–1943), Kristine Bonnevie (1872–1948), and Otto Lous Mohr (1886–1967) on the other.[19]

In Sweden key actors in genetics and medical research initially took up a much less critical attitude toward the value of eugenics than their Norwegian counterparts. Herman Nilsson-Ehle (1873–1949), who introduced and developed Mendelian genetics in Swedish plant breeding and held the first Swedish chair in genetics (1917–1938), wrote popular articles and lectured on the importance of "race biology and race hygiene."[20] Even more important was the influential position taken by physician Herman Lundborg (1868–1943), an early leader in Swedish eugenics. Conservative, racist, and anti-feminist, Lundborg wrote extensively on the threats of degeneration, immigration, and moral decay. At the same time, his scientific work, in which he was able to trace the inheritance of myclonus epilepsy according to Mendelian laws (1913), gave him a respected position, nationally and internationally. From 1916 Lundborg received personal funding from the state budget to conduct "race biological investigations" and in 1922 he was appointed as the first director of *Statens institut för rasbiologi* (the State Institute for Race Biology) in Uppsala. In this position Lundborg continued the anthropological tradition of racial research, initiating wide-ranging studies, including the measurement of hundreds of thousands of individuals describing the "racial character" of the Swedes, of the Sami minority in the Swedish north, and investigating the consequences of "miscegenation." Links were established especially to the German scientific community, and among the visitors and lecturers at the State Institute were geneticists and race ideologists such as Hans F. Günther, Eugen Fischer, and Fritz Lenz.[21]

It was not until the early 1930s that the previously unthreatened position of the Swedish eugenic movement—and of Lundborg personally—began to change. Lundborg's scientific profile, his nationalism, and his pro-German attitude made him increasingly controversial. The simplistic messages spread by proponents of Swedish eugenics were questioned by a new generation of medical and biological researchers. Among them was Gunnar Dahlberg (1893–1956), who was to become Lundborg's successor at the Institute for Race Biology in 1936. As director, Dahlberg picked up his Anglo-American contacts and turned the Institute away from its anthropological focus and German connections.[22]

As Nils Roll-Hansen stresses, the critical attitude toward the popular eugenics movement by medical and biological professionals was "a rejection of what was seen as excesses and unscientific attitudes and not a rejection of the basic ideas of eugenics."[23] There were different views among geneticists about the efficiency of eugenic measures such as sterilization, but at the same time experts such as Bonnevie, Vogt, and Dahlberg maintained that science as such—including human genetics— had an essential role in building a better society. In spite of his attacks on the eugenics movement, Wilhelm Johannsen accepted membership in the Permanent International Commission on Eugenics in 1923, and the following year he entered the Danish commission planning sterilization and castration laws.[24] In Sweden one of the architects of the sterilization program, zoologist and geneticist Nils von Hofsten (1881–1967), expressed caution about expectations of "race improvement." In his standard book on genetics, published in 1919, he stated that "in many cases even the most radical program of racial hygiene cannot wipe out an unfavorable quality in man, and it has less potential to check its spreading than most people, ignorant of the Mendelian laws, believe."[25] Nevertheless, von Hofsten—like many of his contemporary colleagues—was in favor of eugenic policies and contributed to their realization in interwar Scandinavia.

The backing of "sound" eugenic policies by Scandinavian geneticists and other scientists followed three lines of argumentation. Negative eugenics, it was declared, could at least have some impact, especially concerning the number of the "mentally retarded." Second, and irrespective of the effect on the population as a whole, negative eugenics could be important in individual cases in which it could be assumed that an "inferior" child would be born. Third, measures such as sterilization, segregation, and marriage restrictions were defensible socially, morally, and economically: the target groups for eugenics—"mental defectives" in particular—were described as unsuitable parents and a burden to society.[26] A final and unstated motive could be added. Participation in the consolidation of the modern Scandinavian states brought prestige and financial resources to the field of genetics.

EUGENIC POLICIES

Much of the present-day discussion on Scandinavian eugenics focuses on the way sterilization was used in the framework of the Social Democratic welfare states from the 1930s onward. Eugenic polices, however, began in another political context some ten to twenty years earlier. Eugenic thinking inspired early-twentieth-century liberal social reformers when discussing increased state intervention in the fields of poor relief, care of alcohol abusers, or prevention of vagrancy. The first laws clearly to be influenced by eugenics were the marriage act reforms carried out in all the Scandinavian countries in the 1910s and 1920s. Legislation was developed in close transnational cooperation with the explicit aim of producing corresponding Danish, Norwegian, and Swedish marriage acts. In all three countries, the medical profession was involved in their preparation. Medical impediments to marry were confirmed by law throughout Scandinavia in the years 1915–1922. Sweden, however, went furthest by not only including restrictions for persons closely related or mentally ill, but also for the "feebleminded," and for carriers of venereal diseases or inborn epilepsy.[27]

When sterilization laws were introduced in Denmark (1929, 1935), Norway (1934), and Sweden (1934, 1941), the political context had changed both nationally and internationally. Social Democracy had entered the political scene in Scandinavia and large-scale social reforms were being planned. In Germany the National Socialists came to power and gradually turned the country into a "racial state," including "the law for the prevention of genetically diseased offspring," which sanctioned compulsory sterilization (1933). Scandinavian proponents of eugenics now had to perform a delicate balancing act. They wanted to dissociate Scandinavian policies from the blatant racism and eugenic "excesses" in Germany. At the same time, however, they were advocating national sterilization programs that resembled the Nazi-German equivalent, and which furthermore were used by Nazi authorities to show that Germany was not alone in using eugenic sterilization.[28] In Norway medical doctor Karl Evang (1902–1981) condemned German racism in his *Rasepolitikk og reaksjon* (Race Politics and Reaction, 1934). Yet Evang was soon to be director of the national public health service and as such was deeply involved in the administration of the Norwegian sterilization law.[29] In Sweden the parliamentary commission responsible for rewriting the 1934 sterilization act tried to distinguish between Swedish and Nazi German eugenics: "To admit sterilization without consent to the extent of the German law would probably be inconsistent with the Swedish conception of justice."[30] In the end, however, the commission recommended an expanded law in which the target group for sterilization was enlarged to include the "socially" as well as the genetically unfit. While Karl Evang had to flee the country after the German occupation of Norway in 1940, Gunnar Dahlberg in neutral Sweden used his position as director of the State Institute for Race Biology to criticize Nazi race politics and anti-Semitism. Still, although skeptical about what he considered exaggerated belief in the prospects of eugenics, Dahlberg was loyal to, and supported, the Swedish legislation on sterilization.[31]

A distinguishing feature in Scandinavian eugenic policies up to the 1940s is their sociopolitical component. Eugenics, and sterilization in particular, was discussed and supported by influential social policy theorists such as Karl Kristian Steincke (1880–1963) in Denmark in the 1920s, and Alva Myrdal (1902–1986) and Gunnar Myrdal (1898–1987) in Sweden in the 1930s. The sterilization laws were also aimed at persons belonging to the "social problem group" and whose "antisocial behavior" was only loosely regarded as genetically determined. Moreover, sterilizations were initiated not only in mental hospitals and institutions for the mentally disabled, but also by local-level social workers. Accordingly, some historians suggest that the Scandinavian social reforms of the 1930s and 1940s were closely tied to eugenic legislation—the former would hardly have been so ambitious without the latter. Eugenics, in other words, was a necessary counterbalance to a social policy that was to the advantage of all citizens—even the "unfit." Social Democratic welfarism consequently is said to explain the Scandinavian attraction to eugenics.[32]

This interpretation, however, has been contested. Since there was general support for eugenics in the interwar period, and the Scandinavian sterilization laws were decided upon in broad political consensus, sterilization polices most probably would have developed irrespective of the governments in office. Further more, and notwithstanding some Social Democrats' strong support for racial hygiene, eugenics and sterilization were comparatively marginal issues in the wider context of social policy debates and reforms. This is especially true in the postwar era, when the Scandinavian states moved meaningfully toward universal social rights. In fact, the realization of the "Scandinavian model" in the 1950s and 1960s was simultaneous with the *phasing out* of eugenics. In sum, this latter approach recognizes the social policy dimension of Scandinavian eugenics, but relates it to the paternalistic mentality shaped by early-twentieth-century poor relief systems as much as to the welfare discourse and social engineering of the 1930s and 1940s.[33]

To explain the high numbers of Scandinavian sterilizations, historians have also studied the ways in which sterilization became a tool in local-level medical practice and social administration. In Sweden sterilization was used extensively, and sometimes ruthlessly, at some mental institutions and by some regional poor-law boards, backed up by the National Board of Health. This, however, can hardly be ascribed to the "Scandinavian model" or the welfare reforms but should rather be attributed to the values and intentions of bureaucrats and local-level medical practitioners and social welfare officers.[34]

Eugenic sterilization was implemented mainly from the 1930s to the 1950s, a period in which altogether some 35,500 individuals seem to have been sterilized in Scandinavia for eugenic and/or social reasons.[35] The great majority was women, and it can be argued that the history of sterilization was part of a broader control of women's sexuality.[36] In hindsight, and according to today's values, much of the implementation of the Scandinavian laws up to the 1950s may indeed be labeled a practice of compulsory sterilization. On paper, however, the laws were based on voluntariness, and free will was said to be respected, since operations "without consent" (still not mandatory), following third-party applications, were possible only in cases of "severe mental deficiency" or "legal incompetence."[37] In Sweden the great majority of sterilization was formally voluntary and followed from a personal application from the patient. However, sterilizations could still be carried out under pressure, for example as a precondition for discharge from a mental institution, from a home for the "feebleminded," or for permission to get a "eugenic" abortion.[38] In practice a system of deception developed, sanctioned by the Swedish National Board of Health. In instructions published in 1947, the Board advised doctors and other professionals involved to ignore, as long as possible, any refusals or protests from persons considered to be "legally incompetent:"

> As a rule, the best way to treat such patients would seem to be to consider it
> more or less self-evident that the operation is to be performed once the Board
> has given permission; should they ask outright, however, it must not be kept
> from them, of course, that it will not be carried out by force.[39]

Scandinavian and German policies of sterilization clearly were rooted in a common eugenic discourse that had developed within a network of international scientific cooperation from the late nineteenth century onward. Yet the dissociation from Nazi German race politics by many Scandinavians involved in eugenics was not entirely a question of double standards. The German sterilization act, for instance, made sterilization mandatory for certain categories of people defined as carriers of hereditarily determined conditions. The German law also was the starting point for an extensive program of enforced sterilization, which led to operations on hundreds of thousands of Germans up to the outbreak of the war in 1939. The Scandinavian sterilization laws, on the other hand, did not allow for the use of physical force.[40] The most important difference however, between the German and Scandinavian cases, relates to the wider context of eugenics. Only in Nazi Germany did racial hygiene become a cornerstone in national politics. Only in Germany did the sterilization law prove to be "a first step on the road to murder," to quote Diane Paul, while the corresponding Scandinavian legislation "never [was] linked to a broader program of racial discrimination and extermination."[41]

THE POSTWAR PERIOD

The breakdown of the Nazi terror-regime in 1945 and the revelations of its horrifying atrocities made the need to bracket Nazi eugenics even more important. Speaking on national radio in 1946, Nils von Hofsten—now the Swedish expert on "genetic hygiene" at the National Board of Health—dismissed any similarities between Swedish eugenics and German "race doctrines." According to von Hofsten, the German version was dangerous not only because of its terrible consequences, but also because it caused distrust of "real race science:" "Our Sterilization Act is very different from the one the Germans had. In essential respects its principles are entirely the opposite."[42] This failure to make parallels to the Nazi German case, or at least to learn from it, meant that there was no break with eugenic practices in the immediate postwar years. In fact, eugenic sterilization reached its climax in the period 1943–1949 in Sweden, 1944–1950 in Denmark, and 1948–1950 in Norway.[43]

The use of sterilization in Scandinavia changed, however, from the mid-1950s. Operations motivated by eugenics and/or concerns about "anti-social behavior" declined, as did sterilizations of the "feebleminded." The figures for Sweden dropped from the peak 1,034 sterilizations of "feebleminded" in 1944 to 101 in 1959. Similar changes took place in Denmark and Norway. Collective concerns were gradually replaced by individual problems as the motive for sterilization. These "medical" sterilizations, as they were typically labeled, were usually the outcome of negotiated agreements at the local level rather than the coercion characterizing the 1930s and 1940s. From the 1960s, sterilization was also increasingly used as voluntary birth control, especially in Denmark and Norway.[44]

It is important to note that these changes took place without any revision of the laws. Thus the total number of recorded sterilizations during the period of formal eugenic laws (such as the often referred to 63,000 Swedish operations 1935–1975) does not tell us much about eugenic practices. In fact, current historical studies in Denmark, Norway, and Sweden indicate that the use of sterilization in the latter half of the twentieth century comes close to that of many other western countries. As Paul Weindling argues: "What was done legally in Sweden was probably done as a matter of medical discretion in other contexts."[45]

The turnaround of Scandinavian sterilization practices in the 1950s cannot be explained by the exposure of Nazi German atrocities. Neither did it follow from a radically different attitude toward sterilization among key actors in genetic science or the medical bureaucracy. Instead, the fall of eugenic sterilization seems to be connected to a general transformation of the relation between individual and state, together with a shift in attitude in the postwar period toward the rights of people with learning difficulties. Among medical professionals in Sweden there was an increasing sense of unease in the 1960s over sterilization . Letters from women sterilized in the 1940s and early 1950s were beginning to show up frequently at the National Board of Health: "You have ruined our lives forever," two sisters wrote in 1966. "You are the ones that destroyed me," a woman claimed in 1968. Accordingly, the board adopted a more cautious position in its handling of applications for sterilization. At the local level the hesitation to use sterilization grew at institutions and hospitals.[46] Increasingly, eugenic or socially motivated sterilization proved to be an outdated method—ethically as well as scientifically. The eugenic acts were abolished and replaced by sterilization laws based on voluntary consent in Denmark in 1967 and 1973, in Sweden in 1975, and in Norway in 1977.

In parallel with the decline in eugenic sterilization, the discourse on race changed in the postwar period. For years the anthropological concept of man and the discussion of "race differences" survived in textbooks. As sociology moved forward at Scandinavian universities, however, biological determinism was challenged. Geneticists, too, adopted a less reductionist view and stressed the complex interplay between heredity and the environment. This movement away from an older paradigm had more to do with changed values than with changes in scientific knowledge. The anti-racist scientists who, in the 1930s and early 1940s, represented one of many approaches, became dominant after World War II.[47] Gunnar Myrdal wrote in 1944 that "the social definition and not the biological facts actually determines the status of an individual and his place in interracial relations":[48] he became involved in the preparation of the UNESCO statement on race in the early 1950s. So too did Gunnar Dahlberg, who also contributed to the UNESCO campaign against racism.[49]

Race, race hygiene, and eugenics became gradually more contentious concepts. Danish encyclopedias were the first to replace an older terminology with words such as "population" and "hereditary" hygiene in the late 1940s. Derogatory expressions and references to "inferior" human beings were discouraged, although Nazi German eugenics was ignored rather than openly challenged.[50] In 1959 the Swedish Institute for Race Biology was absorbed into Uppsala University and became the Department of Medical Genetics. The new director, Jan-Arvid Böök (1915–1995), declared as one of the goals of the reformed institution: "A total dissociation from the older 'race-hygienic' approach and a shift to medical genetics—that is, the importance of genes for diseases and health."[51]

The decline of eugenic sterilization and the change of vocabulary do not mean that the idea of eugenics totally disappeared. The aims of contemporary applied genetics no doubt correspond with one of the core goals of traditional eugenics: the promotion of health by means of genetic selection. Furthermore, the use of procedures such as genetic counseling and prenatal testing are probably less voluntary than officially stated. For instance: by advising parents in "risk groups," or simply by offering genetic tests, medical expertise influences individual behavior. In both Denmark and Sweden, prenatal diagnosis (PND) has became standard procedure for women over 35. Today this practice is presented as a voluntary choice in the interest of the parent and child. In fact, however, prenatal diagnosis was introduced in the 1970s—in all the Scandinavian countries—after careful cost-benefit analysis of PND compared to the care of handicapped children.[52]

The distance between history and current genetic practices also seems shorter if we consider the multiple aspirations of yesterday's eugenics, some probably regarded as agreeable today. Eugenics was a broad concept and a stage where different ambitions met. It was early described as a movement for the common good, with the problematic potential to fuel paternalistic values and to justify repressive policies. At the same time, however, eugenicists and their allies could emphasize the interests of the individual—the right of children to grow up sound and healthy, for women to be able to control their reproduction. Thus the mixed motives and complex practices of twentieth-century Scandinavian sterilization policies seem worrisome in more than one way. They certainly reveal a history where good intentions and abuses blended. They also reveal, as Lene Koch notes, that "the differences between past and present might be smaller than we would like to believe."[53]

NOTES

1. "Swedish Newspaper Details Sterilizations," *Washington Post*, August 25, 1997; "Time for Austria to Face Facts," *The Guardian*, September 3, 1997.

2. Nils Roll-Hansen, "Eugenics before World War II: The Case of Norway," *History and Philosophy of the Life Sciences* 2, no. 2 (1980): 269–298; Roll-Hansen, "Geneticists and the Eugenics Movement in Scandinavia," *British Journal for the History of Science* 22, no. 3 (1989): 335–346; Gunnar Broberg and Mattias Tydén, *Oönskade i folkhemmet: Rashygien och sterilisering i Sverige* (Stockholm: Gidlunds, 1991); Lene Koch, *Racehygiejne i Danmark 1920–56* (København: Gyldendal, 1996).

3. Gunnar Broberg and Nils Roll-Hansen, eds., *Eugenics and the Welfare State: Sterilization Policy in Denmark, Sweden, Norway, and Finland* (East Lansing, MI: Michigan State University Press, 1996). Quote from Roll-Hansen, "Conclusion: Scandinavian Eugenics in the International Context," in Broberg et al., *Eugenics and the Welfare State*, 267.

4. Peter Weingart, "Science and Political Culture: Eugenics in Comparative Perspective," *Scandinavian Journal of History* 24, no. 2 (1999): 176. Weingart's comparisons of Sweden and Germany were later criticized in Nils Roll-Hansen, "Eugenic Practice and Genetic Science in Scandinavia and Germany," *Scandinavian Journal of History* 26, no. 1 (2001): 75–82.

5. Dorothy Porter, "Eugenics and the Sterilization Debate in Sweden and Britain before World War II," *Scandinavian Journal of History* 24, no. 2 (1999): 145–62; Paul Weindling, "International Eugenics: Swedish Sterilizations in Context," *Scandinavian Journal of History* 24, no. 2 (1999): 179–197.

6. Maija Runcis, *Steriliseringar i folkhemmet* (Stockholm: Ordfront, 1998); Mattias Tydén, *Från politik till praktik: De svenska steriliseringslagarna 1935–1975*, 2nd ed. (Stockholm: Almqvist & Wiksell International, 2002).

7. Lene Koch, *Tvangssterilisation i Danmark 1929–67* (København: Gyldendal, 2000); Per Haave, *Sterilisering av tatere 1934–1977: En historisk undersøkelse av lov og praksis* (Oslo: Norges forskningsråd, 2000). Unlike in Sweden, so-called medical sterilizations were not regulated by law in Denmark and Norway, and thus were not registered in the same way.

8. In this article the term "Scandinavia" is used in a strict sense, whereas "the Nordic countries" refers to Finland and Iceland as well as Denmark, Norway, and Sweden.

9. Nils Roll-Hansen, "Den norske debatten om rasehygiene," *Historisk Tidsskrift* 59, no. 3 (1980): 261; Koch, *Racehygiejne i Danmark*, 44; Gunnar Broberg and Mattias Tydén, "Eugenics in Sweden: Efficient Care," in Broberg et al., *Eugenics and the Welfare State*, 83–84.

10. Quoted in Anna Tunlid, *Ärftlighetsforskningens gränser: Individer och institutioner i framväxten av svensk genetik* (Lund: Lund University, 2004), 106.

11. Bent Sigurd Hansen, "Something Rotten in the State of Denmark: Eugenics and the Ascent of the Welfare State," in Broberg et al., *Eugenics and the Welfare State*, 9–76; Koch, *Racehygiejne i Danmark*; Broberg and Tydén, *Oönskade i folkhemmet*.

12. On Key and social Darwinism, see Mike Hawkins, *Social Darwinism in European and American Thought 1860–1945* (Cambridge: Cambridge University Press), 265–269. Key on euthanasia: Ellen Key, *Lifslinjer*, 6 vols. (Stockholm: Bonnier, 1903–1906), 2: 326, cf. 324, 521–522.

13. Atina Grossmann, *Reforming Sex: The German Movement for Birth Control and Abortion Reform* (New York and Oxford: Oxford University Press, 1995), 15.

14. Tydén, *Från politik till praktik*, 535–546.

15. Michael Freeden, "Eugenics and Ideology," *The Historical Journal* 26, no. 4 (1983): 959–962.

16. Roll-Hansen, "Conclusion," 268.

17. Ibid., 268–269.

18. Johannsen in 1917 quoted in Hansen, "Something Rotten in the State of Denmark," 23.

19. Nils Roll-Hansen, "Norwegian Eugenics: Sterilization as Social Reform," in Broberg et al., *Eugenics and the Welfare State*, 157–161, 163–167.

20. On Nilsson-Ehle and eugenics: Tunlid, *Ärftlighetsforskningens gränser*, 130–142, 218–224.

21. On Lundborg: Broberg and Tydén, *Oönskade i folkhemmet*; Broberg and Tydén, "Eugenics in Sweden."

22. Broberg and Tydén, *Oönskade i folkhemmet*; Broberg and Tydén, "Eugenics in Sweden."

23. Roll-Hansen, "Norwegian Eugenics," 167.

24. Hansen, "Something Rotten in the State of Denmark," 25–26.

25. Nils von Hofsten, *Ärftlighetslära* (Stockholm: Norstedts, 1919), 494.

26. For similar argumentation in the international community of eugenicists, see Diane B. Paul, *The Politics of Heredity: Essays on Eugenics, Biomedicine, and the Nature-Nurture Debate* (Albany, NY: State University of New York Press, 1998), chaps. 6 and 7.

27. On the Scandinavian marriage laws and eugenics, see Kari Melby, Anu Pylkkänen, Bente Rosenbeck, and Christina Carlsson Wetterberg, *Inte ett ord om kärlek: Äktenskap och politik i Norden ca 1850–1930* (Göteborg: Makadam, 2006), chap. 4; Mattias Tydén, "Medicinska äktenskapshinder. Om rashygienens etablering i svensk politik under 1910-talet," in Marika Hedin, Urban Lundberg, Jens Rydström, and Mattias Tydén, *Staten som vän eller fiende? Individ och samhälle i svenskt 1900-tal* (Stockholm: Institute for Futures Studies, 2007), 99–132.

28. On foreign sterilization laws in German propaganda, see Robert N. Proctor, *Racial Hygiene: Medicine under the Nazis* (Cambridge, MA: Harvard University Press, 1988), 96–97.

29. Roll-Hansen, "Norwegian Eugenics," 174.

30. Cited from the 1936 report on sterilization by the Swedish Commission on Population, quoted in Broberg and Tydén, "Eugenics in Sweden," 114–115.

31. Broberg and Tydén, "Eugenics in Sweden," 92–94, 105–107.

32. For example Koch, *Racehygiejne i Danmark*; Koch, *Tvangssterilisation i Danmark*; Runcis, *Steriliseringar i folkhemmet*; Alberto Spektorowski and Elisabet Mizrachi, "Eugenics and the Welfare State in Sweden: The Politics of Social Margins and the Idea of a Productive Society," *Journal of Contemporary History* 39, no. 3 (2004): 333–352.

33. Tydén, *Från politik till praktik*; Per Haave, "Tvangssterilisering i Norge," in Hilda Rømer Christensen, Urban Lundberg and Klaus Petersen, *Frihed, lighed og tryghed: Velfærdspolitik i Norden* (Århus: Jysk Selskab for Historie, 2001); Niels Finn Christiansen, "Racehygiejne og socialpolitik," *Bibliotek for læger* 193, no. 3 (2001): 199–209.

34. Esp. Tydén, *Från politik till praktik*; also Haave, "Tvangssterilisering i Norge.

35. Denmark 1929–1960: ca. 11,000, Norway 1934–1960: ca. 7,000, Sweden 1935–1960: ca. 17,500. These figures, which exclude so-called medical operations, roughly reflect the different size of population in the respective country. However, they are still a matter of interpretation, since operations often were performed with mixed motives and in a twilight zone of voluntariness, pressure, and compulsion. Thus, they should for instance not to be read as the total number of involuntary sterilizations in Scandinavia. Cf. Roll-Hansen, "Conclusion," 263.

36. For a gender analysis of the Swedish history of sterilization, see Runcis, *Steriliseringar i folkhemmet*.

37. The formal grounds for sterilization without consent varied between the three countries.

38. According to the 1936 Swedish abortion law, an abortion performed on "eugenic indication," with the woman being the carrier of the "defected" genes, should be combined with a sterilization.

39. Quoted in Broberg and Tydén, "Eugenics in Sweden," 116. The different ways Swedish sterilization laws opened up for involuntary sterilization are dealt with extensively in Tydén, *Från politik till praktik*, esp. chaps. 4–6.

40. The closest parallel to German practices concerns the Norwegian Sterilization Act of 1942. Based on compulsion, this law was introduced by the Quisling Nazi puppet regime and remained in force until May 1945. The number of sterilizations of mental patients rose sharply, but the total number of operations according to the law—ca. 500—most likely was a disappointment to the local Nazi authorities. See Per Haave, "Sterilization under the Swastika: The Case of Norway," *International Journal of Mental Health* 36, no. 1 (2007): 45–57.

41. Diane B. Paul, *Controlling Human Heredity: 1869 to the Present* (Atlantic Highlands, NJ: Humanities Press, 1995), 90.

42. Nils von Hofsten on Swedish national public radio, March 7, 1946. Quoted in Broberg and Tydén, *Oönskade i folkhemmet*, 162.

43. Broberg and Tydén, "Eugenics in Sweden," 109–110; Koch, *Tvangssterilisation i Danmark*, 136–137; Haave, *Sterilisering av tatere*, 157.

44. Broberg and Tydén, 'Eugenics in Sweden,' 113; Tydén, *Från politik till praktik*, 70–72; Koch, *Tvangssterilisation i Danmark*, 207–208 and chap. 13; Haave, "Tvangssterilisering i Norge," 142–143.

45. Weindling, "International Eugenics," 196.

46. Quotations from Tydén, *Från politik till praktik*, 12.

47. Elazar Barkan, *The Retreat of Scientific Racism: Changing Concepts of Race in Britain and the United States Between the Worlds Wars* (Cambridge: Cambridge University Press, 1992), 341–346; Nils Roll-Hansen, "Eugenics in Scandinavia after 1945: Change of

Values and Growth in Knowledge," *Scandinavian Journal of History* 24, no. 2 (1999): 207–208.

48. Gunnar Myrdal, *An American Dilemma: The Negro Problem and Modern Democracy*, 2 vols. (New York: Harpers & Brothers Publishers, 1944), 1: 115.

49. Broberg and Tydén, "Eugenics in Sweden," 130; Gunnar Dahlberg, ed., *Raser och folk* (Stockholm: Svenska UNESCO-rådet, 1955).

50. Lene Koch, "Past Futures: On the Conceptual History of Eugenics," *Technology Analysis and Strategic Management* 18, no. 3–4 (2006): 339–340.

51. Quoted in Gunnar Broberg, *Statlig rasforskning: En historik över Rasbiologiska institutet* (Lund: Lund University Press, 1995), 81.

52. Lene Koch, "The Meaning of Eugenics: Reflections of Genetic Knowledge in the Past and Present," *Science in Context* 13, no. 3 (2004): 326–327; Christian Munthe, *The Moral Roots of Prenatal Diagnosis: Ethical Aspects of the Early Introduction and Presentation of Prenatal Diagnosis in Sweden* (Göteborg: Centre for Research Ethics, 1996); Mattias Tydén, "Staten och våra gener," in Torbjörn Lundqvist ed., *Den kreativa staten: Framtidspolitiska tendenser* (Stockholm: Institute for Futures Studies, 2006).

53. Lene Koch, "Eugenic Sterilisation in Scandinavia," *The European Legacy* 11, no. 3 (2006): 308.

FURTHER READING

Broberg, Gunnar. *Statlig rasforskning: En historik över Rasbiologiska institutet* (Lund: Lund University Press, 1995).

Broberg, Gunnar, and Mattias Tydén. *Oönskade i folkhemmet: Rashygien och sterilisering i Sverige* (Stockholm: Gidlunds, 1991).

Broberg, Gunnar, and Nils Roll-Hansen, eds. *Eugenics and the Welfare State: Sterilization Policy in Denmark, Sweden, Norway, and Finland* (East Lansing, MI: Michigan State University Press, 1996).

Haave, Per. *Sterilisering av tatere 1934–1977: En historisk undersøkelse av lov og praksis* (Oslo: Norges forskningsråd, 2000).

Koch, Lene. *Racehygiejne i Danmark 1920–56* (København: Gyldendal, 1996).

Koch, Lene. *Tvangssterilisation i Danmark 1929–67* (København: Gyldendal, 2000).

Runcis, Maija. *Steriliseringar i folkhemmet* (Stockholm: Ordfront, 1998).

Scandinavian Journal of History 24, no. 2 (1999) [Special Issue: Eugenics in Scandinavia].

Tunlid, Anna. *Ärftlighetsforskningens gränser: Individer och institutioner i framväxten av svensk genetik* (Lund: Lund University Press, 2004).

Tydén, Mattias. *Från politik till praktik: De svenska steriliseringslagarna 1935–1975*, 2nd ed. (Stockholm: Almqvist & Wiksell International, 2002).

CHAPTER 22

THE FIRST-WAVE EUGENIC REVOLUTION IN SOUTHERN EUROPE: SCIENCE *SANS FRONTIÈRES*

MARIA SOPHIA QUINE

EXISTING accounts of eugenics rarely take cognizance of its critical connective elements. In an era of increasing communication, due to the growth of scientific societies, journals, and congresses, ideas about eugenics were regularly transmitted across national borders. Eugenics was a movement whose international geographic reach, sociocultural infiltration, and diffusion within different branches of scientific knowledge grew enormously in the period before World War II. Eugenics defined itself as the world's first "applied" and universal science. By its very nature as a messianic movement seeking to change government action and private behavior globally, eugenics was first and foremost a "science without frontiers." The transnational character of eugenics coexisted with the rigid nationalism of the interwar period, and, from the outset, geo-cultural determinants of science shaped divergence and difference within worldwide eugenics, along religious, regional, cultural, and scientific lines.

This chapter focuses largely on Italy as a case study of eugenics in Catholic southern Europe. This example amply shows the extent of transnational linkages and interconnectedness within eugenics, not only at the level of international science congresses, but also, perhaps more surprisingly, through the formation of a "Latin" federation of eugenic organizations, spanning Europe and Latin America. This essay also examines Catholic responses to eugenics within a comparative context. The Galtonian imperative of "conscious selection," which some eugenicists used to justify such radical proposals as forced sterilization, euthanasia, and mass murder, contravened the sanctity of human life consecrated in Catholic doctrine, if not always convention. It is notable that Italy, Spain, and Portugal did not follow the path "Toward the Final Solution" traversed by other nations. Nonetheless, an active dialogue between Catholicism and eugenics occurred in these countries, and a compromise position on acceptable forms of "anti-natalism" emerged. For some, then, science and religion were compatible. Within the international movement, a distinct variety of softer "Latin" eugenics evolved, which defined itself in direct opposition to the dominant "Anglo-Saxon," "Nordic," and Nazi types, which were inclined more toward negative solutions to population problems. Through religious, cultural, and institutional ties, the "Latin" eugenics that arose in Italy felt affinity for and reached out to the kindred eugenics of Latin America and of fraternal countries in a family of nations in western and eastern Europe.

ITALY'S PLACE IN WORLD EUGENICS

The First International Congress, held in London from July 24 to 30, 1912, marked the formal inauguration of eugenics as an organized, worldwide movement. Bleecker Van Wagenen, chairman of the organizing committee of the congress, dispassionately outlined the various anti-natalist methods endorsed by eugenicists to preserve racial integrity: life segregation of the unfit (or segregation during the reproductive years); compulsory sterilization, usually of those with an insane or alcoholic inheritance; restrictive marriage laws and customs; eugenic education of the public and of prospective marriage mates; systems of mating purporting to remove defective traits; polygamy; euthanasia; neo-Malthusian information; and artificial interference to prevent conception.[1] Van Wagenen was a leading figure within the American eugenics movement, based at Cold Harbor, New York, a collaborator of Harry H. Laughlin (1880–1943), and the chairman of the committee which, in 1914, produced a key report on the "best practical means of cutting-off the defective germ-plasm" in the population.[2]

Despite the willingness to discuss openly measures that clearly ran contrary to existing law and custom in most countries, delegates at the 1912 gathering in London remained hesitant to endorse the negative eugenic proposals under scrutiny. A noteworthy exception to this cautious approach was evidenced by Agnes Bluhm (1862–1944), an obstetrician from Berlin, whose contribution to the congress explicitly and forcefully made a strong case for compulsory sterilization. She believed that the primary challenge confronting eugenicists was to convince politicians and the public alike that they should embark upon a new type of war, a "Race War," to preserve the racial stock and prevent its extinction. Significantly, however, her opinion represented a minority at the congress. A more hesitant position held sway. Even those who advocated negative eugenics recognized that drastic measures might alienate potential supporters and jeopardize their cause.[3]

Though extremely radical in conception and content, Van Wagenen's preliminary report, for example, concluded on a note of resignation that public interest and public opinion still diverged. He felt that it would be premature to advocate publicly the introduction of laws to weed and wipe out the threat of mental and physical defectiveness from the racial stock. Religion posed a huge obstacle to the spread of eugenic sentiment, in his opinion. With its opposition to birth control, the Catholic Church appeared to pose the biggest threat. But Van Wagenen was encouraged by the fact that the Vatican had still issued no dogma on the subject. He acknowledged that the majority of Catholic opinion was staunchly opposed to any form of sterilization or other means of conscious selection, for the purpose of reproductive fitness, or even on medical or compassionate grounds. Nonetheless, he maintained that there were encouraging signs that a new eugenic morality was awakening greater interest in these urgent matters among social workers, health professionals, and private citizens. Growing numbers of politicians, he maintained, were also increasingly coming around to the idea that drastic measures were necessary to eliminate confirmed degenerates and criminals from the general population. The revolution in attitudes leading toward final victory in the struggle to prevent race suicide would be slow in the coming, but it would, ultimately, happen.

Eugenics set about creating this new and revolutionary racial consciousness. At the 1912 conference, few voices proclaiming the inviolability of reproductive freedoms and the human body could be heard. Nonetheless, members of the Italian delegation took a more sociological than biological view of human evolution; this partly accounted for their divergence from a hard-line position. One of the vice presidents of the congress, Giuseppe Sergi (1841–1936), professor of anthropology at the University of Rome, questioned the certainty of those eugenicists who claimed that they could eliminate biological inferiority from the human race through selective breeding. The causes of variability in human beings, he asserted, remained an unsolved problem and, so long as they did, experiments in genetic engineering remained an impossible dream. Another of the vice-presidents, and the only Italian delegate on the general committee of the conference, Alfredo Niceforo (1876–1960), professor of statistics at the University of Naples, opposed the principle of conscious selection on the pragmatic grounds that it would stymie the forces of social mobility and racial regeneration. He explained that he spent most of his time measuring the demographic characters of the different classes. His research confirmed that the lower classes did, indeed, exhibit differing characteristics from the upper classes, such as their higher death rate and birth-rate, increased frequency of certain causes of death, pronounced precocity of age at marriage and a predilection for certain forms of crime. Inferior traits, he explained, produced inferior men who belonged to the inferior classes. But he also believed that social exchanges between the inferior and the superior classes occurred frequently, blurring socioeconomic distinctions and creating a milieu in which the generation of greater physical variation among people and more beneficial mutations in biotype were possible.[4]

Achille Loria (1857–1943), professor of political economy at the University of Turin, launched such a strong assault against the inherent élitism of the Galtonian position that the ideas presented in his paper became a major talking point in discussions. Loria noted that "no dynamometer of intellect" had yet been invented, so assessing the worthiness to breed of people on a mass scale and on the basis of elusive mental and moral capabilities was impractical for the state. By what criteria, exactly, was "artificial selection of the best specimens" to be guided, he asked. The crux of his argument rested on his unequivocal refutation of the notion that there was a strong correlation between class and fitness. Galton was wrong to maintain that the economic élite were also the "psycho-physical élite," Loria stated. "Great patrimonies are created, not by superior genius, as by shameful and iniquitous practices." Even when "rich men are in some cases superior," moreover, "their descendents would lack these qualities of greatness, because of the return of the mean law which Galton himself developed." Since a high income, particularly that procured by the accident of birth through inherited wealth, did not necessarily guarantee the propagation of superior progeny, eugenics had to aim more broadly at promoting racial improvement through positive health and social reforms, rather than through negative means, like marriage prohibitions.[5] So many of the leading figures of world eugenics, such as Francis Galton himself, as well as Madison Grant (1865–1937), Jon Alfred Mjøen (1860–1939), and Alfred Ploetz (1860–1940), were upper-class men of independent means whose privileged position in society was reflected in their contempt for the lower orders, who seemed to them to be producing an ever-increasing torrent of criminal, abnormal, and idiotic offspring. Italian eugenicists reacted strongly to this sort of class-based eugenics and attempted to offer progressive alternatives to it.

Director of a clinic for mental and nervous disorders at the University of Genoa, Enrico Morselli (1852–1929) was, perhaps, the Italian eugenicist with the greatest propensity to contemplate the necessity of negative measures. Having written extensively, as a dedicated Darwinist, on the problem of "evolutionary regression" and, as a committed racist, on the problem of biological inequality among humans, he would seem to be an ideal candidate for more extreme eugenics. In his lectures in anthropology at the Universities of Turin and Genoa, delivered between 1887 and 1908, Morselli set out to demonstrate that inferior races would perish through natural selection and that the white race would attain human perfection because of their physical and mental superiority. A psychiatrist, Morselli had for years been deeply influenced by the work of Bénédict Morel (1809–1873) on the role of mental deficiency in racial degeneration. In his paper delivered at the first international eugenics conference in London in 1912, Morselli expressed his openness to the possibility that certain forms of selective breeding, such as marriage prohibitions for the unfit, were palatable and even desirable in some cases. Nonetheless, his starting point was a fundamental acceptance of the desirability of human variability and an appreciation of the unique qualities of his own people. Eugenics, he affirmed, should aim to bring the human species to perfection, but it should never strive for the biological uniformity or the equalization of people, races, or nations. Morselli explained that he believed in the Mendelian laws of inheritance which, in his under-standing, postulated that every race possessed certain characteristics which were transmitted to descendants. This hereditary endowment comprised the progeni-tors' germ-plasm, which constituted the building blocks of the racial biotype that was passed down from one generation to the next. In Morselli's opinion, psychological attributes obeyed the same laws that governed bodily characters. Thus, the ancestral intellectual capacities, creative impulses, and emotional disposition of a race per-sisted alongside the primordial physical qualities. Hence, Morselli's commitment to the preservation of the distinctive "ethnic psychology" and physical genotype of his own Italian "race" prevented him from desiring to eradicate biological and psychological difference in others by means of "artificial selection."[6]

Adherence to a Mendelian hereditarian stance did not preclude commitment to an evolutionary perspective compatible with a platform promoting "positive" eugenics. Indeed, at this early stage in the formation of their movement, Italian eugenicists as a whole shared a staunch environmentalist position, positing that health, educational, welfare, and social reforms would produce benefits for the race and nation in the long term. Many of them opposed the class prejudices and blatant élitism of eugenicists in "Anglo-Saxon" and "Nordic" countries. Their vision was of a class-blind, meritocratic eugenic order in which the Italian race's best qualities, already proven by Italy's unequaled contribution to the development of Western civilization, would be encouraged to thrive and to grow. Only partly explained by religion, they also exhibited a collective cultural antipathy toward the principle of "conscious" or "artificial" selection. As the example of France amply demonstrates, Catholicism was not necessarily an obstacle to support for extreme solutions to per-ceived racial defilement. The ferocity of its tradition of anti-Jewish sentiment partly accounts for the apparent exceptionality of France in this regard.[7] The much higher concentration of medical doctors within the eugenic movement in France than in Italy also partly explains the secularism and even anti-clericalism that prevailed within the French variant and the greater propensity of French eugenicists to advocate bio-medical rather than social measures. In Italy, anthropologists, demog-raphers, economists, and sociologists dominated the eugenic society which they formally created within Giuseppe Sergi's Roman Anthropological Society in March 1913–April 1914. Thus the medical and hereditarian perspective, which commonly led to an acceptance of negative eugenics, had less of a footing within the Italian movement.[8]

The strength of the socialist movement in Italy, its immense influence upon med-icine, science, and society more broadly, and the intimate connections between left-wing thought and Darwinism and Social Darwinism there, meant that Italian eugenicists generally considered the working class to be less of a threat to the "race" than did eugenicists in some other countries, especially Britain.[9] A more egalitarian eugenics emerged in Italy, which sought to create a new society where class differen-tials in morbidity, mortality, and criminality would cease to be a problem for the race. Even after the conquest of power by the fascists in 1922, these socialist tendencies within Italian eugenics found expression in the support of the eugenic movement for the regime's willingness to mount eugenically inspired welfare and population policies. While a harsher negative eugenics tended to arise in highly industrialized and urbanized societies, where a large and unruly proletariat and underclass seemed to threaten the social order, Italy, in contrast, shared with more agrarian nations, like Brazil and Romania, a tendency to generate a brand of eugenic argument with strong modernizing and developmental impulses.[10] "Fecund" rural Italy and its highly prolific peasants were, of course, the romanticized ideal of Italian eugenicists. Nonetheless, Italian eugenicists were not anti-modernizers, conservatives, or reactionaries. While they wanted to preserve the fertility of the countryside and its people, they also recognized that the wealth of the nation depended upon workers, both urban and rural, whom they considered to be Italy's chief economic endowment.

Ethical considerations also motivated Italian eugenicists in that they recognized that endorsement of such relatively timid measures as marriage prohibitions opened up the floodgates to more radical and anti-humanist propositions. There was also a latent anarchic spirit among eugenicists in Italy, manifested in their refusal to contemplate the creation of a society singularly geared to the production of uniformly "fit" human specimens. In this regard, the healthy skepticism and irreverence of Italian culture probably played a large part in encouraging Italian eugenicists to question the absolute certainties and collectivist ambitions of some of their colleagues abroad. Italian scientists preferred to embrace biological difference and see society as an exciting mélange of diverse traits and abilities all mixing together and generating new, different, and potentially extraordinarily favorable variations for the human species.

Negative or Positive Routes in the Eugenic Revolution

The 1912 conference in London forced Italian scientists to recognize the potential threat that eugenics posed to reproductive freedoms. A serious discussion about negative eugenics began immediately after the London meeting, as Italian eugenicists struggled to define their own position on the issue of whether society and the state had a right to regulate the fertility of the so-called unfit. In a review of the London meeting that appeared in the national newspaper, the *Corriere della Sera* on September 4, 1912, Alessandro Clerici stated with utter certainty that Italian scientists would never endorse any draconian legislation allowing governmental or medical authorities to infringe upon the basic human right to procreate.[11] Clerici overstated the case somewhat, however, for the position of Italian eugenics was more complex than his bold conclusion would allow. During this formative period in the development of Italian eugenics into an organized movement, members of the incipient society based in Rome, as well as the broader community of scientists throughout the nation who addressed eugenic issues in their work, intensely debated the issue of negative eugenics, generally, and birth control and sterilization, particularly, after 1912.

At a 1913 meeting of the Roman Anthropological Society, in which the role of eugenics was discussed, some of those attending indicated that they might be amenable to the idea that the state should limit the fertility of the unfit. The strongest argument in favor of imposing some form of restriction on personal sexual and reproductive liberties came from Achille Loria, the socialist economist, who regarded Switzerland's recent imposition of premarital medical examinations as an "index of the progress of civilization."[12] Furthermore, Loria maintained that when individuals were a hazard to public health, they should be forcibly prohibited from reproducing. Although he did not endorse compulsory sterilization, he did make his acceptance of the concept of negative eugenic measures quite clear. Those present acknowledged that the question of the social control of the masses lay at the heart of eugenics.

Those most vulnerable to the new forms of social control advocated by eugenicists in some countries were naturally the least powerful members of society. This made it all the more important for Italian eugenicists to get their program right; they felt a tremendous responsibility to the nation to strike the right balance between the freedom of the individual and responsibility toward the collectivity.[13]

Enrico Morselli summed up these debates about negative eugenics in an extraordinary book entitled *Mercy-Killing: Euthanasia.* He listed the various direct measures to control the reproduction of "anti-social elements who threaten the racial constitution": the extermination of "subjects ill-adapted to reproduction or harmful to the social body; the exile or deportation of the unfit; the social segregation and confinement of defectives; sterilization by means of castration, vasectomy, radium and iodine poisoning, hysterectomy and salpingectomy; forced abortions; the creation of a female reproductive cast; legalized polygamy for men with a superior inheritance; and the use of contraception as the eugenic measure." He then went on to describe the various indirect means of limiting the fertility of dysgenic people: marital bans; premarital medical testing (primarily for tuberculosis and syphilis, as well as mental defectiveness); financial incentives for marriage among the most elect; programs for social hygiene to decrease the spread of contagious diseases, like malaria; public health and educational campaigns. Morselli stated that "humanitarians may have a certain repugnance for repressive laws," but society had an "absolute right to protect itself from the harm caused by the propagation of the unfit and the undesirable." Morselli was clearly attracted to the idea that eugenic science might help humanity evolve "more perfect human types" by means of "artificial interference in natural selection." The appeal of eugenics for scientists was this very possibility of human betterment; but this promise opened up all sorts of ethical concerns about how far society should go to alter the course of evolution. Morselli argued that the implementation of negative eugenics in Italy was only a "very remote possibility" because of the scientific community's respect for the country's prevailing customs, laws, and values.[14]

Given the social primacy of the Catholic Church in Italy, Morselli argued, Italian eugenics was compelled to devise a more "bland and moderate" program of action based on "positive neo-Lamarckian" measures to promote racial health. Interestingly, Morselli did not hesitate to endorse immediate and radical measures to prohibit racial intermixing between Italians and their colonial subjects. Although he strongly opposed forms of "racial euthanasia," like "mass alcoholization or murder by means of tuberculosis or syphilis," on the grounds that these "dishonored civilization," he believed that conscious "sexual selection" aimed at preventing intermingling between blacks and whites in the empire was an absolute necessity.[15] This was one area in the dispute about negative measures where most Italian scientists could agree wholeheartedly on a more hard-line approach. Italian eugenics, like Italian fascism, was racist and chauvinist to the core. The "soft" approach only applied to members of their own "race" and nation.

Notwithstanding positions like Morselli's, generally even the most hereditarian of eugenicists, who strongly believed that injurious traits were heritable, could not bring themselves to advocate sterilization. A psychologist trained within the Lombrosian tradition, Giuseppe Sergi, like so many other scientists at the time, found himself drawn to the ideas of Herbert Spencer and became, in fact, one of Spencer's translators in Italy. In much of his early work on human degeneration, published before World War I, Sergi gave full voice to his doubts about whether public and private welfare could help to contain the spread of hereditary ills such as pauperism, prostitution, and criminality. For him, social decay had biological causes, and some elements within the sub-proletariat were irremediable. Nonetheless, he expressed practical reservations about the potential usefulness of negative eugenics. Addressing the call for marriage prohibitions for the epileptic, criminal, tubercular, alcoholic, and the insane, Sergi argued that this sort of measure would only lead to the far graver problem of increasing illegitimacy, an inevitability if people were legally prevented from marrying. On the issue of sterilization, Sergi considered it imprudent to implement social policies whose actual efficacy remained in doubt. Even if, at some time in the future, the truth of the hereditarian thesis were to be established, he contended, a poor country like Italy would never be able to afford the costly mass programs required to eradicate all heritable disease. Rather than endorse measures whose effects were questionable, Italian scientists like Sergi believed that the best way to promote racial progress was by means of positive social intervention improving the housing, health, nutrition, and welfare of the people.[16]

Other Italian hereditarians also proved unwilling to accept the premise that environment had no role to play in producing the psycho-social degenerate. Sante De Sanctis (1862–1935), a neuroscientist and social reformer, thoroughly opposed the notion that the mentally ill should be compulsorily sterilized for the good of the race. He remained an advocate of custodial and curative care for the so-called mentally deficient and degenerate. Only slowly, he lamented, were Italian psychiatrists ceasing to perform post-mortem craniectomies on "idiots" in order to find, as Lombroso had instructed, the cerebral signs or "stigmata" of degeneracy. He felt certain that his profession could never allow a new barbarism to reign by condoning the compulsory sterilization of their patients.[17] Other Italian psychiatrists, such as Benigno De Tullio and Giuseppe Vidoni, expressed doubts about the usefulness of "sexual amputation" as a social prophylactic against those with an "injurious inheritance" because they saw no causal connection between the genitals and the brain. Some American psychiatrists claimed that sterilization had a therapeutic impact upon patients, but the Italian medical community was skeptical. Sterilizing the mentally infirm seemed to them a wasteful exercise whose beneficial effects on society and the individual were largely unproven. They questioned whether Switzerland, where the practice of non-consensual and un-authorized sterilizations had, as in the United States, been secretly taking place within mental asylums since before World War I, would see any benefit in the future from a policy that degraded its perpetrators and its victims alike. The segregation of the mentally infirm from society, they believed, was a far more humane way of protecting the race.

ITALIAN EUGENICS UNDER FASCISM

The American Museum of Natural History in New York City hosted the Second International Congress of Eugenics in the autumn of 1921. In America, "race" was the exclusive focus of eugenicists concerned about the germ plasm. The perceived threat posed by Blacks, Jews, and immigrants stood at the top of their agenda. American delegates at the 1921 conference supported calls for legal sanctions against all detrimental influences upon the White, Anglo-Saxon, Protestant breeding-stock of the nation.[18] By contrast, Italian eugenicists took a soft-line approach to the problem of race contamination. They did contemplate the adoption of some form of negative eugenics, but they again stopped well short of endorsing anything as radical as forced sterilization. In the 1920s, a lively debate about these issues continued to take place in fascist Italy in the pages of specialist medical, public health, and legal journals. Government bodies also participated in discussions about what the desirable and appropriate contours of a eugenic policy might be in Italy.

One of the main loci of discussions about these contentious matters was the Italian Institute of Hygiene, Insurance, and Social Assistance, originally founded in Rome in 1922 as a private charity devoted to the study of problems relating to public health. Its founder was Ettore Levi (1880–1932 [by suicide]), a Jewish intellectual who had been a member of the moderate Left, the birth control movement, and the eugenics society before the rise of fascism. Levi was the leading proponent of social medicine in Italy. As founder of the Institute of Social Medicine, he was instrumental in its establishment as a recognized discipline, backed by university training programs and guidelines. He defined social medicine as the science of those illnesses affecting the health of the collectivity, the purpose of which was the prevention and cure of disease for the benefit of the individual and the nation. Levi was drawn to fascism because of its professed commitment to the health and hygiene of the "stirp" (denoting ethnic Italians); in this regard, he is an interesting example of a Jewish fascist, which was by no means a contradiction before the dissemination of anti-Jewish legislation beginning in 1938. Levi's Institute was committed to the principles of "eutenics" (*eutenica*), which, in contrast to "Anglo-Saxon" or "Nordic" eugenics, advocated improvements to the home and social environment, as well as the protection of motherhood and infancy through welfare reforms, as the best means to promote racial advancement.

Launched in 1922, the Institute's journal, *Difesa Sociale* (Social Defence), began a dialogue with fascist officialdom and a range of health and medical professionals in Italy. One of the most controversial issues under consideration was the so-called "pre-matrimonial certificate." Some eugenicists and their supporters, including members of the government's Royal Commission for the Study of Post-war Problems, believed that medical certification, demonstrating that a couple were free of contagious social and sexual diseases, such as tuberculosis and syphilis, should be a requirement before marriage. Objections to prenuptial health screening were based on the grounds that it would be offensive, intrusive, coercive and impractical. Opponents alleged that any such scheme would create the possibility of medical fraud for gain, would pose the difficulty of actually enforcing the ban on the unfit from getting married, and would cause extramarital unions and illegitimacy to rise. Levi's Institute lobbied for the introduction of a mild negative eugenic program for social prophylaxis and favored the idea of medical certification before marriage.[19]

The fascist regime, however, remained opposed to any measures that deviated from the pronatalist path already being frantically pursued. The preparedness of the dictatorship to control all aspects of its demographic campaign, which was devoted to an increase in the quality and the quantity of the Italian population, is amply illustrated by the fact that it simply subsumed Levi's institute within the organs of the state: it became a public agency under the direction of the National Fund for Social Insurance in 1928. While this gave the Institute a national platform, the change also marked the loss of freedom of that sector within Italian eugenics which veered toward the idea of some sort of selection for the sake of the race. Talk of any kind of restrictions to reproductive freedoms now became an impossibility, as the regime co-opted eugenics and steered population policy towards an unconditional pronatalist, reformist, and environmentalist position. "Positive" health and welfare reforms, the fascist line oft repeated, would gradually bring about beneficial psycho-physiological adaptations to the individual and the race. Grounded in a Lamarckian evolutionary perspective, this thinking ran contrary to the hereditarian and Mendelian paradigm that was perceived to be the doctrinal basis of "Anglo-Saxon" and "Nordic" eugenics. Under state control, the activities of Levi's institute were restricted to the dissemination of "sanitary propaganda" and its research confined to questions relating, in particular, to the government's attempts to contain the spread of tuberculosis.

This unwavering pronatalist and positive stance gained official endorsement from the state in fascist Italy's new penal code, which came into effect in July 1931, and took a tough line against so-called "anti-Malthusianism" or "the procurement of impotence to procreate." It defined as an absolute necessity for the nation the defense of the "continuation and integrity of the race" through strict measures against abortion, birth control, and sterilization. The Pope had spoken specifically on these matters for the first time when Pius XI issued his famous encyclical, *Casti connubii,* on 31 December 1930. This decree affirmed the sanctity of marriage and its procreative purpose and condemned all forms of contraception as acts against God and nature. The Pope broadened the scope of his condemnation when he specifically stated that any artificial intervention to prohibit conception ran contrary to Church doctrine. Moreover, a separate part of the address condemned both compulsory sterilization by the state and voluntary sterilization by the individual. The state had no right whatsoever to sterilize an innocent person. And "self-mutilation" was also unlawful; the "bodily organs should not be rendered unfit for natural functions except when the good of the whole body cannot otherwise be provided for," the Holy Office emphatically decreed.[20]

A wholesale disintegration of liberal and humanitarian values, as happened in interwar Germany, did not occur in fascist Italy. If anything, the unrelenting pronatalism and welfarism of Mussolini's dictatorship helped keep Italy's eugenic movement in check. The eugenicists who came to prominence during this period reflected the priorities of the regime. One immensely influential religious leader, Father Agostino Gemelli (1878–1959), a Franciscan friar, was instrumental in making Catholicism compatible with eugenics. He founded the Catholic University of the Sacred Heart in Milan in 1921 and served as its chancellor for many years. A physician by training, Gemelli devoted his life to the study of psychology and was a major figure in that field. A Lombrosian revisionist, Gemelli criticized the simplistic and rigid positivism of Lombroso and his contemporaries and attacked the biological materialism of his own colleagues within the international eugenic movement. His research affirmed that each human being, defined as a totality of organic matter, emotional responses, and complex behaviors determined by environmental, psychic, and innate forces, was remarkably plastic and changeable. Gemelli believed wholeheartedly that even the most "hopeless" or "useless" individuals could be cured or redeemed by science.[21]

Italian eugenicists responded to the obstacle that Catholicism posed to their cause by adapting their platform to the particular circumstances of their own country. In other Catholic nations too, such as Belgium, eugenics took on a populist, pronatalist guise as a campaign for "family endowment" in order to attract support. Formally established in 1919, the Belgian eugenics society, like the French, had an intense interest in promoting the interests of large families through benefits, incentives, and privileges. This support for *familles nombreuses* was the linchpin of a proposed legislative program revolving around the aim of increased fertility, which included, as in Italy, fierce opposition to birth control and abortion, as well as the single-issue campaign for the so-called "moral" education of youth. The one major negative proposal that Belgian eugenicists contemplated—and advocated far more vociferously and openly than in Italy—was the premarital medical examination. Moderation paid off well, in the sense that official recognition came with the patronage of the Belgian king and the Belgian Red Cross after the war; government support for a eugenic social and population policy also grew in the 1920s.[22]

In Portugal, too, a Catholic context helped shape eugenics. But in Portugal, as in Spain and Latin America, eugenics responded just as much to the socioeconomic realities of the country as it did to the religious affiliation of the population. In an overwhelmingly poor, low-waged, and agrarian nation like Portugal, where mere subsistence was a real difficulty for many peasants, urban factory workers had few rights, and labor and social conditions in general were appalling by European standards, eugenicists (who were slow to organize into a proper society and movement) called chiefly for the extension of basic public health provision and the introduction of even a modicum of government reforms. As state welfare hardly existed at all, and church and charitable institutions struggled to deal with disease and destitution on a mass scale, the severity of social problems dominated native eugenics, while the more esoteric obsessions that could preoccupy some eugenicists in privileged and affluent nations were simply not seen as an option.[23]

In some contexts, culture took precedence over religion in determining the content of a national variety of eugenics. In Austria, for example, where Catholicism remained by a huge margin the largest denomination within the republic throughout the interwar years, the brand of eugenics that finally emerged officially in 1925 had the audacity to campaign loudly for widespread use of birth control (not technically illegal) by the working class, premarital screening for mental defects, and even the abolition of the ban against abortion on the grounds that these would be appropriate social defenses against the wanton procreation of the undesirable subaltern orders. Like any other special-interest group, eugenicists were able to enjoy ful freedom of speech and assembly in Austria's newly formed liberal democracy. Possibly the presence of such vocal anti-clericals, as many Austrian eugenicists were, and their connections to the Socialist Party, contributed to the ferocious clerical reaction and right-wing backlash that occurred in Austria in the 1930s and had such tragic consequences after the *Anschluss* by Nazi Germany in 1938.[24]

Operating within the context of a dictatorship, single-mindedly pursuing its own social agenda, as well as a political policy of pacification of the Vatican, Italian eugenicists were not in a position to dictate their own terms. Insofar as it existed, dissent from the official line endorsed by the alliance of church and state, consecrated in 1929, did not have much of an outlet in fascist Italy. At least one prominent doctor, Cesare Michele, who worked for the fascist regime's welfare organization catering to women and children, was rumored at the time to be violating the law by performing abortions for rich clients in secret. Aware of the potential scandal, Mussolini and his advisors chose not to make an example of the physician because to have done so would have resulted in potentially damaging publicity. His activities, like that of other suspected abortionists, remained underground. Achille Loria, like Mussolini himself, had been in the pre-war period a well-known "Malthusian," or advocate of birth control. There are many examples such as these, but controversial views that ran contrary to fascist dictates were kept quiet. The regime's campaign to increase the birthrate was a major showpiece whose ultimate success, despite its demonstrable failure to reverse demographic trends, was never allowed to be questioned in the media.[25]

By cultivating close ties with fascist officialdom, successfully creating for himself a reputation as the chief expert in the field and securing numerous positions of power and influence in public office through patronage, Corrado Gini (1884–1965) became the leading eugenicist of the period. His position was rigidly pronatalist. A figure of national and international prominence, he helped to broker an alliance between fascism and eugenics and to shape government policy in the 1920s and 1930s. He was also instrumental in steering Italian eugenics away from an "Anglo-Saxon," Nazi, or "Nordic" direction, in making pronatalism its defining dogma, and in bringing it closer in line with other like-minded movements.

THE EMERGENCE OF "LATIN" EUGENICS WITHIN THE INTERNATIONAL MOVEMENT

Held in Milan in September 1924, the first conference ever organized by the Italian Society of Genetics and Eugenics (formed in 1919 from its precursor), together with the Royal Italian Society of Hygiene, emphasized that positive reforms would be the hallmark of Italian eugenics.[26] Despite the inclusion of genetics in the title of their society and the increasing prominence of questions relating to biology and genetics at subsequent national conferences in 1929 and 1937 (the last before 1949), Italian eugenicists preferred to use the term "social eugenics" to describe their aims and to distinguish their movement from those with a more hereditarian, selectionist, or eliminationist orientation. In September and October 1929, they held their second, two-week congress, this time in Rome; over 300 delegates, including many foreigners, attended.[27] Along with Achille Loria and Cesare Artom (1879–1934), a distinguished biologist, anatomist, and Jewish intellectual, Gini served as co-president of the thriving Italian Society of Genetics and Eugenics. His leading role within the international eugenics movement allowed him to make and sustain contacts with foreign scientists. As ideological and policy divergences within the International Federation of Eugenic Organizations (the IFEO, established in 1921) became more pronounced, and the connections between American and German eugenics and their allied movements in Britain and Scandinavia grew more deep and extensive, Gini made moves to found a separate society for those committed to a positive program.

His research activities had also gained notoriety within the International Union for the Scientific investigation of Population Problems (the IUSPP, founded in 1928), whose constitution declared that its work on population questions should not have a moral, religious, or political outlook. Gini took the opportunity of a 1933 Rome conference on population to approach like-minded foreign eugenicists with a view to establishing a break-away organization from the IFEO for those opposed in principle to the variegated platform of negative eugenics. His vision of a Latin International Federation of Eugenic Societies quickly became a reality as countries as diverse as Argentina, Brazil, France, Mexico, Romania, Catalonia (Spain),

Portugal, and French and Italian Switzerland accepted invitations to join. Belgium expressed an interest in joining once it revived its flagging eugenic society.

As the prime mover of the plan to unite eugenic societies with a shared "positive" purpose, Gini served as president of the newly formed Latin international federation, which held its inaugural meeting at the congress of the Eugenic Societies of Latin America in Mexico City in October 1935. A founding address by Gini, who could not be present, was read by Alfredo A. Saavedra, a physician and perpetual secretary of the Mexican Society of Eugenics. Gini's speech emphasized the enthusiastic response that his proposal received. Every single member of the regional Latin federation of eugenic societies, which included those firmly established in Argentina, Peru, and Mexico, as well as those still in formation in Colombia, Cuba, Costa Rica, Uruguay, Honduras, and Panama, agreed to join the new international organization. Membership also included those European societies, in France, Spain, Italy, Portugal and elsewhere, which shared a "Latin" sensibility and style in their eugenic programs. Some of these countries possessed a common cultural, linguistic, historical and ethnic heritage, such as Romania and Italy, whose strong attachment derived from their shared pedigree of *Romanità*. Romanian eugenicists, like their Italian colleagues, were generally less inclined than eugenicists in Germany and the United States to advocate the introduction of coercive and compulsory negative measures, like the sterilization of the unfit. Partly, Gini explained, this had to do with the superior societies of these Latin nations, where, because of the strength of family and community ties, a threatening residuum of hard-core defectives and degenerates imperiling the race did not exist to the same extent as it did in the more atomized and individualistic "Anglo-Saxon" and "Germanic" nations. Romania and Italy, moreover, were kindred nations that would forever be linked by their ancient Roman connection and unbroken ties of blood and history.[28] The myth of a proud Romano-Dacian race as ancestral racial progenitors, forefathers of the nation, and protectors of the "authentic" national identity and folk traditions of the Romanian people informed much of the discourse of nationalists, eugenicists, and fascists in interwar Romania and provided a powerful familial bond with their Italian counterparts.

Religion comprised a key component of Gini's conception of "Latinity." In the case of France, Belgium, Spain, and Portugal, this "Latin commonality" was founded upon a shared Catholicism, which functioned as a cornerstone of nation, state, and society and precluded policies favoring abortion, contraception, and other forms of reproductive restrictions. On scientific, moral, and humanitarian grounds, too, Gini stressed that Latin eugenics was a "regenerative" and "curative" science committed to births, not deaths. The pronatalism at its foundation was the most positive form of eugenics because it sought to protect and promote the essence and the best of the collectivity and the race, without sacrificing individual rights and freedoms. Latin eugenics upheld "human dignity and personal integrity." In their haste to perfect humanity, eugenicists should never forget that they were dealing with human beings and unique individuals, not laboratory "flies or rabbits" to be propagated according to some experimental blueprint of a master race. The hereditarianism of some eugenicists was a dangerous ideology with destructive nihilism as its heart. The "Latin scientist," Gini stressed, would always remain reluctant to destroy "one of the most salient manifestations of what it means to be human"—reproductive and sexual choice—and could never contemplate depriving human beings of their personhood and humanity.[29]

At the International Congress on Population in Paris in 1937, the Italian delegates spoke about the innate "vitality" of fecund populations and the "energy" associated with "reproductivity." They contended that fascist demographic policy had a sound scientific base in modern biology and defended the logic of their government's efforts to protect the race by increasing the birthrate. The underlying assumptions of their arguments were that Italian women and men were distinguished by their "hyperfecundity" and that this was a beneficial characteristic which had to be preserved.[30] Since 1928, Gini had (as part of his work with the IUSPP) been compiling and examining anthropometric data taken from 15,000 Harvard female undergraduates and a random sample of Italian women; his research confirmed to him that Italian women, by virtue of their especially fertile biotype, possessed greater "reproductive potentiality" than their American counterparts; this evolutionary asset was evidenced by the early age of menarche and the late onset of menopause that typified the lives of so many Italian "mothers of the race."[31] A recurring implication in the arguments used by Italian scientists was that a high birthrate positively correlated with male sexual prowess and potency; on that score, Italian men, the reasoning went, had little to fear since they were demonstrably more virile than their "Anglo-Saxon" and "Nordic" counterparts.[32]

The Second International Congress of the Latin Federation of Eugenic Societies was scheduled to take place in Bucharest in September 1939, but was canceled because of Britain's declaration of war against Germany. In September 1940, the National Congress on the Science of Population took place in Oporto, Portugal, and was attended by many foreign delegates. Italy was represented by Gini and Fabio Frassetto, an acclaimed anthropologist and anatomist based at the University of Bologna. Both Frassetto's paper on "biotypology" and Gini's on "denatality" continued to develop what was a formative principle of Latin eugenics—namely, that "hyperfecundity" was a positive force for the race and that "prolificity" was a product of a superior racial constitution.

CONCLUSION

If historians wish to hold eugenics accountable, in some way, for the atrocities committed in the pursuit of racial betterment before and during World War II, then the existence of Latin eugenics within the international movement never amounted to much of an ameliorating force. Undoubtedly, as the twentieth century's first "public science," eugenics of the first wave succeeded, in dramatically different national contexts, in spreading "a new eugenic consciousness," shaping social opinions and ideas, and carving out for itself a prominent role in policy and government. Some eugenicists, like those in the United States and Germany, came closer than others to realizing the aims of their "total revolution" in existing values, statutes, and institutions. Similarly conceived and executed, radical programs of race hygiene by means of mass compulsory sterilization in a Nazi dictatorship and an American democracy were the concrete expression of a cultural crisis, manifest so tragically for so many in the widespread collapse of liberalism and humanism in the first half of the twentieth century, to which eugenics undoubtedly contributed.[33] Others, like Gini, Gemelli, and Pende in Italy, were able to exert tremendous influence over government, while at the same time seeking to accommodate overriding political dictates and public sensibilities.

Historians preoccupied with the problem of explaining the "Dark Side of Progress," Europe's "Descent into Barbarism," and the "Road to Auschwitz" have long held eugenics to account as a peculiarity of Protestant "Anglo-Saxon" and Germanic cultures and a dangerous "pseudo-science" fueling Nazism and resulting in mass murder. Scholars now know that not all eugenicists were reactionary, anti-Jewish, or racist extremists with evil, genocidal intentions. Within the complex, shifting, and heterogeneous world eugenics movement, the strand championed by Italy and its allies represents a more palatable variety than the far more familiar Nazi type. Significantly, however, eugenics, in both its Latin and non-Latin forms, redefined the relationship between the individual, society, and the state. Whether it was pro-life, positive, and pronatalist or more extreme, negative, and antinatalist in orientation, the underlying presupposition of eugenics was that the interests of mere individuals had to be subordinated to the higher ones of the collective, the "race," the nation, and the state. Whatever shape it took, eugenics was fundamentally anti-liberal, anti-humanist, and authoritarian in means and ends. Even proposals to improve health care and welfare benefits were conceived as ways to enhance the quality of the genetic stock and the racial inheritance of the nation, rather than the quality of the lives of individuals and their families. The eugenic ideal was that the private, sexual, and social behavior of human beings could be coordinated and controlled by a masterful and commanding state and its servants of professional experts in eugenic medicine and science.

The racial utopia envisioned by eugenicists everywhere was a totalitarian fantasy that contributed in no small measure to the breakdown of democratic values and parliamentary systems in the interwar period and operated in perfect consonance with the forces of fascism, Nazism, and dictatorship that were responsible for so much misery, death, and destruction. But after the fall of fascism in 1943–1945, eugenics did not disappear in Italy or elsewhere. On the contrary, second-wave eugenics emerged as an offshoot of genetics and biotechnology. Unlike the state-centred, old-style, coercive eugenics, which mainly sought to influence government, the new eugenics primarily aims to give wealthy private individuals reproductive choices and control in the form of enhanced fertility and the ability to manipulate the genetic inheritance that they pass to their offspring.[34]

Until his death in 1965, Italy's premier eugenicist, Corrado Gini, continued to play a major role in a de-racialized, post-fascist version of eugenics. To public acclaim within his own country, he continued research in the newly established field of "genetic demography," which was an attempt by old-style eugenicists to rebrand their product into a socio-biological discipline befitting the post-1946 welfare democracy of the Italian Republic.[35] Gini may not have been the most heinous collaborator around at the time, but elements of his fascist past, sanitized and forgotten after 1945, were decidedly unsavory.

In particular, his racism and his collaboration with the fascist regime's imperial policies should not have been whitewashed. On behalf of the International Labour Organization and other organizations, Gini became a high-profile player on the world eugenic stage after World War I. In particular, his appointment to the presidency of the International Federation of Eugenic Organization's Commission for the Study of the Eugenic and Disgenic Effects of the War in 1927 was a tremendous accolade. After all, the work of the commission comprised one of the chief collaborative and transnational projects of international eugenics in the inter-war period. The outcome of his involvement, however, led to a major controversy that contributed to his desire to break away from the IFEO. One of Gini's own major interests was the subject of so-called "primitive races"; his work in this field allowed him to contribute to the IFEO's committee on "race crossing." It also led to his involvement with the International Union for the Scientific Investigation of Population Problems. Gini was enlisted by the IUSPP to compile vital statistics on so-called inferior races. With the help of the Royal Italian Geographic Society, fifteen scientific expeditions under Gini's command were sent in the 1930s to Africa, America, Asia, and elsewhere in Europe in order to compile anthropometric and demographic data on "the white race" and its interaction with a range of "primitive and decadent ethnic groups." A particular concern of Gini was to elucidate the deleterious effects of miscegenation on the "fecundity" of the white race.

Pushing the confines of demography and population statistics ever closer to biology, eugenics, and genetics, just as Galton himself had done, Gini was also simultaneously preparing the ideological arsenal for the fascist regime's extensive anti-miscegenation legislation, which was implemented in Italian East Africa after the violent conquest of Ethiopia in 1935–1936. So draconian were the laws on cohabitation, "sexual congress," and relations between the conquering and the vanquished "races" that they have been compared to the system of Apartheid in South Africa. Indeed, the rationale was the same—the notion of the necessity of the separate development and the total segregation of the races in order to protect European blood from contagion by inferior elements informed both experiments.[36] From the late 1920s, Gini's research and connections with fascist population policies were becoming increasingly uncomfortable for the IUSPP, which attempted to consider population apolitically. In particular, the IUSPP's honorary general secretary, Captain George H. L. F. Pitt-Rivers, grew increasingly uneasy about Gini's political and scientific biases and intentions. In 1932, he formally censured Gini and then withdrew funding for his commission, before resolving, with the support of the executive committee of the IUSPP, to dissolve his investigative team entirely in 1937. Pitt-Rivers outlined his reasons in an utterly damning critique of Gini's aims and methods. This accused the renowned Italian scientist of conducting work that was entirely unscientific—by any internationally accepted standard of research into population matters, Pitt-Rivers stressed—and that was politically motivated, highly suspect, and sub-standard.[37]

The criticism had no effect upon Gini's reputation at the time or his resuscitation after the war. In fact, the national awards and honors in recognition of his outstanding service to science continued to accumulate in the 1950s and 1960s. Gini did, however, keep a low profile when it came to matters pertaining to his past life as a leading eugenicist. Discredited, eugenics ceased to play much of a role in the first and only postwar conference of the re-formed *Società Italiana di Genetica e di Eugenica* (Italian Genetics and Eugenics Society), which met briefly in September 1949. Although Gini's Latin Federation failed to be revived after World War II, the sentiments that first brought it into existence have continued to have relevance in the postwar period and into the twenty-first century in government and media-generated scares about the low birthrate, a "dying" population, the endangered nation and invading immigrants. At a much deeper level of consciousness and culture as well, Italian pronatalism is alive and thriving within the Italian medical and scientific communities, as issues like abortion, reproductive technology, stem-cell research and "euthanasia," as well as the rights and responsibilities attached to them, remain highly controversial and contested. For example, advocates of scientific "progress" accuse the Catholic Church of undue influence in a secular and democratic society and contend that its position on assisted conception, reproductive technology, and research on human embryos is "medieval" and "backward."[38] In an investigation of the attitudes of physicians toward the assisted death of terminal patients in a palliative context, one of many such studies over the years, the researchers concluded that the majority of doctors questioned were opposed to "euthanasia" and that "the variable most strongly associated with a negative response" was "religious belief."[39] Just as they were in Gini's day, national culture and religion remain determinants of attitudes and anxieties about those issues that have concerned eugenicists, old and new, for well over a century.

NOTES

1. *Problems in Eugenics: Papers Communicated to the First International Eugenics Conference Held at The University of London, July 24–30, 1912*, vol. 1 (London: The Eugenics Education Society, 1912), 460–479.

2. See Harry H. Laughlin, *Report of the Committee to Study and to Report on the Best Practical Means of Cutting Off the Defective Germ-Plasm in the American Population*, vol. 1, *The Scope of the Committee's Work* (New York: Eugenics Record Office, 1914).

3. *Problems in Eugenics*, vol. 1, 387–395.

4. Giuseppe Sergi, "Variazione e eredità nell'uomo," and Alfredo Niceforo, "The Cause of the Inferiority of Physical and Mental Characters in the Lower Social Classes," in *Problems in Eugenics*, vol. 1, 9–15 and 189–194.

5. Achille Loria, "The Psycho-Physical Élite and the Economic Élite," *Problems in Eugenics*, vol. 1, 178–184; see also *Problems in Eugenics*, vol. 2, 50–53.

6. Morselli's lectures were published as the definitive pro-Darwinist textbook in general anthropology: Enrico Morselli, *Antropologia generale: L'Uomo secondo la teoria dell'evoluzione: Lezioni dettate nelle università di Torino e di Genova*, 2 vols. (Turin: Unione Tipografico Editrice, 1911); *Problems in Eugenics*, vol. 1, 60–62.

7. In France, a more pronatalist eugenics prevailed until the advent of the Vichy dictatorship, which swept away all obstacles to the more extremist, anti-Jewish, and racist eugenic proposals already being implemented in America and Germany. See William H. Schneider, *Quality and Quantity: The Quest for Biological Regeneration in Twentieth Century France* (Cambridge and New York: Cambridge University Press, 1990), 281–282.

8. The majority of the 58 founding members of the Italian "Committee for the Study of Eugenics" were social scientists: Atti Della Società Romana Di Antropologia, "Verbali," in *Rivista di Antropologia* 18 (1913) and 19 (1914).

9. See Diane Paul, "Eugenics and the Left," *Journal of the History of Ideas* 45, no. 4 (1984): 567–590.

10. Greta Jones, *Social Hygiene in Twentieth-Century Britain* (Beckenham: Croom Helm, 1986), introduction.

11. Alessandro Clerici, "L"Eugenetica," *Corriere della Sera*, September 4, 1912.

12. Natalia Gerodotti, "From Science to Social Technology: Eugenics and Politics in Twentieth-Century Switzerland," *Social Politics* 13, no. 1 (2006): 59–88.

13. Atti Della Società Romana Di Antropologia, "Adunanza del 21 Marzo 1913," *Rivista di Antropologia*, 18 (1913): 511–514.

14. Enrico Morselli, *L'Uccisione pietosa: L'Euthanasia: In rapporto alla medicina, alla morale ed all'eugenica* (Turin: Bocca, 1923), 227–251, 261–262.

15. Ibid., 236–237.

16. See, for example, Giuseppe Sergi, *Le degenerazioni umane* (Milan: Fratelli Dumolard, 1889). See Sergi's "L'Eugenica dalla biologia alla sociologia," in Atti della Società Romana di Antropologia, *Rivista di antropologia* 19 (1914): 351–379.

17. Sante De Sanctis, *Deboli di mente e criminali* (Milan: Società Editrice Libraria, 1915).

18. B. Mehler, *A History of the American Eugenics Society, 1921–1940* (PhD diss., University of Illinois, 1988).

19. Istituto italiana di medicina sociale, *Difesa Sociale*; published throughout the fascist period and beyond, the journal published its first issue in January 1922 and continues publication to this day.

20. John Thomas Noonan, *Contraception: The History of Its Treatment by the Catholic Theologians and Canonists* (Cambridge, MA: Belknap Press of Harvard University Press, 1966).

21. Agostino Gemelli's two-volume classic, *L'Enigma della vita e i nuovi orizzonti della biologia: Introduzione allo studio delle scienze biologiche* (Florence: Libreria Editrice Fiorentina, 1909; 2nd ed., 1914) became a major textbook in experimental psychology in universities and defined the discipline as a biological science. vol. 2 forcefully challenged hereditarianism directly.

22. M. T. Nisot, *La question eugénique dans les divers pays*, vol. 2 (Brussels: L'Association Internationale pour la protection de l'enfance, 1929), 130–135; Hugh H. R. Vibart, *Family Allowances in Practice: An Examination of the Development of the Family Wage System and of the Compensation Fund, Principally in Belgium, France, Germany and Holland* (London: P. S. King, 1926).

23. Nisot, *La question eugénique*, vol. 2, 432; Richard Cleminson, *Anarchism, Science, and Sex: Eugenics in Eastern Spain, 1900–1937* (Oxford and New York: Peter Lang, 2000); Thomas F. Glick, Miguel Angel Puig-samper, and Rosaura Ruiz, eds., *The Reception of Darwinism in the Iberian World: Spain, Spanish America, and Brazil* (Dordrecht and Boston: Kluwer Academic Publishers, 2001); João Arriscado Nunes and Marisa Matias, *A Regulatory Void?: Reprogenetics in Portugal*, STAGE (Science, Technology, and Governance in Europe) Discussion Paper 20 (European Commission, June 2004); Belén Jiménez-alonso, "Eugenics, Sexual Pedagogy and Social Change: Constructing the Responsible Subject of Governmentality in the Spanish Second Republic," *Studies in History and Philosophy of Biological and Biomedical Sciences* 39, no. 2 (2008): 247–254.

24. Nisot, *La question eugénique*, vol. 2, 92.

25. Maria Sophia Quine, *Italy's Social Revolution: Charity and Welfare from Liberalism to Fascism* (Basingstoke: Palgrave, 2002), part 2.

26. Società Italiana Di Genetica E Di Eugenica, *Atti del Primo Congresso Italiano di Eugenetica Sociale promosso dalla Società Italiana di genetica e di Eugenica e dalla Reale Società Italiana D'Igiene, Milano 20–23 Settembre, 1924* (Rome: Società Italiana di Genetica e di Eugenica, 1927); see A. Gemelli's explanation of the social and moral mission of Italian eugenics in his address to the conference, "Religione e eugenetica," 53–66.

27. Società Italiana Di Genetica E Di Eugenica, *Atti del II Congresso Italiano di Genetica ed Eugenica, proposto dalla Società Italiana di Genetica ed Eugenica, Roma, 30 Settembre-2 Ottobre, 1929* (Rome: Società Italiana di Genetica e di Eugenica, 1932); see the list of attendees, including many members of the government, 5–7.

28. Corrado Gini, "Parole inaugurali del Prof. Corrado Gini letta alla riunione delle Società di Eugenica dell'America Latina tenutasi a Messico il 12 ottobre 1935," *Genus* 2, nos. 1–2 (June 1936): 77–81. The affinity that Gini and other Italian eugenicists (and fascists) felt for their Romanian "brothers" had to do with the myths of origin and ancestry that formed the basis of Romanian nationalism, racism, and fascism. Radu Ioanid, *The Sword of the Archangel: Fascist Ideology in Romania* (New York: Columbia University Press, 1990).

29. Gini, "Parole inaugurali," 80.

30. On the 1937 meeting, see "Comunicazioni," *Genus* 4, nos. 3–4 (1940): 204.

31. Gini achieved truly global acclaim in the 1930s.

32. Just one example of this is Marcello Boldrini's *La fertilità dei biotipi: Saggio di demografia costituzionalistica* (Milan: Vita e pensiero, 1931).

33. Maria S. Quine, *Population Policies in Twentieth-Century Europe: Fascist Dictatorships and Liberal Democracies* (London and New York: Routledge, 1996).

34. See issue 60 of *New Formations: A Journal of Culture/Theory/Politics*, which is devoted to "Eugenics Old and New."

35. See *Genus* 22, nos. 1–4 (1966), a commemorative issue devoted to Gini, to mark the anniversary of his death in 1965.

36. Alberto Sbacchi, *Legacy of Bitterness: Ethiopia and Fascist Italy, 1935–1941* (Lawrenceville, NJ: The Red Sea Press, 1997).

37. Copy of the 1937 report: G. H. L. F. Pitt-Rivers, *Interim Report on Scientific Organization*, in file D. 110, Wellcome Library, London.

38. Gilberto Corbellini, "Scientists, Bioethics, and Democracy: The Italian Case and Its Meaning," *Journal of Medical Ethics* 33 (2007): 349–352.

39. G. Di Mola, P. Borsellino, C. Brunelli, M. Gallucci, A. Gamba, M. Lusignani, C. Regazzo, A. Santosuosso, M. Tamburini, and F. Toscani, "Attitudes Toward Euthanasia of Physician Members of the Italian Society for Palliative Care," *Annals of Oncology* 7, no. 9 (1996): 907–911.

FURTHER READING

Burgio, Alberto, ed. *Nel nome della razza: Il razzismo nella storia d'Italia, 1870–1945* (Bologna: Il Mulino, 1999).

Burgio, Alberto, ed. *Radici e frontiere: Ricerche su razzismo e nazionalismi* (Milan: Associazione Merx centouno, 1993).

Cassata, Francesco. *La Difesa della Razza: Politica, ideologia, e immagine del razzismo fascista* (Turin: Einaudi, 2008).

Cassata, Francesco. *Il fascismo razionale: Corrado Gini fra scienza e politica* (Rome: Carocci, 2006).

Cassata, Francesco. *Molti, sani, e forti: L'eugenetica in Italia* (Turin: Bollati Boringhieri:, 2006).

Ciceri, Massimo. *Origini controllate: L'eugenica in Italia, 1900–1924* (Tesi di Laurea, Università di Milano, 1992/1993). Accessible via www.tesionline.it

Gillette, Aaron. *Eugenics and the Nature-Nurture Debate in the Twentieth Century* (Basingstoke: Palgrave, 2007).

Guarnieri, Patrizia. *Individualità difformi: La psichiatria antropologia di Enrico Morselli* (Milan: Franco Angeli, 1986).

Mantovani, Claudia. *Rigenerare la società: L'eugenetica in Italia dale origini ottocentesche agli anni trenta* (Rubbettino: Soveria Mannelli, 2004).

Pogliano, Claudio. *Bachi, poli, e grani: Appunti sulla ricezione della genetica in Italia, 1900–1953* (Florence: Leo S. Olschi, 1999).

Pogliano, Claudio. *L'ossessione della razza: antropologia e genetica nel XX secolo* (Pisa: Scuola Normale Superiore, 2005).

Quine, Maria Sophia. *Science sans frontières: Darwinism and Social Darwinism in Italy and Elsewhere in the Nineteenth and Twentieth Centuries* (London: Pickering and Chatto, forthcoming).

CHAPTER 23

....

EUGENICS IN EASTERN EUROPE, 1870s–1945

....

MARIA BUCUR

In the late nineteenth century eugenics became a powerful tool used both for imperial control and for nationalist anti-imperial challenges from the Baltic to the Balkans. Starting around that time public health began to develop as an important arena for constructing modern states that emulated "proper" European institutions and intellectual discourses. Doctors, biologists, and even some philosophers, lawyers, and politicians became fascinated with eugenics as the most appealing and "progressive" synthesis to preserve the past while controlling the future in the wider European context. After World War I, eugenicist discourses were reshaped to effect an internal colonization which rendered, for instance, illiterate peasants into active agents of ethnic purification and fulfillment of "biological capital."[1] While some of this activity corresponds to similar developments elsewhere (in South Asia, for instance), the contradictory but simultaneous scientific and political claims to a European cultural allegiance and race hierarchy render the eastern European imperial lands a fascinating case study in the intertwined history of colonialism and eugenics.

In the early nineteenth century the southeastern European borderlands became areas of intense contestation between the Habsburgs and the Ottomans. There has been little attempt to integrate this period of colonial rule inside Europe within the larger literature on colonialism.[2] Recent work on Bosnia-Herzegovina shows that after 1878 this new province became the object of a "civilizing mission" engineered by Viennese colonial administrators bent on modernizing an overwhelmingly premodern society through, among other policies, programs of public health and "social hygiene."[3] This preliminary research suggests the need to further examine the discourses and specific programs that Austria-Hungary sought to implement in

Bosnia, to better understand the sources and effects of bio-political ideas spun in Vienna in the late nineteenth century.

Nationalism as a concept has been at the heart of much of this scholarship, at first implicitly and more recently explicitly, including comparisons with anti-colonial movements elsewhere.[4] But questions regarding the role of race theories and eugenics in particular have only recently become a subject of scholarly engagement. Marius Turda is one of the first historians to identify race theories developed in the nineteenth century as influential in the shaping of public health in Hungary and Romania, and to make a claim for the centrality of this racial discourse in the later development of nationalist discourses.[5] A few historians of Poland, Romania, Austria-Hungary, and Bulgaria are beginning to integrate new research on early eugenics into the rich literature on the nationalist movements in eastern Europe before World War I.[6]

What is particular about the intra-European colonial legacies is the allegiance of anti-imperial nationalist movements (including eugenicists) to European civilization. Nationalists from Poland to Greece conceptualized their people's authentic core, traditions, and claim to sovereignty and legitimacy among the nationalist elites not as a counterweight to the European imperial presence, but as either a precursor to, or as actively constructing, European civilization.[7] The post-imperial discourses in Europe sought integration and acceptance in a larger European home rather than distance and separation from the "civilizing" goals of European colonialism. Eugenics was one of the intellectual discourses through which practitioners in aspiring new professional and intellectual disciplines sought to situate themselves alongside their western European peers, as partners in creating a better European society, a goal they understood as biological.

IMPERIAL AMBITIONS AND ANTI-IMPERIAL CONTESTATIONS: EUGENICS IN EASTERN EUROPE BEFORE 1918

The literature on science in the late nineteenth century clearly places biologists and doctors in Britain, Germany, and France at the forefront of the development of eugenic discourses. In the Habsburg lands and the Balkans, too, eugenics became significant in the 1880s, at the same time that doctors, scientists, and social reformers in western Europe began to embrace Francis Galton's ideas.[8] Vienna became a training ground for many eastern European doctors, some of whom later promoted eugenics in the imperial borderlands. The Balkan (post)-imperial lands figure only marginally in the historiography of science in modern Europe, however. Doctors and scientists here generally had limited institutional support, yet given their training at medical centers in Vienna, Paris, and Berlin, eugenicist discourses were significant among the emerging medical and science elites in Bulgaria, Romania, and elsewhere.[9]

This is not to overstate the centrality of eugenicist discourses in countries barely embarking on the institutionalization of public health. Historians of eastern European eugenics differ on how forceful this movement was, partly because they approach the phenomenon from different entry points—specialized publications, policy-making, policy implementation, versus their echoes in state politics.[10] Historians of science and medicine have generally been even less observant about the impact of eugenics in this region.[11] Yet the fact that medical institutions were quite underdeveloped at a time when doctors and scientists interested in eugenics were returning from western Europe played in these young enthusiasts' favor. Albeit toned down by respect for tradition, eugenics framed modernization persuasively, defining collective identity above individual rights in ways that resonated with the collectivist discourses in their countries.[12]

Recent research on Austro-Hungarian public health policies in the new colony of Bosnia-Herzegovina (1878–1918) shows that advocates of eugenics in Vienna hoped to mobilize and control newly acquired populations through bio-politics. A discourse that blended a biologically determinist view of cultural specificities (especially regarding the Islamic populations in Bosnia) with a desire to make the population healthier catalyzed programs to train doctors in pre- and post-natal care, as well as to develop public health programs from inoculation against epidemics to personal hygiene.[13] It should be stressed that the goal was not the individual well-being of Bosnians, but rather the ability of this population to serve the Austro–Hungarian interests in the area.

Eugenics served as a rationale for separating communities according to their national (read biological) identity and to redistribute resources along ethnocentric lines as part of an imperial discourse. This was the case not only with the more marginalized Magyars and Poles, but also with the German populations. Germanic race-based eugenicist discourses served implicitly as a tool for contesting the imperial cohesion of Austria-Hungary, especially by those who looked toward the *Volksdeutsche* across the border in Germany as their community, rather than to the assimilated Jewry in Vienna.[14] In Vienna, for instance, a number of anthropologists who supported the concept of biological/racial hierarchies conducted anthropometric measurements in the army as a way to separate more clearly (presumably more scientifically) the various ethnic groups serving together in the multi-ethnic military.[15]

In the Habsburg Empire, articulating theories of biological determinism along racial and ethnic lines seemed like a "silver bullet" for sorting out the great linguistic, religious, and overall cultural diversity of the populations that lived in such borderland regions as Transylvania and Vojvodina. Such distinctions had not mattered 50 years earlier, when dreams of independence from or federal autonomy inside the empire had not yet budded. But by the 1880s, Austrians, Italians, Slovenes, Croats, Serbs, Hungarians, Slovaks, Poles, Czechs, Ruthenes, and Romanians had embarked upon contests for legitimate control over resources and territory at the expense of the old idea of loyalty to the dynasty. Historical precedents, linguistic/cultural identity, and legal precedents were the lines of argument employed by most nationalists. But all these arguments proved contestable and led to unsolvable antagonisms among various ethnic groups and vis-à-vis the imperial center. Eugenics promised a way out. By 1914, it played a growing role among doctors and biologists, not just as a ticket for greater professional empowerment, but also as a means to shape nationalist debates. The same theories came to be used for two opposing ends: the imperial dreams of modernizing and controlling a variety of populations, and the desires of the emerging nationalist elites to shape the future by means of biological segregation.

EUGENICS AND INTERNAL COLONIZATION AFTER WORLD WAR I

After the war, when Bulgarians, Hungarians, Poles, Czechs, Serbs, and Romanians acquired independence, they initially welcomed self-determination. Few thought much about the importance of the League of Nations and Minorities Treaties in overseeing their internal affairs. Yet challenges from minorities soon appeared, and these states spent a great deal of effort responding to or trying to cover up violations of the treaties. In this environment of unquestioning acceptance of ethno-nationalism and ethnic tension over the outcomes of the war, eugenics offered an important tool for political legitimation and for embracing modernization in what appeared to be a rational, scientific view of the world.[16]

The array of institutional developments connected to eugenics in this region varied, of course, in each country and among the case studies presented here. The Austro-Hungarian legacies were the oldest in the region. Eugenically inflected courses in biology, medicine, and anthropology had been taught at the University of Vienna since the late nineteenth century, although no formal eugenics society existed prior to World War I. The Viennese Society for Racial Hygiene was founded in 1924 by Otto Reche (1879–1966), director of the Department of Anthropology at the University of Vienna. Other supporters of eugenics included the world-famous psychiatrist Julius Wagner-Jauregg (1857–1940).

In contrast, historians focusing on Poland and Hungary have identified structures embracing eugenicist ideas starting at the turn of the twentieth century. In Poland, the Society for Combating Sexually Transmitted Diseases (1903) began to advocate a biologically–determinist vision of venereal disease and prostitution. The society gradually evolved into the Polish Eugenics Society (1922) under the leadership of Leon Wernic (1870–1952), a physician trained in Warsaw. In Hungary, debates about eugenics and the social utility of this science began around the same time, but a formalized Eugenics Society was created only in 1914; it later grew into the Hungarian Society for Racial Hygiene and Population Policy (1917), under the leadership of József Madzsar (1876–1940), Lajos Dienes (1885–1974), and István Apáthy (1863–1922).

In Romania, there were several important centers for research, teaching, and experimental policy-making: the Institute for Hygiene, affiliated with the Medical School in Cluj, led by Iuliu Moldovan (1882–1966), who trained a new generation of increasingly radically-racist anthropologists, among them Iordachi Făcăoaru and Petre Râmneanțu (1902–1981); the Institute of Anthropology, affiliated with the Medical School in Bucharest, with Francisc Rainer as its leader; and the Institute for Demography, funded by the Ministry of Health, led by Sabin Manuilă (1894–1964). All these state-funded centers coordinated the publishing of research, the popularization of eugenics through textbooks, curricular integration of eugenics in various disciplines (biology, hygiene, anthropology), and the training of public health specialists in the spirit of eugenicist ideas. The extent of the support Romanian eugenics received from the state seems unique in the region.

The Bulgarian Society for Racial Hygiene (1928) capitalized on the interest in eugenics among doctors and anthropologists. Stefan Konsulov (1885–1954) was a prominent figure in this circle, though many others also published treatises on eugenics and sought to connect theoretical scientific debates with policy-making, especially in the realm of eradicating malaria. In Greece, doctors, anthropologists, and lawyers became interested in eugenics around the same time. Stavros Zurukzoglu (1896–1966), a physician, was the first to introduce eugenicist ideas (1925) into the Greek Anthropological Association, whose leader, Ioannis Koumaris (1879–1970), became an ardent supporter of eugenics. Similar discussions around race and biology, and about the need to establish clear scientific hierarchies among ethnically diverse and mixed populations preoccupied physicians and anthropologists in Yugoslavia, where, in 1920, racial biologist Svetislav Stefanović (1874–1944), the president of the Association of Yugoslav Physicians, published *Eugenics: The Hygiene of Human Conception and the Problem of Heredity,* under the official auspices of the Ministry for National Health. But much like in Greece, interest in eugenics did not translate into specific institutional developments and publications dedicated exclusively to eugenics, as had been the case in Romania, for instance.

In most of these cases, where birth control policies with a eugenicist character were passed, the main proponents of eugenics were not the architects of such legislation. Romania was an exception, as Moldovan was the main author of a eugenically inspired comprehensive public health law in 1932. Even there, however, the shape of the legislation and its ultimate implementation were controlled by politicians and bureaucrats with varied understandings of eugenic ideas, sometimes in conflict with the aims of the eugenicist institutions and professional enthusiasts. Alongside these institutional developments, there were characteristic intellectual, social, and political trends in many of these countries.

A New Technocratic Elite

As the medical profession flourished in post-imperial eastern Europe, doctors of the new ethnic majorities saw opportunities open up—professionally, economically, and socially. They were engaged in building new state institutions for medical education and practice, and specific public policies that implied greater need for doctors and greater resources allocated to medical practice. Though welfare measures of the kind contemplated in western Europe were absent in eastern Europe in the 1920s, access to medical services and public health were discussed as measurements of modernization and progress. Historians such as Mária Kovács have emphasized the importance of doctors in the development of the larger field of professional technocrats in postwar eastern Europe.[17]

Doctors in these countries helped construct eugenicist discourses. The experience of the war and the active role many doctors played dealing with the catastrophic effects of epidemics such as typhoid fever, as well as chronic conditions such as sexually transmitted diseases, rendered these health care providers active proponents of the need for the state to manage, if not directly control, the spread of disease as a means to prevent future catastrophes and to augment the biological capital of their own ethnic group.[18]

These developments coincided with an international trend in medicine and social discourse that favored eugenicist views. Such views conveniently (for the doctors) and persuasively (for ethno-nationalist politicians) connected with the interests and practical challenges in the new eastern European states. Thus, it comes as little surprise that many doctors plucked eugenicist ideas out of their medical school education and transferred them to the particularities of their own territories.

As many historians have underscored, eugenicist convictions met with professional opportunism to create a solid alliance, but not one necessarily oriented toward a right-wing ideological position.[19] Turda focuses on the increasingly nationalist racist elements that characterized Romanian eugenics after World War I, which he considers brought about an alliance between eugenicists and radical right-wing parties in Romania.[20] I see both evidence of right-wing radicalism and distance from it: some doctors were politically neutral, or aligned expediently with whichever party lent them greater public authority. In Poland, for instance, there was a wide range of affiliation among eugenicists with existing political parties.[21] This variety of political leanings suggests that, for some eugenicists, political identification was opportunistic, a platform for advancing their technocratic dreams of controlled progress and medical care.[22] For others, eugenics and political party affiliations offered a means for advancing their personal agendas of acquiring social and economic power. And for some, eugenics was part and parcel of a deeper self–identification with a racist-nationalist political ideology.

In their attempt to capture state resources for their own public health agenda, these doctors embraced a form of internal colonization among the populations they treated. At the broadest level, eugenicists connected those least linked to the state—peasants in especially remote areas—to state control through public health policies; and in more localized forms, doctors aimed at, and partly succeeded in, defining populations along ethnic/racial lines in their individual locales, while linking them to a spectrum of "blood" and anthropometric hierarchies. These biologically deterministic hierarchies were tied to ethnic-nationalist notions of state responsibility for the well-being of citizens, and connectedly, the duties of citizens toward the state. Ultimately, eugenicists wanted to reshape the behavior of these populations toward biological separation and to encourage greater rates of reproduction among the "healthy" populations, invariably defined as the ethnic group to which these doctors belonged.

Yet eugenicists also offered a positive vision of progress through public health policies: they sought to acquire greater funding for public health programs as a means to improving the well-being of people across the country.[23] They argued that the new states could achieve their full potential only when their populations were well-educated, healthy, and fully mobilized in the service of the country. The crucial element of their claims was that specific rural populations in remote areas retained essential components of their ethnic group's vitality, which needed to be both found and cultivated, much like turning a precious natural resource into an important source of revenue. Eugenics offered the ideological framework for articulating this desire to mobilize these resources as an organic, naturally desirable process. Hidden in this positive picture of coaxing the "biological capital" was the implicit hierarchization of how public health policies were to be implemented locally, giving priority to the members of the ethnic majority, while ignoring (if not outright excluding) others.[24]

Modernization

Eugenicists in eastern Europe were self-avowed advocates of controlled modernization. Doctors and practitioners of newly recognized professions (for example, lawyers, architects, engineers) were deeply invested in discourses that advocated progress, as was the case elsewhere. Eugenicists often spoke about the encroachment of "social illnesses," from tuberculosis to venereal diseases, in the context of their mostly unmodernized countryside, which they nonetheless described as the fount of strength, the *élan vital* of their nation. Contrasting non-cosmopolitan, provincial sites as places where strength and purity should be preserved against the encroachment of metropolitan vice was common in the anti-colonial movements.

In eastern Europe, this discourse made sense for similar reasons: the countryside was where the majority of the new ethnic majorities were often located, and where there was little ethnic or religious intermarriage;[25] and it was also in the countryside where the lack of public health services and education was most acute and, by many observers' accounts (be they ethnic exclusivists or not), most urgently needed. Thus, for the purposes of making a persuasive argument with the political and social elites, constructing a discourse that focused on preserving and strengthening the potentialities of the underprivileged, poor, uneducated peasants seemed like a noble and necessary dream, and at the same time a politically and socially innocuous one. It fit existing views of the peasantry and of the role educated elites needed to play in the countryside. Two stumbling blocks stood in the way of success, however. First, the peasants, much like those colonized by the British, were human beings with strong cultural roots in religious belief, and not particularly trusting of the science-based view of the world that eugenicists preached. Second, the doctors themselves were more willing to write about the need to do the hard work of education and enlightenment in the countryside than actually to undertake the work themselves.

RACE AND RACISM

In the interwar period, ideas of racial-biological hierarchy became popular all over post-imperial eastern Europe, taking on different meanings in varying locations and resulting in different kinds of policies around controlling or protecting the purported racial hierarchies. Historians of eastern European eugenics seldom agree about the degree of racism in these movements, especially about their relationship with racist politics. Some are quicker to identify the use of race-based theories in these countries as a sign of growing exclusionary social policies and an important force in shaping racist policies, especially in the late 1930s and during World War II.[26] Others view these race-based theories as one of several elements that framed the scientific discourse, especially the policy ideas of the eugenicists.[27]

Following research and measurements developed in western Europe and the United States, many eastern European doctors and biologists attempted to situate their own populations within a continuum of racial/ethnic identities. These researchers also sought to isolate the qualities of ethnic minorities. In some cases, there were efforts to segregate, for instance, Serbs from Croats.[28] There were also efforts to assimilate, for instance, Szeklers into Romanians.[29] As several historians have shown, blood agglutination and anthropometric measurements as uncontestable proof of specific racial/ethnic identities were in vogue in the 1920s and 1930s. These measurements were employed differently, depending on the particular policy intention. For instance, assimilation of the Hungarian-speaking Szeklers seemed more advantageous to Romanian researchers trying to claim Transylvania as part of Romania rather than as part of Hungary.[30] If Szeklers could be proven to be serologically closer to Romanians, one could presumably argue that they, and the territory they inhabited, should remain under the control of the Romanian state, rather than be claimed by revisionist Hungary. Such arguments clashed with the research done in Hungary, which sought to prove that the majority of the population in Transylvania was in fact "biologically" Hungarian.[31]

While the ethnic diversity of eastern European countries made it complicated to construct a unitary, persuasive, and scientifically acceptable theory of racial/ethnic hierarchy by the standards of the time, most of these countries shared one racist assumption recast by eugenicists in biological terms: anti-Semitism.[32] But even this did not have the same force in all eastern European eugenics movements. In Romania, for instance, some eugenicists placed much greater emphasis on where Hungarians were racially situated vis-à-vis the Romanians than on where Jews were to be placed in racial hierarchy. And for ethnic groups that had become minorities overnight in newly formed states, eugenics offered a way of constructing either new strategies for autonomy, or an ideological platform for revisionism. In Romania, for instance, German populations in Transylvania articulated a strong eugenicist discourse that blended cultural and biological attributes to claim the need for this community to remain united and pure (biologically), as an island of Germanness in the Romanian state. The long standing historical precedent of the German (Saxon) communities in this area as autonomous colonists at the border of Christendom since the Middle Ages served as an important argument for their purported biological purity, and also for why the Saxons needed to maintain this unique identity. Theirs, Saxon eugenicists claimed, was a unique and culturally important mission, one that needed to be secured and preserved through self-imposed biological isolation and other public health self-help policies. While this group never made political claims against the Romanian state, they advocated a virtual apartheid.[33]

These examples suggest that while racist ideas espoused by colonial powers in Africa and Asia convinced their own elites of the factual basis of their hierarchies, such ideological victories could not be claimed in eastern Europe. Whether they acknowledged each other across state and ethnic lines or not, eastern European eugenicists were often in conflict with one another regarding the claims of biological purity and superiority on behalf of different ethnic groups.

ILLIBERALISM

One common trait of most eastern European eugenics was their disregard for liberal pluralist parliamentary politics.[34] Parliamentary pluralism had developed in the imperial eastern European lands in a few places (the Austro-Hungarian Empire in particular), but had been rather narrow in its definition of citizenship and the electorate.[35] Thus, even in places such as Czechoslovakia and Poland, where some political parties or factions had existed for half a century, the explosion of political formations and the emergence of universal suffrage after 1918 proved chaotic and resulted in largely unstable political processes. Overall, the newly emerged, more democratic electoral policies of the 1920s brought about fluidity and even instability rather than the solidification of stable institutions and policies. Therefore, it was unsurprising that parliamentary pluralism and democratic electoral policies came under fire with the Great Depression, as historians of eugenics during this period agree.[36] These illiberal voices merged with eugenicist visions of organicist national unity, building on ideas of health, strength, and vitality.[37]

There are two exceptions in this regard. In Poland, scholarship thus far has emphasized the "progressive" angle of the movement and political leanings that embraced change through political negotiation in a parliamentary setting.[38] And in Greece, where interest in eugenics developed much more after World War II than in the rest of eastern Europe, the movement operated largely within the confines of a parliamentary democracy, with doctors and other supporters there focusing on legislative change within this political setting.[39]

LEGISLATION AND IMPLEMENTATION

The most important weakness of the eugenicist movements in eastern Europe was their inability to mobilize and control human energies. For states facing a dizzying array of problems—political, administrative/institutional, economic, and military— the eugenic agenda, especially expressed as an overarching imperative for completely restructuring the state, rather than implementing piecemeal reforms, met with resistance on the part of politicians. Even where there was sympathy for these ideas across the political spectrum, heavy war debt payments in the 1920s and crippling economic crises in the 1930s dictated severe choices that impaired the eugenicist agenda.[40]

Given these problems, governments could turn to a variety of expenditures to see quick returns for their goal of establishing the primacy of the majority ethnic group. The military was foremost on that agenda, followed by education. Eugenicist ideas were partially integrated through courses, textbooks, and student selection, but most politicians directed their educational reforms to focus on linguistic or cultural, rather than biological, unification. Public health lagged behind in political and especially fiscal state support.

It was only during World War II, when Nazi-allied Hungary and Romania participated in the anti-Soviet offensive, that some of these dreams of eugenicist colonization were more directly integrated in state policy and expenditures. The Hungarian government used notions of racial hierarchy in their control of northern Transylvania, and the Romanian government that ruled Transnistria during the war underwrote studies that attempted to uncover the "true" Romanian biological essence of the inhabitants of that region, whether they spoke Romanian, Russian, or Ukrainian. The same administrations also adopted the anti-Semitic views of Nazi Germany and of their own leadership to lead or collaborate in the implementation of the Final Solution. In the wild new racist ideology of *Lebensraum*, "purifying" by means of genocide and incorporating into one's own ethnic group by means of biological measurements were part of the same colonizing quest, abruptly terminated by the end of the war at the hands of the Soviet Armies.

After the war, denazification processes and political realignment along the ideologies and strategic interests of the Soviet Union in Europe meant that most of the supporters of eugenics were either purged from their official positions, regardless of their actual actions on behalf of fascist governments and ideas, or had to make a *volte-face* in their public statements in order to continue to work in a professional capacity.[41] Thus, eugenics as a movement was brought to a halt in all but one country, Greece, where interest in eugenics in fact emerged more strongly in the postwar period.[42]

CONCLUSIONS

The eastern European case offers both similarities and important differences from extra-European colonial/imperial lands, as well as from eugenics in western Europe. The eastern Europeans' self-identification with and aspiration toward inclusion in European civilization is the most important departure vis-à-vis non-European colonized people. The ways in which eugenicist ideas were deployed in the Habsburg and post-Habsburg lands both at the imperial center (Vienna) and on the periphery (for example, in Transylvania) in order to stimulate biologically controlled progress, often using the same ideas and employing the same racial hierarchies, most clearly illustrate this important particularity.

In the realm of eugenics, this region is unique in Europe in terms of the difficulty eugenicists faced in articulating non-self-contradictory theories of racial hierarchy and arguments about the need to modernize, segregate, and mobilize people. If it was easy for British colonizers to claim racial superiority to non-European populations on the basis of race hierarchy, similar racial claims could not be sustained in eastern Europe without a great deal of convoluted explanation about hidden hereditary facts, such as blood agglutination. Some racial hierarchies were easier to "sell" than others, on the basis of already well-established racist clichés, especially regarding Jews. Ultimately, this case stands as an example of both the attempt to criticize the hegemony of western European colonial-eugenicist hierarchies and also the desire to emulate similar developments in these post-imperial states while affirming European racial hierarchies.

NOTES

1. This term was used most prominently in Romania by Iuliu Moldovan and his followers. See Maria Bucur, *Eugenics and Modernization in Interwar Romania* (Pittsburgh, PA: University of Pittsburgh Press, 2002).

2. One important departure is Patrick Zylberman, "Civilizing the State: Borders, Weak States and International Health in Modern Europe," in *Medicine at the Border: Disease, Globalization and Security, 1850 to the Present,* ed. Alison Bashford (Basingstoke: Palgrave, 2006), 21–40.

3. Brigitte Fuchs, "Gender, Religion, and Hygiene in Bosnia–Herzegovina 1878–1914," in *Health, Hygiene and Eugenics in Southeast Europe to 1945,* eds. Marius Turda, Christian Pomnizer, and Sevasti Trubeda (Budapest: Central European University Press, 2010, forthcoming).

4. For an example of the older primordialist scholarship, see Peter F. Sugar and Ivo J. Lederer, eds., *Nationalism in Eastern Europe* (Seattle, WA: University of Washington Press, 1969). For new scholarship reframing the significance and usefulness of nationalism from a constructivist perspective, see Jeremy King, "The Nationalization of East Central Europe: Ethnicism, Ethnicity, and Beyond," in *Staging the Past: The Politics of Commemoration in Habsburg Central Europe, 1848 to the Present,* eds. Maria Bucur and Nancy Wingfield (West Lafayette, IN: Purdue University Press, 2001), 112–152. On nationalism and colonialism in eastern Europe, see Katherine J. Fleming, *The Muslim Bonaparte: Diplomacy and Orientalism in Ali Pasha's Greece* (Princeton, NJ: Princeton University Press, 1999); Maria Todorova, *Imagining the Balkans* (Oxford and New York: Oxford University Press, 1997); and Larry Wolff, *Venice and the Slavs: The Discovery of Dalmatia in the Age of Enlightenment* (Stanford, CA: Stanford University Press, 2001).

5. See Marius Turda, "Heredity and Eugenic Thought in Early Twentieth-Century Hungary," *Orvostörténeti közlemények. Communicationes de Historia Artis Medicinae* 51, no. 1–2 (2007): 101–118; Marius Turda, "The Nation as Object: Race, Blood, and Biopolitics in Interwar Romania," *Slavic Review* 66, no. 3 (Fall 2007): 413–441.

6. See the individual contributions to Marius Turda and Paul J. Weindling, eds., *"Blood and Homeland": Eugenics and Racial Nationalism in Central and Southeast Europe, 1900–1940* (Budapest: Central European University Press, 2006) and Turda et al., *Health, Hygiene, and Eugenics.* The contributors to the latter volume and a few additional scholars presented papers on the themes of the book at a conference held in Berlin in May 2007, entitled "Hygiene—Health Politics—Eugenics: Engineering Society in 20th-Century Southeastern Europe." A related conference entitled "Medicine in the Balkans: Evolution of Ideas and Practice to 1945" was held in London in January 2008.

7. These kinds of claims vis-à-vis the political past and cultural belonging coexist in all the countries cited here, and indeed in all the countries of the area. The comparative weight of these lines of argumentation depends, however, on politics, cultural preferences, and regional contests, as they developed over time from the nineteenth century. For an excellent critical look at the Balkan region in terms of such contests, see, for example, Katherine E. Fleming, "Orientalism, the Balkans, and Balkan Historiography," *American Historical Review* 105, no. 4 (2000): 1218–1233.

8. Turda, "Heredity and Eugenic Thought"; Bucur, *Eugenics and Modernization*; Turda and Weindling, *"Blood and Homeland"*; Turda et al., *Health, Hygiene and Eugenics.*

9. Bucur, *Eugenics and Modernization*; Gergana Mircheva, "Marital Health and Eugenics in Bulgaria, 1878–1940," in Turda et al., *Health, Hygiene and Eugenics*, forthcoming.

10. These differences were reflected best in the lively discussions that took place during the "Hygiene—Health Politics—Eugenics" conference in Berlin, May 2007, and is reflected in both the upcoming volume, Turda et al., *Health, Hygiene and Eugenics*, as well as Turda and Weindling, *"Blood and Homeland."*

11. In my own research on Romania, I found virtually no references to eugenics in the specialized literature focusing on the history of medicine in that country. See Bucur, *Eugenics and Modernization.*

12. Bucur, *Eugenics and Modernization*; Turda, "The Nation as Object"; Turda, "Heredity and Eugenic Thought"; Rory Yeomans, "Of 'Yugoslav Barbarians' and Croatian Gentlemen Scholars: Nationalist Ideology and Racial Anthropology in Interwar Yugoslavia," in Turda and Weindling, *"Blood and Homeland,"* 83–123.

13. Fuchs, "Gender, Religion."

14. See Margit Berner, "From 'Prisoner of War Studies' to Proof of Paternity: Racial Anthropologists and the Measuring of 'Others' in Austria," in Turda and Weindling, *"Blood and Homeland,"* 41–54.

15. Margit Berner, "The Distribution of 'Race' and Types: National Surveys of the Viennese Anthropology Society, c. 1870–WWI," paper presented at the *Council for European Studies Sixteenth International Conference*, Chicago, March 2008.

16. Presented here are what I see as common attributes of the eugenics movements in eastern Europe in the interwar period. Yet there was diversity and even conflict: the same ideas were used for opposite claims, especially between ethnic majorities and ethnic minorities. Therefore, while these attributes describe the shape of eugenics in eastern Europe, they do not accurately define every eugenic movement, or even "eastern European" eugenics.

17. Maria M. Kovacs, *Liberal Professions and Illiberal Politics: Hungary from the Habsburgs to the Holocaust* (Washington, DC: Woodrow Wilson Center Press; Oxford: Oxford University Press, 1994); Bucur, *Eugenics and Modernization.*

18. Turda and Weindling, *"Blood and Homeland"*; Bucur, *Eugenics and Modernization*; Turda, "The Nation as Object"; Christian Pomnizer, "Muslims, Typhus and the Nation: Medicalisation of Ethnic Distance in Bulgaria," in Turda et al., *Health, Hygiene and Eugenics.*

19. Pauline M. H. Mazumdar, *Eugenics, Human Genetics and Human Failings: The Eugenics Society, Its Sources and Its Critics in Britain* (London and New York: Routledge, 1992).

20. Turda, "The Nation as Object."

21. Magdalena Gawin, "Eugenics and Progressivism in Poland, 1905–1939," in Turda and Weindling, *"Blood and Homeland,"* 167–183.

22. Bucur, *Eugenics and Modernization.*

23. See especially Turda et al., *Health, Hygiene and Eugenics*; and Bucur, *Eugenics and Modernization.*

24. Here there is great variety within each country and among countries in the area. Given their dizzying array of ethnic groups, and where each eugenicist movement situated various distinct ethnic/racial groups within their larger race hierarchies, they might seek alliances with some (for example, the Romanians with the Germans in Romania), seek to exclude others (for example, the Jews in Hungary), or ignore some groups (for example, the Serbians with the Muslim Bosnians).

25. This was the case in Poland, Hungary, Yugoslavia, and Romania, but much less so in Bulgaria, or less of a concern in the more urbanized Czechoslovakia.

26. Turda, "The Nation as Object;" Rory Yeomans, "Colonizing the National Body: Demography, Abortion and the Limits of Science in the Independent State of Croatia," in Turda et al., *Health, Hygiene and Eugenics.*

27. Bucur, *Eugenics and Modernization*; Sevasti Trubeta, "Serving the Nation and Race: Physical Anthropology in Greece (1924–1950)," paper presented at the *Council for European Studies Sixteenth International Conference*, Chicago, March 2008; and Vassiliki Theodorou and Despina Karakatsani, "Eugenics and 'Puericulture' in Interwar Greece: Medical Concerns for Ameliorating the Biological Capital," in Turda et al., *Health, Hygiene and Eugenics*, forthcoming.

28. Yeomans, "Colonizing the National Body."

29. Turda, "The Nation as Object;" Bucur, *Eugenics and Modernization.*

30. Romania had acquired Transylvania from Hungary after the Tiranon Treaty (1920).

31. Marius Turda, "From Craniology to Serology: Racial Anthropology in Interwar Hungary and Romania," *Journal of the History of the Behavioral Sciences* 43, no. 4 (2007): 361–377.

32. Kovacs, *Liberal Professions*; Bucur, *Eugenics and Modernization*; Turda, "The Nation as Object."

33. Tudor Georgescu, "In Pursuit of a Purged Eugenic Fortress: Alfred Csallner and the Transylvanian Saxon Eugenic Discourse in Interwar Romania," in Turda et al., *Health, Hygiene and Eugenics.*

34. Kovacs, *Liberal Professions*; Bucur, *Eugenics and Modernization*; Turda, "The Nation as Object." Magdalena Gawin offers a different view regarding the Polish case, as do historians of eugenics in Greece. See Magda Gawin, *Rasa i nowoczesność. Historia polskiego ruchu eugenicznego* (Warsaw: Neriton, 2003) and Trubeta, "Serving the Nation."

35. Universal male suffrage was introduced only in 1907, and property limitations that framed political rights for most of the nineteenth century eliminated most rural populations.

36. Kovacs, *Liberal Professions*; Bucur, *Eugenics and Modernization*; Turda, "The Nation as Object"; Mircheva, "Marital Health"; Trubeta, "Serving the Nation."

37. The illiberalism of eugenics attracted allies from fascists to peasantists and feminists.

38. Gawin, "Eugenics and Progressivism"; Gawin, *Rasa i nowoczesność.*

39. Trubeta, "Serving the Nation."

40. For an overview of eastern Europe in the interwar period, see Ivan Berend, *Decades of Crisis: Central and Eastern Europe before World War II* (Berkeley, CA: University of California Press, 1998).

41. On legacies in the postwar period in Romania, see Bucur, *Eugenics and Modernization.*

42. Trubeta, "Serving the Nation;" Turda and Weindling, *"Blood and Homeland."*

FURTHER READING

Baader, Gerhard, Veronika Hofer, and Thomas Mayer, eds., *Eugenic in Österreich. Biopolitische Trukturen von 1900–1945* (Vienna: Czernin Verlag, 2007).

Bucur, Maria. *Eugenics and Modernization in Interwar Romania* (Pittsburgh, PA: University of Pittsburgh Press, 2002).

Bucur, Maria. "Awakening or Constructing Biological Consciousness? Astra's Role in the Romanian Eugenic Movement," *Colloquia. Journal of Central European History* 2, no. 1–2 (1995): 172–185.

Bucur, Maria. "In Praise of Wellborn Mothers. On Eugenics and Gender Roles in Interwar Romania," *East European Politics and Societies* 9, no. 1 (1995): 123–142.

Bucur, Maria. "From Private Philanthropy to Public Institutions. The Rockefeller Foundation and Public Health in Interwar Romania." *Romanian Civilization* 4, no. 2 (1995): 47–60.

Daskalova, Krassimira. "Foremothers: Fani Popova-Mutafova," *Gender and History* 14, no. 2 (2002): 321–339.

Dugac, Željko. *Protiv bolesti I nesnania: Rockefeerova fondacija u meduratnoj Jugoslaviji* (Zagreb: Srednja Europa, 2005).

Feinberg, Melissa. *Elusive Equality: Gender, Citizenship and the Limits of Democracy in Czechoslovakia, 1918–1950* (Pittsburgh, PA: University of Pittsburgh Press, 2006).

Gawin, Magdalena. *Rasa I nowodzsność. Historia polskiego ruchu eugenicznego, 1880–1952* (Warsaw: Neriton, Instytut Historii PAN, 2003).

Kovacs, Maria M. *Liberal Professions and Illiberal Politics: Hungary from the Habsburgs to the Holocaust* (Washington, DC: Woodrow Wilson Center Press; Oxford : Oxford University Press, 1994).

Turda, Marius, Christian Pomnizer, and Sevasti Trubeda, eds. *Health, Hygiene and Eugenics in Southeast Europe to 1945* (Budapest: Central European University Press, forthcoming, 2010).

Turda, Marius. "'To End the Degeneration of a Nation': Debates on Eugenic Sterilization in Inter-war Romania," *Medical History* 53, no. 1 (2009): 77–104.

Turda, Marius and Paul J. Weindling, eds. *"Blood and Homeland:" Eugenics and Racial Nationalism in Central and Southeast Europe, 1900–1940* (Budapest: Central European University Press, 2006).

Turda, Marius. "From Craniology to Serology: Racial Anthropology in Interwar Hungary and Romania," *Journal of the History of the Behavioral Sciences* 43, no. 4 (2007): 361–377.

Turda, Marius. *Eugenism şi antropologie rasială în România, 1874–1944* (Bucharest: Editura Cuvântul, 2008).

CHAPTER 24

....

EUGENICS IN RUSSIA
AND THE SOVIET UNION

....

NIKOLAI KREMENTSOV

COMPARED to the ever-growing and variegated literature on the history of eugenics in other countries, the history of eugenics in Russia has attracted relatively little scholarly attention and has never inspired a book-length examination. Nonetheless, thanks to the pioneering works of Mark B. Adams, published nearly 20 years ago, the institutional and intellectual developments of Russian eugenics as a science of human heredity have been outlined, particularly in relation to the growth of genetics during the Soviet period.[1] The similarities and differences of these developments to experiences in other countries have been partially examined, along with the role that Western eugenics and genetics communities (particularly in Germany and the United States) played in shaping Russian eugenics.[2] Yet, the history of Russian eugenics as an ideology—a particular way of thinking about human heredity, diversity, and evolution—remains largely uncharted territory.[3] Similarly, public and professional attitudes to eugenics both as a science and as an ideology await careful investigation. One of the largest holes in our knowledge is the influence that eugenic ideas exerted on actual policy-making in a variety of fields, from social hygiene to family planning and from abortion to immigration policies. Although new archival and printed materials have become available during the last 20 years, a comprehensive history of Russian eugenics remains to be written.[4]

THE BEASTLY PHILOSOPHY:
EUGENICS IN IMPERIAL RUSSIA

Although the first Russian translation of Francis Galton's *Hereditary Genius* appeared in 1874, the subsequent quarter century saw little interest in eugenic ideas, and no other works by the founding father of eugenics were ever published in Russia. The Russian empire lacked the socioeconomic conditions—from urbanization to declining fertility, and from immigration to overpopulation—that fueled such interest elsewhere. The huge, sparsely populated, predominately agrarian, autocratic, poly-confessional, and multi-ethnic empire provided neither sufficient data nor receptive audiences for eugenic concerns. Even though some commentators, for example obstetrician Vasilii Florinskii (1834–1899) of the Medical-Surgical Academy, did speak of "improving humankind" as early as 1866,[5] these ideas did not spark a Russian debate, to say nothing of an organized movement.

Around 1900, the advent of industrialization, along with the rapid growth of medical, scientific, pedagogical, and legal professions, began to change the situation. During the first two decades of the twentieth century, when eugenics began its institutionalization in western Europe and North America, eugenic ideas started to filter into Russia. From 1900 to 1917, various publishers issued Russian translations of works by prominent British, Dutch, French, German, and U.S. proponents of eugenics, including Georg Buschan, Charles Davenport, Emile Duclaux, Alfons Fischer, August Forel, Kurt Goldstein, Max von Gruber, Karl Pearson, Elie Perrier, Théodule Ribot, Charles Richet, and Johannes Rutgers.[6] Russia's professional communities of psychiatrists, jurists, pedagogues, anthropologists, hygienists, and biologists considered the ideas of their Western colleagues, addressing various facets of eugenic research, policies, and ideologies in professional and popular periodicals.[7] Russian would-be-eugenicists were well informed of varied approaches to the issues of "human betterment" developed in other countries and picked selectively from the pool of available ideas, liberally mixing French *puériculture* with German *Rassenhygiene,* Anglo-American *eugenics* with French *anthropologie sociale,* and German *Sozialpathologie* with French *eugénetique.* They invented a special name, *antropotekhnika* (anthropo-technique), modeled after the Russian word for animal breeding, *zootekhnika* (zoo-technique), which served as a synonym for Russian translations/transliterations of such corresponding English, German, and French termsaseugenics (*evgenika*), *Rassenhygiene*(*rassovaiagigiena*), *Fortpflanzungshygiene* (*generativnaia gigiena*), and *eugénetique* (*evgenetika*).[8]

Although Russian proponents of eugenics borrowed extensively, several particular features distinguished their approach. Most commentators criticized the "race" and "class" components of eugenic ideas and policies espoused by US, German, and British eugenicists. Many placed strong emphasis on environment/education/nurture, as did their French colleagues. They largely rejected "negative measures" (be it sterilization or segregation) promoted by U.S., German, and

Scandinavian eugenicists, advocating instead the improvement of social conditions, reeducation, and prophylactic medicine.

Russian responses to the First International Eugenics Congress held in 1912 in London displayed these features prominently. Although Russia sent no official representatives to the congress, at least two Russians attended its sessions. The eminent philosopher and theoretician of anarchism, Prince Petr Kropotkin (1842–1921), took part in the congress discussions, and Isaak Shklovskii (1865–1935), a popular journalist (writing under the pen name Dioneo), covered the congress for Russian magazines. Kropotkin delivered a passionate diatribe against the congress's class bias: "Who were unfit?," he exclaimed rhetorically, "the workers or the idlers? The women of the people, who suckled their children themselves, or the ladies who were unfit for maternity because they could not perform all the duties of a mother? Those who produced degenerates in slums, or those who produced degenerates in palaces?" He vehemently opposed proposals to sterilize the "unfit," insisting that such social measures as the abolition of slums "would improve the germplasm of the next generation more than any amount of sterilization."[9] Shklovskii echoed Kropotkin's criticism. The subtitle of his correspondence from the congress—"Beastly Philosophy"— speaks for itself. While Kropotkin attacked the "class" components of eugenic ideas, Dioneo focused his critique on "race:" "All those, purportedly scientific, data, upon which the doctrine of higher and lower races are based, cannot withstand criticism, for the very simple reason that anthropology knows of no pure races."[10]

Indeed, although certain Russian anthropologists, particularly among proponents of "criminal anthropology," did engage in the propaganda of the superiority of the "Great-Russian race,"[11] the majority rejected the "racialization" of their subjects. Nevertheless, many enthusiastically embraced the eugenic vision of "bettering humankind." It was the anthropologist Ludwik Krzywicki (1859–1941) who wrote entries on eugenics for various Russian encyclopedias and apparently coined the Russian term *antropotekhnika*.[12] Eugenics offered anthropologists an opportunity to become not simply the "observateurs de l'homme," but also to play a prominent social role as experts on human diversity and evolution. Yet, as did other Russian anthropologists, Krzywicki cautioned against too hasty application of "negative" eugenic measures, which, in his opinion, "at the present time turn into the instrument of narrow class interests."[13]

Many Russian jurists and criminologists were skeptical of the ideas of "inborn criminality" and proposals to sterilize prisoners, which were quite popular in Western eugenic circles. In 1912, a St. Petersburg jurist, Pavel Liublinskii (1882–1938), published a highly critical assessment of U.S. eugenic laws.[14] Similarly, many Russian pedagogues and psychologists critically evaluated the ideas of "hereditary feeble-mindedness," arguing that so-called "defective children" could be brought up to be normal members of the society.[15] At the First Russian congress on public education in January 1914, Kharkov University professor Isaak Orshanskii (b. 1851) delivered a report on "heredity and degeneration," which prompted the congress to issue a special "resolution on the struggle against criminality, suicide, defectiveness, and degeneration among children," calling for founding specialized schools for the edu-cation of "defective children."[16]

Many Russian physicians were sympathetic to eugenics. For doctors dealing with chronic diseases, psychiatrists and neurologists in particular, eugenics offered a new research methodology (medical family histories, twin studies, and statistical analysis) and a new interpretative framework, replacing the old vague ideas of "inborn constitution" with new principles of heredity (be they Galtonian, Weismannian, Mendelian, or Lamarckian).[17] During this period, several doctoral dissertations on "heredity and disease" were defended in Russia.[18] Some psychia-trists, notably Tikhon Iudin (1879–1950), took up the ideas of degeneration as an explanatory tool in their studies of the mentally ill.[19] Others focused on "hereditary talents," continuing Galton's research program.[20]

Eugenics garnered a warm reception among Russian hygienists and public health doctors.[21] A programmatic statement opening the first 1910 issue of a new journal, *Hygiene and Sanitary Science,* argued that "generative hygiene (eugenics)" ought to constitute an important part of Russian public health agendas.[22] In the same issue, the journal began publishing a series of articles on eugenics and intro-duced a special section featuring reviews of Western books and journals on the subject.[23] As did their Western colleagues, Russian social hygienists focused particu-larly on questions of alcoholism and heredity.[24]

Eugenics also found a receptive audience in the nascent community of experi-mental biologists, especially geneticists, who exploited eugenic rhetoric in order to legitimize their new field. The community's oracle established in 1912, *Priroda* (Nature), regularly featured articles on both genetics and eugenics.[25] Two founders of Russian genetics, Nikolai Kol'tsov (1872–1940) in Moscow and Iurii Filipchenko (1882–1930) in St. Petersburg, were particularly active in this endeavor, publishing translations and reviews of Western works, lecturing, and building alliances with other scientists and physicians interested in genetics and eugenics.[26]

The communities of physicians, anthropologists, psychiatrists, jurists, peda-gogues, and geneticists thus capitalized on the topics that resonated with their own professional interests and that allowed them to use eugenics ideas, research, and rhetoric to bolster their claims to autonomy and authority vis-à-vis the autocratic Russian state and competing professional groups.

Science and ideology:
Eugenics in Bolshevik Russia

In the years prior to the Bolshevik Revolution of October 1917, eugenics failed to spark an organized movement or find an institutional setting. The situation changed dramatically after the revolution. Despite a bloody civil war, famine, epidemics, and economic deprivation, in the course of a few years eugenics boasted a nationwide society, research institutions, and specialized periodicals. It entered teaching curricula and found a grassroots following in the new Soviet Russia.

Of all the disciplinary groups concerned with eugenics during the pre-revolutionary period, one—geneticists—spearheaded the institutionalization of eugenics in Bolshevik Russia. As elsewhere in the world, the institutionalization of eugenics went hand in hand with the institutionalization of genetics. Two leaders of Russian genetics, Kol'tsov in Moscow and Filipchenko in Petrograd, played a pivotal role. The Bolshevik revolution liquidated the private endowments that had supported Kol'tsov's Institute of Experimental Biology (IEB), established in 1916. This forced Kol'tsov to search for new patrons from among the newly created Bolshevik state agencies.[27] Kol'tsov's association with the People's Commissariat of Public Health (Narkomzdrav) proved particularly rewarding. Commissar Nikolai Semashko (1874–1949), a Bolshevik physician, was an active proponent of social hygiene and the leading force of its institutionalization.[28] Eugenics found its first institutional home at the State Museum of Social Hygiene, created by Narkomzdrav in January 1919.

Among its various activities, the Museum established a "consultative group" on "the biological question," which covered general biology, anthropology, and racial hygiene. Kol'tsov became a leading member and with the "consultative group" created the Russian Eugenics Society (RES) in November 1920.[29] Kol'tsov became the chairman, the psychiatrist Iudin and the anthropologist Viktor Bunak (1891–1979) members, and another anthropologist, Mikhail Volotskoi (1893–1944), the secretary of the governing council. With the establishment of the society, Bunak became the head of the IEB eugenics department, Volotskoi an assistant, and Kol'tsov defined the department's "general scientific direction." Kol'tsov also became the editor in chief of the society's oracle—*Russian Eugenics Journal* (REJ)—launched in early 1922.

From the very beginning, Kol'tsov sought the support of Filipchenko, his brother-in-arms in creating Russian genetics, and invited him to head the IEB eugenics department. However, Filipchenko had already organized Russia's first genetics department at Petrograd University and a genetics laboratory within the university's Institute of Natural Sciences. In early 1921, under the auspices of the Russian Academy of Sciences, Filipchenko established a Bureau of Eugenics to study "questions of heredity specifically in application to humans" and launched his own journal, *Proceedings of the Bureau of Eugenics*.[30] In 1924, he joined Kol'tsov on the REJ editorial board.

Having built the institutional bases, the champions of Russian eugenics began to revive their international contacts, reviewing current Western works on eugenics and arranging for their Russian translation.[31] Russian eugenicists were unable to attend the Second International Eugenics Congress in 1921, but the following year the RES joined the Permanent International Commission on Eugenics, with Kol'tsov representing Russian eugenics on its council and several subsequent conferences.

Soviet eugenics did not simply follow the paths of its Western counterparts. It was profoundly shaped by local traditions and institutional and ideological landscapes. In his presidential address to the RES general meeting in October 1921,

Kol'tsov identified three key components of eugenics.[32] The first—"pure science," which he named "anthropogenetics"—was to gather knowledge of human heredity. The second—"applied science," which, echoing his pre-revolutionary predecessors, Kol'tsov termed "anthropotechnique"—was to employ that knowledge to find appropriate methods of improving the genetic quality of future generations. And the third—"eugenic religion," comparable, in Kol'tsov's opinion, to nationalism, Christianity, Islam, and socialism[33]—was to espouse an "ideal" that would "give meaning to [human] life and motivate people to sacrifices and self-limitations." The REJ's second issue carried an article, "On the tasks and paths of anthropogenetics," written by Kol'tsov's most talented student in genetics, Aleksandr Serebrovskii (1892–1948), which outlined the research methodology and agendas of the new science.[34]

Between 1920 and 1925, founders of Russian eugenics published and lectured to professional and lay audiences, organized exhibits and public discussions, and included eugenics in the syllabi of courses on general biology in secondary schools and universities. This propaganda bore plentiful fruits: by the mid-decade, RES membership had more than tripled to include not only geneticists, social hygienists, psychiatrists, and anthropologists, but also gynecologists, pedagogues, public health and education officials, jurists, neurologists, and criminologists. During the early 1920s, RES local chapters, as well as independent eugenic groups, appeared in many provincial centers. Furthermore, eugenics found a grassroots following: in 1926, Kol'tsov received a request for advice and support from "the eugenic society of perfectionists"—a small commune organized by several enthusiasts in southern Russia to put ideas of "eugenic marriage" into practice. Eugenic ideas also became the subject of popular plays and fiction, which generated lively debates in literary and theatrical circles and among the general public.[35]

The geneticists Kol'tsov and Filipchenko initiated the institutionalization of Soviet eugenics, but physicians interested in hereditary diseases also became engaged. In 1922, Kiev University professor Aleksei Krontovskii (1885–1933) established a "bureau for studies in human heredity." Three years later, he published a manual for "studying human pathological heredity and constitution."[36] During the 1920s, physicians debated the role of "hereditary constitution" in the etiology of various diseases, ranging from tuberculosis to schizophrenia.[37] In 1927, the Moscow Society of Neurologists and Psychiatrists established a special "genetic bureau for the study of hereditary diseases" under well-known neurologist, Sergei Davidenkov (1880–1961).[38]

The particularities of the newly created Soviet public health system, with its focus on prevention, the social contexts of health, and the protection of maternity and infancy (usually known by its abbreviations, *Okhmatmlad* or *OMM*) help explain a specific configuration of individuals, disciplines, and institutions involved with eugenics in the 1920s. *Okhmatmlad* became one of the main foci of Soviet public health and social policies. The ideology underpinning *Okhmatmlad* activities, which ranged from the establishment of clinics for pregnant women to the propaganda of breast-feeding, coincided to a great extent with the ideas of French *puériculture,* and eugenicists took special steps to win over OMM officials and researchers. In December 1920, Kol'tsov delivered a keynote address to the first all-Russian conference on *Okhmatmlad,* entitled "Eugenics as a Scientific Foundation for the Work of the OMM Department [of Narkomzdrav]." His talk focused on abortion, providing a natural bridge between eugenic and OMM concerns, and it prompted the conference to acknowledge that "from the points of view of eugenics and of the protection of maternity and infancy the spread of abortions is the greatest evil and cannot be tolerated."[39] Several jurists with a long-standing interest in eugenics, notably Pavel Liublinskii, who in 1925 became a REJ co-editor, developed the legislative basis of *Okhmatmlad,* preparing laws on social support for pregnant women, single mothers, and orphans, and analyzed the "eugenic consequences" of various pieces of legislation in Russia and abroad.[40]

Eugenics found enthusiastic followers among obstetricians and gynecologists: as early as 1922, their societies in Kiev and Moscow held special meetings on eugenics.[41] In June 1924, the Sixth Congress of Gynecologists and Obstetricians devoted a special session to "eugenics and biological questions."[42] Saratov University professor Nikolai Kakushkin (1863–1942) insisted that not only "all the questions of a woman's health pertaining to her child-bearing abilities," but also "all the questions of breast-feeding, child hygiene, preschool and school education, marriage and sex hygiene, struggle against venereal diseases and prostitution," should come under the purview of "the eugenicist-gynecologist."[43] Clearly, for gynecologists, eugenics offered a means of advancement in the competition with other medical specialists over not just *Okhmatmlad,* but the entire field of public health. The congress's participants also hotly debated the eugenic role of contraceptives and abortion (legalized in Russia in November 1920). In subsequent years, the eugenic consequences of birth control continued to command close attention: the 1928 All-Union Congress of Gynecologists and Obstetricians took "the temporary sterilization of women" as its second key topic.[44]

Eugenics also enjoyed wide popularity among social hygienists. Defining their own field as "a science of the future, which studies and shapes the factors that promote the biological well-being of humanity," many social hygienists saw eugenics as "the ultimate goal of all sanitary-medical activities."[45] They included eugenics in the curricula of social and professional hygiene and even physical education courses, since, according to the Commissar Semashko, "physical education is a foundation of eugenics."[46] Social hygienists certainly saw eugenics as a means of advancement in their role as government experts and advisers on public health and social policies. They initiated several pieces of eugenic legislation, including prohibition on marriages before the age of 18 and on marriages between close relatives and between mentally ill persons. They also proposed that a prospective couple inform each other of their medical histories prior to marriage and present a written deposition to that effect to the marriage registration agency.[47] The 1926 Soviet Civic Code put these initiatives into a law.

During the early 1920s, given the scarcity of resources, Soviet eugenic research was limited mostly to the use of questionnaires to construct eugenic and clinical genealogies. A few investigators utilized twin studies for the same purpose, as well as to determine the inheritability of certain physical traits and pathological conditions. As the economic situation in the country improved, eugenicists enthusiastically embraced the mapping of blood groups in various ethnic populations and geographical settings. Indeed, the USSR was the first state where such studies were institutionalized: in 1926, a special "commission to study blood groups" was set up in Kharkov and soon began to issue its own journal.[48]

If in their research methods Soviet eugenicists were indistinguishable from their colleagues elsewhere, the foci of their investigations differed noticeably. To begin with, Soviet eugenicists completely ignored the issues of "mongrelization," even though the country's population offered ample materials to study "mixed marriages" between people of different "races." Second, they conducted practically no research on the "unfit." To the contrary, numerous institutions created in the 1920s to study criminals and criminality took up as their major slogan: "there is no [such thing as] an inborn criminal."[49] With the notable exception of Volotskoi,[50] Soviet eugenicists were highly skeptical of "negative" eugenics and repeatedly criticized restrictive eugenic laws. Continuing the pre-revolutionary tradition, Soviet pedagogues and proponents of "pedology"—the science of childhood—also rejected the sterilization or isolation of so-called "defective children." Instead, they advocated "re-education," searching for suitable methods and organizing special institutions for this purpose.

Although they did study a variety of hereditary medical conditions, Soviet eugenicists paid far more attention to investigations of the "fit," focusing especially on "creative talents." Nearly one-half of all articles published by Soviet eugenic journals analyzed the "inheritance" of literary, musical, mathematical, and artistic abilities. Even in their studies of "pathological heredity" many eugenicists emphasized the links between creativity and certain forms of "hereditary dysfunctions," including epilepsy, schizophrenia, and psychoses. In 1925, a group of psychiatrists, endocrinologists, and anatomists founded a special journal, *The Clinical Archive of Genius-ness and Gifted-ness*, producing "pathographies" of famous Russian writers, poets, and musicians.[51]

Despite its growing popularity in professional and lay circles, by the mid-1920s Soviet eugenics also encountered extensive criticism, mostly from the new institutions of "communist science," which attacked eugenics along three main lines: egalitarianism, Marxism, and Lamarckism. The critics understood the numerous studies of "creative talents" as utterly incompatible with the proclaimed egalitarianism of the Bolshevik state.[52] They branded eugenics a "bourgeois science," some urging the creation of a "socialist" eugenics that would advance the "eugenic interests of the proletariat."[53] Most opponents accused eugenics of ignoring the "environment," particularly social and economic conditions. The emphasis on "environment" led many Marxist commentators to resort to the Lamarckian inheritance of acquired characteristics in their explanations of human heredity, diversity, and evolution. Lamarckism also attracted a number of physicians who tried to reconcile the ideas of "hereditary constitution" with the principles of Mendelian genetics and at the same time to defend the Soviet emphasis on prophylactic medicine that seemed impotent in the fight against diseases rooted in heredity. Much of the debate revolved around the application of the notions of "genotype" and "phenotype" to human heredity and hereditary diseases.[54] According to the founder of the Circle of Materialist-Physicians, Solomon Levit (1894–1938), "the reconstruction of Soviet medicine on a prophylactic basis" would be theoretically unthinkable without the recognition of the inheritance of acquired characteristics.[55]

Eugenicists spent considerable effort in answering these criticisms. Commissar Semashko published an article, tellingly entitled "Eugenics, Theirs and Ours," which called for clear distinction between "Western, bourgeois" and "Soviet, proletarian" eugenics.[56] Kol'tsov and Filipchenko waged a coordinated campaign against Lamarckism in popular and professional periodicals. Serebrovskii went even further: he joined the Communist Academy to oppose the critics from within their main base, claiming that modern genetics represented a "truly Marxist" view of heredity and variability, while Lamarckism was "anti-Marxist."[57] Moreover, to assuage the accusations of elitism, Serebrovskii introduced the notion of a "gene fund" (*geno-fond*) describing the "nation's genetic capital."[58] Following his student's lead, Kol'tsov argued that the country's population possessed "a gigantic gene fund," which contained countless genes of creativity, talent, and genius, and that the utilization of this "genetic wealth" was the primary task of Soviet eugenics.[59]

Following this line of reasoning, two years later, Kol'tsov introduced the notion of "euphenics" (*evfenika*) that studies the "methods of changing the phenotype, without changing the genotype, to obtain the most valuable for us phenotypes of cultivated plants, domesticated animals, and humans."[60] According to Kol'tsov, such social measures as education, prophylactic medicine, and *Okhmatmlad* cannot affect the genotype and, thus, have no direct eugenic consequences. But they do affect the phenotype and thus work as "powerful euphenic instruments," facilitating (or inhibiting) the expression of certain genes.

Eugenicists managed to fend off the criticisms and continued the development of their discipline. In 1928, the "materialist-physician" Levit, who had converted to genetics under Serebrovskii's tutelage, organized an Office of Human Heredity and Constitution at the Medical-Biological Institute (MBI). But in just a few months, eugenicists found themselves under a new attack.

The Rise and Fall of Medical Genetics:
Eugenics in Stalin's Russia

The attack on eugenics reflected profound transformations of Soviet Russia induced by a new "revolution from above": during the late 1920s, Joseph Stalin (1878–1953) began to consolidate his power and the 1928–1929 "Great Break" marked dramatic changes in all facets of life in the country and the launching of the first Five-year Plan. The "revolution from above" greatly diminished the autonomy and authority enjoyed by the scientific community during the 1920s and it led to the rapid "Stalinization" of Soviet science.[61] The "Great Break" spelled an end to the role played by professionals as government advisers and experts in all areas of the country's life. That role was now reserved for party bureaucrats and ideologues.

Already the first wave of "Marxist" criticism during 1925–1927 had made many proponents of Soviet eugenics wary. In late 1925, Filipchenko added the word "genetics" to the name of his Bureau of Eugenics; in 1928, he removed the word "eugenics" from the name of his bureau and his journal altogether. The "Great Break" exacerbated this trend. The first All-Union congress on genetics, which was held in 1929 in Leningrad and brought together nearly 2,000 participants, did not have a single session on human genetics.[62] Just a few months after the congress, in May 1929, Filipchenko declined an invitation to renew the membership of his Bureau in the International Federation of Eugenic Organizations.

But several other eugenicists tried to adjust their enterprise to the new contexts. In late 1929, the first volume of proceedings issued by the MBI Office of Human Heredity and Constitution opened with two programmatic articles by its editors; both aimed at presenting research on human genetics as vital for socialist construction.[63] Serebrovskii identified a "truly socialist" way of achieving eugenic goals: the "separation of love and reproduction" and the artificial insemination of Soviet women with "recommended sperm" from a "talented producer." Of course, to implement this vision, Serebrovskii noted, the country needed to expand research on anthropogenetics considerably. Levit's article advanced the view that anthropogenetics held the key to solving nearly all the major problems facing modern medicine. He followed Kol'tsov in emphasizing the distinction between eugenic and euphenic consequences of medical and social interventions and insisting, contrary to his own earlier opinion, that "it is genetics that provides a scientific foundation for prophylactic medicine."

The timing of Levit's and Serebrovskii's panegyrics to "socialist eugenics" proved most unfortunate: they coincided with major ideological campaigns of the Great Break aimed at placing trusted Stalinists in positions of power. Under these conditions, Serebrovskii's "eugenic manifesto," with its assertion of the role of specialists in human genetics as experts on the Five-year Plan (and the country's future more generally), was bound to provoke a negative response. Indeed, in September 1930, the society "Leninism in Medicine" issued a ten-page exposé, under the telling title "Regarding the production plan of 'socialist eugenics,'" which characterized Serebrovskii's ideas as a "psychotic delusion."[64] Serebrovskii immediately published a repentant letter, admitting that his 1929 manifesto contained a number of "anti-party mistakes," "mechanistic formulas," and suffered from "abstract theorizing." Yet, he defiantly insisted that "these mistaken statements in no way related to the main thoughts developed in the article."[65]

Perhaps, this new attack would have proved insufficient to spell the end for eugenics in Soviet Russia, had it not coincided with certain institutional actions. In early 1930, the party apparatus initiated an "inspection" of all learned societies, and the Russian Eugenics Society was singled out.[66] The society ceased to exist and its journal discontinued with the last issue in 1930. A few months later, preparing the IEB plan for the next year, Kol'tsov renamed his department of eugenics the "department of anthropogenetics" and reformulated its tasks as "studying the various phenomena of human heredity and variability, defined not only by heredity, but also by the influences of external environment."

By the end of 1930, two out of the three key components of eugenics identified by Kol'tsov in 1921—the "applied science" of anthropotechnique and the "religion/ ideology" of bettering humankind—had been ousted from Soviet Russia. Yet its third element—the "pure science" of anthropogenetics—continued. Levit put all his formidable energies toward its advancement. In March 1930, he became MBI director and immediately upgraded his own Office of Human Heredity and Constitution to the status of the institute's major division.[67] By 1934, Soviet eugenicists had cut their losses and regrouped. On May 15, 1934, Levit organized a conference on "medical genetics."[68] And remarkably, the leading members of the now defunct Russian Eugenics Society presented key papers on the interrelation of genetics and medicine. The conference adopted a resolution that fell nothing short of a manifesto of medical genetics, notwithstanding the now obligatory "critique" of "bourgeois eugenic perversions." The resolution called upon Narkomzdrav to "create scientific research centers in medical genetics and cytology" in every large city throughout the entire country and to expand the teaching of genetics in medical schools. The future of Soviet medical genetics seemed bright. The new commissar of public health, Grigorii Kaminskii (1895–1938), enthusiastically supported Levit's enterprise. In the fall of 1935, MBI was renamed the Institute of Medical Genetics (IMG).

But within just a few months, the fortunes of human genetics in Russia turned once more. The beginning of the Great Terror in the summer of 1936 prompted Levit's expulsion from the Bolshevik party and his dismissal from the IMG directorship. The rising political tensions between Nazi Germany and the USSR sensitized the Soviet leadership to the historical and current links among eugenics, medical genetics, and *Rassenhygiene*.[69] Despite the considerable effort of Soviet geneticists to "expose" *Rassenhygiene*—and to dissociate, in the words of one of them, "real genetics" from its "perversions" in Nazi propaganda and policies—human genetics, in the minds of many, retained fascist connotations.[70] Levit and his coworkers were accused of holding "fascist views" on human genetics,[71] and in the spring of 1938, Levit was arrested and executed. With the death of its most active champion and the dissolution of its main research center, the field of medical genetics in the Soviet Union disintegrated. In late 1948, as a result of Lysenko's campaign against genetics, even the few remaining clinical investigations were abandoned, and Soviet medical genetics disappeared from public view for nearly 20 years.

EUGENICS IN A REVOLUTIONARY SOCIETY

Russian eugenics's life span, institutional and disciplinary composition, patronage pattern, and research foci differed substantially from those in other countries. After nearly two decades of "disembodied" existence during the Imperial era, eugenics was quickly institutionalized in Soviet Russia as a scientific discipline. In just ten years, however, the very word "eugenics" became a pejorative term, and its proponents redefined their enterprise as "medical genetics." After a brief period of rapid growth and popularity in the early 1930s, medical genetics was declared a "fascist science" and virtually disappeared from the Soviet scientific scene toward the end of the decade.

Although, as elsewhere, eugenics in Soviet Russia developed rapidly during the early 1920s, the contexts of its institutionalization were quite particular. In contrast to many other settings where eugenics was funded largely by private individuals and institutions, Soviet eugenics enjoyed exclusively state patronage. Unlike central and southern Europe, where eugenics fed into the project of building a nation-state and capitalized on "blood and soil" mythology, the USSR was a multinational state, with every nation of the Union accorded (at least on the level of official pronouncements) equal rights and equal status. Similarly, the ideas of class and race inequality, which to a large degree underpinned the support for eugenics in Britain, Germany, the United States, and elsewhere, were anathema to the proletarian state that aimed at the creation of a classless, multi-ethnic society and that officially denounced nationalism and racism. So the standard justifications for the rise of eugenics in the early 1920s cannot help us to understand the situation in Soviet Russia.

Yet, the USSR had several features in common with other countries. Even though the Bolsheviks were not building a *nation* state, they were nevertheless *building a state*, creating its governing apparatus, laws, institutions, practices, and bureaucracies, and thus establishing and expanding their social control over the population. As many historians of eugenics in other countries have demonstrated, the extensive medicalization connected to eugenic projects became one of the "social control" instruments of state-building and modernization. Certainly, the same was true of Soviet eugenic projects, which explicitly or implicitly afforded a much greater role to medical and public health professionals in social policy-making than they had ever played before. This explains why medical specialists, from social hygienists to gynecologists, enthusiastically promoted eugenics during the 1920s.

But why did the Bolsheviks accord eugenicists that position? Eugenic ideas of "bettering humankind" resonated strongly with the Bolsheviks' early visions of the country's (and ultimately the world's) future: it is telling that Semashko and Kaminskii, both commissars of public health, supported eugenics. Like eugenicists, the Bolsheviks believed in social progress and in the ability of humans to direct it. This congruence of interests allowed Soviet eugenicists quickly to institutionalize their field in post-revolutionary Russia. Eugenics provided an array of meanings, which helped the two groups to develop a common language and to foster the dialogue. This shared language also allowed eugenicists to translate their own, often quite esoteric, interests into a language understood and appreciated by their patrons.

The "end of eugenics" in Russia came much earlier than in any other setting and within entirely different contexts. In 1930, with the Bolshevik party apparatus asserting its own control over decision- and policy-making in all walks of life, Soviet eugenicists were forced to concede to a large degree their expert role to party functionaries and ideologues. This explains the way eugenicists "truncated" their enterprise. They were compelled to give up two key elements of their doctrine most closely associated with social policies—the "applied science" of anthropotechnique and "eugenic religion/ideology." Yet, they were able to hold on to and further develop its third element: the "pure science" of anthropogenetics, quickly rechristened "medical genetics." A few years later, however, the political tensions between Stalin's Russia and Hitler's Germany tainted that "pure science" in the eyes of Bolshevik leaders with "fascist connotations," which led to its demise in the Soviet Union, prefiguring the postwar decline of eugenics in many other countries.

Despite its short life span, eugenics left a lasting footprint on various social policies in Soviet Russia, a footprint that so far both historians of eugenics and historians of Russia have thoroughly neglected. Perhaps blinded by the Soviet official negative attitude toward eugenics in the 1930s, numerous studies on feminism, family, *Okhmatmlad*, demography, civic and criminal justice, prophylactic medicine, abortion, and birth control in Soviet Russia all but ignore eugenics, even during its heydays in the 1920s. In his recent discussion of "Stalinist pronatalism in its pan-European context," David L. Hoffmann referred extensively to the role eugenic ideas played in pronatalist policies adopted by various countries, but failed even to mention eugenics in Russia.[72] However, as the 1926 Soviet Civic Code demonstrates, eugenics certainly affected *Okhmatmlad*, family, and marriage legislation in the 1920s. Similarly, many historians of Russia have analyzed even such a "eugenically charged" issue as abortion with at most a passing remark on eugenics.[73] Yet even a cursory examination reveals the profound impact of eugenic ideas on Soviet abortion policies during the 1920s and, as witnessed by the 1936 anti-abortion law, even after Soviet eugenics had been officially disbanded. Although the law was enacted in June 1936, a debate over possible exceptions, particularly over medically indicated abortions, continued for at least another year. A resulting list of medical conditions deemed sufficient to warrant permission for abortion included a variety of hereditary diseases, and it clearly shows the considerable influence that eugenic ideas still exerted on the minds of the experts and officials involved. As this example indicates, much remains to be done in examining how exactly eugenic ideology penetrated decision-making processes on particular social policies during particular periods.

We can certainly debate the relative weight of structures (the particular directions of Soviet public health, or the entire state system in its Imperial, Bolshevik, and Stalinist forms), ideologies (various trends of Marxism-Leninism-Stalinism), and historic contingencies (the Bolshevik revolution, the Great Break, the Great Terror, or the rise of German Nazism) in shaping the history of eugenics during the three distinct periods of its existence in Russia. We can dispute the relative role of international contacts and local traditions in molding Russian eugenics's institutions and activities. But no matter the outcome of such debates and disputes, a history of eugenics in Russia offers important corrections to customary views on the relationships between science and society, public discourse and state policies, institutions and ideas, professions and disciplines drawn from the history of eugenics in other locales. It provides a whetstone for various generalized hypotheses put forward to explain both the rise and fall of eugenics as a scientific discipline and the lasting influence eugenic ideology exerted (and still exerts) on a variety of social policies and issues around the world.

NOTES

1. Mark B. Adams, "Eugenics in Russia," in *The Wellborn Science: Eugenics in Germany, France, Brazil, and Russia*, ed. Mark B. Adams (Oxford and New York: Oxford University Press, 1990), 153–229.

2. For example, Mark B. Adams, Garland E. Allen, and Sheila Weiss, "Human Heredity and Politics," *Osiris* 20 (2005): 232–262.

3. See Iu. V. Khen, *Evgenicheskii proekt* (Moscow: Institut filosofii RAN, 1993).

4. See V. Babkov, *Zaria genetiki cheloveka* (Moscow: Progress-Traditsiia, 2008).

5. V. M. Florinskii, *Usovershenstvovanie i vyrozhdenie chelovecheskogo roda* (St. Petersburg: Riumon, 1866).

6. For example, Charl'z Davenport, *Evgenika kak nauka ob uluchshenii prirody cheloveka* (Moscow: G. Vuttke, 1913).

7. T. Iudin, "Ob evgenike i evgenicheskom dvizhenii," *Sovremennaia psikhiatriia* 4 (1914): 319–336.

8. L. Krzhivitskii [*Krzywicki*], "Antropotekhnika," in *Entsiklopedicheskii slovar',* 7th ed. (Moscow: Br. A. and I. Granat, 1912), 3: 249–250; K. A. Timiriazev, "Evgenika," *ibid.*, 19: 391–395; L. Krzhivitskii, "Antropotekhnika," in *Novyi entsiklopedicheskii slovar'* (St. Petersburg: Brokgauz and Efron, 1914), 3: 99–101; Anon., "Evgenika," *ibid.*, 17: 173.

9. For Kropotkin's speech, see *Problems in Eugenics* (London: Eugenics Education Society, 1913), 50–51. See also P. Kropotkin, "Eugenics and Militarism," *The Times,* July 30, 1912.

10. Dioneo, "Iz Anglii. Zverinaia psikhologiia," *Russkoe bogatstvo* 10 (1912): 302.

11. See P. I. Kovalevskii, *Vyrozhdenie i vozrozhdenie. Prestupnik i bor'ba s prestupnost'iu* (St. Petersburg: M. I. Akinfiev, 1903); I. A. Sikorskii, *Chto takoe natsiia i drugie formy etnicheskoi zhizni* (Kiev: S. V. Kul'zhenko, 1915).

12. Krzhivitskii, "Antropotekhnika," in *Entsiklopedicheskii slovar'* 3: 249–250.

13. Krzhivitskii, "Antropotekhnika," in *Novyi entsiklopedicheskii slovar'* 3: 100.

14. P. I. Liublinskii, "Novaia mera bor'by s vyrozhdeniem i prestupnost'iu," *Russkaia mysl'* 3 (1912): 31–56.

15. P. I. Kovalevskii, *Otstalye deti (idioty, otstalye i prestupnye deti), ikh lechenie i vospitanie* (St. Petersburg: Vestnik dushevnykh boleznei, 1906).

16. "Khronika," *Gigiena i sanitarnoe delo* 1 (1914): 118.

17. See I. G. Orshanskii, "Rol' nasledstvennosti v peredache boleznei," *Prakticheskaia meditsina* 8–9 (1897): 1–120.

18. N. Kabanov, *Rol' nasledstvennosti v etiologii boleznei vnutrennikh organov* (Moscow: Prostakov, 1899); A. Sholomovich, *Nasledstvennost' i fizicheskie priznaki vyrozhdeniia u dushevno- bol'nykh i zdorovykh* (Kazan': Imperatorskii universitet, 1913).

19. T. Iudin, "O kharaktere nasledstvennykh vzaimootnoshenii pri dushevnykh bolezniakh," *Sovremennaia psikhiatriia* 8 (1913): 568–578.

20. I. G. Orshanskii, "Izuchenie nasledstvennosti talanta," *Vestnik vospitaniia* 1 (1911): 1–41; 2: 95–127.

21. See S. Ukshe, "Vyrozhdenie, ego rol' v prestupnosti i mery bor'by s nim," *Vestnik obshchestvennoi gigieny* 6 (1915): 798–816.

22. Anon., "Programma zhurnala," *Gigiena i sanitariia* 1 (1910): 1–5.

23. K. V. Karaffa-korbutt, "Ocherki po evgenike," *Gigiena i sanitariia* 1 (1910): 41–48, 138–145, 276–281.

24. I. V. Sazhin, *Nasledstvennost' i spirtnye napitki* (St. Petersburg: P. P. Soikin, 1908).

25. See L. P. Kravets, "Nasledstvennost' u cheloveka," *Priroda* 6 (1914): 722–743; Kr. L., "Evgenetika," *Priroda* 10 (1914): 1229.

26. N. Kol'tsov, "Alkogolizm i nasledstvennost'," *Priroda* 4 (1916): 502–505; Iu. Filipchenko, "Evgenika," *Russkaia mysl'* 3–6 (1918): 69–96.

27. See Mark B. Adams, "Science, Ideology, and Structure: The Kol'tsov Institute, 1900–1970," in *The Social Context of Soviet Science*, eds. L. L. Lubrano and S. G. Solomon (Boulder, CO: Westview Press, 1980), 173–204.

28. See S.G. Solomon, "Social Hygiene and Soviet Public Health, 1921–1930," in *Health and Society in Revolutionary Russia*, eds. S. G. Solomon and J. F. Hutchinson (Bloomington, IN: Indiana University Press, 1990), 175–199.

29. V. Bunak, "O deiatel'nosti Russkogo evgenicheskogo obshchestva za 1921 god," *Russkii Evgenicheskii Zhurnal* [hereafter REZh] 1, no. 1 (1922): 99–101.

30. Iu. Filipchenko, "Biuro po evgenike," *Izvestiia Biuro po Evgenike* [hereafter IBE] 1, no. 1 (1922): 1–4. See M. B. Konashev, "Biuro po evgenike, 1922–1930," *Issledovaniia po genetike* 11 (1994): 22–28.

31. For instance, R. R. Gats [Gates], *Nasledstvennost' i evgenika* (Leningrad: Seiatel', 1926). For Russian geneticists' international activities, see Nikolai Krementsov, *International Science between the World Wars: The Case of Genetics* (London and New York: Routledge, 2005).

32. N. K. Kol'tsov, "Uluchshenie chelovecheskoi porody," *REZh* 1, no. 1 (1922): 3–27. All the following quotations are from this source.

33. Kol'tsov obviously used the word "religion" in the sense we use today the word "ideology."

34. A. S. Serebrovskii, "O zadachakh i putiakh antropogenetiki," *REZh* 1, no. 2 (1923): 107–116.

35. See Yvonne Howell, "Eugenics, Rejuvenation, and Bulgakov's Journey into the Heart of Dogness," *Slavic Review* 65, no. 3 (2006): 544–562.

36. A. A. Krontovskii, *Nasledstvennost' i konstitutsiia* (Kiev: GIZ Ukrainy, 1925).

37. Compare M. I. Lifshits, *Uchenie o konstitutsiiakh cheloveka s kratkim ocherkom sovremennogo polozheniia voprosa o nasledstvennosti* (Kiev: GIZ Ukrainy, 1924); T. I. Iudin, *Psikhopaticheskie konstitutsii* (Moscow: Sabashnikov, 1926).

38. S. N. Davidenkov, "Geneticheskoe biuro pri M. O. N. i P.," *REZh* 6, no. 1 (1928): 55–56.

39. *Materialy pervogo Vserossiiskogo soveshchaniia po okhrane materinstva i mladenchestva* (Moskva: OMM Narkomzdrava, 1921), 41–50.

40. P. I. Liublinskii, "Evgenicheskie tendentsii i noveishee zakonodatel'stvo o detiakh," *REZh* 3, no. 1 (1925): 3–29.

41. See E. M. Deliariu, "Evgenika, ee metody i znachenie," *Ginekologiia i akusherstvo*, 5 (1923): 159–160.

42. "Evgenika i biologicheskie voprosy," *Ginekologiia i akusherstvo* 4 (1924): 409–413.

43. N. M. Kakushkin, "Evgenetika i ginekologiia," in *Trudy VI s"ezda obshchestva ginekologov i akusherov* (Moscow: n.p., 1925), 415.

44. G. P. Sakharov, "Protivozachatochnye sredstva i evgenika," in *Protivozachatochnye sredstva v sovremennom nauchnom osveshchenii*, eds. A. P. Gubarev and S. A. Selitskii (Moscow: n.p., 1928), 34–47.

45. T. Ia. Tkachev, *Sotsial'naia gigiena* (Voronezh: Gubzdravotdel, 1924), 11, 153.

46. N. Semashko, "Predislovie," in *Fizicheskaia kul'tura v nauchnom osveshchenii* (Moscow: n.p., 1924), 3.

47. A. N. Sysin, "Pervye shagi evgenicheskogo zakonodatel'stva v Rossii," *Sotsial'naia gigena* 3–4 (1924): 11–20.

48. See *Biuleteni Postiinoi komisii vivchannia krov'ianikh ugrupovani* (Kharkiv, 1927).

49. E. K. Krasnushkin, "Chto takoe prestupnik?" in *Prestupnik i prestupnost'* (Moscow: Moszdravotdel, 1926), 32.

50. See M. Volotskoi, *Podniatie zhiznennykh sil rasy. Novyi put'* (Moscow: Zhizn' i znanie, 1923).

51. *Klinicheskii arkhiv genial'nosti i odarennosti (evropatologii), posviashchennyi voprosam patologii genial'noodarennoi lichnosti, a takzhe voprosam patologii tvorchestva* (Sverdlovsk, 1925–1929). The activity of this group is partially explored in I. Sirotkina, *Diagnosing Literary Genius* (Baltimore, MD: John Hopkins University Press, 2001).

52. G. Shmidt, "Ne iz verkhnikh desiati tysiach, a iz nizhnikh millionov," *Pod Znamenem Marksizma* [hereafter *PZM*] 7 (1925): 128–133.

53. M. Volotskoi, *Klassovye interesy i sovremennaia evgenika* (Moscow: Zhizn' i znanie, 1925).

54. Vas. Slepkov, "Nasledstvennost' i otbor u cheloveka," *PZM* 4 (1925): 102–122.

55. S. Levit, "Problema konstitutsii v meditsine i dialekticheskii materialism," in *Meditsina i dialekticheskii materializm* 2 (1927): 20–21.

56. N. A. Semashko, "Ikh evgenika i nasha," *Vestnik sovremennoi meditsiny* 10 (1927): 639–649.

57. A. S. Serebrovskii, "Teoriia nasledstvennosti Morgana i Mendelia i marksisty," *PZM* 3 (1926): 98–117.

58. For details, see Mark B. Adams, "From 'Gene Fund' to 'Gene Pool': On the Evolution of Evolutionary Language," in *Studies in the History of Biology*, eds. William Coleman and Camille Limoges (Baltimore, MD: Johns Hopkins University Press, 1979), vol. 3, 241–285.

59. N. K. Kol'tsov, "Rodoslovnye nashikh vydvizhentsev," *REZh* 4, no. 3–4 (1926): 103–143.

60. N. K. Kol'tsov, "Evfenika," *Bol'shaia Meditsinskaia Entsiklopediia* 9 (Moscow: Medgiz, 1929): 689–692.

61. For details, see Nikolai Krementsov, *Stalinist Science* (Princeton, NJ: Princeton University Press, 1997).

62. See *Trudy Vsesoiuznogo s"ezda po genetike*, 6 vols. (Leningrad: VIR, 1930).

63. A. S. Serebrovskii, "Antropogenetika i evgenika v sotsialisticheskom obshchestve," *Mediko-biologicheskii zhurnal* 5 (1929): 3–19; S. Levit, "Genetika i patologiia (v sviazi s sovremennym krizisom v meditsine)," *Mediko-biologicheskii zhurnal* 5 (1929): 20–39.

64. "Po povodu proizvodstvennogo plana 'sotsialisticheskoi evgeniki,'" *Moskovskii meditsinskii zhurnal* 9 (1930): 77–87.

65. A. S. Serebrovskii, "Pis'mo v redaktsiiu," *Mediko-biologicheskii zhurnal* 4–5 (1930): 447–448.

66. See G. Sobolev, "Russkoe Evgenicheskoe Obshchestvo," *VARNITSO* 5 (1930): 49–50.

67. S. Levit, "Chelovek kak geneticheskii ob"ekt i izuchenie bliznetsov kak metod antropogenetiki," *Mediko-biologicheskii zhurnal* 4–5 (1930): 273–287.

68. *Konferentsiia po meditsinskoi genetike. Doklady i preniia*, issued as an appendix to the journal *Sovetskaia Klinika* 20, no. 7–8 (1934).

69. See E. A. Finkel'shtein, "Evgenika i fashizm," in *Rassovaia teoriia na sluzhbe fashizma* (Kiev: Gosmedgiz, 1935): 37–88; Z. A. Gurevich, "Fashizm, 'rasovaia gigena' i meditsina," in *Rassovaia teoriia na sluzhbe fashizma* (Kiev: Gosmedgiz, 1935): 89–125.

70. G. Frizen, "Genetika i fashizm," *PZM* 3 (1935): 86–95.

71. E. Kol'man, "Chernosotennyi bred fashizma i nasha mediko-biologicheskaia nauka," *PZM* 11 (1936): 64–72.

72. David L. Hoffmann, "Mothers in the Motherland: Stalinist Pronatalism in Its Pan-European Context," *Journal of Social History* 34, no. 1 (2000): 35–54.

73. See Elizabeth Waters, "The Modernisation of Russian Motherhood, 1917–1937," *Soviet Studies* 44, no. 1 (1992): 123–135.

FURTHER READING

Adams, Mark B. "The Politics of Human Heredity in the USSR, 1920–40," *Genome* 31, no. 2 (1989): 879–884.

Adams, Mark B. "Eugenics as Social Medicine in Revolutionary Russia," in *Health and Society in Revolutionary Russia*, eds. S.G. Solomon and J. F. Hutchison (Bloomington, IN: Indiana University Press, 1990), 200–223.

Adams, Mark B. "Soviet Nature-Nurture Debate," in *Science and the Soviet Social Order*, ed. Loren R. Graham (Cambridge, MA: Harvard University Press, 1990), 94–138.

Flitner, Michael. "Genetic Geographies: A Historical Comparison of Agrarian Modernization and Eugenic Thought in Germany, the Soviet Union, and the United States," *Geoforum* 34 (2003): 175–185.

Graham, Loren R. "Science and Values: The Eugenics Movement in Germany and Russia in the 1920s," *American Historical Review* 82, no. 5 (1977): 1133–1164.

Krementsov, Nikolai. "Eugenics, *Rassenhygiene*, and Human Genetics in the late 1930s," in *Doing Medicine Together: Germany and Russia between the Wars*, ed. Susan G. Solomon (Toronto: University of Toronto Press, 2006), 369–404.

Krementsov, Nikolai. "Marxism, Darwinism, and Genetics in Soviet Russia," in *Ideology and Biology: From Descartes to Dawkins*, eds. Ron Numbers and Denis Alexander (Chicago, IL: Chicago University Press, 2010), 215–246.

Spektorowski, A. "The Eugenic Temptation in Socialism: Sweden, Germany, and the Soviet Union," *Comparative Studies in Society and History*, 46, no. 1 (2004): 84–106.

CHAPTER 25

EUGENICS IN JAPAN: SANGUINOUS REPAIR

JENNIFER ROBERTSON

In a 1968 paper on birth control policy published in English in the *Japanese Journal of Human Genetics,* geneticist Ei Matsunaga (b. 1922) declared that "no eugenic[s] movement has ever existed in Japan." He also alluded to the 1948 Eugenic Protection Law (*Yūsei hogohō*) as "the first of its kind."[1] Not only was there a vibrant eugenics movement in Japan in the early twentieth century, but the 1948 Eugenic Protection Law was in large part a revision of its wartime predecessor, the 1940 National Eugenic Law. How could Matsunaga not have known these facts?

Matsunaga headed the National Institute of Genetics, during which time (1983–1989) he established Japan's DNA Data Bank. He is not alone among Japanese scientists who, after Japan's defeat in 1945, distanced themselves from scientific policies and practices encouraged under the aegis of ultranationalism and colonialism. Unlike its German counterpart, the Japanese state has maneuvered to obscure its history of militarism. The erasure of eugenicists and eugenic practices from the public, and even scholarly, record is one of the many local consequences of the state's inability to deal constructively with its imperial past.[2]

The public sphere in early-twentieth-century Japan was shaped by the discourse of eugenics and was premised on a future-oriented vision of a racially pure nation-state peopled by sturdy and fertile citizens. These people were the so-called New Japanese (*shin'nipponjin*) whose anthropometrically ideal bodies would serve as the caryatids of the expanding Japanese empire. Eugenics offered a grand narrative within which to locate the trajectory of New Japan. Eugenicists, all of whom were nationalists, if not ultranationalists, believed that *only* New Japanese could compete successfully with western Europeans and Americans in international affairs.

The exact genesis of the New Japanese was the subject of heated and divisive debates that continue to shape the discourse of ethno-nationality to this day. Introduced under the auspices of eugenics was a new national premium on "pure blood" (*junketsu*) and "wholesome" (*kenzen*) heredity as a necessary condition of race betterment and modern nation-building. Blood remains an organizing metaphor for profoundly significant, fundamental, and perduring assumptions about Japanese-ness and otherness. Eugenics provided a framework in fin-de-siècle Japan within which blood became a cipher for specifically modern ideas of "disciplinary bio-power."[3] In this connection, my title, "sanguinous repair," refers to the perceived restorative properties attributed to "pure blood" by Japanese eugenicists and colonial administrators alike.

Eugenics, often along with blood type, was used to differentiate, at home and abroad, the "fit" and the "unfit," "us" from "them."[4] The "science of superior birth" was effectively utilized by Japanese eugenicists and others both to pose and answer reflexive questions such as: Who are we? What have we become? What do we know? Where are we going in a greatly changed and changing society and world?[5] In Japan, these kinds of interrogations were first posed in the context of modern science in the late nineteenth century when the methods of "applied biology" were informed by the demographic priorities of the expanding empire. As we shall see, the nascent eugenics movement played a critical role in the discursive formation of a new, *modern* Japanese cultural and national identity, debates that continue to inform the popular perception of postmodern, posthuman Japan.

The aim of this chapter is to spell out the relationships between eugenics, nationalism, and colonialism in Japan, and to highlight the ways in which eugenics was popularized and incorporated into everyday practices and official policies at home and in the colonies. Although I dwell on eugenics-related activities in the late nineteenth and early twentieth centuries, I also address some of their postwar guises. The public record of eugenics in the service of imperialism may have been whitewashed after 1945, but eugenics per se does not have a bad name in Japan. In short, whereas the wartime context of eugenics remains problematic, the "well-born science" continues to thrive in various ways, such as genetic testing and ectogenesis. I refer to some of these guises as "posthuman eugenics," or the biotechnological enhancement of human life and reproduction. As I argue in the conclusion, Japan was only one of many nation-states to employ eugenics as social policy nearly a century ago, but it may be one of the first to implement posthuman eugenics to address looming demographic concerns.

NATIONALISM AND THE NEW JAPANESE

Eugenics was introduced to Japan by Japanese physicians, scientists, and journalists who were familiar with Francis Galton's *Hereditary Genius,* which had been translated into Japanese shortly after it was published in England in 1869. Before the neologism *yūseigaku* (science of superior birth) was coined around the turn of the century, the Japanese referred to eugenics in its romanized form, *yuzenikkusu*. By the 1930s, these two terms were often used interchangeably with *minzoku eisei*, or "race hygiene," after the German *Rassenhygiene*, which, in turn, were used synonymously with two older expressions, *minzoku/jinshu kairyō* (race betterment) and *minzoku/jinshu eisei* (race hygiene). *Minzoku* and *jinshu*, the two Japanese words for "race" in both the social and phenotypical senses, for the most part were used interchangeably, although *jinshu* remains the more clinical, social-scientific term (cf. *Rasse*) and *minzoku* the more popular and populist term (cf. *Volk*). When prefixed with names, such as Nippon and Yamato, the latter an ancient and nationalistic appellation for Japan, *minzoku* signified the conflation of phenotype, geography, culture, spirit, history, and nationhood. All of these semantic and semiotic inventions were part of the ideological agenda of the Meiji Restoration (1868) and were incorporated into the postwar (and current) constitution of 1947, which retained the definition of nationality and citizenship as a matter of blood, or *jus sanguinus* (as opposed to citizenship determined by place of birth, or *jus solis*).

Eugenics was perhaps the most influential of the new ideologies of the body that were formulated in the late nineteenth and the early twentieth centuries in nation-states around the world. As chapters in this volume show, these new ideologies, which included public hygiene and lifestyle reform, emphasized the links between physical and mental fitness, nutrition and physiology, and basically identified the corporeal body as a central locus for human well-being and development. In 1920s Japan, when eugenics had become a regular topic in the popular media and scholarly literature, some proponents of the "well-born science" proclaimed that it had been an inherent feature of Japanese marriage customs since at least the eighth century. Ikeda Shigenori (1892–1966), a German-trained eugenicist and founder of one of Japan's several eugenics associations,[6] claimed in a 1928 article that premodern "eugenic truths" (*yūseigakuteki jijitsu*) were evident in ancient Buddhist prescriptions for selecting a marriage partner, namely, that the partner should appear healthy, have no obvious deformities, and no family history of insanity, criminal behavior, addictions, and so forth.[7]

The defeat by imperial sympathizers of the 250-year military rule of the Tokugawa shogunate (1603–1867) enabled the restoration of the Meiji emperor in 1868 to a ruling position within a parliamentary system. An imperial policy of selective and controlled Westernization was introduced together with unprecedented social reforms.[8] These included the joint institutionalization in the Civil Code of monogamy and the patriarchal household, which was designated the smallest legal unit of society, a status it maintained until the promulgation in 1946 of the postwar constitution, which granted sovereignty to the individual. The concept of a family-state (*kazoku kokka*) system was invented by late-nineteenth-century ideologues to create a familiar and modern community—the nation—where one had not existed before. Prior to this time, the majority of Japanese claimed an affinity with a locality or a circumscribed region, and not the "imagined community" of the nation. Although the Japanese state was consolidated by the eighth century, a distinctive Japanese national identity was forged over a thousand years later, largely through the new systems of universal education and a conscription-based military.[9] Some pundits stretched out the family metaphor and likened Japanese nationality to membership in an exceptional "bloodline" (*kettō*). The familial conception of the nation-state profoundly influenced the nascent idea of the uniqueness of *the* Japanese as a distinct race.[10]

Beginning with the colonization of Okinawa in 1874, the state consolidated through military force a vast Asian-Pacific domain, the so-called Greater East Asia Co-Prosperity Sphere (*daitōa kyōeiken*)—a rubric coined in August 1940. The need to "propagate and multiply" (*umeyo fuyaseyo*) taller and heavier Japanese bodies that could "properly oversee the nation's global expansion" was quickly recognized by public and private sector institutions alike. Ikeda Shigenori, along with his contemporaries, contributed to public debates about the efficacy of applying eugenics as social, national, and colonial policy, and helped to fuel an ambitious national campaign to grow the population from roughly 70 million to 100 million persons— a goal that was finally reached in 1967.

Inspired by the German Wandervogel and Czech Sokol physical fitness organizations, and with the support of leading politicians, scholars, physicians, and military officials,[11] Ikeda founded the Yūsei undō (Eugenic Exercise/Movement Association) in 1926. That, along with a eugenics journal of the same name, aimed to foster among the general public an interest in incorporating hygienic and eugenic practices into everyday life practices. The journal ceased publication in January 1930. It is significant that both movement and journal incorporated the word exercise (*undō*), which means more than just a physical activity that is undertaken in order to improve one's health. Exercise alludes to the development of bodily skills as well as to the kinesthetic experience of a performance. Unlike "discipline," which connotes a teleology of control, "exercise" is more open-ended, naming the movement or action through which the body becomes something else and actively participates in making meaning.[12] Ikeda established the coed Legs and Feet Society (Ashi no kai). in 1927, as a subgroup within his association, in part to promote New Japanese self-fashioning through physical fitness regimens and outdoor activities.

Ikeda alluded in his speeches and articles to the bio-performativity—the exercise or exercising—of blood as a unique bio-cultural resource. Thus, in his 1927 eugenic manifesto, "Yūsei nippon no teishō," (Manifesto for Eugenic Japan) he declared:

> Blood talks. Japanese are, in the end, Japanese. Blood binds with blood. Japanese are, in the end, Japanese. There is nothing that talks more substantively than blood. There is nothing that binds together human being more intrinsically than blood. Even if [Japanese] are born in America, speak American [sic], have American nationality, pay taxes in America, work in America, or live in America, Japanese are, in the end, Japanese. As compatriots, [we] do not regard [Japanese-Americans] as foreign nationals or a foreign people.
>
> It is said that the spirit of charity and equality can only be achieved if the nationality of blood is broken. However, it is fundamentally impossible to break the nationality of blood.

> We are all anticipating the construction of Eugenic Japan (*yūsei nippon*). This island nation is a eugenically blessed country. Because we do not share borders with another country our contacts with foreign peoples have been superficial and thus our blood has been divinely protected [from mixing]. The unbroken and integral three-thousand year history of our imperial people and our blood ties as a grand family-state are unique in the world. With our innate good fortune, we must once more, from our position as cultured persons creating culture, elevate culturally, scientifically, rationally, and substantively, the truth of our ethnic superiority.[13]

Blood, according to Ikeda, was a substance that possessed superlative and irreversible binding properties and was a valuable resource that enabled the vigorous continuity of Japanese culture.[14]

FROM HYBRID VIGOR TO PURE BLOODEDNESS

In Japan, the discourse of eugenics clustered around two essentially incommensurable positions concerning blood: the "pure-blood," or *junketsu,* position, and the "mixed-blood," or *konketsu,* position. The proponents of each position acknowledged the "mixed-blooded," or multiethnic, ancient history of Japan, an idea developed in the late nineteenth century by the German physician and genealogist, Erwin von Baelz (1849–1913), who had spent thirty years in Japan (1876–1906) studying the racial origins of the Japanese people. Baelz, applying the then dominant teleological evolutionist paradigm, proposed that the so-called Yamato stem-race, associated with the Imperial household and its allegedly unbroken lineage stretching back over 2,500 years, had, by the sixth century, conquered and subjugated the different racial groups coexisting on the islands. These groups, he maintained, were assimilated selectively and slowly, so that by the nineteenth century, "Yamato blood" was a refined and superior substance.[15] Japanese pundits favoring the pure-blood position were eager to preserve the eugenic integrity of the pristine Yamato stem-race; those promoting the mixed-blood position enumerated the eugenic benefits of hybrid vigor through the mixing of Japanese and non-Japanese blood.[16]

The "mixed-blood" position was first articulated in an 1884 essay, *A Treatise on the Betterment of the Japanese Race* (*Nippon jinshu kairyōron*), penned by the Keio University-educated journalist Takahashi Yoshio. Invoking a Social Darwinist scenario, Takahashi argued that Japan was undergoing a transition from a "semi-civilized" to a "civilized" status represented, in his view, by northern European countries and their "physically superior" populations. This "civilized" status could be expedited through the marriage of Japanese males and Anglo females, or, as he phrased it, the "mixed-marriage of yellows and whites" (*kōhaku zakkon).*[17] Anglo females were viewed as superior birthing vessels. Mixed-blood marriages, Takahashi hypothesized, would be an expedient way of creating a taller, heavier, and stronger, in short "a physically superior Japanese race, thereby making it possible for the Japanese to compete successfully with Europeans and Americans in international affairs."[18] The complicated logistics of the "mixed blood" position were never addressed.

The "pure-blood" position was advocated by Katō Hiroyuki (1836–1916), a veteran politician, imperial advisor, and chancellor of Tokyo University. Katō's scathing critique of the mixed-marriage plan was published in 1886 in both an academic journal, *Tōyō Gakugei* (Oriental Arts and Sciences) and the *Tōkyō Nichinichi Shinbun,* a leading daily newspaper. To summarize, Katō first of all objected to the notion that the Japanese were less civilized than Europeans.[19] Second, he argued that interbreeding "yellows" and "whites" would create a completely new hybrid category of person whose political and social "status" would be unclear and perplexing. Miscegenation, Katō concluded, would result in race *transformation* and not race betterment, and would, over the course of several generations, seriously dilute the pure blood—or racial and cultural essence—of the Japanese. He declared emphatically that whereas mixed-blood marriages between yellows and whites would insure the "complete defeat" (*zenpai*) of Japan by Westerners, pure-bloodedness would insure for eternity Japan's distinctive racial history, culture, and social system.[20]

Although the pure-blood position came quickly to dominate, the pluses and minuses of both arguments were hotly debated in the eugenics literature through 1945. In fact, these debates were so antagonistic that in 1892, (Baron) Kaneko Kentarō (1853–1942)—the trusted aide of Prime Minister (Count) Itō Hirobumi (1841–1909) who had also served as Japan's first prime minister 1885–1888)—wrote to Herbert Spencer (1820–1903) requesting advice, among other things, about how to settle the rancorous debates in Japan over the issue of "mixed-blood" marriages. Spencer's response both supported and underscored the dominance of the pure-blood position. Excerpts from Spencer's August 26, 1892, letter in response to Kaneko's queries reveals what was to be a persistent tendency in eugenic thinking to meld inherited and acquired characteristics, and Darwinian and Lamarckian principles:

> To your…question respecting the intermarriage of foreigners and Japanese, which you say is "now very much agitated among our scholars and politicians" and which you say is "one of the most difficult problems," my reply is that, as rationally answered, there is no difficulty at all. It should be positively forbidden. It is not at root a question of social philosophy. It is at root a question of biology. There is abundant proof, alike furnished by the intermarriages of human races and by the interbreeding of animals, that when the varieties mingled diverge beyond a certain slight degree *the result is inevitably a bad one* in the long run…By all means, therefore, peremptorily interdict marriages of Japanese with foreigners.[21]

One cannot but wonder whether the Anglocentric Spencer was concerned about Japanese "purity" or about banishing even the thought of Anglo-Japanese offspring. These apprehensions about "mixed-blood" marriages continue today in Japan, cloaked as debates about citizenship, blood-donation guidelines, and the desirability of so-called international marriages.

In an article published in the May 1911 issue of *Jinsei-Der Mensch* (Humankind), the first eugenics journal published in Japan, zoologist Oka'asa Jirō scoffed at the proposal of "yellow-white marriages," dismissing this as one example of the "maniacal fascination with the West" (*seiyōshinsui*) that defined the early Meiji period.[22] Over 25 years later, in 1939, political theorist Ijichi Susumu published an article in *Kaizō* (Reconstruction), a popular, generally liberal, literary periodical, advocating the intermarriage of Japanese males and "carefully selected" Manchurian females. He referred to his proposal as a "racial blood transfusion" (*minzoku yūketsu*) and argued that "mixing superior Japanese blood with inferior Manchurian blood would stimulate the development and civilization of inferior peoples by producing hybrid offspring who would mature as natural political leaders."[23]

Ijichi's ideas in turn were rebuffed by Tōgō Minoru, an eminent theorist of colonialism, whose ideas about blood informed state policy. Tōgō reiterated Katō's earlier objections to mixed-blooded offspring, arguing that they constituted a "new race" (*shinminzoku*); miscegenation by definition could only fail to produce the cultural objective of colonial assimilation, namely Japanization (*nipponka*). Mixed marriages between Japanese and non-Japanese Asians, he asserted, would effectively corrupt and "dissolve the soul (*tamashii*) of the pure Japanese race and national body" and thwart the imperial expansion of the Japanese people.[24]

POPULARIZING EUGENICS

Fujikawa Yū, a physician and medical historian, was among the dozens of Japanese medical students who, having studied in Germany, were eager to apply western European ideas about eugenics and race hygiene to the general project of "improving the Japanese race." In 1905, Fujikawa published the journal *Jinsei-Der Mensch* (Humankind), which he modeled after German eugenicist Alfred Ploetz's (1860–1940) *Archiv für Rassen- und Gesellschafts-Biologie* (Journal for Racial and Social Biology) founded a year earlier. Articles by an international array of scholars interested in these same issues were translated into Japanese and included in each issue, along with reviews and synopses of books and articles on race science as a form of social medicine and public policy.

From around 1905 onward, eugenics was popularized countrywide through the daily newspapers and weekly magazines. Because of Japan's historically high rate of literacy, established scientists like Fujikawa were able to use the burgeoning mass media to foster an appreciation of race betterment through selective and self-conscious procreation. Not only did eugenicists contribute regularly to the media, but the various eugenics journals, *Jinsei-Der Mensch* (1905), *Yūseigaku* (Eugenics, 1924), *Yūsei Undō* (Eugenic Exercise/Movement, 1926) and *Minzoku Eisei* (Race/Ethnic Hygiene, 1931), all featured columns and articles devoted to summarizing the coverage of eugenics themes in the news.[25]

By the early 1930s, detailed "eugenic marriage" questionnaires were printed in or inserted into popular magazines for public consumption. Housewives especially were encouraged to administer the surveys, and an exemplary eugenic-marriage questionnaire was published in 1933 in the *Fujin Kōron* (Women's Review), a leading mainstream women's magazine. The insert was titled, "A Marriage Survey That Amateurs Can Undertake" (*shirōto de dekiru kekkon chōsa*). There were nine categories of investigation: personal history; disposition and character; personal conduct; health status; hobbies, tastes, and habits; religious beliefs; political orientation; lifestyle; and financial status. Clearly, the successful completion of these eugenic-household questionnaires was ultimately contingent upon the literacy and diligence of the surveyor; namely, an urban, middle-class educated woman with enough free time to devote to the task.[26] If necessary, however, detective agencies could be commissioned to assist. In fact, one historian of science, Fujino Yutaka, claims that the first detective agencies (*kōshinjo*) were founded in Osaka in 1892 to conduct background checks on potential marriage partners, a service that remains in high use today.[27]

The popularization of eugenics was further fostered through traveling exhibitions of hygienic practices, organized along with better baby contests and "healthy body beauty" contests. Eugenic marriage counseling centers were opened, some in department stores.[28] Beginning in 1883, numerous "hygiene exhibitions" (*eisei tenrankai*) were staged countrywide, sponsored first by a Buddhist temple in Tokyo and subsequently by the Japanese Red Cross, and after 1938, by the newly created Welfare Ministry. By the late 1920s, the theme and content of many of these exhibitions were based on public opinion polls, and the relationship between heredity and marriage practices proved to be one of their most popular themes.[29]

Through networks of modern institutions and industries, such as the army, schools, hygiene exhibitions, immigration training programs, the press, fashion, advertising, popular genealogies, and so forth, the Japanese people were encouraged to think in totally new and different ways about their bodies. They were to think of their bodies as plastic—capable of being molded—and as adaptable, pliable, and transformable through new hygienic regimens of nutrition and physical exercise.

For males, these regimens were part of their military training, which had begun in 1873, when a modern conscription army was established, replacing the hereditary warrior (samurai) class that epitomized the Tokugawa period (1603–1867). Females, exempt from military service, were exposed to these regimens at the many private sector schools and academies that competed to enroll girls and women whose education was more or less neglected by the Meiji government, at least initially. Clothing also fell under the eugenic gaze. Whereas boys and men were encouraged to wear crewcuts and Western-style outfits to symbolize the modernity of New Japan, girls and women were to represent through costume and hairstyle a nostalgically reimagined traditional Japanese culture, although they were urged to loosen the normally tightly cinched *obi,* or sashes, of their kimono, and to simplify the traditional chignon to facilitate the regular cleaning and combing of their hair. All Japanese were advised by public health agents to learn how to walk properly, to use chairs whenever possible, and to avoid kneeling for long lengths of time, which was thought to cause bowed legs and pigeon-toedness.[30] The desirable corporeal results and aesthetic effects of these new hygienic practices were perceived as transmittable by blood through "eugenic marriages" (*yūsei kekkon*).

EUGENIC MARRIAGES

At the time that eugenics was introduced in Japan, heredity (*iden*) was understood in a general sense as whatever one received from one's parents and ancestors, making them morally as well as medically culpable should their offspring be less than wholesome. Japanese race scientists thus also worked to reform marriage and sexual practices more generally because it was through sex, regulated by the institutions of marriage—as well as licensed prostitution—that either positive or negative eugenic precepts, or both, were most effectively implemented.[31]

The tenacious persistence of "blood marriages" despite private and state efforts to condemn their transaction provoked intensified efforts to eliminate that tradition. Some villages were even known as "blood-marriage hamlets" (*ketsuzoku kekkon buraku*) because the vast majority of inhabitants had married their first cousins, half cousins, second cousins, uncles, or nieces. A demographer employed by the government noted that the proportion of consanguineous marriages in Japan averaged 16 percent in the 1920s.[32]

Dismissing the folk belief that the familiarity shared by married blood relatives insured household diplomacy and stability, Ikeda Shigenori lectured throughout Japan on the need to shift the basis of and for desirable familiarity between females and males from close kinship per se to the modern alternative of equal coeducation and shared hobbies. In his lectures and essays, delivered and written in an often folksy style, Ikeda repeated the slogan of his association, "superior seeds, superior fields, superior cultivation" (*yoi tane, yoi hatake, yoi teire*). This, he explained, was a metaphor for "superior genes, superior society, superior education" (*yoi iden, yoi shakai, yoi kyōiku*).[33] Coeducational programs and leisure activities, such as those offered by his Legs and Feet Society, and not consanguineous marriages, were promoted by Ikeda as a healthier way to foster familiarity and intimacy among potential spouses.[34]

One of the first lines of offense against consanguineous unions was the "eugenic-marriage counseling centers" (*yūsei kekkon sōdansho*) that were opened in Tokyo and regional cities from 1927. The earliest centers were sponsored and staffed by Ikeda's Eugenic Exercise/Movement Association. Citing the evolutionary categories proposed by Lewis Henry Morgan in *Systems of Consanguinity and Affinity of the Human Family* (1871), Ikeda argued that monogamous marriage practices, together with the systematization of physical education, were the key to improving the Japanese race and modernizing Japan.[35] Ikeda and his colleagues followed Francis Galton in emphasizing the dialectical relationship between eugenics and marriage.

A number of the eugenic marriage counseling centers, including Ikeda's, were opened in department stores—such as Shirokiya in the elegant Nihonbashi section of Tokyo—in order to make information about social and race hygiene and associated behaviors and practices easily available to consumers. Women especially were targeted, for "female citizenship" was defined not in terms of legal rights but in terms of procreation and consumption.[36] Modern scientific—specifically hygienic and eugenic—knowledge was dispensed as a commodity. The staff of the eugenic-marriage counseling centers also provided matchmaking services, introducing potential spouses to each other based on the autobiographical health certificates they had completed and filed at the centers.

According to the health profile (*shinshin kensahyō*) of a eugenic couple appearing in *Shashin Shuho Shūhō* (Photograph Weekly) in April 1942, by which time the centers were well established throughout Japan, the ideal woman was 154 centimeters tall, weighed 51 kilograms, and had a chest size of 80 centimeters. The ideal man was 165 centimeters tall, weighed 58 kilograms, and had a chest size of 84 centimeters. Both were free from disease and had "normal" genealogies. As the quintessential eugenic couple, they were committed to observing the "ten rules of marriage:" choose a lifetime partner; choose a partner healthy in body and mind; exchange health certificates; choose someone with normal genes and wholesome heredity and ancestry; avoid marriage with blood relatives; marry as soon as possible; discard superstitions and quaint customs; obey your parents; have a simple and economical wedding; and, reproduce for the sake of the nation. The health profile was accompanied by photographs of the couple and their health certificates, scenes of a simplified, eugenic marriage ceremony, and a cartoon of the desired outcome of eugenic marriage counseling; namely, a family of eight children.[37]

Ikeda regarded the ostracism and sterilization of the unfit as a crude and simplistic approach to the project of race betterment. His views stood in stark contrast to those of Nagai Hisomu (1876–1957), a German-trained physician who expounded on the benefits of "race hygiene" (*minzoku eisei*) in part through sterilization. Nagai founded the Japanese Race Hygiene Society (*Nippon minzoku eisei gakkai*) in 1930. By 1939 the Society had a membership of thirteen hundred; the list of its founding sponsors includes the names of two future postwar prime ministers: Yoshida Shigeru (1878–1967) and Hatoyama Ichirō (1883–1959).[38] Its monthly journal, *Minzoku eisei* (Race Hygiene), served to broadcast Nagai's proposals for race improvement, which included marriage and fecundity among so-called superior persons and the segregation and sterilization of so-called abnormal persons, namely, the mentally infirm, physically handicapped, and sexually alternative.[39] Nagai played a role in the popularization of eugenics by serving as a judge in a nationwide beauty contest, designed to select from among thousands of contestants a young woman who epitomized the modern ideal of "healthy-body beauty" (*kenkōbi*).[40]

Nagai helped to draft the National Eugenics Law (Kokumin yūseihō) which was passed in May 1940 and activated in July 1941. This law was modeled after the first German racial hygiene law of 1933, which in turn had been informed by earlier U.S. sterilization laws.[41] The overarching purpose of this law was to insure the betterment of the Japanese ethnic nation (*minzoku*) by preventing (through sterilization) the reproduction of "unfit" people with an allegedly hereditary disease, and by promoting the reproduction of genetically healthy people.[42] Even then eugenicists knew that hereditary diseases may be hidden in "normal-looking" carriers. They echoed and cited their foreign counterparts, such as eugenicist Ethel Elderton (1878–1954), Galton's assistant, in warning about the dangers of "latent defects," especially with respect to consanguinity.[43]

Comparatively few sterilizations were performed in Japan following the passage of the National Eugenics Law in 1940. Between 1941 and 1945, 15, 219 persons (6,399 females and 8,820 males) were targeted for sterilization, although 435 (243 females and 192 males), or about 29 percent of the total, were actually sterilized.[44] One critic of sterilization even argued that the divine origins and purity of the "Yamato race" raised serious doubts in his mind about the validity of that procedure: "one must not equate a divine people with livestock."[45] Other critics of eugenics and sterilization, like the sexologist Yasuda Tokutarō, stressed instead the importance of the physical and social environment on human development, and the complexity of human motives to reproduce or not.[46]

EPILOGUE: POSTWAR AND POSTHUMAN EUGENICS

The 1948 Eugenic Protection Law (Yūsei hogohō) that geneticist Ei Matsunaga claimed to be the "first of its kind" was passed in July 1948 and activated two months later. Like that of its predecessor, the National Eugenics Law, the explicit purpose of the Eugenic Protection Law was to prevent the birth of "unfit offspring" (*furyō na shison*) with the additional proviso to protect maternal health and life. This law was amended several times: in 1949 to include economic hardship as a valid reason to induce abortion;[47] in 1952 to eliminate the need for women seeking an abortion to obtain the permission of a regional eugenic protection committee; in 1955 to allow nurses and midwives to sell birth control devices and drugs; and so forth. Whereas the law originally allowed abortions up to 28 weeks into the pregnancy, in 1976 and in 1990, this period was reduced to 24 weeks and 22 weeks, respectively, in response to new medical technologies that made it possible to keep alive younger neonates.[48] According to the statistics generated in 1995 by the Ministry of Health and Welfare, from 1949 to 1994, 16,520 sterilizations were performed without the patient's own consent; 11,356 of these involuntary sterilizations were performed on women, and 5,164 on men.[49]

Parliamentary debates on the 1948 law continued through the spring of 1996, when it was abolished in June and replaced in September of that year by the current Maternal Protection Law (*Botai hogohō*) from which references to "eugenically inferior offspring" were omitted. Political scientist Tiana Norgren notes that "the impetus for the 1996 revision came from the small, politically weak groups of handicapped activists who sought to eliminate the eugenic content of the law," aided by pressure from the international community.[50] Actually, Norgren is not entirely accurate, for the eugenic content was not so much eliminated as obscured by a more concentrated focus on maternal and infant health, which had always been an important facet of the eugenics practiced in Japan. The historical debates about blood and maternity that I have reviewed help us to understand why in Japan (unlike in Germany, Israel, and the United States), "eugenics" is neither an avoided nor negatively charged term.

A century ago, eugenics constituted a synergistic nexus of theory, ideology, and practice that blurred and even fused any hypothetical boundary between the street and the laboratory. In several respects, little has changed in this respect in Japan. The postwar eugenics law may have been renamed and revised in 1996, but the term "eugenics" itself was never disowned. Thus, the journal *Minzoku Eisei* (literally, Race Hygiene) continues to be published under that title, although its English title was changed in the mid-1970s to the *Japanese Journal of Health and Human Ecology*.

Ideology and demography were intertwined motives for the application of eugenics as social policy in late-nineteenth and early-twentieth-century Japan. In order to grow a "pure blooded" population, both in terms of sheer numbers but also in height and weight, females, as reproducers of the nation, especially were targeted by early eugenicists for the purposes of "sanguinous repair." Today, the Japanese state is again anxiously invested in raising the birthrate, which now stands at about 1.3 children per married woman, and since 2005, essentially on par with the mortality rate. The latest estimates produced by the health ministry show that the current population of approximately 128 million will shrink to less than 111 million in 2035, and to less than 90 million in 2055.[51] This dire demographic forecast is compounded by the rapid aging of Japan. Over 21 percent of the current population of 127.8 million people (which includes permanent foreign residents) is over 65 years of age, and that percentage is expected to increase by 2050 to over 40 percent.[52]

Despite the fact that, according to a 1995 government report, 600,000 immigrants were needed to maintain the labor force, the Japanese state for the most part has continued a postwar precedent of pursuing automation over replacement migration.[53] As former prime minister Koizumi declared, when presented with the report, "If [foreign workers] exceed a certain level, it is bound to cause a clash."[54] At the same time, the state continues to disregard women as a talented and vital labor force, especially at the corporate level, although its agents are quick to blame women alone for the low birthrate.[55]

The Japanese state was not the first to embrace eugenics as social policy in the early twentieth century, but it may very well be the first to employ what I call "posthuman eugenics" both to compensate for the declining and aging population and to make replacement migration less necessary (or even unnecessary). Posthuman generally refers to humans whose capacities are radically enhanced by biotechnological means so that they surpass those of ordinary—or unenhanced—humans. The posthuman condition already is a staple of Japanese *manga* (comics) and *anime* (animated films). Much of current Japanese robotic technology is geared toward literally empowering the human body—for example, Honda's new "walk assist" wearable robot—as well as improving the conditions of and for childbearing—for example, the child care and household robots under development that are imagined by the state to lighten the workload of married women, making them more receptive to multiple pregnancies.[56]

Perhaps the most obvious and problematic biotechnical feature of posthuman eugenics is the artificial uterus, or ectogenetic chamber; that is, an external means of gestation.[57] Japanese scientists have gone farther than their counterparts elsewhere in creating a "womb" for incubating IVF embryos.[58] Dubbed "the better surrogacy argument,"[59] ectogenesis would replace surrogacy and its legal complications.[60] Coupled with pre-implantation genetic testing, an artificial uterus would enable selective, even customized, reproduction.[61] Proponents argue that the ability to select genetic variations for offspring will make reproduction more appealing, lower the possibility of various disabilities, and "enhance" the mental faculties of the developing fetuses.[62] Japanese eugenicists made essentially the same arguments over 70 years ago in promoting "eugenic marriage" (Ikeda Shigenori) and sterilization (Nagai Hisomu).[63]

Whereas early eugenics owes much to animal husbandry, posthuman eugenics is the invention and beneficiary of the newest biotechnologies and has the potential not only to expand the range and possibilities of reproductive practices, but also to enhance the capabilities of humans at every stage of existence, including the cellular. Early eugenics did not simply target discrete individuals; rather, as a component of social policy and public hygiene, eugenics was deployed to create new and reinforce old categories of so-called fit and unfit individuals and groups. A new wave of eugenic practices continues today in the guise of increasingly taken-for-granted biotechnologies. Genetic testing, gene-mapping, prenatal screening, selective (for example, sex-specific) abortion, technologically assisted or enabled reproduction, pre-implantation genetic diagnosis, and surrogacy are some of the "health" services and commodities already offered in countries around the world, including Japan, often under the authority of the state and legitimate medical institutions.

Eugenics as a set of ideological positions and practices continues to be pursued in various ways, perhaps more overtly in Japan than elsewhere. Both the presence of a eugenics movement in Japan and the emergence there of a posthuman eugenics initiative dispel popular notions that eugenics was an early-twentieth-century perversion of science exploited by the Nazis alone. Moreover, an investigation of the applications of eugenics in Japan, past and present, helps to decenter the dominance of Euroamerican narratives of the well-born science and to draw attention to current manifestations around the world of selective social and biological reproductive strategies.

ACKNOWLEDGMENTS

I would like to offer my thanks to the following individuals and institutions: to Alison Bashford and Philippa Levine for inviting me to participate in this project and shepherding the manuscript through several phases; to Alexandra Stern and Celeste Brusati for offering sage feedback at different intervals; to Jeannine Baker for her assistance in formatting the manuscript; and to the many colleagues who have listened to or read my work on Japanese eugenics. Research for this project was provided by: the National Endowment for the Humanities/Advanced Research in the Social Sciences on Japan Fellowship (2008); a visiting professorship in the Department of Anthropology, University of Tokyo (2007); a research grant from the Office of the Vice President for Research, University of Michigan (2003); a faculty research grant from the Center for Japanese Studies, University of Michigan (2003–2004); and a Japan Foundation Research Fellowship (2002).

NOTES

1. Ei Matsunaga, "Birth Control Policy in Japan: A Review from Eugenic Standpoint [sic]," *Japanese Journal of Human Genetics* 13, no. 3 (1968): 189, 199. It is highly unlikely that Matsunaga was unfamiliar with pre-1948 eugenics. After all, he was a college student during the 1940s, graduating at age 23 in 1945 from the Faculty of Medicine, Tokyo Imperial University, five years after the passage of the National Eugenics Law. Throughout his article, Matsunaga uses the term "eugenics" without qualms or qualification.

2. The inability of the Japanese state to engage with its wartime past is the subject of Manichean debates in Japan and the topic of a gigantic, multilingual literature. I address the matter of the state's "willful amnesia" in the context of eugenics in "Dehistoricizing History: The Ethical Dilemma of 'East Asian Bioethics,'" *Critical Asian Studies* 37, no. 2 (2005): 233–250. Following Corrigan and Sayer, I am using "the state" in the singular for reasons of convenience, although I recognize that the term refers to a repertory of agencies and institutions that reinforces and reproduces dominant ideologies and normalizes everyday practices. See Philip Corrigan and Derek Sayer, *The Great Arch: English State Formation as Cultural Revolution* (Oxford: Basil Blackwell, 1985).

3. "Disciplinary bio-power," as elaborated by Michel Foucault, refers to a state's or dominant institution's politicization of and control over biology and biological processes, including recreational and procreational sexual practices, as a powerful means of assimilating and claiming people as subjects. Although the applications of bio-power can be both positive and negative, Foucault focuses especially on its misuses and perversions. See Michel Foucault, *The History of Sexuality,* vol. 1, *An Introduction,* trans. Robert Hurley (New York: Pantheon, 1978) and Foucault, *Discipline and Punish: The Birth of the Prison,* trans. Alan Sheridan (New York: Pantheon, 1979).

4. For further information on the politics of blood type in Japan, see Yuehtsen Juliette Chung, *Struggle For National Survival: Eugenics in Sino-Japanese Contexts, 1896–1945* (New York and London: Routledge, 2002); Michael Kenny, "Blood, Race, and Personality: Origins of Racial Serology and the Search for Genetic Markers of National Difference," paper presented at the 2007 American Anthropological Association Meeting, Washington, DC; and Jennifer Robertson, "Blood—in All of Its Senses—as a Cultural Resource," in *Cultural Resources,* eds. Shinji Yamashita and Jerry Eades (Oxford: Berghahn Books, forthcoming).

5. Renee C. Fox and Judith P. Swazey, "Medical Morality Is Not Bioethics: Medical Ethics in China and the United States," *Perspectives in Biology and Medicine* 273 (1984): 360.

6. Born in Akita prefecture, Ikeda attended college in Tokyo. Following his graduation from Tokyo Foreign Language University (Tokyo Gaigodai), he was employed by Kōdansha, a prominent publishing house, to edit the magazine *Taikan* (Outlook). He later

joined the *Hōchi Shinbun*, a major daily newspaper, and served as a special correspondent to Germany from 1919 to 1924, where he earned doctorates in eugenics and women's history. He was transferred to Moscow in 1925 before returning to Japan and founding his eugenics movement. Ikeda rekindled his journalism career in 1933 by assuming the editorship of the *Keijō Nippō* (Seoul Daily News), based in Seoul. He returned to the *Hōchi Shinbun* as an editor in 1939, and from 1941 through the end of the war worked for Naval Intelligence. After the war he became a prominent "social commentator" (*hyōronka*).

7. Ikeda Shigenori, "Hi no shita ni atarashiki mono nashi [There's nothing new under the sun]," *Yūsei Undō* 3, no. 3 (1928): 26; Ikeda, "Kekkonsha no mimoto chōsahyō [Background survey of marriage candidates]," *Yūsei Undō* 3, no. 9 (1928): 58–61. Similarly, in a lecture published in 1916, Rabbi Max Reichler asserted that "Jewish eugenics" long predated Galton's neologism, arguing that many eugenic rules were certainly incorporated in the large collection of Biblical and Rabbinical laws. Rabbi Max Reichler, "Jewish Eugenics," in Max Reichler, ed., *Jewish Eugenics, and Other Essays: Three Papers Read Before the New York Board of Jewish Ministers, 1915* (New York: Bloch Publishing Company, 1916), 1.

8. For an overview of the modernization of Japan, see Carol Gluck, *Ideology in the Late Meiji Period* (Princeton, NJ: Princeton University Press, 1985), and Marius B. Jansen, *The Making of Modern Japan* (Cambridge, MA: Belknap Press of Harvard University Press, 2000).

9. See Gluck, *Japan's Modern Myths*.

10. As Tessa Morris-Suzuki notes, "the imagery of the family was particularly apposite because it created the ideal framework for asserting the paramount place of the emperor in Japanese society" as the head of the family-state. Tessa Morris-Suzuki, *Reinventing Japan: Time, Space, Nation* (Armonk, NY: M. E. Sharpe, 1998), 84–85.

11. Suzuki Zenji, *Nihon no yūseigaku—sono shisō to undō no kiseki* [Japanese eugenics—the legacy of eugenic thought and the eugenics movement] (Tokyo: Sankyo Shuppan, 1983), 123.

12. Mary Thomas Crane, "What Was Performance?," *Criticism* 43, no. 2 (2001): 177.

13. Ikeda Shigenori, "Yûsei nippon no teisho [Discourse on eugenic Japan]," *Yūsei Undō* 2, no. 1 (1927): 2–3.

14. This continues to be the case, as illustrated most recently by heated debates in the Japanese blogosphere about whether or not Dr. Yoichiro Nambu, the 2008 Nobel Prize winner in physics and a naturalized American citizen, should be claimed by the Japanese news media as "Japanese." Thanks to Junko Teruyama, a PhD candidate in anthropology at the University of Michigan, for bringing this to my attention.

15. Cullen Hayashida, *Identity, Race and Blood Ideology of Japan* (PhD diss., University of Washington, 1976), 24. Yamato is an ancient, and since the Meiji period, chauvinistic name for Japan. Baelz did not support mixed-blood marriages—although he married and had children with a Japanese woman—and proposed instead a "negative" eugenics approach to race betterment by segregating the fit from the unfit. See Fujino Yutaka, *Nihon fuashizumu to yūsei shisō* [Japanese fascism and eugenic thought] (Kyoto: Kamogawa Shuppan, 1998), 388. Similar arguments about pure-blood and mixed-blood were waged in China, where one advocate of mixed marriages attempted to strengthen his case by claiming that the Japanese government had sanctioned the practice of intermarriage between "whites" and "yellow," which of course was not accurate. See Frank Dikötter, *The Discourse of Race in Modern China* (London: C. Hurst; Stanford, CA: Stanford University Press, 1992), 88; for additional general information about the discourse of race and eugenics in China, see also Dikötter, *Imperfect Conceptions: Medical Knowledge, Birth Defects, and Eugenics in China* (New York: Columbia University Press, 1998). Although

aware of their Chinese counterparts, a number of whom visited and studied in Japan, Japanese eugenicists did not cite their work, favoring in contrast the publications of Europeans and North and South Americans. Doubtless Japanese imperial aggression in China since the Sino-Japanese War (1894–1895) also had a negative effect on scholarly exchanges between Japanese and Chinese nationalists and eugenicists. For an informative analysis of the status of China in Japanese scholarship during the late nineteenth and early twentieth centuries, see Stefan Tanaka, *Japan's Orient: Rendering Pasts into History* (Berkeley, CA: University of California Press, 1993).

16. Jennifer Robertson, "Japan's First Cyborg?: Miss Nippon, Eugenics, and Wartime Technologies of Beauty, Body, and Blood," *Body and Society* 7, no. 1 (2001): 1–34.

17. "Marriage" was used as a euphemism for "procreative sexual intercourse."

18. Suzuki, *Nihon no yūseigaku*, 32–34, 39.

19. Weiner states incorrectly that Takahashi's ideas were shared by Katō. See Michael Weiner, "'Self' and 'Other' in Prewar Japan," in *Japan's Minorities: The Illusion of Homogeneity*, ed. Michael Weiner (London and New York: Routledge, 1997), 7.

20. Fujino Yutaka, *Nihon fuashizumu*, 385; Katō Hiroyuki, "Nippon jinshu kairyō no ben [Discussion of the betterment of the Japanese race]," in *Katō Hiroyuki bunsho* [Collected writings of Katō Hiroyuki], eds. Ueda Katsumi, Fukushima Hirotaka, and Yoshida Kō 3 vols. (Tokyo: Dōhōsha Shuppan, 1990), 1: 33, 40–47; Suzuki, *Nihon no yūseigaku*, 35–38.

21. Herbert Spencer, "Herbert Spencer's Advice to Japan," *Eugenical News* 11, no. 11 (1926): 168–169.

22. Oka'asa Jirō, "Jinshukairyō wa jikkō ga dekiru ka [Is it possible to implement race betterment?]," *Eisei Sekai* 2, no. 3 (1915): 2.

23. Ijichi Susumu, "Kōateki konketsuron [Treatise on Asian mix-bloodedness]," *Kaizō* 3 (1939): 86. Years earlier, some colonial administrators had considered a similar policy with respect to Korea and Koreans under the tautological rubric *dōbun dōshu no minzoku*, or "people of the same culture and race"—"tautological" because the alleged sameness was proposed by Japanese colonial ideologues who supported assimilation, or *dōka*, literally "same-ization," that is, Japanization. Support for assimilation and pacification through intermarriage waned as Korean hostility toward the occupiers grew more intense, especially after the anti-Japanese uprising of 1919. The very few "mixed marriages" that were officially condoned were those strategically arranged between Japanese and Korean royalty. See Peter Duus, *The Abacus and the Sword: The Japanese Penetration of Korea, 1895–1910* (Berkeley, CA: University of California Press, 1995), 413–423. Ijichi's views paralleled the dominant position of the state's assimilation policy toward the aboriginal Ainu of Hokkaido, who, since the Meiji Restoration of 1868, had been categorized as "proto-Japanese." Assimilation, it was believed, would accelerate their evolution as "civilized people." See, for example, Takakura Shin'ichirō, *Ainu seisakushi* [History of Ainu policy] (Tokyo: Hyōronsha, 1942).

24. Tōgō Minoru, *Jinkō mondai to kaigai hatten* [The population problem and overseas expansion] (Tokyo: Nihon Seinenkan, 1936), 142–144; Tōgō, "Dai tōa kensetsu to zakkon mondai [The construction of Greater East Asia and the problem of miscegenation]," *Shin Jawa (Djawa Baroe)* 2, no. 1 (1945): 30–34.

25. For example, see "Shinbun ni arawareta yūsei mondai [Eugenics in the daily newspapers]," *Yūsei* 1, no. 5 (1936): 18–22; and "Shinbun ni arawareta yūsei yūsei mondai [Eugenics in the daily newspapers]," *Yūsei* 1, no. 9 (1936): 15–16.

26. cf. Amy Sue Bix, "Experiences and Voices of Eugenics Field-Workers: 'Women's Work' in Biology," *Social Studies of Science* 27, no. 4 (1997): 625–668; see also Jennifer

Robertson, "Blood Talks: Eugenic Modernity and the Creation of New Japanese," *History and Anthropology* 13, no. 3 (2002): 191–216; and Robertson, "Dehistoricizing History."

27. Fujino, *Nihon fuashizumu*, 392.

28. Jennifer Robertson, "Les 'bataillons fértiles': sexe et la citoyenneté dans le Japon impérial [Fertile-Womb Battalions: Sex and Citizenship in Imperial Japan]," in *New Critical Approaches to Twentieth-Century Japanese Thought*, ed. Livia Monnet (Montréal: University of Montréal Press, 2001), 275–301; Robertson, "Blood Talks."

29. Fujino, *Nihon fuashizumu*, 140–141.

30. Irizawa Tatsuyoshi, *Ikaga ni shite nipponjin no taikaku o kaizen subeki ka* [What can be done in order to improve the physiques of the Japanese people] [1913] (Tokyo: Nisshin shoin, 1939), 17–21, 34, 61.

31. For definitive research on the history of sexology in Japan, see Sabine Frühstück, *Colonizing Sex: Sexology and Social Control in Modern Japan* (Berkeley, CA: University of California Press, 2003).

32. Imaizumi Yoko, "Parental Consanguinity in Two Generations in Japan," *Journal of Biosocial Science* 20 (1988): 235; Shinozaki Nobuo, "Ketsuzoku kekkon buraku no jinruiga-kuteki chōsa gaihō [Summary of an anthropological survey of blood-marriage hamlets]," *Jinruigaku Zasshi* 60, no. 3 (1949): 97–100.

33. Ikeda, "Yūsei nippon no teisho."

34. Ibid.; Fujino, *Nihon fuashizumu*, 88; Jennifer Robertson, "Talking Feet: Performance and Performativity in Japanese Eugenics," paper presented at Kalamazoo College, Stanford University, and the University of California at Davis, April 2004.

35. Ikeda Shigenori, *Bunmei no hōkai* [The collapse of civilization] (Tokyo: Hōbunkan, 1925), 31–38, 386; Ikeda, "Yūseigakuteki shakai kairyō undō ni tsuite [On the eugenic social reform movement]," *Yūsei Undō* 4, no. 10 (1929): 19; Miwata Motomichi, "Atarashii kekkon kikan [A new marriage system]," *Yūsei Undō* 2, no. 6 (1927): 29–32.

36. Robertson, "Japan's First Cyborg?"; Robertson, "Les 'bataillons fértiles.'"

37. "Kore kara no kekkon wa kono yō ni [How marriages should be transacted henceforth]," *Shashin Shūhō Shūhō* 218 (April 29, 1942): 18–19.

38. Morris-Suzuki, *Reinventing Japan*, 21; Suzuki, *Nihon no yūseigaku*, 148.

39. Chung, *Struggle For National Survival*; Frühstück, *Colonizing Sex*; Sumiko Otsubo and James Bartholomew, "Eugenics in Japan: Some Ironies of Modernity," *Science in Context* 11, no. 3–4 (1998): 545–565.

40. Robertson, "Japan's First Cyborg?," 23–24.

41. Frühstück, *Colonizing Sex*; see also Tiana Norgren, *Abortion before Birth Control: The Politics of Reproduction in Postwar Japan* (Princeton, NJ: Princeton University Press, 2001).

42. I use "unfit" as shorthand for a variety of terms used by Japanese eugenicists, such as *furyō* (depraved, bad, inferior), *retsujaku na soshitsu* (inferior or feeble constitution), *ijō* (abnormal), *akushitsu na iden* (inferior or bad genes), *rettō* (feebleminded, low caliber), and so forth. The vocabulary and vectors of eugenics were also used to pathologize and contemporize historical constructions of radical otherness, as in the case of Burakumin ("outcastes"). Their stigmatized status was eugenically respun as the consequence of defective germ-plasm. Curiously, of the several articles I read by eugenicists dismantling superstitions surrounding marriage practices, not one made an argument *against* the systematic discrimination of Burakumin in all arenas of Japanese society. Moreover, eugenic discourse was instrumental in creating a caste-like category of "stigmatized other." For more details, see Robertson, "Blood Talks."

43. Ethel Elderton, *On the Marriage of First Cousins* (London: Cambridge University Press, 1911).

44. Suzuki, *Nihon no yūseigaku,* 166; Tanaka Satoshi, *Eisei tenrankai no yokubō* [The ambition of hygiene exhibitions] (Tokyo: Seikyūsha, 1994), 164.

45. Makino Chiyozō, "Danshuhō hantairon [An argument against a sterilization law]," *Yūseigaku* 15, no. 4 (1938): 18–21; see also Suzuki, *Nihon no yūseigaku,* 163; and Takagi Masashi, "Senzen Nihon nihon ni okeru yūsei shisō no tenkai to nōryokukan, kyōikukan [Views on IQ and education in the development of eugenic thought in prewar Japan]," *Nagoya Daigaku Kyōikugakubu Kiyō* 40, no. 1 (1993): 41–52.

46. Suzuki, *Nihon no yūseigaku,* 162–163.

47. Citing the 1993 *Eugenic protection statistical report* (Yūsei hogo tōkei hōkoku), Norgren points out that "[s]ince the 1949 revision, 99 to 100 percent of Japanese women cited 'economic reasons' on the paperwork that must be filled out when an abortion is performed." See Norgren, *Abortion before Birth Control,* 46.

48. Yonezu Tomoko, Nagaoki Akiko and Ōhashi Yukako "Dataizai/yūseihō o meguru nenpyō [Timeline account of contraceptives, abortifactants, and eugenics laws]," *Inpakushon* 97 (1996): 70–77.

49. Takashi Tsuchiya, "Eugenic Sterilizations in Japan and Recent Demands for Apology: A Report," *Newsletter of the Network on Ethics and Intellectual Disability* 3, no. 1 (1997): 4.

50. Norgren, *Abortion before Birth Control,* 77.

51. "19 prefectures to see 20% population drops by' 35," *Japan Times,* May 30, 2007.

52. Ibid.

53. *Policy Brief: Economic Survey of Japan, 2006,* OECD (July 2006), www.oecd.org/dataoecd/50/23/37148463.pdf; Atsushi Kondo, "Development of Immigration Policy in Japan," *Asia and Pacific Migration Journal* 11, no. 4 (2002): 415–436, www.ip.kyusan-u.ac.jp/keizai-kiyo/dp12.pdf.

54. Quoted in Chikako Kashiwazaki and Tsuneo Akaha, "Japanese Immigration Policy: Responding to Conflicting Pressures," Migration Information Source (November 2006), Migration Policy Institute, www.migrationinformation.org/Profiles/print.cfm?ID=487.

55. Suvendrini Kakuchi, "Japan: Dwindling Workforce Forces a Rethink on Role of Women Workers," May 16, 2005, Inter Press Service News Agency, www.ipsnews.net/interna.asp?idnews=28692; Kalyani Mehta, *Untapped Resources: Women in Aging Societies Across Asia* (Singapore: Marshall Cavendish Academic Press, 1997).

56. "Walking Assist," Honda Motor Co., world.honda.com/Walking-Assist/ (accessed December 1, 2008); "Inobēshon 25 [Innovation 25]," www.kantei.go.jp/jp/innovation/index.html. (accessed December 1, 2008); Jennifer Robertson, "*Robo sapiens japanicus:* Humanoid Robots and the Posthuman Family," *Critical Asian Studies* 39, no. 3 (2007): 369–398.

57. Irina Aristarkhova, "Ectogenesis and Mother as Machine," *Body and Society* 11, no. 3 (2005): 43–59; Stephen Coleman, *The Ethics of Artificial Uteruses: Implications for Reproduction and Abortion* (Farnham: Ashgate, 2004); Francesca Dolendo, "Baby Machines: The Birth of the Artificial Womb," *The Triple Helix: The National Journal of Science, Society, and Law at MIT* 2, no. 2 (2006): 4–8; Christopher Kaczor, "Artificial Wombs and Embryo Adoption," in *The Ethics of Embryo Adoption and the Catholic Tradition: Moral Arguments, Economic Reality and Social Analysis,* eds. Sarah-Vaughan Brakman and Darlene Fozard Weaver (Dordrecht: Springer Verlag, 2007), 307–322; Christine Rosen, "Why Not Artificial Wombs?," *The New Atlantis* 3 (Fall 2003), 67–76, www.thenewatlantis.com/archive/3/TNA03-Rosen.pdf.

58. Linda Geddes, "Womb-on-a-chip May Boost IVF Successes," *New Scientist* 2614 (2007): 28; Tan Ee Lyn, "Japan Scientists Devise 'Womb' for IVF Eggs," Reuters, July 27, 2007, www.reuters.com/article/scienceNews/idUSHKG27427920070727

59. David James, "Ectogenesis: A Reply to Singer and Wells," *Bioethics* 1 (1987): 80–99.

60. Peter Singer and Deane Wells, *The Reproduction Revolution: New Ways of Making Babies* (Oxford: Oxford University Press, 1984).

61. Amel Alghrani, "The Legal and Ethical Ramifications of Ectogenesis," *Asian Journal of WTO & International Health Law and Policy* 2, no. 1 (March 2007): 189–212, available at Social Science Research Network, www.ssrn.com/abstract=1019760.

62. Susumu Shimazono, "Why We Must Be Prudent in Researching Human Embryos: Differing Views of Human Dignity," in *Dark Medicine: Rationalizing Unethical Medical Research,* eds. William LaFleur, Gernot Bohme, and Susumu Shimazono (Bloomington: Indiana University Press, 2008), 201–216; Randall Parker, "Embryo Eugenics Finds New Uses," *Future Pundit,* May 9, 2007, www.futurepundit.com/archives/004241.html.

63. It should be noted here that Ikeda Shigenori, like many Japanese scientists and professionals, removed from his postwar résumé all references to his pre-1945 pro-eugenics activism. Nagai Hisomu, a physician who helped draft the 1940 National Eugenic Law, effectively erased from his postwar résumé his fervent and very public pro-sterilization lobbying during the 1930s and 1940s.

FURTHER READING

Chung, Yuehtsen Juliette. *Struggle For National Survival: Eugenics in Sino-Japanese Contexts, 1896–1945* (New York and London: Routledge, 2002).

Frühstück, Sabine. *Colonizing Sex: Sexology and Social Control in Modern Japan* (Berkeley, CA: University of California Press, 2003).

Hayashida, Cullen. *Identity, Race and Blood Ideology of Japan* (PhD diss., University of Washington, 1976).

Norgren, Tiana. *Abortion before Birth Control: The Politics of Reproduction in Postwar Japan* (Princeton, NJ: Princeton University Press, 2001).

Otsubo, Sumiko, and James Bartholomew, "Eugenics in Japan: Some Ironies of Modernity," *Science in Context* 11, no. 3–4 (1998): 545–565.

Robertson, Jennifer. "Japan's First Cyborg?: Miss Nippon, Eugenics, and Wartime Technologies of Beauty, Body, and Blood," *Body and Society* 7, no. 1 (2001): 1–34.

Robertson, Jennifer. "Blood Talks: Eugenic Modernity and the Creation of New Japanese," *History and Anthropology* 13, no. 3 (2002): 191–216.

Robertson, Jennifer. "Dehistoricizing History: The Ethical Dilemma of 'East Asian Bioethics,'" *Critical Asian Studies* 37, no. 2 (2005): 233–250.

Shimazono, Susumu. "Why We Must Be Prudent in Researching Human Embryos: Differing Views of Human Dignity," in *Dark Medicine: Rationalizing Unethical Medical Research,* eds. William LaFleur, Gernot Bohme, and Susumu Shimazono (Bloomington, IN: Indiana University Press, 2008), 201–216.

Tsuchiya, Takashi. "Eugenic Sterilizations in Japan and Recent Demands for Apology: A Report," *Newsletter of the Network on Ethics and Intellectual Disability* 3, no. 1 (1997): 1–4.

CHAPTER 26

EUGENICS IN INTERWAR IRAN

CYRUS SCHAYEGH

THROUGHOUT the first half of the twentieth century, modern educated Iranians expressed great concern about a two-tiered demographic problem besetting their country. This problem's fundamental, and most worrying, dimension was quantitative: estimated at around 10–12 million, Iran's population was considered too small.[1] The reason was not—as in some European countries—fertility decline, but a high mortality rate. A related second dimension was qualitative: of those Iranians who did survive into adulthood, a certain section was not healthy enough—or, in the more strict sense of "quality," purportedly suffered from a deficient hereditary disposition.[2]

The Iranian debate over eugenics was set in the larger framework of this double demographic concern. The importance of this anxiety notwithstanding, it is crucial, at this early point, to emphasize the limits of eugenics in Iran. The few Iranians proposing eugenic solutions identified themselves not as eugenicists, but as physicians with a social-reformist agenda. Moreover, there were in Iran no eugenic organizations or associations. What did exist, then, were mostly advisory texts, using eugenic ideas, a small number of newspaper articles and medical treatises directly referring to *puériculture* (a French term for positive eugenics) and to negative eugenics; and a much larger mass of texts (and a few laws) directed at the relation between health and demographics. In both categories, positive eugenics was dominant (*puériculture* explicitly mentioned only occasionally); nonetheless, some negative eugenic solutions *were* recommended, and a few legally implemented in all but name in the late 1930s.

In this chapter, I will first outline the "hygiene" roots of eugenics and *puériculture* in Iran and point out the social and political reasons why both arose in the 1920s. I will explain Iran's demographic problem, and list the variety of measures intended to tackle it, and demonstrate eugenics' explicit role in, and implicit effects on, these measures. In a second, analytical section, I will explain why modern middle-class ("modernist") physicians were the dominant socio-professional group responsible for the adaptation particularly of *puériculture*; and show how Iran's semi-colonial position affected its adaptation of eugenics. This placed Iran at the margins of international networks of scientific research and, at the same time, turned France into its paramount source of bio-medical education and social reformism.

HISTORICAL BACKGROUND, POLITICAL CONTEXTS, AND THE ROLE OF HYGIENE

In Iran, eugenics was not seen to be separate from or in conflict with hygienic measures. This firm link had historical and logical reasons: eugenics was adopted decades after the onset of a modern discourse about, and certain measures taken in favor of, hygiene and sanitation; in Iran as elsewhere, dominant positive eugenics pursued the same basic objective as hygiene, the improvement and growth of a population deemed weak and small.

The first serious institutional step in introducing modern medicine and hygiene in Iran was the foundation, in 1851, of a school of higher education. The Dar ol-Fonun included a medical section soon dominated by French physicians (Tehran University, including a Medical Faculty, was founded in 1935). Moreover, throughout the second half of the nineteenth century, Western powers pressured Iran's Qajar dynasty (1794–1926) to introduce sanitary controls at their borders. Since the late nineteenth century, modern-educated Iranian physicians started to take particular interest in national and international hygiene and sanitary control.[3] Thus, in the first decade of the twentieth century, some medical dissertations discussed both fields.[4] Likewise, in the later nineteenth century, European and Iranian Dar ol-Fonun professors of modern medicine had started to produce medical treatises.[5]

Historians tend to agree that in Qajar Iran, attempts to improve hygiene (as well as other reforms) were intermittent and fell short of the neighboring Ottoman Empire's more sustained policies. Administratively, for instance, the Iranian Conseil de Santé, founded in 1870 by the French physician and Dar ol-Fonun professor Tholozan, convened only at moments of crisis and soon fell into disuse. It was resuscitated, with the support of Muzaffar al-Din Shah Qajar (r. 1896–1907), only in 1904, as Conseil Sanitaire (CS).

It was only after World War I that bio-medical sciences, medicine, and hygiene really consolidated in Iran and, as importantly, were fed into a new vision of national progress. Various political and social processes explain this change. The new Pahlavi dynasty, founded by Reza Shah (r. 1921/1926–1941), and an emerging modern middle class wished to distance themselves, both from the presumably ineffective Qajars and from the Constitutional Revolution (1905–1911). The modernists acknowledged this political revolution's success in establishing a parliament, but deplored that it "confirmed that the dominance of an ignorant majority is the source of Iranian backwardness."[6] In their view, this sorry state of affairs—peaking with enemy armies' invasion of neutral Iran during World War I—could be corrected only by science-based sociocultural reforms. Both the social and the political conditions for such reforms materialized following World War I, when the end of Russian and British meddling in Iran—part of the nineteenth-century Great Game in Central Asia—created a political vacuum. It was filled by Reza Shah's increasingly autocratic modernist state, which was staffed by modernists—that is, the very class clamouring for encompassing science-based sociocultural reforms. It was under these circumstances that in the 1920s, the older science of hygiene (*'ilm-i bihdasht*) was invigorated and paired up with eugenics as part of a larger attempt to modernize Iran through the application of bio-medical knowledge.[7]

IRAN'S DEMOGRAPHIC PROBLEM

In 1908, Mohammed Hassan Khan *Hakim-ad-Dowleh* argued in his Paris medical dissertation *Grossesse, accouchement, et puériculture en Perse* that

> Children's *puériculture* still needs to be introduced to Persia. Children nurture themselves, so to say. It is not that parents are not attached to their children. Far from it: especially the Persian woman adores her child. But she has no clue about the rules of hygiene and takes care of her child through a routine condemned by the facts: it is the certain cause of an enormous infant mortality depopulating our country. *Persia's population is not increasing because of that infant mortality.* The Persian woman is an excellent reproducer, fortunately does not know Malthusian or neo-Malthusian methods, and thus has many children. But this advantage is destroyed by the fact that fifty per cent—and more—of children die in their early years.[8]

What is interesting, at this juncture, is not so much that Mohammed Hassan Khan *Hakim-ad-Dowleh* trained at the Parisian clinique Baudelocque—workplace of Adolphe Pinard, who reintroduced the concept of *puériculture* in 1895—but the way he linked *puériculture* to hygiene, and both to demographic issues. His central concern—the neutralization of high birthrates by high mortality rates—remained at the core of demographic debate into the 1940s; infant mortality was a particular worry.[9] Iran's problem of underpopulation distinguished it from another Middle Eastern country, Egypt, already concerned about overpopulation in the interwar period.[10] Iranians, on the other hand, feared that their country's population was too small in relation to its vast surface and a grave threat to its social and economic viability.[11] Authors regularly underlined the difference between demographic problems in Iran and most Western countries, that is, between high mortality in Iran and low fertility elsewhere. They commented on Malthus and on the absence of demographic (neo)-Malthusianism in Iran; on demographic reasons for Western colonialism, the West's

low mortality but parallel falling birthrate, and European measures against depopulation; and, not least, on non-Western countries (for example, Japan's) success in
decreasing mortality and increasing population.[12] Overall, they agreed that Iran's
demographic question could only be solved through change. As Dr. Rizazadih Shifaq
commented in 1933, "As long as a country's conditions of life and its bases of
subsistence do not progress...the more the number of persons (alive) rises, the more
distress, pain, and diseases rise, too."[13] In the eyes especially of the modern middle
class, Iran needed better informed parents and a correction of the high mortality rate
by various reforms.[14]

Hygienic and Eugenic Countermeasures to the Demographic Problem

It was here that eugenics and hygiene entered the frame, clustered around two measures. The measures of the first cluster guided women during and following pregnancy. Epitomizing hygiene and occasionally referring to *puériculture,* experts
wedded self-monitoring (nutrition, breast-feeding, infant hygiene) with intervention by an external party (regular medical checkups by a physician) and put emphasis
on demographic quantity as well as quality. The second cluster included medical
examination of prostitutes and two negative eugenic measures: marriage health certificates and support for sterilization (sterilization, however, never became official
policy). Both measures involved a high degree of coercion by state agencies and by
the medical profession, and focused on demographic quality.

It should be noted that texts on sterilization particularly addressed negative
eugenics more often than *puériculture,* which was mostly found in texts on, and for,
child-bearing women. However, maternally focused measures were more important: they preceded the second cluster, were written about much more often, and
had a considerably wider effect. In *this* sense, *puériculture* had a greater, though
more implicit, effect in Iran than negative eugenics—a fact that made sense in the
context of modernist Iranians' concern about small population.

Positive Eugenics: *Puériculture* and the Particular Role of Women

The credo regularly underlined by authors of medical texts was that women were in
greater need of hygienic education and had more responsibility toward their body
and mind than men. Highlighting women's duty to monitor their sexual organs and

visit a physician for regular checkups, they argued that a woman's womb and her sexual organs are "first, the child's initial nurture ground…and, second, have a total and general influence on women's health."[15]

The demographic context of women's health becomes even more obvious in texts on pregnancy, which often featured in general texts on women's health.[16] On the other hand, articles on demography, stressing the role of hygiene in lowering the high mortality rate, often emphasized the particular responsibility of pregnant women for their health. Syphilis was cited as a major risk, especially for the fetus and for new-born children; pregnant women's poor constitution and bad social conditions were seen as a major factor for miscarriages and high mortality during childbirth; weak women were said to run high risks during pregnancy.[17] Obviously, such dangers called for prevention. Sports was one method to keep women fit; more important yet was correct nutrition and mental and physical rest:

> If the pregnant woman belongs to the working class, she should minimalize her
> work as much as possible, especially during the last two months of pregnancy,
> because a mother's work impedes a foetus' natural development, and the child
> who does see the light of the earth is weak and often dies soon…Public gatherings,
> theatres, cinema, and the like have a negative influence on the pregnant woman.
> For some (pregnant women) travel is harmful, causing miscarriages.[18]

The general view that pregnant women should abstain from work and agitation was tuned to a key aspect of Pinardian *puériculture, l'hérédité utérine.* Unlike "*l'hérédité conceptionelle*…transmitted by the parents" to the child, "*hérédité utérine*…[is] transmitted from the mother to the embryo.…That second form, which [Pinard] judged to be as important as the first one, can be significantly improved by the pregnant woman [being allowed to] rest."[19] A number of Iranian physicians adhered to the thesis of *hérédité utérine* and Pinard's recommendations to pregnant women.[20]

Mohammed Hassan Khan *Hakim-ad-Dowleh*'s *Grossesse, accouchement, et puériculture en Perse* was an early text recommending Pinard. While stressing the importance of *puériculture*'s third, postnatal phase, he also addressed its pregnancy-related phase, and the effects of work as well. On the one side, he complained that "pregnancy is considered to be such a natural and banal physiological state that no [type of] hygiene is especially devoted to it. The Persian woman is treated like a woman from the early ages [of humankind]." On the other side, he held that the lack of "fatigue" provided the Persian woman "with good conditions for the normal development of her pregnancy."[21] This assurance did not stand the test of time, however. In a 1940 medical thesis submitted at Tehran University, M.-H. Vahidi lamented that in Iran, most pregnant women were unable to rest.[22] In a newspaper series on health and demographics, Dr. Mirkhani made the same lament and gave pregnant women advice that explicitly referred to *puériculture.*[23]

Better care and knowledge of women during pregnancy was complemented by improved conditions during birth. Mohammed Hassan Khan *Hakim-ad-Dowleh* discussed the risks of birth in early-twentieth-century Iran,[24] and his recommendations were often reiterated in later years. For him, the establishment of schools for midwives was "an overriding public and national interest," particularly because birth was normally handled by women. In the late 1920s, the women's journal *Piyk-i sa'adat-i nisvan* still deplored the shortage of modern midwives and reviled the traditional *qabilih*, lamenting that "after giving birth, many of our dear [women] have died due to the lack of a knowledgeable midwife."[25] By 1935, however, *Danishkadih-yi qabiligi* (College for Midwifery, established in 1930) had become a vital part of Tehran's *Marizkhanih-yi nisvan* (Women's Hospital). Other institutions focusing on educating midwives and assisting women in childbirth complemented the picture.

Enhanced infant care constituted a third component of the cluster of measures directed at women. In general, it was argued that most mothers were insufficiently informed about the hygienic needs of their newborn and infant children.[26] Many authors sought to redress this situation. They paid special attention to nutrition, and particularly to the advantages and conditions of breast-feeding, severely criticized wet nurses, and went so far as to define a woman's refusal to breast-feed as "treason" to both the child and the nation.[27] Breast-feeding highlights the link between health care and demography, and the role of positive eugenics and *puériculture*. Thus, Dr. Mirkhani provided an explicit analysis of the third (post-natal) stage of *puériculture*, providing painstakingly detailed descriptions of the chemical composition of mother's milk, the vitamins it contained, its difference from cow's-milk, and the dangers of trusting a wet nurse to replace the mother.[28] In this view, postnatal *puériculture* was instrumental in Iran's demographic progress.

NEGATIVE EUGENICS: MARRIAGE HEALTH CERTIFICATES AND STERILIZATION

A second cluster of countermeasures to Iran's demographic problem included medical supervision of prostitutes and two negative eugenics measures: marriage health certificates and support for sterilization, which, although directly referring to negative eugenics, never became official policy. Crucial differences separated the first from the second cluster. Measures in the former were meant to boost the number of Iranians surviving pregnancy, birth, and childhood, and thus targeted women and the fetus/newborn after conception; the latter were meant to improve future children's genetic quality and thus concentrated on parents before conception.

Several debates informed the championing of negative eugenics. First, there was a scientific understanding that defective parental genetic setup was liable to damage a child. Venereal diseases and alcoholism were key factors understood to damage parents and injure their offspring. A second context was the awareness of European syphilophobia, arising around 1880, and the related measures—mainly mandatory pre-matrimonial health certificates—that were at least partly implemented, in some European countries, to combat venereal diseases. Recurrent remarks about Western ways of dealing with venereal diseases appear to indicate that Iranians' perception of the problem in Iran was influenced by awareness of the apprehension it was causing in Europe.[29] A third debate concerned the relative importance of social/environmental milieu versus genetic heredity in shaping the human being, as well as the link between different genetic theories and divergent eugenic approaches. The Iranian modernists—while generally underwriting the neo-Lamarckian thesis that milieu and heredity hold equal weight, and that the milieu's effects on a person's genetic structure are heritable to his or her offspring—in certain cases attributed greater weight to heredity. However, this approach was all but marginal. It appeared in only a small number of texts, and solely in the context of the application of genetics for eugenics; even there, it was never wholeheartedly endorsed. Mandatory marriage medical certificates were advocated in many different texts, including newspaper articles, medical treatises, and commentaries published in women's journals. An example of the last is the story, by Mrs. Mihran, a contributor to the Tehrani weekly, *Ittila'at-i haftigi,* of her marriage:

> Since [our marriage],…we knew how grave and responsible a duty the establishment of a family is.…We used to talk together about…(our future) children…[and] both of us, without the slightest excuse or evasion, visited the physician, asking him to subject us to a complete examination, and to assure us about our health.[30]

The women's journal *'Alam-i nisvan* had been calling for medical certification since the early 1920s.[31] Women's organizations helped to promote certificates, and some women's societies lobbied for such laws in the highest political circles.[32] While the issue was raised during the preparation of a new marriage law in the mid-1930s, respective endeavors bore fruit only in October 1938, with the introduction of a law ordering bridegrooms and brides to obtain a certificate of wellness from a state-licensed physician.[33]

Physicians themselves advanced the idea of a pre-marital health check. Some stressed the danger of hereditary diseases; others referred to European countries, where mandatory or voluntary pre-marital health checks headed the list of measures suggested or adopted to impede the further spread of venereal diseases and to advance the "quality" of the population.[34] Often, they emphasized individual responsibility in obtaining certificates. They called on spouses to seek examination from a trustworthy physician, and held that a syphilitic person could marry only if he had enjoyed medical treatment for at least 18 months and had thereafter not suffered from a new attack for another 18 months. Physicians called on heads of family to obtain health certificates before the wedding and to allow physicians to check their family's younger members at least twice a year. They even appealed to men's "honor," asking them to defer marriage as long as they suffered from venereal diseases.[35]

In the late 1930s, newspaper articles on marriage health certificates were published with increasing frequency, mostly in connection with the October 1938 law.[36] Authors emphasized the role of health certificates in preserving a healthy individual and shaping a strong nation and race. The underlying claim held that individuals' strength or weakness directly influenced the nation.[37] However, measures to fortify an individual were seen to benefit both individuals and their offspring—a point that occasionally escalated into open attacks on syphilitic children and the need to prevent syphilitic parents from procreating.[38] Another argument highlighted the state's role in creating the legislative and administrative conditions for the introduction of mandatory marriage health certificates,[39] but at the same time continued to underline the importance of the individual's cooperation.[40] Authors also called on sick parents to abstain from procreating until they had been successfully medically treated. In this context, "eugenic" abortion was also discussed[41] but did not become law.

While texts rarely recommended the introduction of sterilization to Iran, authors did express support for the sterilization policies adopted in some Western countries. In 1921, for example, 'Ali Dashti advocated the idea of "active euthanasia" (by which he probably meant sterilization, since euthanasia in the sense of killing people considered to procreate "deficient" children and thereby damage society was not discussed in the West in the early 1920s). He argued that euthanasia is "an ethical theory which is dictated by the principle of the common good: after all, 'will the tuberculous, the weak and infirm, the hysterical people, and those suffering from anaemia have any other effect on society but to damage and weaken further generations and to impair the race?' "[42]

Other authors referred to sterilization in the context of mostly English and (since 1933 radicalized) German negative eugenics. Although a few mentioned that sterilization was practiced in some American states and in Sweden,[43] it was Nazi Germany that was foregrounded. In July 1933, a new German law had laid the legal grounds for radical negative eugenic actions, inter alia lifting Weimar Germany's prohibition of compulsory sterilization, now managed by medical committees.[44] One Iranian author highlighted the "negative" eugenic nature of this new law preventing mentally retarded and so-called "natural" criminals from procreating in order to improve the population's quality, and underlined their difference from the "positive" eugenic Weimar laws that had encouraged population growth. The author then related the idea and practice of sterilization to the development and aims of negative eugenics and concluded that "there evidently is no doubt that this movement, based on a reform of social life, is crucial [and] will, over time, profoundly affect [humankind]."[45] However, not everyone was confident about the glories of a eugenically organized society. One physician who theoretically supported abortion on negative eugenic indications ended up rejecting it because genetics was not yet able to provide reliable information on the "quality" of a fetus.[46]

EUGENICS AND SOCIAL CLASS

Two decades ago, Mark Adams drew a comparative map "uncovering the diversity of historical eugenics.... In the decades between 1890 and 1930, eugenics movements developed in more than thirty countries.... In some places, eugenics was dominated by experimental biologists, in others by animal breeders, physicians, pediatricians, anthropologists, demographers, or public health officials."[47] In Iran, physicians—an influential profession in the modern middle class, emerging since around the 1920s—were the main advocates of eugenics. This was unsurprising given their generally important role, as private individuals and often as state functionaries, in using bio-medical knowledge for social reforms.

Physicians discussed positive eugenics not only in professional texts like Mohammed Hassan Khan *Hakim-ad-Dowleh*'s *Grossesse, accouchement, et puériculture en Perse*. They did so also in newspapers. Texts on positive eugenics like Mirkhani's series "The Need of Healthy People for Population Increase" had a crucial element in common with articles on negative eugenics (and, for that matter, hygiene): they evinced a clear and public bias by Iran's modern middle class against the country's lower classes.

Indeed, the debate about negative and positive eugenics as well as hygiene had a larger context: whether explicitly (sterilization, *puériculture*) or implicitly (marriage medical certificates), it formed part of the modernists' mission, together with the state, to educate the lower social strata about their health. This undertaking involved crucial questions about what "the people" (*tudih*) should know. Although health education progressed in the interwar period, it had clear limits. Reaching out to and educating the urban and rural lower classes in a short time was no easy task: distances were large, finances short, manpower limited, and political will weak. While municipalities expanded their networks of free medical dispensaries and hospitals from the 1920s, Reza Shah had priorities other than health, especially the armed forces. As for the modern middle class, extremely few physicians wished to practice outside the larger cities or indeed in lower-class districts. Modernist authors often argued that although the lower social strata should be better informed about questions of health, they needed only basic practice-oriented advice to allow them to correct their habits. Detailed knowledge and the theoretical foundations of modern scientific health had to remain the privilege of the modern middle class— key to their cultural distinction, access to professional markets, and social status: "[O]ne must make the *bases of hygiene* understandable to the people."[48]

CONCLUSION

Since the nineteenth century, the presence of European educational, scientific, and medical specialists in Iran was both more limited and less exploitative than in fully colonized countries. Iran's semi-colonial position saved it from the kind of institutional, administrative, political, and budgetary control that European powers exercised in their colonies; at the same time, however, due to that position, Iran could not play an active role in unequal but nonetheless integrated metropolitan-colonial networks of scientific exchange.

Eugenics in Iran reflected this basic fact: internal debates never formed an active part in international discussions about eugenics. And yet, Mohammed Hassan Khan's medical training with Adolphe Pinard, as well as the references to European and American eugenics in medical and popular texts exemplify that Iranians were aware of developments in the world of European science, in "applied" sciences like eugenics, and in related models of social reform.

The acculturation of French *puériculture* (rather than, say, full-fledged negative eugenics) was conditioned partly by the dominant role of French medicine since the mid-nineteenth century, both in Iran in the form of French physicians, and in France in the form of Iranian students. But *puériculture* did not "reach" Iran as part of a mechanical process of diffusionism:[49] it was appropriated because its underlying logic—the need for population growth—suited Iran's particular demographic problems. In this sense, then, the story of eugenics in Iran, although minor compared to most countries, illustrates how even at the fringe of international scientific and social-reformist networks, (semi)-colonial modernist elites were able to make certain choices about the nature and composition of their specific agendas of modernization.

NOTES

1. In the 1950s, population *increase* became Iran's principal demographic worry.

2. For example see Muhammad-ʿAli Tutya, "Maram-i ma" [Our platform], *Sihhat-nama-yi Iran* 1, no. 1 (March 1933): 2–3.

3. Amir Afkhami, *Iran in the Age of Epidemics: Nationalism and the Struggle for Public Health, 1889–1926* (PhD diss., Yale University, 2003); Firoozeh Kashani-Sabet, "Hallmarks of Humanism: Hygiene and Love of Homeland in Qajar Iran," *American Historical Review* 105, no. 4 (2000): 1171–1203.

4. Ardachir Khan Nazare-Aga, *Contribution à l'étude des conférences sanitaires internationales dans leurs rapports avec la prophylaxie des maladies pestilentielles en Perse* (Paris: Vigot Frères, 1903); Ali Khan, *Choléra en Perse, Prophylaxie et traitement* (Paris: Imprimérie de la Faculté de médecine, 1908); Mirza Abbas Khan Alam ol-Molk, *Taoun (Peste). Étude sur la peste en Perse* (Paris: Imprimérie des Facultés, 1908).

5. Hormoz Ebrahimnejad, *Medicine, Public Health, and the Qājār State: Patterns of Medical Modernization in Nineteenth-Century Iran* (Leiden: Brill, 2004), especially about the complex relationship between traditional and modern medicine. For references to medical treatises, see Mariam Ekhtiar, *The Dār ol-Fonun: Educational Reform and Cultural Development in Qajar Iran* (PhD diss., New York University, 1994) and Willem Floor, *Public Health in Qajar Iran* (Washington, DC: Mage, 2004).

6. Mushfiq Kazimi, "Inqilab-i ijtimaʿi," *Farangistan* 1, no. 1 (1924): 6.

7. Cyrus Schayegh, *Who Is Knowledgeable Is Strong: Science, Class, and the Formation of Modern Iranian Society, 1900–1950* (Berkeley, CA: University of California Press, 2009).

8. Mohammed Hassan Khan *Hakim-ad-Dowleh, Grossesse, accouchement, et puériculture en Perse* (Paris: Imprimérie des facultés, 1908), 55 ["La puériculture de l'enfant est à créer en Perse; les enfants s'élèvent pour ainsi dire tout seuls; ce n'est pas que les parents ne soient pas attachés à leur enfants, loin de là; la femme persane en particulier adore son enfant, mais elle ignore les règles d'hygiène, et

soigne son enfant d'après une routine que les faits condamnent, parce qu'elle est cause certainement de l'énorme mortalité infantile qui dépeuple notre pays. *La Perse n'augmente pas de population à cause de cette mortalité infantile*; la femme persane est une excellente reproductrice, elle ignore heureusement les méthodes malthusiennes ou néo-malthusiennes; elle a donc de nombreux enfants; mais cet avantage est détruit par ce fait que 50% des enfants et plus meurent dans la première enfance." My translation; italics in original].

9. For a paradigmatic statement about the importance of infant mortality for the general demographic predicament, see S. Anvari, *Marg-i atfal dar Iran va rahha-yi jilu-giri-yi an [Infant mortality in Iran and methods for its prevention]* (PhD diss., Tehran University, 1937), 7.

10. Omnia El-Shakry, *The Great Social Laboratory: Subjects of Knowledge in Colonial and Postcolonial Egypt* (Stanford, CA: Stanford University Press, 2007).

11. "Ayandih-i Tehran" [Tehran's future], *Ayandih* 1, no. 6 (125): 378–79; A. Malekpur, *Die Wirtschaftsverfassung Irans* (PhD diss., Universität Berlin, 1935), 100, 104; A.-H. Bahriman, *Vasa'il-i afsaiyish-i nufus dar Iran [Methods for population increase in Iran]* (PhD diss., Tehran University, 1937/38), 24, 50; "Himayat-i kudakan" [Protecting the children], *Ittila'at*, February 16, 1935.

12. "Taqlil-i nufus" [Population decline], *Ittila'at*, September 2, 1937; Dr. Rizazadih Shifaq, "Mas'alih-yi izdiyad va sihhat-i nufus," [The problem of the population's increase and health] *Sihhat-nama-yi Iran* 1, no. 3 (1933–1934): 56–58; "Izdiyad-i nufus-i Zhapun" [The increase of Japan's population], *Ittila'at*, February 21, 1934; Dr. Mirkhani, "Luzum-i afrad-i salim bara-yi taksir-i jam'iyat" [The need for healthy people for population increase], *Ittila'at*, December 25, 1937; "Siyasat-i taqviyat va taksir-i nufus" [The politics of population reinforcement and increase], *'Asr-i iqtisad* year 2, no. 132 (1944): 3.

13. Shifaq, "Mas'alih," 54–55.

14. M. Chiluiāns, *Siqt-i mukarrar dar Iran* [Recurring abortion in Iran] (PhD diss., Tehran University, 1946), 1.

15. "Rahnama-yi sihhi bara-yi banuvan" [Health guide for ladies], *Ittila'at*, February 6, 1936; cf. the feminist Sadiqih Dawlatabadi, "Jahan-i zanan" [Women's world], *Iranshahr* 2, no. 1 (1923): 18–19.

16. Mrs. Tarbiyat, "Khatabih-yi Khanum-i Tarbiyat" [A speech by Mrs. Tarbiyat], in *Khatabihha-yi kanun-i banuvan dar sal-e 1314s* [Speeches at the Women's Society in the year 1935/36] (Tehran: Majles, 1936), 43.

17. Dr. A. A'lam, "Bihdasht-i khanivadigi" [Family hygiene], *Ittila'at*, August 26, 1940; M. Kazim-Khatami, *Bihdasht-i ijtima'i-yi kudakan dar bachegi-yi nakhust* [The social hygiene of children during the first phase of infancy] (PhD diss., Tehran University, 1937), 18–21.

18. "Nasaih-i sihhi bih nisvan-i hamilih" [Health advice for pregnant women], *Salnamih-yi Pars* 6 (1931–1932): 108.

19. Anne Carol, *Histoire de l'eugénisme en France: Les médecins et la procréation, XIX-XX siècles* (Paris: Seuil, 1995), 47–48.

20. Bahriman, "Vasa'il," 43; M.-H. Vahidi, *Ravish-i 'amali-sakhtan-i parvarish-i kudakan dar Iran* [A method for the practical realization of puériculture in Iran (French title: *La puériculture en Iran*)] (PhD diss., Tehran University, 1940), 6; H. Basiqi, *Bihdasht-i nuzad [Hygiene of the newborn]* (PhD diss., Tehran University, 1945), 17; Dr. Mirkhani, "Luzum," *Ittila'at*, December 22, 1937.

21. Mohammed Hassan Khan, *Grossesse*, 37; for Pinard, see idem, 96.

22. Vahidi, *Ravish*, 6–7; cf. Basiqi, *Bihdasht*, 16–17, 34.

23. Mirkhani, "Luzum," *Ittila'at*, December 20, 22, 1937.

24. Mohammed Hassan Khan, *Grossesse*, chaps. 3–5.

25. "Qismat-i hifz al-sihhih. Hayat-i nisvan" [Health section. Women's life], *Piyk-i sa'adat-i nisvan* 1, no. 2 (1927/1928): 44.

26. Vahidi, *Ravish*, 53–57, 59; "Rahha-yi 'amali bara-yi bihbud-i nesl-i kishvar va jilugiri az talafat-i kudakan" [Practical measures for the improvement of the race and the prevention of children's mortality], *Jahan-i pizishki* 2, no. 2 (1948): 8–9.

27. A. Quli-ala, *Shir-dadan dar Iran va ta'sirat-i an [Breastfeeding in Iran and its effects]* (PhD diss., Tehran University, 1936), 3. Cf. Bahriman, *Vasa'il*, 45; Kazim-Khatami, *Bihdasht*, 39–59.

28. Dr. Mirkhani, "Luzum." His argument [about digestion and nutrition as the main causes of post-natal infant death can be consulted in the text published in *Ittila'at*, December 23, 1937. The articles about *puériculture* after birth begin at that date, too.

29. "Muzu'-i amraz-i tanasuli va tariqih-yi jilugiri-yi an" [The issue of venereal disease and their prevention], *Ittila'at*, October 19, 1934; Dr. Puya, "Marz-i sifilis," [Syphilis] *Ittila'at*, October 20, 1931.

30. Munir Mihran, "Chira farzandan-i man ziba hastand?" [Why are my children beautiful?] *Ittila'at-i haftigi*, no. 44, January 16, 1941.

31. Jasemin K. Rostam-Kolayi, *The Women's Press, Modern Education, and the State in Early Twentieth-Century Iran* (PhD. diss., University of California, 2000), 230.

32. Masturih Afshar, "Sihhat-i zan va atfal" [Women's and children's health], *'Alam-i nisvan* 12, no. 4 (1932): 198; "Tandurusti va zanashu'i" [Health and marriage], *Mihrigan* 1, no. 13 (1935): 14.

33. Also, a law for the prevention and fight of infectious diseases, passed in June 1941, included the compulsory treatment of venereal diseases, free medication available to needy patients, punishment for spreading venereal diseases, and periodic inspections of brothels.

34. Dr. 'A. Rashti, "Tavarus dar amraz va ta'sir-i an dar tavalud va tanasul" [(The impact of) heredity in diseases, and its influence on birth (rates) and reproduction], *Darman* 1, no. 1 (1936): 63–64; H. Reza'i, *Bimariha-yi maghz va ravan* [Cerebral and mental diseases], 3 vols. (Tehran: Taban, 1944), 1: 23.

35. Dr. 'Ali Khan Mustashfi, "Sifilis aya mu'alijih mishavad?" [Is there a cure for syphilis?], *Sihhat-nama-yi Iran* 1, no. 4 (1933): 102; Dr. Puya, "Kesani kih khud-ra az asib-i sifilis masun midanand?" [People who believe that they are immune against the damages of syphilis], *Ittila'at*, December 24, 1931. Cf. M.-'A. Tutya, *Amraz-i zuhravi [Venereal diseases]*, (Tehran: Fardin, 1931/32), 140–41; E. Nuzari, *Usul-i mu'alijat-i sifilis, va tariq-e jilugiri az sariyat-i an* [The bases of the treatment of syphilis, and methods for the prevention of its transmission], (Tehran: Ittihadiyih, 1931), 20–22.

36. Dr. Najat, "Guvahinamih-yi tandurusti" [Health certificate], *Ittila'at*, December 1, 1938); Dr. 'Abbas Adham A'lam al-Mulk, "Daftar-i sihhat, ya namih-yi tandurusti" [A (personal) health register], *Ittila'at*, 9 April 1936.

37. "Nisl-i salim" [A healthy progeny], *Ittila'at*, October 10, 1938; "Nizhad-i qavi va barumand" [A strong and fertile race], *Ittila'at*, October 12, 1938.

38. "Guvahinamih-yi tandurusti bara-yi zanashu'i" [A health certificate for marriage], *Ittila'at*, October 11, 1938.

39. M. [Probably Ittila'at's editor Mas'udi], "Tasdiq-sihhat-i mazaj" [Health certificate], *Ittila'at*, August 3, 1931; "Nisl-e salim"; "Nizhad-i qavi va barumand"; Najat, "Guvahinamih-yi tandurusti."

40. For state action, see Tutya, "Pishnihadat-i ma" [Our recommendations], *Sihhat-nama-yi Iran* 1, no. 6 (1933); for individual behavior, see Najat, "Guvahinamih-yi tandurusti"; "Dar piramun-i guvahinamih-yi tandurusti" [Concerning the health certificate], *Ittila'at*, October 15, 1938.

41. Dr. Gh. Musaddiq, "Mavarid-i javaz-i asqat-i jinin, az lihaz-i qaza'i, ijtima'i, mazhabi" [The issue(s) of the permission of abortions from legal, social, and religious points of view], *Darman* 2, no. 2 (1937): 53. Cf. Dr. Mustashfi, "Sifilis," 102; "Tandurusti va zanashu'i" [Health and marriage], *Mihrigan* 1, no. 13 (1935/36): 14; Dr. Mirkhani, "Luzum," *Ittila'at*, December 22, 1937.

42. Jutta Knörzer, *Ali Dashti's Prison Days: Life under Reza Shah* (Costa Mesa: Mazda, 1994), 78, citing the fifth edition of *Ayyam-i mahbas*, 108.

43. "'Aqim-kardan-i zan va mard" [The sterilization of women and men], *Ittila'at*, September 9, 1933; "'Aqim-kardan-i maraza va mujrimin" [The sterilization of sick people and criminals], *Ittila'at*, 2 September 1933. With regard to the United States, see also Knörzer, *Ali Dashti*, 78, showing how Dashti argued that in the name of social welfare, certain materialist philosophers have advocated the euthanasia of patients of contagious or congenital diseases, and that for this reason, some U.S. states require a medical examination prior to marriage.

44. "'Aqim-kardan-i maraza va mujrimin"; Az majallih-yi Spectre [From the magazine Spectre], "Ta'qim va qat'-i nisl-kardan-i maraza" [Sterilization or the interruption of sick person's procreation], *Ittila'at*, January 1, 1934.

45. "'Aqim-kardan-i maraza va mujrimin."

46. Musaddiq, "Mavarid," 53; cf. "'Aqim-kardan-i mard va zan."

47. Mark Adams, "Towards a comparative history of eugenics," in *The Wellborn Science: Eugenics in Germany, France, Brazil, and Russia*, ed. Mark B. Adams (New York: Oxford University Press, 1990), 217, 215.

48. "Ta'lim-i bihdasht bih mardum" [Educating the people about hygiene], *Ittila'at*, June 2, 1940.

49. George Basalla, "The Spread of Western Science," *Science* 156 (1967): 611–622.

FURTHER READING

Afkhami, Amir. *Iran in the Age of Epidemics: Nationalism and the Struggle for Public Health, 1889–1926* (PhD diss., Yale University, 2003).

Ebrahimnejad, Hormoz. *Medicine, Public Health, and the Qājār State: Patterns of Medical Modernization in Nineteenth-Century Iran* (Leiden: Brill, 2004).

El-Shakry, Omnia. *The Great Social Laboratory. Subjects of Knowledge in Colonial and Postcolonial Egypt* (Stanford , CA: Stanford University Press, 2007).

Floor, Willem. *Public Health in Qajar Iran* (Washington, DC: Mage, 2004).

Hakim-ad-Dowleh, Mohammed Hassan Khan. *Grossesse, accouchement, et puériculture en Perse* (Paris: Imprimérie des facultés, 1908).

Kashani-Sabet, Firoozeh. "Hallmarks of Humanism: Hygiene and Love of Homeland in Qajar Iran," *American Historical Review* 105, no. 4 (2000): 1171–1203.

Mirkhani, Dr. "Luzum-i afrad-i salim bara-yi taksir-i jam'iyat," [The need for healthy people for population increase] *Ittila'at*, December, 20, 21, 22, 25, 1937.

Schayegh, Cyrus. *Who Is Knowledgeable, Is Strong: Science, Class, and the Formation of Modern Iranian Society, 1900–1950* (Berkeley , CA: University of California Press, 2009).

CHAPTER 27

....

EUGENICS AND THE JEWS

....

RAPHAEL FALK

PROBLEMATIC as defining eugenics may be, defining Jews is even more so. According to Jewish law (Halachah), a Jew is one born to a Jewish mother or who lawfully converts to Judaism. The hereditary element of the laws indicates that those belonging to the Jewish religious-cultural sphere enumerate among their ancestors the ancient Jews of Biblical time. However, conversion to Judaism introduces other ancestral elements, the extension and sources of which are widely disputed. Jews have been for centuries rather isolated. Their persecution in and by many sectors of the Christian and Muslim world meant that they formed, or were forced to form, ethnically and socially separated communities. This semi-isolation led to inbreeding, although gene exchange with the surrounding non-Jews on the one hand, and with distant Jewish communities on the other, also occurred. Only in the recent past have Jews partly been emancipated and accepted into non-Jewish society, ostensibly as equal members. This did not diminish discrimination against them, however, and with the emergence of nationalism and the increasing biologization of interhuman relationships characteristic of the second half of the nineteenth century, claims that Jews were a different *race,* with distinct and inborn properties, grew in popularity.[1]

It was the German journalist and commentator Wilhelm Marr (1819–1904) who introduced the term "anti-Semitism" in his 1880 booklet *Der Weg zum Siege des Germanentums über das Judentum* (The Way to the Victory of Germanity over Jewishness). Subsequently, the traditional religious and sociocultural prejudices against Jews were increasingly reinterpreted as linked to inherent biological properties of the Jewish people as an alien, Semitic race. Many Jews, hoping to assimilate into non-Jewish societies, denied any distinct inborn qualities. Other Jews agreed that they may have distinct inherent characteristics, and the greater the opposition to their integration, the more the consciousness of their distinctiveness ignited their Jewish national flame. Following Volkist slogans of *Blut und Erde,* the Zionists insisted on the immanent right of people with distinct blood to claim a distinct homeland.

The role that eugenics has played in Jewish life, especially in shaping how Jews confronted the world when they left the ghettos, engaged Jewish and non-Jewish researchers alike. It was generally accepted that Jewish law had inbuilt regulations about reproduction that could be (and were) thought of as eugenic, and that the socioeconomic conditions in which Jews lived also had specific eugenic consequences. But it was the issue of the hereditary nature of the so-called Jewish traits and properties that made the difference between the expectations of the future fate of the Jews and of Judaism. Whereas in Nazi Germany Jewish life was systematically destroyed in the name of eugenics, Zionists in the Land of Israel conceived of eugenics as part of their mission to restore the Jewish people.

JEWISH EUGENICS

There was considerable enthusiasm for eugenics among Jewish scholars at the beginning of the twentieth century, many claiming a central role for eugenics in Jewish tradition since ancient times. Indeed, breeding problems have always occupied an important role in Jewish life: the need to secure the continuity of Judaism often gave community considerations priority over the interests and needs of individuals, and rabbis and physicians explicitly linked this tradition to the new "science" of eugenics. On the other hand, Jewish tradition and regulations were deeply committed to the care and welfare of individuals, and consequently also encouraged explicit dysgenic means. In a talk to the New York Board of Jewish Ministers on "Jewish eugenics" in 1915, for example, Rabbi Max Reichler (1885–1957) declared that "Jews, ancient and modern...have always understood the science of eugenics, and have governed themselves in accordance with it; hence the preservation of the Jewish race." Eugenic rules were incorporated, he thought, into the large collection of Biblical and Rabbinical laws. Conscious efforts were made to "improve the inborn qualities of the Jewish race, and guard against any practice that might vitiate the purity of the race."[2]

The attempt to limit the multiplication of "undesirable" elements resulted in prohibiting the marriages of "defectives by reason of heredity," and consanguineous marriages. The Talmud also forbade marrying into a confirmed leprous or epileptic family, or to a woman who had buried three husbands. Reichler considered that

> [t]he distinctive feature, however, of Jewish eugenics lies in the greater emphasis
> laid on the psychical well-being of posterity, in contradistinction to merely
> physical well-being which is the chief concern of modern eugenists.[3]

The marriage between the offspring of what Reichler called "inferior" and "superior" stock, for example the marriage between a scholar and the daughter of an *am-haarez* (ignorant), was condemned as extremely undesirable. Thus the rabbis "endeavored by direct precept and law, as well as by indirect advice and admonition, to preserve and improve the inborn, wholesome qualities of the Jewish race."[4] Rabbis' ideal was "a race healthy in body and in spirit, pure and undefiled, devoid of any admixture of inferior protoplasm," although they were "willing to concede that 'a pure-bred individual may be produced by a hybrid mated with a pure bred'" as in the case of Ruth the Moabitess, among whose progeny was King David.[5] Reichler's ideas were extensively reported in the March 1917 issue of the *Journal of Heredity*:

> Throughout its history, the Jewish race has been subject to vicissitudes greater than those which have caused the disappearance of many another people…Racial survival under such difficulties, and racial continuity in so varied environments, must permit explanation in terms of eugenics, and Rabbi Max Reichler…has attempted such an interpretation.[6]

The philosopher Rabbi Noam Zohar believes that Reichler's paper gives voice to certain understandings of lineage and of Jewish identity that are not uncommon in Jewish circles even today.[7]

In 1911, Maurice Fishberg (1872–1934), a Russian-born American physician and anthropologist, published a book on *The Jews: A Study of Race and Environment*.[8] As Fishberg examined the popular understandings of the Jews, he concluded that Jews were in no way fundamentally different, except insofar as their religious practices and social environment (produced by their persecutions, he argued) created a difference in appearance. Indeed, Fishberg, as reported by the *New York Times,* was "at pains to prove that the Jews, so far from being a pure race, have throughout their history intermingled with the races among whom they dwelt."[9] In the December 1917 issue of the *Journal of Heredity,* Fishberg reiterated his notion of eugenics in Jewish life. Referring explicitly to Reichler's work, he commented:

> I do not know of any other social or religious aggregate that encouraged and practiced positive eugenic life to such an extent as the Jews did in the Ghetto. Most of the Rabbinical teachings are teeming with positive eugenic suggestions and one is inclined to say that the rabbis anticipated Galton by about sixteen hundred years.[10]

But in addition to medieval Jews' ideals of marriage, centered on an interest in intellect in considering marriage and reproduction, Fishberg also noted "strong and active dysgenic tendencies" which "encourag[ed] the proliferation of an enormous number of physical and mental defectives among the children of the Ghetto."[11]

The physician J. Snowman also emphasized that "Judaism and Eugenics are in complete accord, in encouraging the marriage of the fit." He claimed eugenics to be "an ultra-modern form" of Jewish wedding ceremony, "conducted on principles of careful selection."

> Although ancient Jewish practice did not demand a certificate of good health from the parties contracting a marriage, as present-day Eugenists advocate, the old records show that the Rabbis entertained opinions which certainly tended in that direction.[12]

As late as 1939, W. M. Feldman, senior physician at St. Mary's Hospital in London, proclaimed the virtues of "ancient Jewish eugenics." Contrary to Greeks and Romans who, according to Feldman, applied to the human race methods of animal breeding (including eugenic infanticide), the ancient Hebrews

> infused a humanitarian spirit into their system, and by tempering their eugenics with mercy, and combining judicious selective mating with intelligent antenatal and postnatal care, they succeeded in rearing a race...which is the most virile that ever lived, and which has survived at times when many other...races, not subjected to anything like the same persecution and physical as well as mental stress and torture, have perished.[13]

Feldman enumerated in detail the eugenic practices and precautions of the ancient Jews, from the rabbis' opinion that there was no "animation" in the fetus before the 40th day (so that induction of abortion at this stage was not a criminal offense), to the Talmudic commentator according to whom a woman could be sterilized if she was likely to bear children with mental or physical disease.[14] He stressed, however, that although these principles were recommended, they were not sufficiently accurate to be ritually enforced.

Feldman noted that of the 613 Talmudic precepts, those dealing with reproduction were the most important. Jews were wiser than the Greeks, he thought, in encouraging early marriages, "since not only do early marriages tend to obviate impure living, with all its dysgenic consequences...but there is some statistical evidence to the effect that the children of mothers who married young are stronger than the average." Although purposeful avoidance of pregnancy for other than eugenic reasons was condemned, Feldman explained, contraception was permitted when a pregnancy was considered harmful to the mother or to an infant she was nursing.[15]

Feldman declared that his was an attempt to assess the genetic principles of "Rabbinical eugenics" both with respect to earlier Rabbinical thought, and in the light of "modern knowledge."[16] Yet Zohar concludes that these views were one-sided, and, particularly, that they suppressed "traditional critiques of lineage and of the notion of 'Jewish race.'"[17] Thus claims for the eugenic spirit of the ancient Jewish law must be considered more as latter-day interpretations than any immanent expression of eugenic insights.

Jewishness: Nature or Nurture?

The rationale of eugenics in Jewish life depended on the extent to which social, political, religious, or cultural distinctiveness was considered to reflect biological-racial factors. The breakdown of religious and to some extent social ties among Jews, along with attempts to find an "enlightened" and "scientific" definition of Jews, encouraged Jewish intellectuals to participate in studies of the anthropological status of their brethren. But the agenda of Jewish and non-Jewish scholars was different: the latter usually established the distinct racial uniqueness of the Jews, whereas many Jewish scholars argued that Jews were the products of cultural-social, rather than racial-biological processes. In central Europe of the 1820s, a new "Science of Judaism" (*Wissenschaft des Judentums*) was introduced. Its founder, Leopold Zunz (1794–1886), was convinced that Jews' low status was a consequence of non-Jewish ignorance of the cultural richness of Judaism. Abraham Geiger (1810–1874), the founder of the Berlin School of the Science of Judaism in 1872, insisted on a universal conception of Judaism, rejecting Jewish biological distinctiveness and any national implications from his teachings.[18] Other Jewish researchers, however, insisted that Jews were biologically distinct. For example, the anthropologist and researcher of Jewish folklore, Joseph Jacobs (1854–1916), claimed that the Jews' poor physical condition and characteristics were inherited consequences of persecution and the dire living conditions of the ghetto. Indeed, Jacobs cooperated with Galton in producing composite images of the "Jewish type."[19] Significantly, although they agreed that there was something intrinsic in the image of the Jew, for Galton this confirmed the impressions that "every one of them was coolly appraising me at market-value without the slightest interest of any kind." Jacobs, however, conceived an image of a dreamer or thinker rather than that of a cold-blooded merchant.[20] Galton insisted that eugenics was a purely rational manifestation of the science of heredity, without subjective or moral foundations. When interviewed in 1910 by the *Jewish Chronicle*, Galton claimed that many of the laudable properties of the Jews were the consequence of persecutions. Asked: "Is it not rather immoral to look with satisfaction to persecution as an aid to race culture?" his answer was: "It is not immoral but unmoral—it has nothing to do with morals."[21]

Other Jewish scholars accepted that Jewish physical and psychical properties were inherited. Redcliffe Nathan Salaman (1874–1955), a British doctor and plant virus researcher, was an ardent eugenicist. In the first volume of the *Journal of Genetics* he claimed that tracking the progeny of Jewish-Gentile marriages demonstrated that Jewish facial features were inherited and transmitted as simple monogenic Mendelian property.[22] Salaman campaigned against other eugenicists for convincing the British people of the eugenic benefits of Jewish immigration from eastern Europe.[23]

The Warsaw neurologist Shneor Zalman Bychowski (1865–1934) also believed in the biological uniqueness of the Jews and in the need to take strict eugenic measures to avoid degeneration. However, in an article published in Hebrew in 1918 on "Nervous Diseases and the Eugenics of the Jews," Bychowski categorically denied the hereditary nature of the typical Jewish neuroses, despite the claims by "famous neurologists" that Jews tended to suffer from nervous diseases more than any other peoples. Bychowski rejected French neurologist Jean-Martin Charcot's suggestions of an inborn Jewish neurosis that he named "the Wandering Jew" (*le Juif errant*).[24] In addition to exogenic and endogenic factors for nervous disease, he identified perigenic causes—"factors that depend on the environment":

> Among the Jews of Russia and Poland we do not find the usual kind of struggle for existence encountered all over Europe. Their lives were a specific "Jewish" struggle for each piece of bread, for a sip of water to drink, and for some air to breath. This was a struggle for the privilege to overnight outside a goods-truck, for the right to enroll to school and even for the right to be healed.[25]

Evidence that these Jewish neuropathies were linked to the immediate living circumstances of eastern European Jews was that their progeny in New York were not afflicted by these diseases, although they fell prey instead to alcoholism and syphilis.[26]

As noted above, Maurice Fishberg's agenda was different. In his comprehensive study of race and environment, he contended that Jews were, in no essential way, different from other people. In his final chapter he strongly advocated assimilation which, by his own showing, "would practically result in the disappearance of the Jewish race within a comparatively few generations."[27] Fishberg did not doubt the disproportionally large number of Jewish individuals who gained distinction. But he was also immensely interested from the standpoint of eugenics in the fact that hereditary and degenerative defects were more frequent among Jews than among people of other faiths living under similar social and economic circumstances: "It is a matter of common observation that the Jews are physically puny—a large proportion are feeble, undersized; their muscular system is of deficient development with narrow flat chests, and of inferior capacity."[28] While conditions in the medieval ghetto placed a premium on intellect, an especially dysgenic precept, of which Fishberg was critical, was the tradition that "[e]very physical and mental cripple was...encouraged to marry and bring legitimate offspring into the world."[29] Nevertheless, Fishberg concluded that "'race' cannot be considered the cause for the social, economic, and pathological differences between the Jews and the peoples among whom they live."[30]

Compare Fishberg's conclusions with those of his contemporary, Arthur Ruppin (1876–1943), who in 1908 became the head of the Palestine Office of the Zionist Federation: "Have the Jews a right to a separate existence?...Can the Jews do more for humanity by remaining a separate nationality than by becoming absorbed in other nations?"[31] Ruppin's answer was that "Jews have not only preserved their great natural racial gifts, but through a long process of selection these gifts have become strengthened...The rich Jews of the Ghetto vied with one another for the most learned Talmudic scholars as husbands for their daughters, and thus insured the mental progress of the race. The result is that in the Jew of to-day, we have what is in some respects a particularly valuable human type."[32]

Many who claimed that the Jews did comprise a distinct biological-racial entity searched for the Jewish archetype (*Urjude*). But it was German anthropologists who adopted the notion most widely that a distinct Jewish archetype could be identified, and that accordingly eugenic implications may be drawn.

Starting in 1937 in a series of volumes titled *Forschungen zur Judenfrage* (Researches on the Jewish Problem), various aspects of this alleged "problem" were examined from a Germanic, more specifically, a Nazi perspective. In his "Racial Origin and Oldest History of the Hebrews," Eugen Fischer (1874–1967), the German professor of anthropology and eugenics, claimed that by racial cross-breeding "it was shown beyond doubt that the characteristics in question are transmitted without exception in accordance with Mendel's genetic laws... These racial characteristics, like all other inherited characteristics, are thus based on... 'genes.'" Qualifying this determinist eugenic position by noting that "the hereditary predisposition permits a certain range of reaction for its realization in actual development," Fischer overcame the hurdle of the obvious racial variability: "Races are groups of people with quite specific hereditary dispositions, which are purely hereditary in them, and which are lacking in other races."[33] Accordingly, he purported to trace the descent of the Semites and the Hebrews from prehistoric humanity.

Fischer's racial prejudices are hardly disguised by his so-called scientific phrasing: the *Nordisch* race which, according to Fischer, was caught up in the climatic change of the glacial periods in an extremely selective process under unfavorable conditions, became a battle-accustomed, special race of strong character.[34] Further to the south, however, Fischer traced the Mediterraneans, among whom the Orientals emerged, who in their turn contributed to the Jewish people:

> Considering the race as a whole, certain traits will become dominant here which are the inherent chief components of the racial mixture. Hence even in the early history of the Jewish people are seen the emotion, the hatred and the cruelty often developing into bloodlust of the part of the sheep raiser of the Orientaloid race along with the skill, adaptability, cunning and desire to dominate the city founder of the Near Eastern race. In this regard one must not forget the fanatic aspect of the monotheistic belief in Jehovah and the concept of being the chosen people, conceived and retained fanatically by desert nomads.[35]

As to the eugenic aspect, Fischer thought that only a concerted and active selection process following "racial interbreeding" could eliminate the genetics of race. "Without this strong selective process the individual racial elements that went into the mixture remain extant indefinitely."[36]

Otmar Freiherr von Verschuer (1896–1969), Fischer's colleague and successor at the Kaiser Wilhelm Institute for Anthropology, Human Heredity and Eugenics, contested Fishberg's conclusion that Jewishness was a religion rather than a race, and he rejected the claim of another Jew, Felix A. Theilhaber (1884–1956), that inbreeding "guarantees the only objective Jewish identification and maintains the racial nature of Jews, while the adherence to the Jewish religion represents the subjective aspect of belonging to the Jewish entity." Von Verschuer referred to Fischer, who showed that Jews "consist of a number of races which are contrasted as a foreign element to the races of our nation."[37] However, contrary to "characteristics that are absolutely typical of a race" which "clearly establishes the membership of a human being" such as "the black skin color of the Negro races" and "the slanting upper eyelid fold of the Mongolians," the variability among Jews and Germans overlaps, and "an individual characteristic by which a Jew could be recognized with absolute certainty is not known." A description of the Jews living in Central Europe, one that could "separate the genetic from the non-genetic characteristics in order to reach the objective of recognizing the genetic between Germans and Jews" was impossible. Nonetheless, he remained confident of the capacity to "diagnose" race correctly.[38]

Consideration of the purportedly dysgenic consequences of Jewish assimilation in the non-Jewish population, especially the threat of massive immigration of Jews from eastern Europe, was not limited to Germany and German experts. In England Karl Pearson published an intensive study on "The Problem of Alien Immigration into Great Britain, Illustrated by an Examination of Russian and Polish Jewish Children,"[39] the aim of which was to determine the desirability of indiscriminate further immigration into Britain. Noting the centrality of immigration to the project of national eugenics, Salaman, on the other hand, brought evidence that "would seem to show perhaps unequivocally that it is nature rather than nurture which is on the side of the Jewish suckling":[40]

> There has been a tendency to raise barriers against their admission. There would appear to be no question more suitable for the consideration of eugenics than this. The whole problem is a relatively simple one: are these emigrants people of value to the state or not? Do they bring promise of greater gifts beneath their tattered garments than the jaundiced eye of a relieving officer can appreciate?[41]

When A. G. Hughes contrasted Jews and Gentiles in 1928, he pointed out that his term "race" was not intended "to imply more than that the Jews have been a relatively inbreeding group for a long space of time." Nonetheless, he was interested in the differential incidence of certain disease between Jews and non-Jews, suggesting that Jews inherited a distinct physical constitution, probably dependent, he thought on "glandular balance" which produced particular "mental qualities." Turning to special abilities, he commented that Jews were credited with capacity in music, mathematics, and languages, but less in handwork, drawing and painting.[42] As to Pearson and Moul's claim to carry "no political, no religious and no social prejudices,"[43] Hughes found grave methodological problems with their study. It was based on teachers' estimates of the intelligence data of the children of recent immigrants, who spoke little English, and in any case different teachers assessed different children, making comparisons unreliable.[44] In Hughes's own comparative study of Jewish and non-Jewish children (boys and girls, age 8–13, at three different schools), the former proved to be superior to the latter in "intelligence and in attainments in English and arithmetic."[45]

ZIONISM AS EUGENICS

> Ever since Herzl…Jewish race feeling has received a new impetus all the world over. The Jewish problem, far from being, as hitherto, a mere sectarian question of a "peculiar people," has assumed a much wider, national importance, as behoves a race which once played such a great rôle among the nations of the world.[46]

A foremost preacher of degeneration at the fin-de-siècle was Max Nordau (1849–1923), the author of *Entartung* (Degeneration).[47] In this best seller, Nordau warned of the impacts of the industrial revolution—trains running at the mind-boggling speed of 35 kilometers per hour—and of urbanization—mayors having to handle populations of a size that had been the responsibilities of national ministers only a generation earlier. Nordau joined Theodor Herzl, the founder of political Zionism, in calling for a "New Jew" skilled in physical activities. He endorsed a Jewish *Sportsverin* and the turn to agriculture, rather than the traditional learning and business occupations of Jews.

Contrary to the assimilationists, the keepers of traditional Judaism, especially the Zionists, accepted that there were immanent Jewish characteristics, whether inherited from the ancient forefathers, or selected through living isolated for generations as persecuted communities. They argued that special efforts must be made to eliminate such characteristics, on the way to "becoming a Normal People" (a common expression in Zionist literature). Thus from its beginnings the Zionist effort to settle in the Promised Land was conceived as an explicit eugenic effort of the Jewish *Volk*. Most eloquent in perceiving these eugenic efforts were the settlers themselves. The educator Israel Rubin published a letter to physicians and educators in 1934, in the periodical of the Hebrew Authors' Association in Palestine, entitled "The ingathering of the exiles from a eugenic perspective."[48] Rubin viewed "our life in the homeland, in its very essence" to be "a great and courageous national effort in the eugenic sense."

> Anyone, who does not recognize the return of the sons to the land of their forefathers as a great *eugenic* revolution in the life of the nation, does not discern the "forest" from the individual trees...The essence is the sum total: *The production of a New Hebrew type* restored and improved. Thus, a *psychobiological approach to the problem of the settlement of Land of Israel* is a duty to us all![49]

And the physician Joseph Mayer, chief executive of the Labor Organization Sick Fund, the major health insurance fund for the Jews in Palestine, was explicit in his demand for eugenic measures, writing in 1934:

> Who has the right to give birth to children? Eugenics, the science for the improvement of the race and keeping it from degeneration, is concerned with searching for proper answers to this question...Now our nation is resurrected to life in nature in the homeland...For us "eugenics," and especially the prevention of transfer of hereditary diseases, is of even greater importance than it is for other nations!...Do not procreate children if you are not sure that they will be healthy in body and mind.[50]

But it was not only the settlers who were thoroughly imbued in the notions of eugenics. Bychowski, the Warsaw Zionist doctor who denied the genetic basis of eastern European Jews' neuroses, was explicit with respect to the proliferation of proven hereditary diseases and the threat to the settlers' community in Palestine, unless strict eugenic measures were introduced. He went so far as to recommend introducing immigration laws to Palestine that were similar to the infamous U.S.

regulations that became the nightmare of innumerable eastern Europeans who flocked to America:

> It is deplorable that we must mention here the habit spread among Polish and Lithuanian Jews, not to let a man remain bachelor even when he is sick and may transmit the disease to his progeny...This must be especially noted by those who construct the future of the nation—the Zionists. The resurrection of the nation in its homeland will be possible only if the "human material" that will go there will be healthy. In this respect it will be necessary to apply from the beginning strict means, like the "law" against immigration that has been introduced in the United States.[51]

In his function in the Zionist Federation, Arthur Ruppin endeavored to construct the Jewish population in Palestine on rational and sound foundations. He also sought careful regulation of "human material" for Palestine "so new generations will arise in the country that are healthy and strong."[52] As early as the 1920s, a network of physicians carried out medical inspections of immigration candidates. Young immigrants found to suffer from an illness that might adversely affect their chances of economic or social integration were (until the raise of the Nazis to power) denied immigration to Palestine.[53]

All this changed after World War II and the Holocaust.

EUGENICS OF THE JEWS TODAY

Although explicit eugenic efforts were abandoned after World War II, the interest in eugenics in general, and among Jews in particular, did not diminish. Neil Holtzman identifies a distinct continuity in the general perception of eugenics: "The old eugenics used sterilization of those individuals who it was presumed would transmit undesirable traits to their offspring. New eugenics depends on screening healthy carriers, prenatal diagnosis, and selective determination of affected fetuses."[54] Nonetheless, he does signal major differences. In the second half of the twentieth century, prenatal genetic counseling was performed on a strict personal basis: "Selective termination of fetuses that are predicted by prenatal diagnosis to develop future disease is more likely to be accepted by all segments of society than was the old eugenics of sterilization, which was disproportionately foisted on the poor."[55] As opposed to coercive eugenic measures,

> today's reproductive genetics or what Wertz has termed "voluntary eugenics" does not build on violence. Rather it builds on what is often understood to be the individual mothers' "autonomous" decision....The strategies of governmentality lead individuals to police themselves, as normal subjects that pursue their own interests, who seek self improvement, self-satisfaction, and health and happiness.[56]

When genetic screening for detection of carriers of single doses of gene-alternatives (alleles) that need both maternal and paternal contributions for the offspring to become involved in severe diseases introduced in the 1970s, they were often applied in populous Jewish centers in the United States and Canada. The allele related to Tay-Sachs is relatively frequent among Ashkenazi Jews, and these were also the communities in which "education, coercion, peer pressure, a captive audience or something else"[57] promised the best contribution to the success of the screening program.

The interest of present-day Jewish culture in eugenics is most clearly apparent in the juxtaposition of German and Israeli attitudes toward fertility-control technologies. Hashiloni-Dolev argues that German reception and implementation of new reproductive technologies is cautious and highly regulated, while Israeli medical and legal systems "welcome prenatal medical genetics in an almost completely uncritical manner."[58] Although some claim that this generous acceptance of fertility-control technologies emerged from the Zionist movement, "which strove for the rehabilitation of the weak Jewish body, and the Jewish religious tradition, which is intolerant toward physical disability,"[59] others insist that it is a reaction to the fatal loss of a third of the Jewish people in the Holocaust. "For most of the Israeli public and the vast majority of Israeli professionals, this kind of eugenics that was condemned in the past is seen to be in no relation whatsoever to contemporary practices."[60]

Hashiloni-Dolev believes that Israeli "secular" counselors are much more affected by Jewish tradition in their way of reasoning than they themselves imagine. She also reminds us that "Jewish religion is more supportive of reproductive genetics than may appear." Although most orthodox rabbis oppose selective abortions, they *do not* oppose measures that would avoid, to start with, the risk of producing pregnancies of disabled people.[61] As pointed out at the beginning of this chapter, the Talmud positively forbade what were considered to be high-risk marriages.

With respect to contemporary liberal regulations in Israel concerning embryonic stem cell research and human cloning, even when one takes into consideration political arguments like that of the "demographic threat" that the Jewish majority population in Israel will soon be outnumbered by non-Jews, there seems little doubt that these are related to a religious conception that deems such considerations as "morally unproblematic."[62] Indeed, Israeli genetic counselors made an exception to the usual screening ethics in a program designed for screening the ultra-Orthodox Ashkenazi Jewish community. The worldwide Dor-Yesharim organization aims to prevent the marriage of Orthodox couples who are carriers of genetic disorders. In these communities "marriages are between families as much as between individuals, and are prearranged by the parents, often with the help of a matchmaker."[63] Since "no information on carrier status but only on the 'genetic compatibility' of both partners is revealed, a notion of 'genetic couplehood' arises which conceptualizes 'genetic risk' not individually but as a matter of genetic jointness."[64]

Jewish tradition has always stressed the importance of the continuation of the Jewish people as well as of Jewish culture. It is for this reason that reproduction and its regulation has played a significant role in core Jewish practices and debates. Its interpretation through eugenic terms, especially in the late nineteenth and early twentieth centuries, represented accordance to the spirit of the time. But eugenic notions of the Jews prosper today, as ever before.

NOTES

1. Raphael Falk, "Zionism, Race and Eugenics," in *Jewish Tradition and the Challenge of Darwinism*, eds. Geoffrey Cantor and Marc Swetlitz (Chicago, IL: University of Chicago Press, 2006), 137–165.

2. Max Reichler, *Jewish Eugenics* (New York: Block Publishing Company, 1916), 1–2.

3. Ibid., 7–8.

4. Ibid., 10–12.

5. Ibid., 12.

6. "Jewish Eugenics," *The Journal of Heredity* 8, no. 2 (1917): 72–74.

7. Noam J. Zohar, "From Lineage to Sexual Mores: Examining 'Jewish Eugenics,'" *Science in Context* 11, no. 3–4 (1998): 576. Eugenic readings of the Old Testament, the Talmud, and later Sages must, however, be conceived in line with the tradition always to interpret the scripts in relevance to current vagaries of life. "The problem here, as with many other aspects of Jewish bioethics, is one of eliciting, from the tradition going back more than two thousand years, implications for issues raised by modern science and technology." Zohar, "From Lineage to Sexual Mores," 575.

8. Maurice Fishberg, *The Jews: A Study of Race and Environment* (London: Walter Scott Publishing, 1911).

9. "A Study of the Jewish Race: Dr. Maurice Fishberg Seemingly Denies Their Claim to Be a Peculiar People," *New York Times*, February 12, 1911.

10. Maurice Fishberg, "Eugenics in Jewish Life," *The Journal of Heredity* 8, no. 12 (1917): 545.

11. Ibid., 546.

12. J. Snowman, "Jewish Eugenics," *Jewish Review* 4 (1913–1914): 172–173.

13. W. M. Feldman, "Ancient Jewish Eugenics," *Medical Leaves* 2 (1939): 28.

14. Ibid., 29.

15. Ibid., 31–32.

16. Ibid., 37.

17. Zohar, "From Lineage to Sexual Mores," 575.

18. Rachel Livne-Freudenthal, "From 'a Nation Dwelling Alone' to 'a Nation among the Nations' or: 'the Return to History—Between Universalism and Nationalism,'" in *Streams into the Sea: Studies in Jewish Culture and Its Context*, eds. Rachel Livenh-Freudenthal and Elchanan Reiner (Tel-Aviv: Alma College, 2001).

19. Francis Galton, "Composite Portraits," *Nature* 18 (1878): 97–100. See also John M. Efron, *Defenders of the Race: Jewish Doctors and Race Science in Fin-de-Siècle Europe* (New Haven, CT: Yale University Press, 1994), 58–90.

20. Mitchell B. Hart, *Social Science and the Politics of Modern Jewish Identity* (Stanford, CA: Stanford University Press, 2000), 178.

21. Francis Galton, "Eugenics and the Jew," *The Jewish Chronicle*, July 29, 1910.

22. Redcliffe N. Salaman, "Heredity and the Jew," *Journal of Genetics* 1 (1911): 273–292.

23. Todd M. Endelman, "Anglo-Jewish Scientists and the Science of Race," *Jewish Social Studies* 11, no. 1 (2004): 52–92; Raphael Falk, "Three Zionist Men of Science: Between Nature and Nurture," in *Jews and Sciences in German Contexts: Case Studies from the 19th and 20th Centuries*, eds. Ute Deichmann and Ulrich Charpa (Tübingen: Mohr Siebeck, 2007), 129–154.

24. See Jan Goldstein, "The Wandering Jew and the Problem of Psychiatric Anti-semitism in Fin-de-Siècle France," *Journal of Contemporary History* 20, no. 4 (1985): 521–552.

25. Bychowski, quoted in Raphael Falk, "Nervous Diseases and Eugenics of the Jews: A View from 1918," *Korot* 17 (2003–2004): 43.

26. Ibid., 42.

27. Fishberg, *The Jews: A Study of Race and Environment*.

28. Fishberg, "Eugenics in Jewish Life," 543.

29. Ibid., 546.

30. Ibid., 546, 544.

31. Arthur Ruppin, *The Jews of To-Day* (New York: H. Holt, 1913), 212–213 (translated from the German by Margery Bentwich).

32. Ibid., 217.

33. Eugen Fischer, "Rassenentsehung und älteste Rassengeschichte der Hebräer," in *Sitzungsbereiche der Dritten Münchner Arbeitstagung des Reichsinstituts für Geschichte des neuen Deutschlands von 5. bis 7. Juli 1938* (Hamburg: Hanseatische Verlagsanstalt, 1938), 121–136, (translation by Charles E. Weber for the Liberty Bell), 122.

34. Ibid.

35. Ibid., 135.

36. Ibid., 135.

37. Otmar Freiherr von Verschuer, "Rassenbiologie der Juden," in *Sitzungsbereiche der Dritten Münchner Arbeitstagung des Reichsinstituts für Geschichte*. In spite of the translator's vitriolic Introduction, the translation is competent.

38. Ibid., 138.

39. Karl Pearson and Margaret Moul, "The Problem of Alien Immigration into Great Britain, Illustrated by an Examination of Russian and Polish Jewish Children," *Annals of Eugenics* 1 (1925): 5–55.

40. Redcliffe N. Salaman, "Some Notes on the Jewish Problem," in *Eugenics in Race and State: Second International Congress of Eugenics*, eds. Charles B. Davenport, Henry F. Osborn, Clark Wissler, and Harry H. Laughlin (Baltimore, MD: Williams & Wilkins, 1923), 149.

41. Ibid., 152.

42. A. G. Hughes, "Jews and Gentiles: Their Intellectual and Temperamental Differences," *Eugenics Review* 20 (1928): 90.

43. Pearson et al., "The Problem of Alien Immigration into Great Britain," 8.

44. Hughes, "Jews and Gentiles," 90.

45. Ibid., 91.

46. Solomon Herbert, "The Making of a Nation," *Jewish Review* 1 (1910–11): 446.

47. Max Nordau, *Degeneration* (London: William Heinemann, 1895).

48. Raphael Falk, "Zionism and the Biology of the Jews," *Science in Context* 11, no. 3–4 (1998): 587–607.

49. Rubin, quoted in Falk, "Zionism, Race and Eugenics," 151; Falk, "Zionism and the Biology of the Jews," 598. Original emphasis.

50. Mayer, quoted in Falk, "Zionism, Race and Eugenics," 153.

51. Bychowski, quoted in Falk, "Three Zionist Men of Science," 135.

52. Arthur Ruppin, "Die Auslese des Menschenmaterials für Palästina," *Der Jude* 3 (1918–1919): 373–383.

53. Nadav Davidovitch and Shifra Shvarts, "Health, Zionism and Ideology: Medical Selection of Jewish European Immigrants to Palestine," in *Facing Illness in Troubled Times: Health in Europe in the Interwar Years, 1918–1939*, eds. Iris Borowy and Wolf D. Gruner (Berlin: Peter Lang Verlag, 2005), 409–424; see also Falk, "Zionism, Race and Eugenics," 155.

54. Neil A. Holtzman, "Eugenics and Genetic Testing," *Science in Context* 11, no. 3–4 (1998): 398.

55. Ibid., 409.

56. Yael Hashiloni-Dolev, *A Life (Un)Worthy of Living: Reproductive Genetics in Israel and Germany* (Dordrecht: Springer, 2007), 8.

57. Neil A. Holtzman, "Genetic Screening: For Better or for Worse?" *Pediatrics* 59, no. 1 (1977): 132.

58. Hashiloni-Dolev, *A Life (Un)Worthy of Living*, 4.

59. Ibid., 14.

60. Ibid., 34.

61. Ibid., 48.

62. Barbara Prainsack, "'Negotiating Life': The Regulation of Human Cloning and Embryonic Stem Cell Research in Israel," *Social Studies of Science* 36, no. 2 (2006): 173–205.

63. Michal Sagi, "Ethical Aspects of Genetic Screening in Israel," *Science in Context* 11, no. 3–4 (1998): 425–426.

64. Barbara Prainsack and Gil Siegal, "The Rise of Genetic Couplehood? A Comparative View of Premarital Genetic Testing," *BioScience* 1 (2006): 17–36.

FURTHER READING

Biale, David. *Eros and the Jews: From Biblical Israel to Contemporary America* (New York: Basic, 1992).

Cantor, Geoffrey, and Swetlitz, Marc, eds. *Jewish Tradition and the Challenge of Darwinism* (Chicago, IL: University of Chicago Press, 2006).

Efron, John M. "Scientific Racism and the Mystique of Sephardic Racial Superiority," in *Leo Baeck Institute Year Book* 38 (1993): 77–96.

Entine, Jon. *Abraham's Children: Race, Identity, and the DNA of the Chosen People* (New York: Grand Central Publishing, 2007).

Falk, Raphael. *Zionism and the Biology of the Jews* [in Hebrew] (Tel-Aviv: Resling, 2006).

Goldstein, David B., *Jacob's Legacy: A Genetic View of Jewish History* (New Haven, CT: Yale University Press, 1994).

Hart, Mitchell B. "Racial Science, Social Science and the Politics of Jewish Assimilation," in *Science, Race, and Ethnicity: Readings from Isis and Osiris*, ed. John P. Jackson Jr. (Chicago, IL: Chicago University Press, 2002).

Kahn, Susan Martha. *Reproducing Jews: A Cultural Account of Assisted Conception in Israel* (Durham, NC: Duke University Press, 2000).

Kirsh, Nurit. "Population Genetics in Israel in the 1950s: The Unconscious Internalization of Ideology," *Isis* 94, no. 4 (2003): 631–655.

Lorenz, Konrad. "Durch Domestikation verursachte Stürungen arteigene Verhaltens," *Zeitschrift für angewandte Psychologie und Charakterkunde* 59, no. 2 (1940): 2–81.

Müller-Hill, Benno. *Murderous Science: Elimination by Scientific Selection of Jews, Gypsies, and Others, Germany 1933–1945* (Oxford and New York: Oxford University Press, 1988) (translated from the German by George R. Fraser).

Singerman, Robert. "The Jew as Racial Alien: The Genetic Component of American Anti-Semitism," in *Anti-Semitism in American History* ed. David A. Gerber (Champaign, IL: University of Illinois Press, 1986), 103–128.

CHAPTER 28

EUGENICS POLICY AND PRACTICE IN CUBA, PUERTO RICO, AND MEXICO

PATIENCE A. SCHELL

IN the 1898 Treaty of Paris, ending the Spanish-American War, Cuba gained independence from Spain, only to become a "neocolony" of the United States with the 1902 Platt Amendment, which gave the United States the authority to intervene in Cuban affairs; the same treaty ceded Puerto Rico, the "Gibraltar of the Caribbean," to the United States.[1] In spite of U.S. military and political intervention, Mexico marked its centenary of independence with a social revolution (1910–1917). In these three places, eugenics provided the inspiration and justification for a range of health and social policies, rooted in local contexts and history, while engaging with international intellectual currents, demonstrating the diversity of Latin American eugenics.

Across Latin America, the 1920s and 1930s were a booming period for welfare and health legislation, the foundation of health services, protective legislation for women and children, and consideration of eugenics-related issues.[2] Latin American eugenics has been seen within a neo-Lamarckian French-inspired environmentalist eugenics,[3] and we will see a range of influences and eugenics measures in Cuba, Puerto Rico, and Mexico. Because of the importance of the Cuban concept of homiculture on the Latin American movement, this chapter begins with a discussion of that country. The chapter then focuses on Puerto Rico, in which colonial and domestic modernizing eugenics interacted. Finally, the chapter examines the influence of eugenics on Mexico after the triumph of a socially progressive revolution.

CUBA

Although Galton's work was addressed on the natural history curriculum at the University of Havana in the late 1880s, the Cuban eugenics movement was a twentieth-century phenomenon. Lawyers, sociologists, teachers, and other professionals were involved, but most eugenicists were medical professionals, whose interest arose through their study of heredity or social medicine, and who tended to be left-leaning with government links. The first genuine eugenics publication in Cuba was an A. F. Tredgold translation "El estudio de la eugénica," published in the general interest *Cuba Contemporánea* in 1913. Eugenics was also a topic for discussion at the First National Medical Congress held in Havana in 1914. One of the key publications to disseminate these local and international debates was the *Crónica Médico-Quirúrgica de la Habana* (Medical-Surgical Chronicle of Havana).

In this early period, French influence on Cuban medicine, and thus Cuban and Latin American eugenics, was crucial. Two students of Adolphe Pinard (1844–1934), physician Domingo F. Ramos Delgado (1881–1961) and obstetrician and independence struggle veteran Eusebio Hernández Pérez (1854–1933), expanded Pinard's concept of *puériculture,* or the scientific cultivation of the child, to address the adult life cycle and conceptualize the role of heredity in shaping human populations. In their 1911 publication, *Homicultura,* Ramos and Hernández took a holistic view of influences on human development, linking "human fitness to a nation's capacity for peace, order, and prosperity." Their ideas circulated through the National Homiculture League, founded in 1913. Its members included leading intellectuals like Francisco Carrera y Justiz and Maria Luisa Dolz (1854–1928). Ramos and Hernández also published for a non-specialist audience in the journal *Vida Nueva.* Further seeking to popularize their views, Hernández taught a course on homiculture and preventive sexual health at the José Martí Workers' Popular University. The government, meanwhile, made gestures of support, such as the beautiful baby contests, held by the Ministry of Hygiene and Welfare between 1915 and 1933. The homiculture approach spread throughout Latin America as medical practitioners used it to link issues of public health, the environment, heredity, and reproduction in an effort to improve national populations.[4] In Cuba, homiculture approaches led to proposals for prenuptial medical examinations, legal protection for pregnant women, campaigns to improve the employment and living conditions of the working class, and programs to better children's nutrition. These initiatives, however, were not great in number and generally did not reach beyond Havana province, where the capital was located.[5]

In 1921, Ramos turned away from a *puériculture*/homiculture version of eugenics to promote a eugenics of scientific racism with close ties to the U.S. movement. Particularly influential in this regard was leading eugenicist Charles B. Davenport (1866–1944). Before attending the Second International Congress of Eugenics in New York, Ramos traveled to visit Davenport at his laboratory at Cold Spring Harbor, Long Island.[6] This first face-to-face meeting started a long professional association.

During the 1920s, Ramos sought to coordinate and promote eugenics, of the sort Davenport championed throughout the Americas; under the auspices of the Pan American League, he founded the Pan American Central Office of Eugenics and Homiculture, in Havana,[7] which hosted its first international conference in 1927. Disappointingly for Ramos, only 28 official delegates, many of whom were diplomats already based in Havana, represented 16 countries of the Americas; many more people attended unofficially. Armando García González and Raquel Alvarez Peláez speculate that the high costs of travel to Cuba and the official nature of the discussion prompted nations to send their consular staff.[8] But noted eugenicists did attend, including Davenport himself and the Peruvian professor of hygiene at San Marcos University in Lima, Carlos Enrique Paz Soldán (1885–1972).

Ramos and Davenport's goal for the conference was to approve a "Code of Eugenics and Homiculture" that Ramos had drafted with Davenport's input. The code mandated the classification of all inhabitants of the Americas as "good," "bad," or "doubtful" and the restriction of the reproduction of the "bad" or "doubtful" through sterilization or some form of isolation. Immigration would only be allowed for the eugenically fit, and each nation could enact measures to protect its "racial purity." The code reflected, in part, the U.S. concern regarding the racial composition of the Americas because of potential and actual emigration. When Ramos opened debate on the code, he noted the "superiority" of the "white race," to which he attributed such virtues as altruism. Ramos further argued that eugenics should determine national immigration policy, suggesting that existing U.S. laws showed how to classify people and favor "white" immigration. The mixed-race populations of many Latin American countries, which included indigenous, European, African, and Asian peoples, were far removed from the pure eugenic nations that Ramos and Davenport imagined. To improve Latin American populations, Ramos suggested a U.S. model of segregation and forced sterilization.[9]

Ramos and Davenport represented a minority view, however. Peruvian Paz Soldán argued that science was not yet capable of accurately labeling immigrants, and such measures were totalitarian; moreover, racial or national/ethnic mixing (as in the U.S.) strengthened, rather than weakened that country. Paz Soldán proposed rejecting the code. Other delegates challenged the suggestion that Latin American populations were not eugenically sound. Through reference to Mexico's history of conquest, colonization, and racial mixing, that country's delegate, Rafael Santamarina (1884–1966) denied the inferiority of indigenous peoples. He argued that Mexico's population was improving through measures such as investment in rural schools and child labor laws. An expert in child development, Santamarina challenged the reliability of physical and mental tests that had been used to claim the inferiority of Mexican child immigrants in the United States. Thanks in part to these challenges, a homiculture-oriented version of eugenics prevailed. Eugenic sterilization was rejected outright, with the Argentinian and Costa Rican delegates both speaking strongly against it, while delegates had no desire or authority to cede national sovereignty on immigration. The code as a whole was defeated. Compromise was reached on mandatory prenuptial examinations.[10]

Nonetheless, within Cuba itself, immigration became a main concern for eugenicists.[11] According to the 1899 census, Cuba's population of 1,573,000 was two-thirds "white" and one-third Afro-Cuban, with a tiny percentage of Chinese immigrants. This census alarmed some; for the first time since the 1850s, the proportion of whites had fallen, and this data fed into a discourse of a threatening African presence, which, during the nineteenth century, reinforced colonial links with Spain. Yet after independence, elites hoped that through intermarriage and a whitening immigration policy, the Afro-Cuban third would disappear. A whitening policy betrayed the vision of a raceless Cuba that had motivated the nineteenth-century independence struggles, in which Afro-Cubans were vital participants; in their aspirations to create a new, unified, national polity, Cuba's creole elite imagined the nation as founded on its Spanish past alone.[12] This imagined white Cuba is evident in Cuban immigration restrictions enacted during the first decades of the twentieth century. In 1902, the U.S.-imposed Military Order 155 restricted non-white immigration generally, and prohibited the entry of Chinese immigrants as well as people deemed mentally inferior or to be carrying infectious diseases. Contentious debates about the 1906 immigration law meant that racial exclusions were not reiterated, but European (especially from Sweden, Norway, Denmark, and Northern Italy) and Canary Islands immigration was encouraged through funds earmarked for their passage alone. In 1916, the government required that all Jamaican, Puerto Rican, and Haitian immigrants have blood tests before being allowed into the country: while ostensibly this measure was anti-malarial, it was in fact prompted by fears of a growing black population. Spanish immigrants, the vast majority, were not subjected to health checks.[13]

Immigration fears redoubled as the economy faltered. From 1920, an economic crisis caused the deterioration of living conditions, diminishing the appeal of European immigrants. The Second International Conference of Emigration and Immigration, held in Havana in 1928, recommended medical certificates, vaccinations, prenatal care, professional selection of immigrants before departure, and measures to prevent the clandestine immigration of "undesirables." The 1929 U.S. stock market crash prompted further calls to limit or even stop immigration altogether. In the same year, Dr. Francisco María Fernández (1886–1937), president of the Cuban Academy of Sciences, head of the eugenics and homiculture office, and member of the house of representatives, proposed a total prohibition on all immigration for two years. The proposal itself was rejected, but tightening up of requirements did follow. By 1931, 11 percent of Cuba's population was foreign-born, including 79,838 Haitians, 40,471 Jamaicans, and 24,480 Chinese. In 1933, the "50 percent" law required that Cubans must make up that percentage of any workforce. Unemployed foreigners could be forcibly repatriated, most directly affecting Haitians and Jamaicans. Yet there were conflicting demands, as the sugar planters needed this low-wage work force for the seasonal harvest. Racism against these minority populations increased dramatically during the economic difficulties of the 1930s, eventually prompting Dr. Octavio Montoro (1891–1960) to address the issue in front of the Academy of Sciences, suggesting that racial concerns hid structural economic problems.[14]

Ramos himself continued to be actively involved in these debates. Attending the 1932 Third International Congress of Eugenics in New York, he pushed for the study of home populations and prospective immigrant groups to indicate how successful any mixing would be. He further argued that countries should be able to expel undesirable immigrants and their children. To facilitate this process, he also called for the creation of international treaties, working in conjunction with eugenics organizations.[15]

Ramos's views continued to be extreme within the Latin American eugenics movement more broadly. In 1930, the Catholic Church had condemned any eugenic measures that sought to intervene directly in human reproduction, limiting the activities of devout Catholic eugenicists. Moreover, at the Second Pan American Conference of Eugenics and Homiculture, held in Buenos Aires in 1934, the negative eugenics agenda was rejected even more decisively than it had been in Havana. Delegates voted for a children's code proposed by Uruguay and already enshrined in national law there, which reflected a broad public health and social welfare approach to eugenics that U.S. delegates to the meeting rejected. Ramos sought a discussion about sterilization, or at least consideration of voluntary sterilization, but delegates refused to address the issue, much less vote on it. They determined that knowledge of genetics was not yet clear enough to undertake these drastic measures; they also had concerns about morality, individual liberty, and the role of social factors. Responding to the Church's condemnation of eugenic regulation of reproduction and the practical difficulties of implementing prenuptial certificates, the conference actually amended its 1927 approval of them, endorsing only voluntary measures.[16]

PUERTO RICO

While the Pan American delegates refused to countenance sterilization measures, the women of Puerto Rico regularly underwent sterilization, as the island became a laboratory for birth control research. The gendered and racialized debates around birth control and sterilization tied into political debates about the U.S. role on the island, while making poor women and their family formation fundamental to these same debates.[17] Women's sexuality had been key to wider debates during the Spanish colonial period, too. Nineteenth-century hygienists had debated the regulation of prostitution and argued that poor women's sexuality led to "dangerous" racial heterogeneity. But after World War I, the "'problem' of working-class women shifted from prostitution to reproduction and birth control."[18] These concerns about sexuality also fed into the "overpopulation" debate.

From the beginning of U.S. colonization, low standards of living convinced the United States military that the size of the population was the cause of the island's troubles.[19] Yet the exact meaning and utility of "overpopulation" evolved. During World War I, condemning the working class and poor for having too many children, for example, helped to justify the practice of attracting Puerto Ricans into very low wage labor in the United States. Puerto Rican socialists also used the term to express their concern about a ready supply of labor making too many competitors for jobs. By the mid-1920s and 1930s, the term implied that "excessive sexuality" and high fertility caused poverty, crime, disease, and prostitution on the island. In both public debates and political circles, birth control emerged as a possible solution, but support was not widespread. Eugenicists within the U.S. movement also lobbied for birth control in Puerto Rico, depicting Puerto Rican families as "over breeding" and causing widespread social problems.[20]

Yet the currency of "overpopulation" was not based on empirical data. The reasons for poverty and a low standard of living were actually structural and, in part, caused by U.S. policies. A combination of the plummeting peso and small-scale farmers losing out to U.S. sugar interests meant that, by 1925, 70 percent of the population was landless, while 2 percent of the population held 80 percent of the land. Meanwhile, increased concentration on sugar production pushed tenant farmers and peasants into the wage economy. The island's per capita income increased in the late 1920s, yet by 1930 overall unemployment was 60 percent. Thus, economic and political policies, not "overpopulation," were to blame for the fact that Puerto Ricans' health and living conditions did not improve during those first four decades of U.S. administration. Nevertheless, the "population problem" continued to be imagined and acted upon from the 1940s to the 1960s.[21]

Puerto Ricans, too, took up this discourse, especially as limited support for the U.S. presence and living conditions both deteriorated. By the 1930s, doctors, the island's legislature, feminist social workers, and nurses supported birth control to address the "surplus" population and their poor health. Laura Briggs argues that this discourse, shared with social and public health workers from the United States, was integral to a modernizing current of nationalism that argued for reducing family size, improving public health, and encouraging marriage. While birth control was illegal under the Puerto Rican criminal code's version of the Comstock Laws, which prohibited the "dissemination of contraception knowledge and practices," the island's attorney general chose to contort a legal interpretation that allowed birth control clinics, albeit not many, to function.[22]

But other versions of eugenics are evident in the public health initiatives that sought to improve the well-being of communities and modernize the island. Mostly women, and some men, working for the public health department implemented milk feeding points for infants and children, put nurses in schools to reduce tuberculosis, opened dental clinics, and supported visiting nurses. Meanwhile, access to and acceptance of birth control grew. Under the patronage of Clarence Gamble (Procter and Gamble heir), the Association for Maternal and Infant Health promoted birth control as part of the Puerto Rican Reconstruction Administration (within the New Deal). Because Gamble did not believe that poor women had the mental capability to use the diaphragm, which had been the method adopted earlier, unreliable spermicides were now distributed. His concern was not for individual women's reproductive choice, as long as the birth control method was in widespread use and population reduced overall. Explicitly targeting poor women, Gamble sought to diminish the number of poor people on the island; importantly, his shift from a reliable method of birth control to an unreliable method later helped create a wide-spread demand for and use of surgical sterilization.[23]

In 1937, in response to "overpopulation" and with the eugenic goal of eliminating "undesirable elements" of the population, Puerto Rico's legislature formally legalized birth control. Additionally, a new sterilization law cited poverty as a legitimate justification and made provision for involuntary sterilizations under a Eugenics Board. Only 97 such sterilizations were actually ordered, but under this legislation, which remained in force until 1960, many women were voluntarily sterilized, and, unusually in international terms, sterilization became the principal form of birth control on the island. Strong Catholic opposition to birth control prompted a test case that upheld the law and, from 1939, birth control in Puerto Rico became part of a permanent federally funded program; thus birth control was legal in Puerto Rico long before it was in the United States. The public health department offered these services. Moreover, a range of birth control methods were tested on Puerto Rico's poor women, including the pill, as the island offered the attraction of a "cage of ovulating females," according to Katharine Dexter McCormick (1875–1967), the U.S. philanthropist funding the bulk of oral contraceptive research.[24]

The large numbers of sterilizations caused controversy. The Catholic Church condemned the procedure as a heavy-handed response to unemployment and, between the 1940s and 1960s, charged that the widespread sterilizations were part of a secret genocidal plan. Joining the Catholic Church was the Nationalist Party, which sought independence. They also condemned sterilization and birth control as part of a plan to eliminate Puerto Ricans through intentional poverty, emigration, and the introduction of disease into the population (a Rockefeller Foundation doctor, Cornelius Rhoads (1898–1959), had recounted in a personal letter the "introduction" of cancer into seven patients and the killing of several others; he dismissed the letter as a "joke" and was cleared).[25] Challenging negative views on Puerto Rican mothers, these conservative, patriarchal groups depicted women as heroines who gave birth to new Puerto Ricans. The support of U.S. eugenicists for sterilization as a solution to "overbreeding" inadvertently helped these arguments of genocidal policy, although there is no evidence of such a secret plan. Yet in 1960, when the Catholic Action Party ran a candidate against the island's governor, Luis Muñoz Marín (1898–1980), as a de facto referendum on the sterilization policy, it lost decisively. In 1963, the government and church agreed that, as long as the rhythm method was included in a range of birth control techniques discussed with patients, the church would not oppose these measures. Public pressure from some Catholic laity, however, forced Archbishop James P. Davis (1904–1988) to retreat from this agreement, although crucially maintaining that the Catholic Church could not dictate to non-Catholics. By 1970, the Puerto Rican bishops stated that contraception and childbirth were choices made between individuals and God; unusual statements in Latin America interpreted to be tacit approval of government family planning programs.[26]

The statistics on sterilization make clear why this issue was so polemical. By 1955 estimates suggested that 16.5 percent of all women of childbearing age had been sterilized, rising to 34 percent a decade later. By 1976, the U.S. Department of Health, Education, and Welfare found a 37.4 percent sterilization rate. A combination of sterilization policies and emigration to the United States reduced Puerto Rico's birthrate to 30.8 per 1,000 in 1961, one of the lowest in the Caribbean. Sterilization of men, however, was not widespread, as much as U.S. eugenicists might have promoted early sterilization of both men and women to stem population growth.[27]

Considering the tiny number of eugenic sterilizations and the large number of voluntary sterilizations, debates rage over their actual nature. Briggs argues that the widespread use of birth control, especially sterilization, was not in fact due to state-sponsored promotion but because middle-class Puerto Rican professionals, teachers, social workers, nurses, mayors, and newspaper editors, in their professional capacity, linked poverty to large families and pushed contraception as the solution.[28] Still, from the 1930s until the 1960s, surveys indicated that sterilized women were happy with their choice. A survey in 1982 of women who had been sterilized as early as 1954 reported that the vast majority had made their own decision. Another study, based on women who had been sterilized between 1956 and 1961, found that 94 percent remained satisfied. Those who regretted the operation did not imply that they had been forced. But this data cannot be understood without recognizing that these women chose surgical sterilization within limited choices. Women underwent surgical sterilization, in part, due to inadequate availability of non-permanent and safe methods of birth control. A 1953–1954 study concluded the women chose sterilization because alternatives were ineffective and less convenient, as well as due to ready information about and the prestige of the procedure.[29]

MEXICO

Mexico's eugenics movement emerged amid the massive population decline and dislocation of the revolution (1910–1917) that overthrew a regime whose intellectuals had embraced social Darwinism, Spencer's condemnation of hybrid humans, and Auguste Comte's positivism. Thus, as in Cuba and Puerto Rico, eugenics fitted into and responded to a long-standing debate about race, and, in the case of Mexico, about its indigenous and mixed-race population.[30] Unlike the previous regime, however, the post-revolutionary government sought to integrate Mexico's indigenous and mestizo (indigenous and Spanish) majority into the nation through an ambitious health and social policy program that was informed by eugenics.

Eugenics' influence on post-revolutionary policy was evident early on. In 1917, the law of family relations that legalized divorce had clear eugenic tones. Marriage was to be regulated for the benefit not only of the couple themselves, but also for the "benefit of the species," which included preventing marriages among incurable alcoholics and those with infectious diseases. Throughout the 1920s and into the 1930s, *puériculture* and eugenics contributed to the public health, education, and welfare policies of the Mexican state, focusing especially on mothers and children. While men were envisaged as little more than inseminators, women's reproductive choices were understood to contribute to national development and improvement.[31] The First Mexican Congress of the Child, held in Mexico City in 1921, discussed maternal health, the forced sterilization of criminals (narrowly approved), and state-supported whitening of the indigenous population.[32] Many of the conclusions of this first child congress and the second, held in 1923, were implemented through the School Hygiene Service, under the Ministry of Education's Department of Psycho-Pedagogy and Hygiene, which engaged in *puériculture* and eugenics-based research. The remit of the new department was to understand Mexican children's minds and bodies, while improving their overall health. Its director, Rafael Santamarina (1884–1966), had presented work at both Mexican child congresses; he had also attended the 1927 Havana congress, where he challenged Davenport's racism, as noted above. Alexandra Stern argues that the service turned the "public domain" into a "eugenics laboratory."[33]

Many employees of the ministry of education's health and psychology services were members of the Mexican Puériculture Society. The *puériculture* society had a eugenics wing, whose members became the founding members, in autumn 1931, of the Mexican Eugenics Society for the Betterment of the Race (*Sociedad Eugénica Mexicana para el Mejoramiento de la Raza*). Membership included men and women from the inner circles of Mexican politics and public health, as well as recognized biologists, well-known medical professionals, judges, and criminologists. Its founder, secretary, and a leading figure in the movement thereafter was Dr. Alfredo Saavedra (1893–1973). Felix Palavicini (1881–1952), who had organized the first child congress, as well as biologists Fernando Ocaranza (1876–1965) and José Rulfo (1895–1962), the latter of whom introduced Mendelian genetics and experimental techniques to Mexico, were all members. Among the 20 original members, 5 were women, although their numbers did not grow proportionally with the organization, likely because of the limited numbers of women in these fields.[34] This roster of membership indicates how eugenics influenced policy and practice in law, health care, the sciences, and education.

An important aspect of the organization's work was to disseminate eugenics theories more widely among Mexico's professionals and citizens. For example, the society offered courses on reproductive health to nurses and social workers. It hosted "eugenics weeks" and published its own journal, *Eugenesia*, which ran from 1931 to 1954, as well as books, brochures, and magazines aimed at various audiences. Working with the government, it created radio campaigns against alcoholism and venereal disease. In 1932, Saavedra argued for a minimum wage law, a lower cost of living, temperance campaigns, and more physical education. Other members of the society, meanwhile, promoted sex education programs and campaigns against pornography and feminism.[35]

The eugenics society also supported sterilization laws, in part to keep up with such leading eugenic countries as Norway, Sweden, and the United States. In 1932, the only eugenic sterilization law in Mexico came into force in the Gulf state of Veracruz, under the radical anticlerical governor Adalberto Tejeda (1883–1960). Salvador Mendoza, a sociologist and economist, had written the law in consultation with the eugenics society. Sterilization was to be a service provided by a new office within the state's health department, the Bureau of Eugenics and Mental Hygiene. The bureau had under its authority issues of inheritance, alcoholism, prostitution, *puériculture,* and criminality. Included within the law, as well, were measures for sex education, free birth control for the poor, eugenic grounds for divorce, and restrictions on bars and the sale of alcohol (while encouraging "the use of beer and soft beverages, a real relief in the tropical climate of his state," as Mendoza explained). In cases of "idiocy," mental illness, delinquency, and chronic disease, forced sterilization was allowable with the authorization of three physicians. There is no evidence that this law was implemented, however, and it was certainly out of step with much of the eugenics movement by the time it came into force. Nancy Leys Stepan notes that the Nazi eugenic sterilization law, enacted a year later, was roundly condemned by Mexican eugenicists at the "Second Eugenics Week" held in Mexico City in 1934, on the grounds that there was inadequate knowledge of genetic inheritance to justify the measures.[36]

Yet even with the condemnation of sterilization, there were still negative eugenic ideas in circulation among influential Mexicans. Mexican psychiatrists, who had studied in Germany under Dr. Emil Kraepelin (1856–1926), brought the influence of National Socialist doctrines to their work. Dr. Matilde Rodríguez Cabo (1902–1967) was one such psychiatrist. In 1935, as the head of the Child Psychology Department at the National Asylum, Rodríguez endorsed euthanasia of the "less apt" and socially useless who would burden the state. The concerns of the eugenicists chimed with the assumptions in the social sciences more broadly, including sociology, anthropology, and legal medicine, about inheritance. These professionals followed Lombroso's view of born criminals, believing in an inherited predisposition to prostitution, homosexuality, and alcohol abuse. These beliefs, in part, indicate the continued influence of Lamarck. In the early and mid-1930s, Mexican eugenicists did not support Mendel's genetics, but rather believed in the inheritance of acquired characteristics. Thus Mexican eugenicists feared the long-term consequences of such "racial poisons" as tuberculosis, syphilis, and alcoholism. By the end of the 1930s, Lamarckian inheritance had been so discredited in international science that Mexican eugenicists began to accept Mendelian ideas. Concurrently, and in response, the focus of eugenics moved away from sexual and reproductive behavior. Nonetheless, the influence of Lamarck's concepts remained strong and helps to explain the subsequent interest in constitutional medicine (*biotipología*), which allowed for a Mendelian understanding of genetics, while still emphasizing the importance of environmental factors.[37]

Still, a variety of expert opinions about Mexico's diverse population jostled for supremacy. Some members of the Mexican Eugenics Society for the Betterment of the Race depicted Mexico as a heterogeneous nation in which the mixing of different ethnic groups was beneficial; in so doing, they picked up on a discourse dating from the end of the regime of Porfirio Díaz (1876–1911), exemplified by the writer Andrés Molina Enríquez (1865–1940) "who hailed the mestizo as the beacon of national progress" in his widely read *Los grandes problemas nacionales* (1909).[38] Dr. Eliseo Ramírez argued that separation of races was against Mexican eugenics and that hybrids were being proved stronger than the "pure" lines, thanks in part to the genetic work of Nicolay Ivanovich Vavilov (1887–1943) of Russia. Saavedra pushed for the study of Mexico's racial map, in order to determine which groups could be more easily assimilated into Mexican society, by which he meant its creole society. Like the nineteenth-century French anthropologist Paul Broca (1824–1880), Saavedra argued that the "nearer" races made for stronger mixes, while the "far" mixes resulted in inferior children. Meanwhile, biologist Ocaranza suggested that mestizos were a problematic population, as they united the defects of both their Spanish and indigenous ancestors. These debates about race were at the heart of national policy. Yet underpinning even this glorification of the mestizo as the national race was the little-articulated view that eventually mestizos, too, would disappear, due to the superiority of "whites." Unlike Cuban eugenicists, however, Mexican eugenicists never moved beyond debates to involvement in making laws based on race. The Mexican Eugenics Society and the Pro-Race Committee for Mexico City, which pushed for legislation that stigmatized Chinese immigrants and later Jewish refugees, had only one member in common.[39]

These debates about race were part of the new post-revolutionary nationalism and a national debate about the meaning of being Mexican. The 1930 census, unlike previous ones, did not include racial categories.[40] José Vasconcelos (1882–1959), minister of education from 1921–1924, also glorified the mestizo, but for him the mestizo was a "spiritual beacon of Hispanic civilization" and was Mexico's link to the future. He contended that mestizos incorporated the best qualities of the contributing peoples, and would create a eugenics based not on science but on aesthetics. His spiritual eugenics would create a fifth or "cosmic" race, which was superior to the others because it united the beautiful elements within the other four. But he, too, continued to see the superiority of the Europeans.[41]

Contrasting were the views of Manuel Gamio (1883–1960), a noted anthropologist with a degree in archaeology from Columbia University, where he worked with Franz Boas (1858–1942). Gamio had close involvement with the eugenics movement, having been president of the Mexican delegation to the 1921 New York eugenics congress and vice president of the event. He was a regular contributor to the eugenics society journal, *Eugenesia,* as well as being involved in their activities. As much as he endorsed the assimilation of Mexico's indigenous population, he inverted eugenics' racial categories. For Gamio, mestizos were a "pure" race, strengthened by the resistance of indigenous people to years of colonization, and strong due to adaptation and natural selection. The high rates of mortality among the indigenous population were due to external factors, not natural weakness. But his promotion of Mexico's indigenous population was not without caution. Gamio described the mestizo as Mexico's "national" race, its leaders, and the group through which a national culture would develop. Moreover, he suggested that it was culture, not biology, which determined indigeniety; through cultural assimilation, Mexico's indigenous population would decline, forging a more homogenous population.[42] The post-revolutionary glorification of the mestizo was still underscored by centuries of racism.

CONCLUSION

In this comparison of the history of eugenics in Cuba, Puerto Rico, and Mexico, it is readily evident how adaptable eugenic concepts were to local political, social, and cultural contexts. In Mexico, a central concern was to increase and improve the population after the decimation of the revolution. In a majority mestizo and indigenous nation, to which large-scale European immigration was not realistic, *puériculture* and homiculture approaches had obvious appeal. Eugenic discussions about race also fit into new attempts to understand the essence of the Mexican nation, and to depict mestizos as nation-building stock. Likewise, in Puerto Rico, eugenics was originally a movement of liberals and feminists endorsing a modernizing program, to improve working-class families. Eugenics appealed to some Puerto Ricans because of the potential for reform and improvement of the island's population, through healthy reproduction.[43] Yet at the same time, Puerto Rico's colonial relationship with the United States gave great scope for birth control experimentation. The U.S. concerns for "overpopulation" were fears that the island's racially mixed, Catholic poor were not reproducing responsibly and were thus creating problems of crime, unemployment, and disease. For the United States, there was serious anxiety about political responsibility for such a dysgenic society. The influence of the United States on Cuban eugenics is also clear, especially through the collaboration between Ramos and Davenport and their attempts to create a consensus on hemispheric eugenics; the consensus they sought, however, had little to do with the ethnic makeup or versions of eugenics of the majority of Latin American countries. Cuba, like the United States, depicted itself as a "white" nation and attempted to use immigration policy to make the island more so. Rejecting the Cuban approach, in general, Latin Americans sought to offer alternative understandings of eugenics and solutions to eugenic problems; understandings that depicted their heterogeneous populations as able to contribute to national development.

ACKNOWLEDGMENTS

My thanks to the editors for their invitation to contribute to this volume and their helpful criticisms, and to Paulo Drinot, Stuart Durkin, David T. Scott, and Alexandra Minna Stern for their comments on earlier drafts.

NOTES

1. Annette B. Ramírez de Arellano, and Conrad Seipp, *Colonialism, Catholicism, Contraception: A History of Birth Control in Puerto Rico* (Chapel Hill, NC: University of North Carolina Press, 1983), 4.

2. Anne-Emanuelle Birn, "'No More Surprising than a Broken Pitcher?' Maternal and Child Health in the Early Years of the Pan American Sanitary Bureau," *Canadian Bulletin of Medical History* 19, no. 1 (2002): 32.

3. Peter Wade, "Race and Nation in Latin America: An Anthropological View," in *Race and Nation in Modern Latin America*, eds. Nancy P. Appelbaum, Anne S. Macpherson, and Karin Alejandra Rosemblatt (Chapel Hill, NC: University of North Carolina Press, 2003), 274, addressing Nancy Leys Stepan, *"The Hour of Eugenics": Race, Gender and Nation in Latin America* (Ithaca, NY: Cornell University Press, 1991).

4. Alejandra Bronfman, *Measures of Equality: Social Science, Citizenship and Race in Cuba, 1902–1940* (Chapel Hill, NC: University of North Carolina Press, 2004), 119, quotation 118; Armando García González, "El desarrollo de la eugenesia en Cuba," *Asclepio: Revista de la Historia de la Medicina y de la Ciencia* 51, no. 2 (1999): 86–87; Armando García González and Raquel Alvarez Peláez, *En busca de la raza perfecta: Eugenesia e higiene en Cuba (1898–1958)* (Madrid: Consejo Superior de Investigaciones Científicas, 1999), 4–11, 118–121; Consuelo Naranjo Orovio and Armando García González, *Medicina y racismo en Cuba: La ciencia contra la inmigración canaria en el siglo XX* (La Laguna, Tenerife: Centro de la Cultura Popular Canaria, 1996), 137; Stepan, *"The Hour of Eugenics,"* 76–77, 80–81.

5. García and Alvarez, *En busca*, 136; and Naranjo and García, *Medicina y racismo*, 162.

6. Bronfman, *Measures of Equality*, 120; Lynne M. Getz, "Biological Determinism in the Making of Immigration Policy in the 1920s," *International Science Review* 70, no. 1–2 (1995): 27; Naranjo and García, *Medicina y racismo*, 143; Stepan, *"The Hour of Eugenics,"* 172.

7. Armando García González and Raquel Alvarez Peláez, *Las trampas del poder: Sanidad, eugenesia y migración. Cuba y Estados Unidos (1900–1940)* (Madrid: Consejo Superior de Investigaciones Científicas, 2007), 127, 137; García and Alvarez, *En busca*, 155–56, 159; Stepan, *"The Hour of Eugenics,"* 124, 175.

8. García and Alvarez, *En busca*, 175.

9. Birn, "'No More Surprising,'" 33; García and Alvarez, *En busca*, 184–87, 190, 306; Nancy Leys Stepan, "The Pan American Experiment in Eugenics," in *Science and Empires: Historical Studies about Scientific Development and European Expansion*, eds. Patrick Petitjean, Catherine Jami, and Anne Marie Moulin (Dordrecht, Boston, MA, and London: Kluwer Academic Publishers), 201, 203; Stepan, *"The Hour of Eugenics,"* 175, 179; Naranjo and García, *Medicina y racismo*, 140–143.

10. García and Alvarez, *En busca*, 191–193, 197; Naranjo and García, *Medicina y racismo*, 140–141, 144; Stepan, *"The Hour of Eugenics,"* 178, 180–181; Stepan, "The Pan American Experiment," 204.

11. Naranjo and García, *Medicina y racismo*, 162.

12. Alejandro de la Fuente, "Race, National Discourse, and Politics in Cuba: An Overview," *Latin American Perspectives* 25, no. 3 (1998): 30; García and Alvarez, *En busca*, xvii; Aline Helg, "Race in Argentina and Cuba, 1880–1930: Theory, Policies, and Popular Reaction," in *The Idea of Race in Latin America, 1870–1940*, ed. Richard Graham (Austin, TX: University of Texas Press, 1990), 47. See also Aviva Chomsky, "'Barbados or Canada?' Race, Immigration, and Nation in Early-Twentieth-Century Cuba," *Hispanic American Historical Review* 80, no. 3 (2000): 417, n3.

13. Chomsky, "'Barbados,'" 439–441; De la Fuente, "Race, National Discourse, and Politics," 32–33; Helg, "Race in Argentina and Cuba," 54; García and Alvarez, *Las trampas*, 189–190; Lillian Guerra, "From Revolution to Involution in the Early Cuban Republic: Conflicts over Race, Class, and Nation, 1902–1906," in Appelbaum et al., *Race and Nation*, 152–156.

14. Bronfman, *Measures of Equality*, 124; García, "El desarrollo de la eugenesia," 90–92; García and Alvarez, *En busca*, 136; and Naranjo and García, *Medicina y racismo*, 144–146, 155, 158, 164.

15. Naranjo and García, *Medicina y racismo*, 147–148.

16. García and Alvarez, *En busca*, 429; Stepan, "The Pan American Experiment," 205–206; Stepan, *"The Hour of Eugenics,"* 184, 186–187.

17. Laura Briggs, *Reproducing Empire: Race, Sex, Science and U.S. Imperialism in Puerto Rico* (Berkeley, CA: University of California Press, 2002), 51, 108.

18. Briggs, *Reproducing Empire*, 74; Eileen J. Suárez Findlay, *Imposing Decency: The Politics of Sexuality and Race in Puerto Rico* (Durham, NC: Duke University Press, 1999), 88.

19. Ramírez and Seipp, *Colonialism, Catholicism, Contraception*, 13–14. See pp. 8–9 for a brief overview of Puerto Rico's legal status.

20. Briggs, *Reproducing Empire*, 83–84, 90–94, quotation 83; Bonnie Mass, "Puerto Rico: A Case Study of Population Control," *Latin American Perspectives* 4, no. 4 (1977): 68; Nancy Ordover, *American Eugenics: Race, Queer Anatomy, and the Science of Nationalism* (Minneapolis, MN: University of Minnesota Press, 2003), 150; Ramírez and Seipp, *Colonialism, Catholicism, Contraception*, 16–23, 29.

21. Briggs, *Reproducing Empire*, 84–86, 120; Ordover, *American Eugenics*, 150; Ramírez and Seipp, *Colonialism, Catholicism, Contraception*, 12–13, 23.

22. Briggs, *Reproducing Empire*, 75, 90–94; Mass, "Puerto Rico," 68; Ramírez and Seipp, *Colonialism, Catholicism, Contraception*, 16–23, 29, quotation 49.

23. Briggs, *Reproducing Empire*, 101–105; and Ordover, *American Eugenics*, 151.

24. Briggs, *Reproducing Empire*, 106–107; and Ramírez and Seipp, *Colonialism, Catholicism, Contraception*, 51–56. Katherine Dexter McCormick's phrase gives the title to Lara Marks, "'A Cage of Ovulating Females:' The History of the Early Oral Contraceptive Pill Trials, 1950–59," in *Molecularizing Biology and Medicine: New Practices and Alliances, 1910s–1970s*, eds. Soraya de Chadarevian and Harmke Kamminga (Amsterdam: Harwood Academic Publishers, 1998), cited in Briggs, *Reproducing Empire*, 135.

25. On Rhoads see Briggs, *Reproducing Empire*, 76–77.

26. Briggs, *Reproducing Empire*, 76–77, 81, 149–151; Roberto Mac-Lean y Estenós, *La eugenesia en América* (Mexico, DF: Biblioteca de Ensayos Sociologicos, Institute de Investigaciones Sociales, Cuadernos de Sociología, Universidad Nacional, 1952), 45–46; Mass, "Puerto Rico," 68–69; Ordover, *American Eugenics*, 151; Ramírez and Seipp, *Colonialism, Catholicism, Contraception*, 27, 49–51, 138, 158, 164 and chap. 9 on clinical trials of the pill carried out in Puerto Rico. See also Laura Briggs, "The Discourses of 'Forced Sterilization' in Puerto Rico: The Problem with the Speaking Subaltern," *differences* 10, no. 2 (1998): 30–66.

27. Although both the Health Department and the Family Planning Association promoted vasectomies, very few men underwent the procedure because of gendered views of male sexuality. Mass, "Puerto Rico," 71–72; Ordover, *American Eugenics*, 151; Ramírez and Seipp, *Colonialism, Catholicism, Contraception*, 135–138, 178.

28. Briggs, *Reproducing Empire*, 149–158.

29. Briggs, *Reproducing Empire*, 152–153, 155; Mass, "Puerto Rico," 73; Ramírez and Seipp, *Colonialism, Catholicism, Contraception*, 140–144.

30. Alan Knight, "Racism, Revolution, and *Indigenismo*: Mexico, 1910–1940," in *The Idea of Race*, ed. Graham, 78, 80–82.

31. Alexandra Minna Stern, "Responsible Mothers and Normal Children: Eugenics, Nationalism, and Welfare in Post-revolutionary Mexico, 1920–1940," *Journal of Historical Sociology* 12, no. 4 (1999): 369–370, 375, 377–378; Stern, "Mestizofilia, biotipología y eugenesia en el México posrevolucionario: Hacia una historia de la ciencia y el estado, 1920–1960," *Relaciones* 21, no. 81 (2000): 68; Laura Suárez y López Guazo, "La influencia de la Sociedad Eugénica Mexicana en la educación y en la medicina social," *Asclepio* 51, no. 2 (1999): 54–55. Suárez quotes the legislation at length.

32. Stepan, *"The Hour of Eugenics,"* 56, 131. See also Helen Bowyer, "Child Welfare in Mexico," *Bulletin of the Pan American Union* 55, no. 6 (1922): 563–565, and Laura Suárez y López Guazo, "Medicina y mejoramiento racial: La eugenesia en México," *Boletín Mexicano de Historia y Filosofía de la Medicina* 3, no. 1 (2000): 5–6.

33. Stern, "Responsible Mothers," 373, quotation 383; Patience A. Schell, "Nationalizing Children through Schools and Hygiene: Porfirian and Revolutionary Mexico City," *The Americas* 60, no. 4 (2004): 576–577.

34. Stepan, *"The Hour of Eugenics,"* 57, 109–110; Suárez, "La influencia," 57, 59, 65; Suárez, "Medicina," 7; Laura Suárez y López Guazo, "Eugenesia, salud mental y tipología psicológica del mexicano," *Asclepio* 54, no 2 (2002): 34.

35. Mac-Lean y Estenós, *La eugenesia,* 17; Suárez, "Eugenesia," 31; Suárez, "La influencia," 66, 83; Stepan, *"The Hour of Eugenics,"* 55, 100.

36. Stepan, *"The Hour of Eugenics,"* 131–133; and Suárez, "La influencia," 60. Salvador Mendoza, "Regulations on Eugenics and Mental Hygiene in the State of Veracruz (Mexico)," *American Journal of Psychiatry* 90 (1933): 277–283 includes the full text of the law. Quotation on 278.

37. Stern, "Mestizofilia," 63, 76–78, 81; Suárez, "Medicina," 9–10, n 23.

38. Alexandra Minna Stern, "From Mestizophilia to Biotypology: Racialization and Science in Mexico, 1920–1960," in Appelbaum et al., *Race and Nation,* 190.

39. Stepan, *"The Hour of Eugenics,"* 138; Stern, "Mestizofilia," 63–64, 66; Stern "From Mestizophilia," 192–193; Suárez, "La influencia," 62, 80.

40. Stern, "Mestizofilia," 67–68.

41. Anne Doremus, "Indigenism, Mestizaje, and National Identity in Mexico During the 1940s and the 1950s," *Mexican Studies/Estudios Mexicanos* 17, no. 2 (2001): 379–380; Knight, "Racism, Revolution, and *Indigenismo,*" 86, 92; Stepan, *"The Hour of Eugenics,"* 150; Stern, "Mestizofilia," 61–62; and quotation Stern, "From Mestizophilia," 191.

42. Doremus, "Indigenism, Mestizaje, and National Identity," 380–381; Knight, "Racism, Revolution, and *Indigenismo,*" 85; Stern, "Mestizofilia," 61; Stern, "From Mestizophilia," 191; Suárez, "Eugenesia," 24, n15; Suárez, "La influencia," 55–56, 74–75.

43. Briggs, *Reproducing Empire,* 99–100.

FURTHER READING

Briggs, Laura. *Reproducing Empire: Race, Sex, Science and U.S. Imperialism in Puerto Rico* (Berkeley, CA: University of California Press, 2002).

García González, Armando. "El desarrollo de la eugenesia en Cuba," *Asclepio: Revista de la Historia de la Medicina y de la Ciencia* 51, no. 2 (1999): 85–100.

García González, Armando, and Raquel Alvarez Peláez. *En busca de la raza perfecta: Eugenesia e higiene en Cuba (1898–1958)* (Madrid: Consejo Superior de Investigaciones Científicas, 1999).

García González, Armando, and Raquel Alvarez Peláez. *Las trampas del poder: Sanidad, eugenesia y migración. Cuba y Estados Unidos (1900–1940)* (Madrid: Consejo Superior de Investigaciones Científicas, 2007).

Glick, Thomas F., Rosaura Ruiz, and Miguel Angel Puig-Samper. *El Darwinismo en España e Iberoamérica* (Madrid: Universidad Nacional Autónoma de México, Consejo Superior de Investigaciones Científicas and Ediciones Doce Calles, 1999).

Ramírez de Arellano, Annette B., and Conrad Seipp. *Colonialism, Catholicism, Contraception: A History of Birth Control in Puerto Rico* (Chapel Hill, NC: University of North Carolina Press, 1983).

Stepan, Nancy Leys. *"The Hour of Eugenics": Race, Gender and Nation in Latin America* (Ithaca, NY: Cornell University Press, 1991).

Stern, Alexandra Minna. "Responsible Mothers and Normal Children: Eugenics, Nationalism, and Welfare in Post-revolutionary Mexico, 1920–1940," *Journal of Historical Sociology* 12, no. 4 (1999): 369–397.

Stern, Alexandra Minna. "Mestizofilia, Biotipología y eugenesia en el México posrevolucionario: Hacia una historia de la ciencia y el estado, 1920–1960," *Relaciones* 21 (2000): 59–91.

Suárez y López Guazo, Laura. "La influencia de la Sociedad Eugénica Mexicana en la educación y en la medicina social," *Asclepio: Revista de la Historia de la Medicina y de la Ciencia* 51, no. 2 (1999): 51–84.

Suárez y López Guazo, Laura. "Medicina y mejoramiento racial: La eugenesia en México." *Boletín Mexicano de Historia y Filosofía de la Medicina* 3, no. 1 (2000): 4–15.

CHAPTER 29

THE PATH OF EUGENICS IN BRAZIL: DILEMMAS OF MISCEGENATION

GILBERTO HOCHMAN, NÍSIA TRINDADE LIMA, AND MARCOS CHOR MAIO

SOCIOLOGIST Gilberto Freyre's 1933 book *Casa Grande e Senzala* is considered a landmark in the changing perspectives on the historical formation of Brazil, in particular because of his positive vision of racial mixing and his emphasis on cultural explanations of Brazilian society. In the preface to his work, Freyre (1900–1987) explored his own racial prejudices, referring to one of the most important debates during the First Brazilian Congress of Eugenics in Rio de Janeiro in 1929, then the capital of the Republic:

> Once, after being absent from Brazil for almost three years, I saw a group of Brazilian sailors—mulatos and *cafuzos*—making their way [...] through the soft snow in Brooklyn. They gave me the impression of caricatures of men and the phrase of an English or American traveler about Brazil which I had just read came to mind: "The fearfully mongrel aspect of population." Miscegenation resulted in this. I needed someone to tell me then, like Roquette-Pinto said to the Aryanizers at the Brazilian Congress of Eugenics, that the individuals that I believed represented Brazil were not simply mulatos or *cafuzos*, but diseased mulatos or *cafuzos*.[1]

Freyre's memories of these Brazilian sailors in New York drew on the predominant position of eugenics in Brazil and other Latin American countries, foregrounding the physician, anthropologist, educator, director of the National Museum (Museu

Nacional) and president of the 1929 Brazilian Eugenics Congress, Edgard Roquette-Pinto (1884–1954). In his work Roquette-Pinto refuted the inferiority of Brazilian *mestiços*, attributing the problems of the country, such as low rural productivity, illiteracy, and disease to social rather than biological causes. The 1929 Congress signaled the defeat—but not the disappearance—of the most hard-line, racist, and orthodox ideas of the so-called Aryanists, led by the great disseminator of eugenics, Renato Kehl (1889–1974). It was the Congress that shaped the future path of eugenics in Brazil.[2]

In the 1920s, eugenics made its name internationally as a scientific theory of human heredity and as a movement that was simultaneously intellectual and political. Its wide appeal created a heterogeneous body of explanations and great variation in the different national contexts in which it developed.[3] The most influential work on the history of eugenics in Latin America, that of Nancy Stepan, has called attention to this diversity, which was most evident in the Brazilian eugenics movement in the 1920s when important scientists began to defend Mendel's laws and widen the distinction between eugenics and sanitation, challenging the then hegemonic neo-Lamarckism.[4] For Stepan the control of reproduction rather than the reform of the social environment was the prescription to be derived from Mendelism.[5]

We argue that in the Brazilian case the negative and racialized implications that characterized Mendelian-influenced eugenics in the Anglo-Saxon context did not occur in the same form or with the same intensity. Brazilian exponents of eugenics, such as Roquette-Pinto, were both defenders of Mendel's theories of inheritance and advocates of social reforms: they opposed negative eugenics. For some of these scientists and doctors it was necessary to separate the problems of inheritance, belonging to eugenic discussion, from those resulting from the social environment, which could be resolved by government policies. Sanitation and education were seen in Brazil (and some other countries in the region) as important objectives, since according to some Mendelian scientists the Brazilian people were not degenerate, but rather diseased and illiterate. The defense of the primacy of sanitation, hygiene, and education over eugenics, then, was not restricted to doctors influenced by neo-Lamarckism and French eugenics.[6]

The diffusion of eugenics in Brazil also occurred in the context of the social and economic problems associated with widespread infectious and parasitic diseases, often regarded as a serious obstacle to Brazil's successful transformation into a nation.[7] It was this association between race and health that we see in Freyre's image of "diseased mulatos and *cafuzos*." The politically organized demands for sanitation in Brazil in the 1910s are thus central to an understanding of eugenics in the region. Eugenics coexisted with nationalist movements, which bloomed during this decade, and which generally demanded greater state welfare activism.[8]

Since the end of the nineteenth century, the intellectual and political elites of the country, influenced by deterministic and pessimistic positions in relation to climate and race, had been faced with an important question: How would it be possible to construct a civilized nation in tropical lands (inhospitable for some) with a mixed population (whom some regarded as degenerate)?[9] This question, formulated in the late nineteenth century, structured the anxiety of Latin American intellectuals regarding the future of the region and underlies the local paths followed by eugenics in the early twentieth century.[10] The same question, rephrased in different combinations of elements and images, structured other experiences in South America.

In the Argentinian case, historians stress the hegemony of positive eugenics, expressed as education and public hygiene policies (in particular, school and urban hygiene), as instruments for broader idea of population "improvement."[11] This eugenic perspective also favored European immigration policies that looked at certain nationalities in a more positive way. Some authors have emphasized the role of negative eugenics, focusing on the ties to fascism, as well as social control and political and police repression.[12] The incorporation of indigenous populations, whose cultures and practices were often considered backward and uncivilized, was—and continues to be—the great dilemma of Andean countries such as Peru and Bolivia. The elites of European background—a minority in demographic terms—proposed solutions ranging from health and education reforms and the revaluation of a native past imagined as glorious to population control and exclusion of indigenous people.[13]

As elsewhere, Brazilian eugenics brought together a wide range of professionals—physicians, journalists, anthropologists, biologists, educators, and lawyers—and involved a series of different and sometimes contradictory responses to local challenges of national identity. Eugenics was a type of lingua franca within Brazilian and Latin American scientific and intellectual circles in the 1920s and 1930s; it was never a homogenous political and intellectual movement with an organized and consensual agenda. To the contrary, precisely because of the fluidity of its meaning and its near omnipresence in the scientific debate, eugenics, like the idea of race, could be shared by many as a general ideal for "improving populations." Cleavages always emerged in relation to the view of the place of blacks, indigenous natives, *mestiços,* immigrants, and those deemed socially incapable. Differing ideas about the problems of the country produced markedly different solutions ranging from sterilization and selective immigration to matrimonial control, education, health, and sanitation. Like other experiences in Central America and the Caribbean, eugenics below the Panama Canal was also marked by adaptations and even by reinventions based on social, political, ethnic, and cultural conditions imposed by local contexts.[14]

RACIAL THEORIES AND BRAZILIAN DILEMMAS AT THE END OF THE NINETEENTH CENTURY

Since independence from Portugal in 1822, segments of the Brazilian intellectual elite had sought solutions for the two factors pervasively perceived as obstacles to a civilized Brazil: climate and race. Pessimistic visions of the Brazilian people and the future of the nation were initially produced by foreign scientists and intellectuals who deemed the population backward in evolutionary terms. The principal influences were the English historian Henry Buckle (1821–1862), author of *History of*

Civilization in England (1861) and defender of the argument that the more exuberant nature was in a country, the more difficult it would be for the country to become civilized: Count Arthur Gobineau (1816–1882), author of the famous *An Essay on the Inequality of the Human Races* (1853) and a French diplomat who served in Brazil for a little over a year between 1869 and 1870; and Louis Agassiz (1807–1873), a Swiss naturalist based in the United States who founded and directed the Museum of Comparative Zoology at Harvard University and who visited Brazil to collect species of fauna and flora in 1865. These three authors and their assessments of Brazil raised questions and dilemmas relevant for any project of national and state building in the later nineteenth century. For Buckle, who dealt only briefly with Brazil in his book, Brazilian nature was so splendid that it ended up producing apathetic and mentally hindered people who needed the assistance of Europeans in order to develop fully, an argument shared by Gobineau. However, for the French aristocrat, the principal deficiency of the country was to be found in its people, whom he considered ugly and inferior due to their high level of racial miscegenation, which produced degenerate types among both the elites and the poor. The emphasis on intense Brazilian racial intermixing and its characterization as negative and an obstacle to civilization was also present in the reflections of Agassiz.[15]

Invested with the authority of scientific laws, racial theories were also used by some Latin American intellectuals as starting points to diagnose a dim future for the former European colonies because of their racial composition and unconquerable nature. One of the main considerations of Brazilian intellectuals consisted of the formation of a national community, among whom were some they considered to be non-citizens and threatening, largely indigenous peoples and African slaves. The end of slavery in May 1888 and the creation of a republican regime in November 1889 were political landmarks that underscored the dilemmas of the Brazilian Empire. The demand for paid labor to replace slaves in the expansion of agriculture directly raised the problem of which immigrants were desirable. And the dawn of the Republic gave rise to concerns over national unity, increasingly perceived as the need for a "Brazilian people," now seen as a racial unit to be created in the middle of diversity. These changes help us to understand the context of the emergence of eugenics in Brazil from the 1910s.

Between the end of the Empire and the first two republican decades, Brazilian intellectuals sought to deal with racial and climatic determinism in an original manner. Three writers are exemplary: the essayist Sílvio Romero (1851–1914), the physician Raimundo Nina Rodrigues (1862–1906), and the engineer Euclides da Cunha (1866–1909).

Romero was critical of the complacency with which the old imperial elite regarded both itself and Brazil. He advocated scientific studies on the population from both a biological and a cultural perspective, with an emphasis on miscegenation. Romero believed that the racial mixture of the population would produce a new Brazilian literary and cultural expression. For Romero, "every Brazilian is *mestiço*, when not in the blood, then in the ideas."[16] His vision was of a process of racial intermixing leading toward whitening, which would foster a homogenous national type.

Starting from the same racialist reference as Romero, Nina Rodrigues, a doctor and professor in the Medical School of Bahia, proposed a divergent description of the Brazilian people. According to Rodrigues, Brazil was characterized by racial diversity, not just in its origin and current state, but also in its future. Instead of a process of miscegenation through which a progressively amalgamated Brazilian people would be produced, he argued that biology demonstrated that racial inter-mixing would not eliminate differences between the races, since these were ontological. Racial mixing would not produce a homogenous *mestiço* type, but rather would create varied individuals, many of whom would be contemptible in comparison with the original races.[17] He interpreted mixing with "inferior" races as a tragedy that not even large-scale miscegenation with whites could alleviate.[18]

Euclides da Cunha also made use of racial and climatic categories in his inter-pretation of the Brazilian people. An engineer, military officer, and journalist, he enthusiastically greeted the new regime established in 1889. However, his optimism suffered a setback with the Canudos War (1896–1897), a popular rebellion in the interior of the state of Bahia. His reflections on the episode marked a dividing point in the debate about what Brazil and its people were and should be.[19] Cunha's starting point was a pessimistic synthesis of evolutionism and climatic and racial explana-tions. However, he changed his perspective, coming to understand race as a histor-ical category and not as absolute or definitive. For Cunha the transformation of race did not occur solely through miscegenation, but through a relationship with the environment and the historical events in which populations were involved. This approach is expressed in his explanation of the place of the *sertanejo* (the "back-lander") in the national project. The isolation of the *sertanejo* in the interior and their struggle and slow adaptation to the environment had produced a reasonably stable and strong "sub-race" where humans and nature were conflated. In Cunha's vision this was a backward population, but not a degenerate one. In fact, he thought that the population of the interior was the bedrock on which Brazilian nationality would be built.[20]

These three authors were typical in the way they made use of European deter-ministic racial theories and constructed interpretations and proposals for the problem of the construction of nationality. They, among others, formulated the matrix for reflection on the possibilities of a civilized country with a *mestiço* population.

HEALTH AND EDUCATION POLICIES AS EUGENICS

The debate over national identity in Brazil was vigorous during the First Republic (1889–1930), since many intellectuals associated republican government with the idea of progress and the civilizing process, in a country troubled by its colonial and slave-holding past, and with what many saw as the racial inferiority of its population.

During and after World War I, stimulated by the political and intellectual environment it shaped, alternatives for the construction of nationality began to emerge in Brazil.

"Brazil is still a great hospital."[21] This statement, issued in a public addresses in October 1916 by Miguel Pereira (1871–1918), a prominent associate of the Faculty of Medicine of Rio de Janeiro and former president of the National Academy of Medicine, was the trigger for a political movement promoting rural sanitation and was one of the recurrent images highlighting the social problems of the country.[22] This strong image, simultaneously a denunciation and diagnosis, was also a therapeutic proposal for Brazil—the "overwhelming" power of the idea of sanitation, to use the expression of the writer Monteiro Lobato (1882–1948).[23] Pereira's statement was based both on the dramatic reports of disease, illiteracy, and poverty by doctors and scientists from the Oswaldo Cruz Institute,[24] who traveled into the interior of Brazil in the 1910s, and by the repercussions of the discovery in 1909 of a new "tropical disease" by the Brazilian scientist Carlos Chagas (1879–1934)—*Trypanosomiasis Americana* or Chagas disease—which left rural populations unable to work.[25] The political repercussions of Pereira's position contributed to the establishment of a consensus about the equation "*sertão* (backlands) of Brazil equal to disease and abandonment."[26] Health and education policies were considered the pillars of a project to modify this context, along with the occupation of the vast territory of the country and the integration of rural populations into the nation.[27]

The creation of the Pro-Sanitation League of Brazil (*Liga Pró-Saneamento do Brasil*) in February 1918 was the organized expression of this political movement, with its message that rural endemic diseases (ancylostomiasis, malaria, and Chagas disease—"the unholy trinity") were the principal problems facing Brazil. The League demanded that the government address the sanitary and public health conditions of the interior. Led by the doctor Belisário Penna (1868–1939), this "medical crusade for the *patria*"[28] converted many intellectuals to the creed of hygiene and brought together scientists, doctors, journalists, military officers, and lawyers, many of whom were influenced by eugenic ideas. As well as successfully establishing health services and rural sanitation between 1918 and 1920, this political movement interpreted disease and illiteracy in rural Brazil as resulting from the absence, neglect, or indifference of public authority. It thus ruled out race and climate as the determinants of backwardness. The League saw state action as the best way to restore the health of the rural population and to integrate them into the nation.

It was in this context that eugenic ideas began to circulate with greater intensity in the 1920s. Despite the persistence of stereotypes and ideas associated with racial differences among the intellectuals who adhered to the sanitation campaign in Brazil (including those who participated in the diffusion of eugenics), there was a clear predominance of a discourse that refuted the idea that ethnic difference made nationhood unfeasible. A country that some considered "condemned by race," could now be "absolved by experimental medicine, by the laboratory," and through public campaigns related to sanitation, public health, vaccination, and medical care.[29]

The strong association between eugenics and hygiene, with its emphasis on intervention in the environment and the regulation of, among other practices, alcoholism and sexual behavior, was notable in the 1910s and 1920s. At one of the conferences of the Eugenics Society of São Paulo (founded in 1918: see below), the physician Olegário de Moura, claimed: "sanitation is eugenics."[30] The same phrase was used in a broader Latin American context by the Peruvian doctor Carlos Enrique Paz Soldán (1885–1972), one of the most important public health and social medicine leaders in the region. Concerned with the incorporation of indigenous populations, he defended the "re-peopling of America with its own races, selecting them for their health and the fight against endemics diseases and vices."[31] Thus, this strong association between eugenics and sanitation can be explained not only by the influence and circulation of international eugenic ideas but also by new responses to the problem of the racial composition of the population, which had been discussed since the end of the nineteenth century and which was now raised in a markedly nationalist context in which public health came to play a leading role. In this way, as Nancy Stepan has argued, eugenics became "a metaphor for health."[32]

EUGENICS INSTITUTIONS IN BRAZIL, 1917–1930

Until 1917 there were few explicit reference to eugenics in the Brazilian press or medical periodicals. In São Paulo that year, Renato Kehl gave his first lecture, calling on the press and "men of science" to become engaged in eugenic propaganda as the only way to save the population from degeneration. This conference was a landmark in the institutionalization of eugenics in Brazil, gaining considerable coverage in the press.[33]

The Eugenics Society of São Paulo (Sociedade Eugênica de São Paulo) was created on January 25, 1918, in Santa Casa de Misericórdia, a traditional hospital charity institution. The new association, the first of its kind in Latin America, was in a state that bloomed economically and politically under the First Republic (1889–1930). Its president was Arnaldo Vieira de Carvalho (1867–1920), director of the recently created Medical School of São Paulo. Its principal intent was to prevent the approval of an amendment of an article in the Civil Code that would allow marriage between uncles/aunts and nieces/nephews. The Institutes of Lawyers of São Paulo and Rio de Janeiro and the National Academy of Medicine shared the Society's position against these marriages.[34] The Society also organized conferences whose themes extended the strong association between sanitation and eugenics. The death of Carvalho and the transfer of Renato Kehl to Rio de Janeiro resulted in the demise of the society at the end of 1919.

The diffusion of eugenics was continued by other organizations, notably the Brazilian Mental Hygiene League (Liga Brasileira de Higiene Mental), which from its inception in 1923 campaigned for mandatory prenuptial medical examinations and against alcoholism and syphilis.[35] Many bills requiring the compulsion of pre-nuptial medical examination were presented to the National Congress during the 1920s, described by the doctor and representative, Amaury de Medeiros (1893–1928), as a form of constructive eugenics.[36] Other representatives with medical expertise, such as Oscar Penna Fontenelle (1898–1963), proposed bills criminalizing contagion by transmissible disease, and creating sex education in schools. None of these initia-tives for compulsion was successful in the 1920s, because of the strong opposition on the part of both liberal politicians and parliamentarians influenced by Catholic thinking. The League also included on its agenda debate on the necessity for the control of immigration and the sterilization of the "mentally deficient." While ster-ilization measures were defended by many of its members,[37] there was much con-troversy within the League, and its official periodical, *Archivos Brasileiros de Higiene Mental,* indicated that there was no consensus in this period about the adoption of such radical eugenic measures.[38]

A shift from "constructive eugenics" to more radical measures like steriliza-tion is evident in the ideas and work of Renato Kehl. Until the end of the 1920s, Kehl was strongly influenced by the vision that associated eugenics, health, and sanitation. He was very close to doctors and intellectuals active in the Pro-Sanitation League of Brazil and had a strong relationship with his father-in-law, Belisário Penna, leader of the rural sanitation movement. This association influ-enced his work as head of the propaganda and hygienic education service of the Leprosy and Venereal Disease Service (Inspetoria da Lepra e Doenças Venéreas), linked to the National Department of Public Health (Departamento Nacional de Saúde Pública), between 1920 and 1927. After leaving the public health service and assuming the position of medical director of Bayer Industry in Brazil (1927) Kehl's position changed, and he moved closer to the radical ideas of negative eugenics. On a trip to Germany in 1928, he established contacts with biologists, doctors, and anthropologists sympathetic to eugenics. He visited Hermann Muckermann (1877–1962), director of the Institute of Eugenics of Berlin, and made contact with the anthropologist Hans Haustein and with Eugen Fischer (1874–1967), director of the Kaiser-Wilhelm Institute for Anthropology, Human Genetics, and Eugenics in Berlin, and one of the principal enthusiasts of Germanic Aryanism. Kehl also established relations with Austrian and Scandinavian eugenicists, maintaining regular correspondence with them. It was through these contacts that Kehl's attention was drawn to the work on inheritance and families carried out by Charles Davenport (1866–1944) at the Eugenics Record Office in the United States, from which he derived proposals for compulsory sterilization, racial segregation, and prohibiting entry to the country of individuals from races considered inferior.[39]

In 1929, shortly after returning from a trip to Germany and more than a decade after creating the first Latin American eugenics society, Kehl returned to eugenic propaganda with his periodical, *Boletim de Eugenia.* Published monthly with an average print run of 1,000 copies, the periodical was progressively expanded,

becoming a supplement of the medical journal *Medicamenta.* The journal circulated until 1933.[40] In 1929 Kehl published *Lições de Eugenia,* a book in which he condemned racial intermixing and proposed the prohibition of marriage between
different racial groups. By this point, Kehl's adherence to negative eugenics was
clear:

> In the first place negative eugenics stipulates educational propaganda, the appeal
> to those who, naturally, "have a conscience," in order not to propagate their
> perversions and deformities....Other resources advocated by negative eugenics to
> avoid indigent paternity consist of legal measures to make degenerates and
> criminals unable to reproduce themselves....Another measure proposed by
> negative eugenics is the sterilization of degenerates and criminals. The simple
> prohibition of the marriage of these individuals will only constitute an
> "attenuating measure," capable of being bypassed, while sterilization will
> represent a "radical measure," that is often necessary.[41]

Kehl's proposals were never put into practice and were strongly contested in
scientific and intellectual circles in the country. Nevertheless, his was not an isolated
voice in the eugenics debate. Others adopted a similar position in relation to the
sterilization of the unfit and "those with perversions," including psychiatrists in the
Brazilian League of Mental Hygiene and some delegates to the 1929 Brazilian
Congress of Eugenics. More conciliatory strategies were formulated by others, such
as the biologist Octávio Domingues (1897–1972), who suggested to Kehl the possibility of assimilating Catholic intellectuals to the eugenist campaign.[42] Palpably, the
Catholic tradition in Latin American countries was an important factor in the unfavorable attitudes toward negative eugenics.

Proponents of other initiatives favored Mendelism over sanitation eugenics but
distanced themselves from negative eugenics. Roquette-Pinto carried out studies of
the "Brazilian ethnic types" through the National Museum of Rio de Janeiro, and
Octávio Domingues began genetic investigations of plants and animals at the Luiz
de Queiroz Higher School of Agriculture (Escola Superior de Agricultura Luiz de
Queiroz) in Piracicaba (São Paulo state). Domingues had cordial relations and regular correspondence with Kehl and sat on the editorial board of *Boletim de Eugenia*
in 1932–1933.[43] Roquette-Pinto, on the other hand, was Kehl's principal antagonist,
and his ideas and actions indicate that there was no necessary relationship between
Mendelism and negative eugenics. Influenced by Comtean positivism, Roquette-
Pinto argued that since all peoples belonged to the same humanity, their only
difference was their level of civilization. His experience with indigenous Brazilians
living isolated in the interior and in the Amazon region laid the foundations of his
vision of Brazilian races and types.[44] He argued for action on health and living conditions, emphasizing that "alongside fatalistic eugenics that preaches that outside
inheritance there is no salvation, another eugenics has been established, concerned
with favoring the acquisition of the best somatic characters on the part of those
who are living."[45] These positions were at the center of debate at the First Brazilian
Congress of Eugenics.

THE BRAZILIAN CONGRESS OF EUGENICS
AND THE FUTURE OF A *MESTIÇO* PEOPLE

Four integrated medical and scientific events were held in Rio de Janeiro between June 30 and July 7, 1929 under the auspices of the centenary of the National Academy of Medicine. Among them were the First Brazilian Congress of Eugenics, where a broad range of eugenics topics was discussed: race and immigration; maternal and child health; age at marriage; child rearing; the teaching of physical education; venereal disease prevention; child mortality; feminism; maternity; and the investigation of paternity. There were also discussions of negative eugenic practices, such as prohibition of marriage between individuals from different races, and sterilization of the so-called "*tarados*" (literally, perverts), who included the blind, the deaf and dumb, the mentally disabled, epileptics, drug addicts, the alienated, and beggars.[46]

The agenda of the congress, divided into sections, is indicative of the polysemia of eugenics in Brazil, with the inclusion of themes that in principle were not directly related to inheritance. Still, the conference placed considerable emphasis on the association between eugenics and race, and there was intense controversy about the dysgenic character of racial intermixing.[47] One of the most heated discussions took place in the section on Legislation and Education, chaired by the educator Levi Carneiro (1882–1971), about relations between races and immigration. The journalist Azevedo Amaral (1881–1942), in a paper entitled "The Eugenic Problem of Immigration," recommended restriction of immigrants with antisocial tendencies. His proposal was defeated by only three votes.[48] Another of his controversial recommendations proposed the restriction of the entrance of immigrants, especially black immigrants, from non-white countries. Oscar Penna Fontenelle defended this recommendation based on the indicators of labor productivity in Latin American countries. He argued that in countries such as Argentina, where there was only a minimal black presence, productivity was much higher than in Brazil. In opposition to Fontenelle and Amaral, Roquette-Pinto said that the low levels of health of the Brazilian population were a consequence of the incidence of diseases such as malaria and ancylostomiasis and could not be attributed to racial factors. Much more forceful was the argument of the doctor Fernando de Magalhães (1878–1944), according to whom Amaral's proposal was unjust and even suicidal, since the Brazilian past was based on miscegenation, while those taking part in the Congress of Eugenics were also *mestiços*. In his own words: "There is an injustice here, because all our past is based on racial intermixing, and there is a suicide, because *we are all mestiços* and thus we exclude ourselves."[49]

Azevedo Amaral's proposal to restrict black immigrants was defeated by 25 votes to 17, but the result indicated a division between the members of the Congress. This defeat was an important moment for the eugenics movement and the medical community, but principally for the government and for deputies and senators who discussed these themes in the National Congress. The discussion about race and immigration was not restricted to forums such as the Eugenic Congress. It was also present in proposed laws on the settlement and colonization of the interior of the country, as well as being debated in newspapers and in medical and scientific journals. Due to the oligarchical nature of the Brazilian republic until 1930, which restricted the access of the vast majority of the population to both political citizenship and higher education, doctors were inevitably a part of the intellectual and political elite of the country's politics (at both a regional and national level), while many had simultaneous political and professional careers. Medical institutions, congresses, journals, and opinions had an influence on the political arena.

In the 1920s, there were some efforts to make race a criterion in immigration policy. One of the greatest controversies occurred following the announcement of a project in 1921 for a group of African Americans to emigrate to Brazil.[50] One result of this proposal was the unsuccessful presentation of a bill to prohibit the immigration of "individuals from the black race." In 1923 another bill—also defeated—proposed the same restriction, but added a curb on Japanese immigrants. The National Society of Agriculture, which defended the interests of large farmers, mobilized in favor of Japanese immigration, along with such important scientists and doctors as Roquette-Pinto and Olímpio da Fonseca Filho (1895–1978).[51]

In the Anthropology section of the Congress, the debate on race and eugenics figured prominently, and one of the high points of the conference was Álvaro Fróes da Fonseca's (1890–1988) talk on "The Great Problems of Anthropology." He pointed out the absence of a scientific basis to justify racial inferiority or the dysgenic character of racial intermixing, referring to research on *mestiços* carried out by anthropologists from different countries, and emphasizing the contribution of Franz Boas (1858–1942). He criticized the common confusion between race and species, and he opposed racist derivations from scientific theory on the inheritance or origin of humans. Fonseca, like Roquette-Pinto, thought it necessary to avoid "the unconscious or intentional confusion between *mestiços* raised in healthy conditions and those at the margin of society."[52]

Roquette-Pinto's paper, "Notas sobre os tipos antropológicos brasileiros" (Notes on the Brazilian anthropological types) was one of the principal counter-positions to negative eugenics and the thesis of the dysgenic character of racial intermixing. It described an anthropometric study of racial groups and racial intermixing in Brazil. After concluding that all the racial types in Brazil were eugenic, he pointed to the history of the country and specifically to slavery as one of the causes of poverty and inequality: "a critical study of the historical development of Brazil demonstrates that these evils are a consequence of an entanglement of factors, the consequence of a slave holding society. The cause of the evils was not race; it was slavery...Anthropology proves that man in Brazil needs to be educated and not substituted."[53]

The 1929 Eugenics Congress was important because it clearly defined the terms of the dispute that divided the Brazilian eugenics movement. There were those, on the one hand, who denied any future for racially intermixed peoples and prescribed their gradual replacement via reproductive control and selective immigration. And on the other hand, there were those who, whether Mendelian or Neo-Lamarckian, relied on government action to transform the same peoples. The latter position was accepted by the majority and drew on a more optimistic vision of the future of a racially intermixed people: the population did not need to be replaced, but rather educated, fed, and given proper infrastructure for hygiene. The problem was not racial composition, but the absence of good government policies. It is revealing, and perhaps the result of this irreconcilable division, that this was the first and only Eugenics Congress held in Brazil.

Eugenics in the 1930s: Final Considerations

In October 1930, following the so-called 1930 Revolution, *gaúcho* Getulio Vargas (1882–1954) came to power as president of the Republic. From 1937 to 1945, he held that position in the explicitly authoritarian form of the Estado Novo, governing as a dictator. The modernizing and centralizing government of Vargas signified the end of the first republican experience that was based on a controlled and exclusionary political participation and an almost complete absence of social policies. The 1930–1945 period is a landmark in the establishment of industrial and social policies in Brazil. A range of institutional changes molded Brazilian politics, establishing a legal and material framework that shaped the system of social protection for many decades, including labor legislation, the regulation of the working day, medical assistance, vacations and retirement for urban workers, minimum wage, and protection for mothers, infants, and the family. Some of the long-held demands of eugenicists for more state activism were met through Vargas's projects, particularly through actions related to maternal and child protection, which were central for a government that articulated the special role of infancy, a general idea of race, and the construction of the nation.[54] The policies of the Vargas government were not immune to the ambiguities of a centralizing and authoritarian government in the 1930s that extended social protection to the world of urban labor at the same time that it implemented actions of political and social control through bio-typological identification and political repression.

Prompted by this commitment to state intervention, eugenicists under the leadership of Renato Kehl created the Brazilian Central Commission of Eugenics (Comissão Central Brasileira de Eugenia) in 1931, to promote a "hard-line" eugenics agenda as part of the new judicial framework of the Brazilian state.[55] The National Assembly, which approved a new Brazilian Constitution in 1934, discussed negative eugenic proposals to legalize abortion in exceptional cases and birth control for eugenic reasons, but they were not approved. On the other hand, the Assembly did approve a prenuptial medical examination—physical and mental—for potential husbands and wives.[56]

Continuing earlier dissent, Roquette-Pinto, along with influentials intellectuals like Gilberto Freyre and Arthur Ramos (1903–1949), signed in October 1935 the "Manifesto of the Brazilian Intellectuals against Racism" (Manifesto dos Intelectuais Brasileiros contra o Preconceito Racial) that argued against the ideas of the racial inferiority of the Brazilians, in particular the mulatos and blacks, as well as against negative eugenics.[57]

The use of racial criteria for immigration policy through the creation of the category of *desirable immigrants* continued to be debated during the creation of the new constitution. Racial restrictions were presented in bills such as those by representative and doctor Miguel Couto (1865–1934), who proposed the prohibition of African immigration and by representative and doctor Arthur Neiva (1880–1943), whose bill permitted entry of white immigrants only.[58] In the end, the proposal that was approved dispensed with racial criteria, using instead the classification of nationality as an alternative. This principle, enshrined in the 1934 Constitution, survived in the authoritarian 1937 constitution. Brazilian immigration policy became increasingly restrictive from the middle of the 1930s to the end of World War II. And while from a legal and constitutional perspective Brazil did not adopt racial criteria to restrict "undesirables," discriminatory positions and actions based on racist visions were nonetheless in practice during this decade, as in the case of Jews.[59]

Despite the decline of the eugenics movement after the war (in which Brazil was directly involved on the side of the Allies from 1942), the dilemmas of a *mestiço* nation persisted in the intellectual and political agenda, albeit in a different form. The terms of discussion of the racial problem were radically transformed in the 1950s, moving from the question of *race and national identity* to an understanding of social inequalities centered on *race relations*. Indeed, intellectuals and international agencies saw Brazil as a possible laboratory of racial democracy. During the 1950s, for example, the United Nations Educational, Scientific and Cultural Organization (UNESCO) sponsored a cycle of research on racial relations in Brazil, which was seen as a positive national case. In the years that followed, race nonetheless persisted as a socially material category and as one of the basic causes of social discrimination in a society still marked by profound inequality. Relations between race, racism, and poverty in the explanation of inequalities are still on the Brazilian contemporary political agenda.[60]

In the period covered by this chapter, eugenics presented itself as a heterogeneous intellectual and political movement, but this was not unique to the Brazilian experience, since it can be identified in other South American countries. Eugenics incorporated diagnoses and propositions related to environmental and social questions, as well as proposals for the control of reproduction, racial discrimination, and immigration. One issue in particular predominated in this region: there were constant attempts to find a solution to the dilemma first identified in the late nineteenth century concerning the possibilities of constructing a national state through the incorporation of a population characterized by large-scale miscegenation, as in the case of Brazil, or the significant presence of indigenous peoples, as in the Andean countries. These characteristics were considered by many as obstacles to any attempt to shape civilized nations on the continent.

Were *mestiços* degenerate on the one hand, or diseased and uneducated on the other? In the 1920s and 1930s, eugenics was characterized as the scientific lingua franca that would solve this dilemma. For this reason it became impossible to dissociate it from debate on the two key and interdependent questions: the national and the racial question. After the political agenda of the former Spanish and Portuguese colonies became monopolized by the theme of the unity of territory, the formation of their populations was at the heart of the recurring discussions of national identity. In interaction with these contextual and historical factors, eugenics acquired local specificity in Brazil in particular, and in South America more generally.

ACKNOWLEDGMENTS

Our thanks to the editors, Philippa Levine and Alison Bashford, for their suggestions and criticisms, and for their generous, detailed, and careful review of the English translation. We are grateful also to Diego Armus and Ricardo Ventura Santos for their comments.

NOTES

1. Gilberto Freyre, *Casa-Grande & Senzala: Formação da Família Brasileira sob o Regime de Economia Patriarcal* (Rio de Janeiro: Maia & Schmidt, 1933), xii. Published in English as *The Masters and the Slaves: A Study in the Development of Brazilian Civilization* (New York: Alfred A. Knopf, 1946).

2. Vanderlei S. Souza, "As Leis da Eugenia na Antropologia de Edgard Roquette-Pinto," in *Antropologia Brasiliana: Ciência e Educação na Obra de Edgard Roquette-Pinto*, eds. Nísia Trindade Lima and Dominichi Miranda de Sá (Belo Horizonte; Rio de Janeiro: Editora UFMG; Editora Fiocruz, 2008), 213–244.

3. Mark B. Adams, *The Wellborn Science: Eugenics in Germany, France, Brazil, and Russia* (Oxford and New York: Oxford University Press, 1990).

4. Nancy Stepan, "Eugenics in Brazil, 1917–1940," in Adams, *The Wellborn Science*, 110–152; Stepan, "*The Hour of Eugenics*": *Race, Gender, and Nation in Latin America* (Ithaca, NY: Cornell University Press, 1991).

5. Stepan, "*The Hour of Eugenics*", chaps. 3, 4.

6. Evidence that corroborates this argument can be found in works such as Lima and Sá, *Antroplogia Brasiliana*; Stepan, "*The Hour of Eugenics*"; Ricardo V. Santos, "A Obra de Euclides da Cunha e os Debates sobre Mestiçagem no Brasil no Início do Século XX: Os Sertões e a Medicina-Antropologia do Museu Nacional," *História, Ciências, Saúde-Manguinhos* 5, supplement (1998): 237–254; Marcos Chor Maio, "Raça, Doença e Saúde Pública no Brasil: Um Debate Sobre o Pensamento Higienista do Século XIX," in *Etnicidade na América Latina: Um debate sobre raça, saúde e direitos reprodutivos*, eds. Simone Monteiro and Livio Sansone (Rio de Janeiro: Editora Fiocruz, 2004), 15–44.

7. Nísia T. Lima and Gilberto Hochman, "'Condenado pela Raça, Absolvido pela Medicina': O Brasil Descoberto pelo Movimento Sanitarista da Primeira República," in *Raça, Ciência e Sociedade*, eds. Marcos C. Maio and Ricardo V. Santos (Rio de Janeiro: Editora Fiocruz/CCBB, 1996), 23–40; Luiz Antônio de Castro Santos, "O Pensamento Sanitarista na Primeira República: Uma Ideologia de Construção da Nacionalidade," *Dados-Revista de Ciências Sociais* 28, no. 2 (1985): 237–250.

8. Lúcia Lippi de Oliveira, *A Questão Nacional na Primeira República* (São Paulo: Editora Brasiliense, 1990).

9. For a broader discussion of the idea of degeneration in Brazil, see Dain Borges, "'Puffy, Ugly, Slothful and Inert': Degeneration in Brazilian Social Thought, 1880–1940," *Journal of Latin American Studies* 25, no. 2 (1993): 235–256.

10. See Antonello Gerbi, *La disputa del nuevo mundo: Historia de una polémica, 1750–1900*, 2nd ed. (Mexico: Fondo de Cultura Econômica, 1982) and Patience Schell's chapter on Cuba, Puerto Rico, and México in this volume.

11. Stepan, "*The Hour of Eugenics*"; Diego Armus, *La Ciudad Impura: Salud, Tuberculosis y Cultura en Buenos Aires, 1870–1950* (Buenos Aires: Edhasa, 2007); María Silvia Di Liscia, "Los Bordes y Límites de la Eugenesia, Donde Caen las Razas Superiores: Argentina, Primera Mitad del Siglo XX," in *Políticas del Cuerpo: Estrategias Modernas de Normalización del Individuo y La Sociedad*, eds. Gustavo Vallejo and Marisa Miranda (Buenos Aires: Siglo XXI, 2007), 377–409; Eduardo A. Zimmermann, "Racial Ideas and Social Reform: Argentina, 1890–1916," *The Hispanic American Historical Review* 72, no. 1 (1992): 23–46.

12. Marisa Miranda, "La Antorcha de Cupido: Eugenesia, Biotipología y Eugamia en Argentina, 1930–1970," *Asclepio* 55, no. 2 (2003): 231–255; Gustavo Vallejo, "El Ojo del Poder en el Espacio del Saber: Los Institutos de Biotipología," *Asclepio* 56, no. 1 (2004): 219–244.

13. Walter Mendoza and Oscar Martínez, "Las Ideas Eugenésicas en la Creación del Instituto de Medicina Social," *Anales de la Facultad de Medicina* 60, no. 1 (1999): 55–60; Marcos Cueto, *The Return of the Epidemics: Health and Society in Peru During the Twentieth Century* (Burlington, VT: Ashgate, 2001); Ann Zulawski, *Unequal Cures: Public Health and Political Change in Bolivia, 1900–1950* (Durham, NC: Duke University Press, 2007).

14. Peter Fry, "Politics, Nationality and the Meaning of 'Race' in Brazil: Border of the Past, Promise of the Future," *Daedalus* 129, no. 2 (2000): 83–118.

15. On Agassiz, see Thomas E. Skidmore, *Black into White: Race and Nationality in Brazilian Thought* (Oxford and New York: Oxford University Press, 1974); Stephen Jay Gould, *The Mismeasure of Man* (New York: W. W. Norton, 1981).

16. Silvio Romero, *História da Literatura Brasileira*, 5 vols., 5th ed. (Rio de Janeiro: Garnier, 1888; Rio de Janeiro: José Olympio, 1953), 1: 56.

17. Mariza Corrêa, *As Ilusões da Liberdade: A Escola Nina Rodrigues e a Antropologia no Brasil* (Bragança Paulista: Editora da Universidade São Francisco, 1998); Julyan G. Peard, *Race, Place, and Medicine: The Idea of the Tropics in Nineteenth-Century Brazilian Medicine* (Durham, NC: Duke University Press, 1999); Lilia Moritz Schwarcz, *The Spectacle of the Races: Scientists, Institutions, and the Race Question in Brazil, 1870–1930* (New York: Hill and Wang, 1999); Raimundo Nina Rodrigues, "Os mestiços brasileiros," *Brazil Medico* 4 (1890) 51, 59, 67, 77; Rodrigues, *As Raças Humanas e a Responsabilidade Penal no Brasil*, 3rd ed. (1894; Salvador: Progresso, 1957).

18. Skidmore, *Black into White*, 57–62.

19. Euclides da Cunha, *Os Sertões* (Rio de Janeiro: Laemmert & Cia, 1902). Published in English as *Rebellion in the Backland* (Chicago, IL: University of Chicago Press, 1944).

20. Ibid.

21. Miguel Pereira, "'O Brasil é ainda um Imenso Hospital'—Discurso Pronunciado pelo Professor Miguel Pereira por Ocasião do Regresso do Professor Aloysio de Castro, da República Argentina, em Outubro de 1916," *Revista de Medicina—órgão do Centro Acadêmico "Oswaldo Cruz"/Faculdade de Medicina e Cirurgia de São Paulo* 7 (1922): 3–7.

22. Castro Santos, "O Pensamento Sanitarista na Primeira República;" Lima and Hochman, "'Condenado pela Raça, Absolvido pela Medicina'"; Simone P. Kropf, *Doença de Chagas, Doença do Brasil: Ciência, Saúde e Nação (1909–1962)* (Rio de Janeiro: Editora Fiocruz,

2009); Nísia Trindade Lima, "Public Health and Social Ideas in Modern Brazil," *American Journal of Public Health* 97, no. 7 (2007): 1209–1215. For a general view of the relations of eugenics, education, and hygiene in Brazil, see Vera Regina Beltrão Marques, *A Medicalização da Raça: Médicos, Educadores e Discurso Eugênico* (Campinas: Editora da Unicamp, 1994).

23. Monteiro Lobato, *Mr. Slang e o Brasil e Problema Vital*, 8th ed. (1918; São Paulo: Brasiliense, 1957).

24. The Oswaldo Cruz Institute, previously named Instituto Soroterápico, was established in Rio de Janeiro in 1900 during the bubonic plague epidemic. Under the direction of Oswaldo Cruz (1872–1917), the scientist who headed the institute from 1903 to 1917, it had become an important research and training center for public health professionals. From 1917 to 1934, its director was Carlos Chagas. On the role of the institute in Brazilian science, see Nancy Stepan, *Beginnings of Brazilian Science: Oswaldo Cruz, Medical Research and Policy, 1890–1920* (New York: Science History Publications, 1976); Jaime Benchimol, ed., *Manguinhos do Sonho à Vida—a Ciência na Belle Époque* (Rio de Janeiro: Casa de Oswaldo Cruz–FIOCRUZ, 1990).

25. Lima and Hochman, "'Condenado Pela Raça, Absolvido Pela Medicina;'" Lima, *Um Sertão Chamado Brasil—Intelectuais e Interpretações Geográficas da Identidade Nacional*; Kropf, *Doença de Chagas, Doença do Brasil*.

26. Gilberto Hochman, *A Era do Saneamento—as Bases da Política de Saúde Pública no Brasil* (São Paolo: Hucitec, ANPOCS, 1998), 59–71.

27. Ibid.; Castro Santos, "O Pensamento Sanitarista na Primeira República;" Lima, *Um Sertão Chamado Brasil*.

28. Miguel Couto, "Alocução de paraninfo da turma de doutorandos de 1916," *Revista Médico-Cirúrgica do Brasil* 25 (1917): 13.

29. Lobato, *Mr. Slang e o Brasil e Problema Vital*, 298; Lima and Hochman, "'Condenado pela Raça, Absolvido pela Medicina.'"

30. Olegário de Moura, "Saneamento-Eugenia-Civilização," in *Annaes de Eugenia*, ed. Sociedade Eugênica de São Paulo (São Paulo: Editora da Revista do Brasil, 1919), 80–92.

31. Original expression in an article in the Peruvian journal *La Reforma Medica*, republished in the periodical *Saúde*, official organ of the Pro-Sanitation League of Brazil. Carlos E. P. Soldan, "Eugenização da América," *Saúde*, no. 4 (1919): 95–96.

32. Stepan, "Eugenics in Brazil, 1917–1940," 22.

33. Stepan, *"The Hour of Eugenics"*, 46–50. See also Vanderlei S. de Souza, "La Eugenesia de Renato Kehl y la Formación de una Red Internacional en el Período de Entre-Guerras," in *Políticas del Cuerpo: Estrategias Modernas de Normalización del Individuo y la Sociedad*, eds. Gustavo Vallejo and Marisa Miranda (Buenos Aires: Siglo XXI Editora, 2007), 428–429.

34. Vanderlei S. Souza, *A Política Biológica como Projeto: A 'Eugenia Negativa' e a Construção da Nacionalidade na Trajetória de Renato Kehl (1917–1932)* (MA diss., Fundação Oswaldo Cruz, 2006); Souza, "La Eugenesia de Renato Kehl."

35. Sergio Carrara, *Tributo À Vênus—a Luta Contra a Sífilis no Brasil, Da Passagem do Século aos Anos 40* (Rio de Janeiro: Editora Fiocruz, 1996).

36. Renato Kehl, *Lições de Eugenia* (Rio de Janeiro: Francisco Alves, 1929).

37. José Roberto F. Reis, "Raça, Imigração e Eugenia: O Projeto de 'Regeneração Nacional' da Liga Brasileira de Higiene Mental," *Estudos Afro-asiáticos* 36 (1999): 29–55; José Roberto F. Reis, "'De Pequenino é que se Torce o Pepino:' A Infância nos Programas Eugênicos da Liga Brasileira de Higiene Mental," *História, Ciências, Saúde-Manguinhos* 7, no. 1 (2000): 135–157; Jurandir Freire Costa, *Ordem Médica e Norma Familiar* (Rio de Janeiro: Graal, 1979).

38. Reis, "Raça, Imigração e Eugenia: O Projeto de 'Regeneração Nacional;'" Reis, "'De Pequenino é que se Torce o Pepino.'"

39. Vanderlei S. de Souza, "Em Nome da Raça: A Propaganda Eugênica e as Idéias de Renato Kehl nos anos 1910 e 1920," *Revista de História Regional* 11, no. 2 (2006): 29–70; Souza, "La Eugenesia de Renato Kehl."

40. Souza, *A Política Biológica como Projeto*, 132.

41. Kehl, *Lições de Eugenía*, 151–152.

42. Letter from Octávio Domingues to Renato Kehl, Piracicaba, São Paulo, January 15, 1933, Renato Kehl papers, Casa de Oswaldo Cruz-Fundação Oswaldo Cruz.

43. Souza, "A Política Biológica como Projeto," 132.

44. Nísia Trindade Lima, Ricardo V. Santos, and Carlos E. A. Coimbra Jr., "Rondonia de Edgard Roquette-Pinto: Antropologia e Projeto Nacional," in Lima and Sá, *Antropologia Brasiliana*, 99–121.

45. Edgard Roquette-Pinto, *Seixos Rolados (Estudos Brasileiros)* (Rio de Janeiro: Mendonça, Machado, 1927), 203.

46. Bulhões de Carvalho, *Anais e Trabalhos do I Congresso Brasileiro de Eugenia* (Rio de Janeiro: 1929), 225.

47. Stepan, "*The Hour of Eugenics*"; Souza, "'As Leis da Eugenia' na Antropologia de Edgard Roquette-Pinto."

48. *Anais e Trabalhos do I Congresso Brasileiro de Eugenia*, 20.

49. Ibid., emphasis added.

50. Jeff H. Lesser, *Negotiating National Identity: Immigrants, Minorities, and the Struggle for Ethnicity in Brazil* (Durham, NC: Duke University Press, 1999); Lesser, "Are African-Americans African or American? Brazilian Immigration Policy in the 1920s," *Review of Latin American Studies* 4, no. 1–2 (1991): 115–137; Teresa Meade and Gregory Alonso Pirio, "In Search of the Afro-American Eldorado: Attempts by North American Blacks to Enter Brazil in the 1920s," *Luso-Brazilian Review* 25, no. 1 (1988): 85–110.

51. Lesser, *Negotiating National Identity*.

52. *Anais e Trabalhos do I Congresso Brasileiro de Eugenia*, 77.

53. Edgard Roquette-Pinto, "Notas Sobre os Tipos Antropológicos do Brasil," in *Anais e Trabalhos do I Congresso Brasileiro de Eugenia*, 147.

54. Boris Fausto, *A Concise History of Brazil* (Cambridge: Cambridge University Press, 1999), 198–237.

55. Stepan, "*The Hour of Eugenics*", 163.

56. Stepan, "Eugenics in Brazil, 1917–1940," 140.

57. Arthur Ramos, *Guerra e Relações de Raça* (Rio de Janeiro: Departamento Editorial da União Nacional dos Estudantes, 1943, 171–174).

58. Lesser, *Negotiating National Identity*, Jair de Souza Ramos, "Como Classificar os Indesejáveis? Tensões e Convergências entre Raça, Etnia e Nacionalidade na Política de Imigração das Décadas de 1920 e 1930," in Lima and Sá, *Antropologia Brasiliana*, 179–211; Endrica Geraldo, *O "Perigo Alienígena:" Política Imigratória e Pensamento Racial no Governo Vargas (1930–1945)* (PhD diss., State University of Campinas, 2007).

59. Jeff H. Lesser, ed., *Welcoming the Undesirables: Brazil and the Jewish Question* (Berkeley, CA: University of California Press, 1994); Maria Luiza Tucci Carneiro, *O Anti-Semitismo na Era Vargas: Fantasmas de uma Geração (1930–1945)* (São Paulo: Editora Brasiliense, 1988).

60. See Marcos Chor Maio, "UNESCO and the Study of Race Relations in Brazil: Regional or National Issue?," *Latin American Research Review* 36, no. 2 (2001): 118–136. On racial inequalities in Brazil, see Ricardo V. Santos and Marcos Chor Maio, "Race, Genomics, Identities and Politics in Contemporary Brazil," *Critique of Anthropology* 24, no. 4 (2004): 347–378.

FURTHER READING

Corrêa, Mariza. *As Ilusões da Liberdade: A Escola Nina Rodrigues e a Antropologia no Brasil* (Bragança Paulista: Editora da Universidade São Francisco, 1998).

Gerbi, Antonello. *La disputa del nuevo mundo: Historia de una polémica, 1750–1900*, 2nd ed. (Mexico: Fondo de Cultura Econômica, 1982).

Hochman, Gilberto, and Diego Armus. *Cuidar, Controlar, Curar: Ensaios Históricos Sobre Saúde e Doença Na América Latina e Caribe* (Rio de Janeiro: Editora Fiocruz, 2004).

Lima, Nísia Trindade, and Dominich Miranda de Sá, eds. *Antroplogia Brasiliana—Ciência e Educação na Obra de Edgard Roquette-Pinto* (Belo Horizonte; Rio de Janeiro: Editora UFMG; Editora Fiocruz, 2008).

Maio, Marcos Chor, and Ricardo V. Santos, eds. *Raça, Ciência e Sociedade* (Rio de Janeiro: Editora Fiocruz/CCBB, 1996).

Marques, Vera Regina Beltrão. *A Medicalização da Raça: Médicos, Educadores e Discurso Eugênico* (Campinas: Editora da Unicamp, 1994).

Oliveira, Lucia Lippi de. *A Questão Nacional na Primeira República* (São Paulo: Editora Brasiliense, 1990).

Schwarcz, Lilia Moritz. *The Spectacle of the Races: Scientists, Institutions, and the Race Question in Brazil, 1870–1930* (New York: Hill and Wang, 1999).

Skidmore, Thomas E. *Black into White: Race and Nationality in Brazilian Thought* (Oxford and New York: Oxford University Press, 1974).

Stepan, Nancy Leys. *"The Hour of Eugenics": Race, Gender, and Nation in Latin America* (Ithaca, NY: Cornell University Press, 1991).

Vallejo, Gustavo, and Marisa Miranda, eds. *Políticas Del Cuerpo: Estrategias Modernas de Normalización del Individuo y la Sociedad* (Buenos Aires: Siglo XXI Editora, 2007).

CHAPTER 30

....

EUGENICS IN THE UNITED STATES

....

WENDY KLINE

LIKE many controversial historical topics in US history, American eugenics has undergone a scholarly transformation over the past 50 years. Though the movement held enormous sway during the first half of the twentieth century, historians did not openly critique the movement until the 1960s. A new generation of scholars, influenced by the social upheavals of the decade, approached past events in American history with greater skepticism than their forebears. Mark Haller's *Eugenics: Hereditarian Attitudes in American Thought,* published in 1963, became the first of many comprehensive studies on the impact of the eugenics movement in the United States.[1] Just as biology textbooks were finally renouncing the legitimacy of eugenic principles, scholars began their attack on the insidious role of progressives bent on curbing the population of the so-called "unfit" in the early twentieth century. And for the first time, as Mark Largent recently noted in his history of coerced sterilization in the United States, scholars including Haller linked the American eugenics movement to the Holocaust.[2]

While the "Nazi connection" drew greater attention to the abuse of power in the U.S. eugenic movement, it also, unfortunately, distorted the local history. Linking American eugenics to genocide in Germany provided fodder for sensational histories and the occasional journalistic frenzy, but prevented most from integrating the story into mainstream social history. In other words, rather than ask why so many Americans embraced eugenic and hereditarian ideals in the first half of the twentieth century, many scholars vilified a small number of individual racists as responsible for generating an embarrassing mistake.

Despite this somewhat limiting approach to the history of eugenics, intellectual debates over the role of nature versus nurture in human development (or heredity versus environment) kept eugenics in the spotlight. If anything, such interest has only increased over the past few decades, as the human genome project and other technological developments have raised the bar of genetic engineering and its implications for society's future. Thus, trying to understand the history of the nature/nurture debate became of great interest to both intellectual and social historians. In addition to Haller's study, studies such as Carl Degler's *In Search of Human Nature: The Decline and Revival of Darwinism in American Social Thought* introduced these ideas to a wider audience and blurred the boundaries between eugenics and other ideas about American character.[3]

Scholarship in the 1980s and 1990s

In the 1980s, scholars presented more in-depth studies of influential organizations and individuals. Biologist and historian of science Garland Allen published an institutional study of the Eugenics Record Office at Cold Spring Harbor, as well as essays and articles stressing the relationship between genetics and class. He remains active in the field, asking, for example, "Is a New Eugenics Afoot?" as the title of an essay in the October 2001 volume of *Science* magazine. Though he stresses to *Science* readers that the context of early-twentieth-century eugenics was different from that of the twenty-first, he warns that "we are poised at the threshold of a similar period in our own history and are adopting a similar mind frame as our predecessors."[4] Daniel Kevles published the oft-cited *In the Name of Eugenics: Genetics and the Uses of Human Heredity*, a comparative history of eugenics in the United States and Britain. Kevles delved into biographical sketches of influential figures such as Karl Pearson and Charles Davenport, convincingly demonstrating their influence on issues such as immigration restriction and coercive sterilization.[5] As historians of science, Allen, Kevles, and others who began publishing in eugenics applied a particular lens and interpretive framework common to their field. They were predominantly interested in the scientific theories and training of the scientists involved in promoting hereditarian ideas.

By the 1990s, scholars outside the history of science introduced new approaches to the study of eugenics. Rather than studying the specific flaws in scientific thinking that led to eugenics and its increasing distance from the science of genetics, these scholars approached eugenics as a social movement. This shift effectively widened the parameters of study, the sources used, and the questions asked of the impact of eugenics on American culture. Scholars discovered that eugenic ideology and social programs affected earlier Americans at multiple levels—from the fiction they read, to the movies they viewed, to the biology textbooks they learned from, to the exhibits they viewed at county fairs. While connections to racism and nativism had been evident from the pervasive racist language of eugenicists, a new generation of scholars revealed that gender, too, was a major concern of many eugenicists, and that "race" was far more nuanced in use than had previously been acknowledged. Studies of institutions—such as prisons, mental hospitals, and homes for the "fee-bleminded" (what would be termed "developmentally disabled" today) revealed the impact of eugenic policies on patients, as well as (to a limited extent, due to lack of sources) patient responses to such treatment. Others have looked at a particular region of the United States to understand how eugenics worked on the local level—why, for example, there were relatively few sterilizations in the Deep South, despite the region's reputed racism.

Eugenics and Mental Health

Because those targeted for eugenic segregation or sterilization were frequently insti-tutionalized, historians drew connections between mental health, institutional his-tory, and eugenics. James W. Trent Jr.'s *Inventing the Feeble Mind* is a history of mental retardation in the United States, but it focuses specifically on the shifting ideas of mental health and how it overlapped with eugenics. As Trent demonstrates, intelligence testing had a profound effect on institutionalized patients as well as ideas about eugenics, because of the eugenic assumption that intelligence was an inherited trait.[6] Joel Braslow, with training in both history and psychiatry, investi-gates institutional psychiatric treatment in the first half of the twentieth century by looking at California state institutions for the insane. Analyzing both patient and doctors' records, Braslow delves into the doctor-patient relationship and how psy-chiatrists employed somatic methods such as sterilization for therapeutic reasons. Thus, he argues that although sterilization was purported to be a eugenic procedure (eliminating the possibility of reproduction), institutional psychiatrists viewed it as medically appropriate for their patients.[7] Ian Robert Dowbiggin furthers this line of thought in *Keeping America Sane: Psychiatry and Eugenics in the United States and Canada, 1880–1940*. His study reveals that psychiatric support of eugenics stemmed at least in part from a desire for professional authority. These doctors had their own reasons for adhering to eugenic treatments and did not necessarily embrace eugenic principles.[8]

Eugenics and Religion

The relationship between religion and eugenics has also drawn the attention of scholars, most notably Christine Rosen, who published *Preaching Eugenics* in 2004. Utilizing the records of the American Eugenics Society, along with the personal papers of religious leaders, she argues that eugenics "flourished in the liberal

Protestant, Catholic, and Jewish mainstream," as ministers joined eugenic organizations, lobbied for legislation, and corresponded with eugenic leaders.[9] Her study attempts to explain the appeal of the movement to organized religion, as well as to illuminate the challenges it posed.

Though primarily an intellectual history of religious leaders involved in the movement, *Preaching Eugenics* also draws on sources such as popular novels, vaudeville song lyrics, and eugenics fairs to illustrate the widespread popularity of the movement, even among the religious. Rosen argues that although eugenicists were reluctant to allow amateurs to promote the cause, they quickly saw the benefits of an alliance. Although eugenics was seen as a scientific enterprise, amateur enthusiasts frequently drew metaphors and references from the Bible. Placing eugenics within a religious framework both familiarized congregations with this new science and assured them of its noble causes. Beginning in the 1920s, the American Eugenics Society capitalized on this religious interest, embracing religious metaphors (inscribing their fitter family medal with "yea, I have a goodly heritage," from Psalms 16) and even promoting a eugenics sermon contest. Those religious leaders who contributed to the movement did more than just preach to the converted; they also forced eugenicists to consider the spiritual nature of race betterment.

Not all religious leaders supported the movement, however. Not surprisingly, many Catholics argued that eugenics violated natural law and actively opposed the movement. But Rosen reveals a "spectrum of Catholic opinion" in the early twentieth century, ranging from staunch opposition to active involvement in the American Eugenics Society.[10] Before the growth of public support for eugenic sterilization and the increased involvement of birth control activists, some Catholics viewed eugenics as a legitimate and important avenue of social reform.

EUGENICS, FAIRS, AND FAMILIES

Many historians already established in other fields of U.S. history delved into eugenics to illustrate wider social trends and changes beginning in the 1990s. For example, Robert Rydell, a historian of technology and an expert in world's fairs, devotes a chapter of his book *World of Fairs* to the "Fitter Families for Future Firesides" contests that emerged at county fairs between the wars. What started as "better baby" contests (to counter infant mortality) morphed into the more decidedly eugenic fitter family contests in the 1920s. When founder Florence Sherborn moved from working with the Children's Bureau to become professor of child care at the University of Kansas, she applied her contest expertise to a new setting. As a result of her efforts, at the 1920 Kansas State Fair human subjects were for the first time judged alongside the "Pet Stock" and "Milch Goat" categories. At this and subsequent rural fair contests, judges evaluated family history, mental condition, physical condition, and health habits (the entire testing process took over three hours). Rydell uses this example to illustrate the emergence of an "exhibitionary culture" in the 1920s, one that embraced modernity and progress.[11] More recently, Laura Lovett builds on Rydell's work to make a very different argument about the significance of these contests. According to Lovett, the fitter family contests symbolized the culmination of a long-standing agrarian tradition. They successfully popularized notions of eugenics and encouraged pronatalism (at least in "fit" families) and did so in a rural setting (always taking place at state fairs). As such, she argues, they represented the most blatant form of social pressure to reproduce.[12]

A eugenic-inspired fascination with family occurred not only at county and world's fairs, but also through the Eugenics Record Office at Cold Spring Harbor, New York. Here, noted eugenicist and founder Charles Davenport, along with superintendent Harry Laughlin, trained and employed eugenics field workers (usually middle-class educated young women) to conduct family studies. Between 1910 and 1924, they conducted summer courses and then sent the workers out to collect data or administer fitter family contests. Others were sent to institutions to conduct family pedigrees. Eugenic interest in family pedigrees stemmed from claims that degeneracy and genius were inherited qualities, and that one could trace the roots of both. Exemplars such as the Juke and Kallikak family case studies were used to promote eugenic policy. Nicole Hahn Rafter collected these and nine other family studies, publishing them with an introduction in *White Trash*. Many of the studies were conducted by the Eugenics Record Office, and all of them, according to Rafter, represented a form of propaganda to promote the professional self-interest of the organization.[13] More recently, Daylanne English and Nathaniel Deutsch have offered fresh and more complex analyses of family studies. Deutsch's *Inventing America's "Worst" Family* is a multilayered history of the "Ishmael tribe": a group of poor people settled around Indianapolis who became infamously portrayed in eugenics circles in the late nineteenth and early twentieth centuries.[14] Deutsch tracks the invention of this tribe by Congregationalist minister Oscar McCulloch in 1878, its further denigration in the 1920s by eugenicist Arthur Estabrook, and its celebration as a source of African American Islam by social activist Hugo Leaming. Deutsch ends his study with his own research into the origins and experiences of the so-called tribe, pronouncing them well-established if poor people who deserve a place next to Daniel Boone in the celebration of hardscrabble frontiersmen. Literary scholar Daylanne English analyzes the writings of female eugenics field workers in the early twentieth century. Of the 258 workers trained by the Eugenics Record Office between 1910 and 1924, 240 were women. Most were college graduates who had majored in biology, sociology, or social work. While Rafter and Deutsch draw on the more limited published family studies, English points out that they represent only a fraction of the total number of studies conducted. Drawing on the papers of the Eugenics Record Office housed at the American Philosophical Society Library, she argues that the unpublished female field workers created a new literary genre. "Combining personal narrative, travel narrative, interviews, genealogical data, and statistical analysis," English writes, "the eugenics field workers wrote quintessentially modern national family stories."[15]

EUGENICS, RACE, AND PLACE

English's other contribution to the field of eugenics history comes from her analysis of how eugenics crossed racial lines. Some African American writers of the Harlem Renaissance, including W.E.B. DuBois and Alice Dunbar-Nelson, embraced racial uplift through selective breeding. English argues that DuBois's and Dunbar-Nelson's "intraracial version of eugenics, while it may have been elitist, was not racist or regressive."[16] Likewise, Gregory Dorr's recent work on eugenics in Virginia includes an analysis of the hereditarian attitudes of three notable African Americans—Dubois, Thomas Wyatt Turner, and Marcus Garvey—to suggest that eugenic ideas (and their dissemination) are far more complex than historians have noted. Dorr and English challenge the assumption that African Americans were merely victims or critics of eugenics. Instead, they were sometimes key players who were able to subvert the discourse and reinterpret eugenics as a science that would uplift blacks as well as whites—a science that would, in effect, end racism rather than foster it.[17]

Dorr's study addresses not only race, but also regionalism. *Segregation's Science: Eugenics and Society in Virginia,* contributes to the literature by studying the impact of eugenics in the state of Virginia, and as Dorr demonstrates, it is a crucial state to study in order to understand the intellectual, social, cultural, and legal developments in the eugenics movement. The state was second only to California in the number of eugenic sterilizations performed and was the location of the influential Supreme Court decision *Buck v. Bell* (1927), which upheld Virginia's eugenic sterilization law. Dorr situates his study within southern history, explaining why eugenic and hereditarian ideas held such promise to Virginia's elite—or, in his words, revealing "how Virginians used eugenics to navigate between the extremes of New South 'modernism' and Old South 'traditionalism.'" What he finds emerging from these sources "is a sense of the persistent power of eugenic thought throughout the twentieth century."[18]

Dorr was not the first scholar to suggest the importance of local and regional studies of eugenics in the United States. In 1995, two books were published on eugenics in the South: Edward J. Larson's *Sex, Race, and Science: Eugenics in the Deep South* and Steven Noll's *Feeble-Minded in Our Midst: Institutions for the Mentally Retarded in the South, 1900–1940.* Larson argues that despite the region's early-twentieth-century notoriety for racist public policy, it did not embrace eugenics to the same extent as other regions, and it did so much later. He looks at local legislation alongside women's clubs and institutional records to decipher the distinctive nature of eugenics in the south.[19] Noll analyzed the treatment of the so-called "feeble-minded" in southern institutions, emphasizing the conflicting goals of progressives who wanted to protect society from social deviants and asylum officials who envisioned a very different clientele—those of the severely developmentally disabled.[20]

Nancy Gallagher's study of eugenics in Vermont aimed to "write eugenics history into Vermont history" and to place Vermont's eugenic story within the context of the wider eugenics movement. She looks at the work of zoologist Henry F. Perkins, who directed a eugenics survey of the state from 1925 to 1936. The survey, although privately funded, was modeled on the family studies conducted by the Eugenics Record Office.[21]

More recently, the state of California has been the subject of research—which is not surprising, given the fact that more coerced sterilizations were performed in the state than any other, representing over a quarter of the nation's total of 63,000 sterilized.[22] My study of California, *Building a Better Race*, began as a research paper on the Sonoma State Home for the Feebleminded, where a disproportionate number of young women were sterilized for supposed immoral defects.[23] I began to wonder how and why eugenics became a powerful solution in that region to the problems of social and sexual disorder. Later, Alexandra Stern continued this trend with her book, *Eugenic Nation*. As one of a number of scholars seeking to "push the bounds of what has been considered eugenics," she includes environmentalists, public health officials, and marriage counselors among those who played a role in shaping attitudes about heredity and progress.[24] Perhaps more importantly, she approaches eugenics from a number of different fields, including "new Western" history, the history of medicine, science and public health, and gender.

This interdisciplinary approach is most evident in Stern's chapter on quarantine at the U.S.-Mexican border. Here, she effectively links eugenic concerns about race betterment with concerns about Mexican immigration, arguing that in the early twentieth century, the U.S. Public Health Service (USPHS) and the Border Patrol shaped the "complicated process of racialization in the U.S.-Mexican borderlands."[25] The USPHS instituted quarantines, delousing, and fumigation along the border, affecting hundreds of immigrants daily and contributing to an anti-Mexican sentiment centered upon dirt and disease. No such policies were instituted along the Canadian border, Stern points out, suggesting the "racialized lens" through which these immigrants were viewed.[26] Meanwhile, the Border Patrol, established in 1924 but with roots in centuries-old military patterns, established lines of defense to prevent unauthorized entry into the United States, playing a "critical role in the delimitation of the northern and southern boundaries."[27] These two processes—medicalization and militarization—altered the landscape in the American West and played a crucial role in the development of eugenics. Concerns about race and health shaped both immigration and eugenic policies in twentieth-century California and help to explain why the state performed the highest number of eugenic sterilizations.

Another important state that has recently received attention is North Carolina. Johanna Schoen became the first, and possibly the last, researcher granted access to the state's 8,000 sterilization petitions received by the Eugenics Board between 1934 and 1966. "I felt as if eight thousand strangers were confiding their individual misfortunes to me and pleading for the public recognition of the wrongs done to them," she writes. "I was outraged by what I read, and I struggled to figure out how to give this history the public recognition it deserved."[28] *Choice and Coercion* is the result. Dramatic stories abound in Schoen's narrative, such as that of Estelle, an African

American woman who struggled to control her fertility in the mid-twentieth century. After the birth of her first child, she tried to obtain contraceptives but learned she was ineligible because she was single. By her fourth pregnancy, she tried to get an abortion but was unable; now married and pregnant again, she took birth control pills despite her husband's opposition; when these threatened her health, she tried an IUD, which gave her an infection. After seven children, her request to be sterilized turned down, she had an abortion. Schoen uses stories such as Estelle's to argue that reproductive technologies—namely, birth control, sterilization, and abortion—had the potential to liberate or constrain women, depending on the context. Focusing primarily on North Carolina, she demonstrates that four groups of people influenced the outcome of reproductive policies: scientists, health and welfare professionals, state and county officials, and female clients. All were concerned about reproductive health, but disagreed about how it should be managed. And each group struggled with internal disagreements as well, resulting in "a patchwork of programs with great disparities and contradictions between them."[29] Schoen's in-depth research at the local level demonstrates the importance of incorporating all of these competing voices, for they influenced the effectiveness of reproductive services in North Carolina and elsewhere as well. Although North Carolina was exceptional in some respects—for example, it was one of the first states to introduce state-supported birth control—Schoen suggests that its history has much to tell us about reproductive politics on a broader scale.

GENDER, SEXUALITY, AND PERIODIZATION

While Stern and I focused primarily on California and Schoen on North Carolina, all three authors shared a concern that sexuality and gender had not been adequately analyzed by scholars of the eugenics movement. Much had been written on the impact of eugenics on immigration restriction—most notably, the role of eugenicists in pushing for the 1924 Immigration Restriction Act, which targeted supposedly "dysgenic" immigrants from eastern and southern Europe—but almost nothing had appeared on the ways in which eugenics also spoke to concerns around gender roles in modern America. Other studies have continued and expanded upon this topic, challenging not only the lack of attention to gender, but also the periodization of eugenics. I argued that eugenics continued long after many claimed it had been dismantled—certainly well beyond World War II. I looked at individual eugenicists who moved from negative eugenics—segregation and sterilization of the so-called "unfit"—to positive eugenics—encouraging more children from the "fit" through new pronatalist strategies such as marriage counseling. While this still remains in dispute, others have pushed those boundaries even further, suggesting a continuation of eugenic ideas into the twentieth century. Rebecca Kluchin's work on sterilization and "neoeugenics," Nancy Ordover's analysis of the quest for a gay gene, and Matthew Connelly's study of population control are all recent examples of this kind of work.[30]

EUGENICS AND POPULAR CULTURE

Another way in which scholars have challenged the periodization of American eugenics is through its manifestation in popular culture into and beyond the 1920s. A good example of this trend is *Eugenic Design: Streamlining America in the 1930s*. In this provocative study, art historian Christina Cogdell links eugenic ideology with streamline industrial design in twentieth-century America. As she explains, "streamline designers approached products the same way that eugenicists approached bodies."[31] An interest in efficiency, hygiene, and progress shaped the views of both designers and eugenicists. Though there was little overlap in membership (few architects identified themselves as eugenicists), similar ideas about progress, evolution, and control allow for interesting comparisons. For example, both eugenicists and industrial designers frequently used the word "stream" as a metaphor for evolution, suggesting the importance of purity and progress. Twentieth-century bodies, like products, could be managed and manipulated to create a more perfect race. There are fascinating images in *Eugenic Design*, which include oddities such as the "Criterion" toilet, designed to enforce the hygienically correct posture during evacuation ("the sloped seat angled backward, achieving the natural position every time") in a chapter that links concern for biological efficiency with streamlining.[32] Advertisements, comic strips, industrial design plans, and photographs from eugenic exhibits contribute to her analysis by suggesting the myriad ways in which Americans were exposed to ideas about streamlining, eugenics, and progress.

After publishing *Eugenic Design*, Cogdell co-edited the volume *Popular Eugenics: National Efficiency and American Mass Culture in the 1930s* with Susan Currell. These fourteen essays promote the idea that, in Currell's words, "rather than killing off eugenic thought, the Depression extended and transformed it. In that period," she writes, "the popular press disseminated a version of eugenics to readers that cast it as a renewed topic for social debate."[33] The first half of the volume focuses on popular writing and eugenics; the second on visual culture, from comic strips to popular films such as Dracula and Frankenstein. A less well-known film, *The Black Stork*, is the subject of Martin Pernick's book of the same name. Pernick discovered the only surviving print of this eerie 1916 silent film in a film collector's garage in New Jersey. He declared it a "startling and provocative long-lost motion picture that illuminates many otherwise dark and unknown dimensions of American medicine and culture."[34] The film describes (and stars) prominent Chicago surgeon Dr. Harry Haiselden dramatizing his recommendation to withhold treatment on a burned infant who also had severe physical abnormalities. Pernick uses the film and its reception to address larger questions about how eugenics and heredity were defined and understood within both public health and popular culture.

EUGENICS AND DISABILITY

Questions of the value of a disabled body raised by *The Black Stork* have become the subject of a whole new discipline in history: that of disability history. Scholars working in this new field argue that disability is a category of analysis as important as race, class, or gender in understanding the past. Determining what is "normal" and what is "abnormal" is a social construction that has been used to discriminate against those who do not meet that social norm. Susan Burch and Hannah Joyner have recently published *Unspeakable: The Story of Junius Wilson.*[35] In 1932, Wilson, a deaf African American 24-year-old, was castrated at the North Carolina State Hospital for the Colored Insane. He had been sent there at the age of seventeen after a neighbor accused him of attempted rape, and his inability to make himself understood to the hearing community led to his institutionalization. He remained there for a total of 76 years; he was finally released and was awarded $226,000 for wrongful incarceration in 1997. This story rightly complicates our understanding of eugenics, for it suggests that the categories of difference go beyond race or class, and that even within notions of *disability,* the cultural meaning assigned to deafness throws certain assumptions about so-called "normal behavior" out the window. The intersections of race, eugenics, and disability (specifically, deafness) in the Jim Crow South could isolate one man from both communities that might have protected him: that of the white deaf and that of the black hearing.

The Story of Junius Wilson suggests how far the field has come in the last two decades. Eugenics is no longer a forgotten relic of the past, but a vibrant field that addresses controversial issues from a variety of fields and standpoints. Art historians and literary scholars have joined social and cultural historians in recognizing the significant impact of eugenics on American life. Recent events, such as formal state apologies in California and Indiana for eugenic sterilizations performed, have raised public awareness of the history of eugenics. Books published in the popular press, such as Harry Brunius's *Better for All the World* and Edwin Black's *War against the Weak,* though sensationalist, ensure that more readers will encounter the eugenic past.[36] Public history programs, eugenics exhibits, and educational development organizations such as *Facing History and Ourselves* ensure that teachers and students of history will continue to critically examine the role of eugenics in American history.

NOTES

1. Mark H. Haller, *Eugenics: Hereditarian Attitudes in American Thought* (New Brunswick, NJ: Rutgers University Press, 1984).

2. Mark A. Largent, *Breeding Contempt: The History of Coerced Sterilization in the United States* (New Brunswick, NJ: Rutgers University Press, 2008).

3. Carl N. Degler, *In Search of Human Nature: The Decline and Revival of Darwinism in American Social Thought* (Oxford and New York: Oxford University Press, 1991).

4. Garland Allen, "Essays on Science and Society: Is a New Eugenics Afoot?," *Science* 294, no. 5 (2001); Allen, *The Eugenics Record Office at Cold Spring Harbor, 1910–1940: An Essay in Institutional History* (Philadelphia, PA: University of Pennsylvania, 1986).

5. Daniel J. Kevles, *In the Name of Eugenics: Genetics and the Uses of Human Heredity* (New York: Knopf, 1985).

6. James W. Trent, *Inventing the Feeble Mind: A History of Mental Retardation in the United States* (Berkeley, CA: University of California Press, 1994).

7. Joel T. Braslow, *Mental Ills and Bodily Cures: Psychiatric Treatment in the First Half of the Twentieth Century* (Berkeley, CA: University of California Press, 1997).

8. Ian Robert Dowbiggin, *Keeping America Sane: Psychiatry and Eugenics in the United States and Canada, 1880–1940* (Ithaca, NY: Cornell University Press, 1997).

9. Christine Rosen, *Preaching Eugenics: Religious Leaders and the American Eugenics Movement* (Oxford and New York: Oxford University Press, 2004), 4.

10. Ibid., 139.

11. Robert W. Rydell, *World of Fairs: The Century-of-Progress Expositions* (Chicago, IL: University of Chicago Press 1993).

12. Laura L. Lovett, *Conceiving the Future: Pronatalism, Reproduction, and the Family in the United States, 1890–1938* (Chapel Hill, NC: University of North Carolina Press, 2007).

13. Nicole Hahn Rafter, *White Trash: The Eugenic Family Studies, 1877–1919* (Boston, MA: Northeastern University Press, 1988).

14. Nathaniel Deutsch, *Inventing America's "Worst" Family: Eugenics, Islam, and the Fall and Rise of the Tribe of Ishmael* (Berkeley, CA: University of California Press, 2009).

15. Daylanne K. English, *Unnatural Selections: Eugenics in American Modernism and the Harlem Renaissance* (Chapel Hill, NC: University of North Carolina Press, 2004), 175.

16. Ibid., 17.

17. Gregory Michael Dorr, *Segregation's Science: Eugenics and Society in Virginia* (Charlottesville, VA: University of Virginia Press, 2008).

18. Ibid., 7.

19. Edward J. Larson, *Sex, Race, and Science: Eugenics in the Deep South* (Baltimore, MD: Johns Hopkins University Press, 1995).

20. Steven Noll, *Feeble-minded in Our Midst: Institutions for the Mentally Retarded in the South, 1900–1940* (Chapel Hill, NC: University of North Carolina Press, 1995).

21. Nancy L. Gallagher, *Breeding Better Vermonters: The Eugenics Project in the Green Mountain State* (Hanover, NH: University Press of New England, 1999), xiii. Her study is largely limited to the biography of Perkins and an overview of his survey.

22. Largent, *Breeding Contempt*, 7.

23. Wendy Kline, *Building a Better Race: Gender, Sexuality, and Eugenics from the Turn of the Century to the Baby Boom* (Berkeley, CA: University of California Press, 2001).

24. Alexandra Minna Stern, *Eugenic Nation: Faults and Frontiers of Better Breeding in Modern America* (Berkeley, CA: University of California Press, 2005), 18.

25. Ibid., 80.

26. Ibid., 66.

27. Ibid., 75.

28. Johanna Schoen, *Choice and Coercion: Birth Control, Sterilization and Abortion in Public Health and Welfare* (Chapel Hill, NC: University of North Carolina Press, 2005), 243.

29. Ibid., 5.

30. Matthew Connelly, *Fatal Misconception: The Struggle to Control World Population* (Cambridge, MA: Harvard University Press, 2008); Rebecca Kluchin, *Fit to Be Tied: Sterilization and Reproductive Rights in America, 1950–1980* (New Brunswick, NJ: Rutgers

University Press, 2009); Nancy Ordover, *American Eugenics: Race, Queer Anatomy, and the Science of Nationalism* (Minneapolis, MN: University of Minnesota Press, 2003).

31. Christina Cogdell, *Eugenic Design: Streamlining America in the 1930s* (Philadelphia, PA: University of Pennsylvania Press, 2004), 4.

32. Ibid., 141.

33. Susan Currell and Christina Cogdell, *Popular Eugenics: National Efficiency and American Mass Culture in the 1930s* (Athens, OH: Ohio University Press, 2006), 4.

34. Martin S. Pernick, *The Black Stork: Eugenics and the Death of "Defective" Babies in American Medicine and Motion Pictures since 1915* (Oxford and New York: Oxford University Press, 1996), viii.

35. Susan Burch and Hannah Joyner, *Unspeakable: The Story of Junius Wilson* (Chapel Hill, NC: University of North Carolina Press, 2007).

36. Edwin Black, *War Against the Weak: Eugenics and America's Campaign to Create a Master Race* (New York: Four Walls Eight Windows, 2003); Harry Bruinius, *Better for All the World: The Secret History of Forced Sterilization and America's Quest for Racial Purity* (New York: Knopf, 2006).

FURTHER READING

Currell, Susan, and Christina Cogdell, *Popular Eugenics: National Efficiency and American Mass Culture in the 1930s* (Athens, OH: Ohio University Press, 2006).

Degler, Carl N. *In Search of Human Nature: The Decline and Revival of Darwinism in American Social Thought* (Oxford and New York: Oxford University Press, 1991).

Deutsch, Nathaniel. *Inventing America's 'Worst' Family: Eugenics, Islam, and the Fall and Rise of the Tribe of Ishmael* (Berkeley, CA: University of California Press, 2009).

Dorr, Gregory Michael. *Segregation's Science: Eugenics and Society in Virginia* (Charlottesville, VA: University of Virginia Press, 2008).

Dowbiggin, Ian Robert. *Keeping America Sane: Psychiatry and Eugenics in the United States and Canada, 1880–1940*, (Ithaca, NY: Cornell University Press, 1997).

Haller, Mark H. *Eugenics: Hereditarian Attitudes in American Thought* (New Brunswick, NJ: Rutgers University Press, 1984).

Kevles, Daniel J. *In the Name of Eugenics: Genetics and the Uses of Human Heredity* (New York: Knopf, 1985).

Kline, Wendy. *Building a Better Race: Gender, Sexuality, and Eugenics from the Turn of the Century to the Baby Boom* (Berkeley, CA: University of California Press, 2001).

Larson, Edward J. *Sex, Race, and Science: Eugenics in the Deep South* (Baltimore, MD: Johns Hopkins University Press, 1995).

Rosen, Christine. *Preaching Eugenics: Religious Leaders and the American Eugenics Movement* (Oxford and New York: Oxford University Press, 2004).

Stern, Alexandra Minna. *Eugenic Nation: Faults and Frontiers of Better Breeding in Modern America* (Berkeley, CA: University of California Press, 2005).

CHAPTER 31

EUGENICS IN CANADA:
A CHECKERED HISTORY,
1850s–1990s

CAROLYN STRANGE AND
JENNIFER A. STEPHEN

HISTORIANS' growing sensitivity to transnational phenomena confirms what eugenics proponents of the early twentieth century took for granted: eugenics was a scientific and cultural movement that crisscrossed the globe, as leaders attending conferences of experts and policy-makers exchanged ideas and kept abreast of strategies adopted in other countries. Nevertheless, the character of eugenics as well as the characters who advocated it varied, even in neighboring nations and those with similar histories. This is certainly true of Canada, whose eugenic past was connected closely to that of the United States and to a lesser extent England, about which historians of eugenics have written a great deal more. Yet eugenics in Canada was not simply derivative of Anglo-American thought and practice, nor was Canada's eugenic past a gentler version of its American counterpart.[1]

Considering the vigor and wide appeal of eugenics in Canada, historians were slow to chart its past. Angus McLaren's *Our Own Master Race,* published in 1990, remains the sole overview.[2] Drawing largely on medical, public health, and mental hygiene journals, as well as the publications and papers of organizations that promoted eugenic policies, McLaren analyzed the motives of the medical professionals, business leaders, and politicians, who led Canada's eugenics movement and garnered widespread popular support for the cause of "race betterment." His characterization of eugenics as a popular force awakened Canadians to a dark past that most had associated with other nations. More disturbingly, McLaren revealed that several famous Canadians, celebrated for their contributions to social justice, had been leading eugenicists.[3] Pioneering feminists and social democrats supported eugenics, and so did prominent Protestant Canadians in academia and business. Over the first half of the twentieth century, eugenics in Canada was modern, scientific, and respectable.

In Canada the temporal course of eugenics followed that of other countries, such as Sweden, where science, progressivism, and the nascent welfare state brought mixed benefits. University-trained professionals challenged philanthropists as new experts peddled new solutions for the management of problem people—criminals, prostitutes, paupers, Aboriginals, immigrants, and persons judged mentally and physically subnormal. Their reasoned rather than philanthropic or religious appeals elevated scientists, physicians, psychologists, educators, and public health professionals to positions of influence over public policy by the early twentieth century. Eugenics gained momentum in Canada, as it did in the United States, as mass immigration reduced the proportion of native-born Euro-Canadians in the country's population, particularly in the western provinces. By the 1910s, racially coded definitions of fitness found their way into immigration act amendments, designed to reject all but the fittest Anglo-Celts and Anglo-Saxons. Eugenics made its greatest impact, however, in provincial law, specifically the statutes passed in British Columbia and Alberta, that legalized sterilization of the "unfit." French-Canadians in Quebec and Catholics across the country resisted and rejected calls to control the breeding of "subnormal" persons. Despite these objections, poor young women, the physically and mentally disabled, incarcerated offenders, and Aboriginal people— those most likely to be judged unfit—became the individuals most vulnerable to involuntary sterilization.

Numerous case studies have appeared since McLaren's landmark study, many using previously untapped institutional records, including patient files from institutions where sterilizations took place, many without patients' consent. This body of research paints a checkered history of eugenics in Canada. It was a cluster of ideas and a disparate set of solutions that responded to local concerns, inflected by uniquely Canadian demographic, legal, political, and economic conditions. In two key respects, its history puts a distinct national cast on the wider shared course of eugenics (particularly in the United States and Australia): its radically incommensurate provincial and regional character, shaped by the French-Catholic and English-Protestant cultural divide; and its close association with the federally administered regulation of immigration and program of Aboriginal assimilation.[4]

Selective breeding was a modern idea foreshadowed in nineteenth-century colonial population policies designed to isolate some Aboriginal people and to assimilate others, in an attack against characteristics that Euro-Canadian legislators defined as markers of Aboriginal racial inferiority. By separating children from their families and forcing them to adopt "civilized" habits, so-called residential schools discouraged students from returning to their communities where they might propagate. Furthermore, the now-infamous Gradual Civilization Act of 1857 and the Indian Act of 1876 and its subsequent amendments authorized Indian agents and missionaries to police unions likely to result in the birth of children. Canadian eugenicists rarely addressed the question of Aboriginal peoples in part because the far greater number of suspected inferior immigrants preoccupied them, but also because the colonial "civilizing" regime imposed on the indigenous was already firmly in place decades before eugenicists proposed similar forms of selective breeding for non-native Canadians.[5] Thus race-based reproduction management efforts established a prior logic for eugenic policies concerned to shore up the fitness of Canada's Euro-Canadian majority.

How a Menace was Made

English biomedical politics and the notion of expert-directed human betterment rooted quickly in Canada, where scientists held British and European expertise in high regard. More significantly, eugenics appealed to a coterie of thinkers alive to the challenges facing a young country of vast territory and a tiny population, concentrated overwhelmingly in the cities of the east. Politicians and religious leaders articulated those anxieties and proposed solutions, both spiritual and secular, and so did many of Canada's leading scientists and medical practitioners.[6]

Psychiatrists were among the first academics to embrace eugenics and pronounce it a public issue. In 1890 Nova Scotia's Superintendent of the provincial Hospital for the Insane, Dr. A. P. Reid (1836–1919), called for improved "sanitary" education to reduce the risk of producing the sorts of "diseased ulcerous growths on society" who populated his wards. Reid had trained at McGill University, the country's most prestigious university, which turned out and attracted many of Canada's leading eugenics exponents.[7] Another asylum superintendent, C. K. Clarke (1857–1924), was influenced by European understandings of degeneracy and expounded a crude creed of hereditarianism. As he advised a member of the National Council of Women, "fully fifty percent of the admissions to our asylums are the outcome of bad heredity."[8]

A key McGill advocate was Carrie Derrick (1862–1941), the first woman hired as a McGill professor (of botany) and the founder of the Montreal Suffrage Association. She championed compulsory schooling and educational streaming as a way to preserve children healthy in mind and body from "contamination," and she addressed women's and church groups and even lectured the provincial premier on the topic (albeit to no effect). Derrick had more success with the Montreal Women's Club. To "improve the race" required that "persons with serious hereditary defects, who become wards of the state, [...] be segregated." Protecting society "from a repetition of hereditary blunders" would be costly, but failing to act was far costlier. Echoing women in other jurisdictions, she warned that inaction would lead to "successive generations of the feeble-minded in jails, penitentiaries and other institutions, ill adapted to dealing with them wisely and humanely."[9]

Although the concentration of eugenicists at McGill made Montreal the intellectual center of eugenics in Canada, Quebec's French-Catholic culture limited its influence. The church largely governed education and health care, both of which are provincial responsibilities in Canada, and it preserved its authority in spite of scientific eugenicists' attempts to usurp it. Catholic authorities considered English Protestant experts (particularly those who linked feeblemindedness to large families) as threats to Catholicism and to French-Canadian culture.[10] Theologians countered materialist science with Church doctrine, based in scripture and, after 1930, the papal encyclical, *Casti Connubii*, which expressly condemned "all the inventions of modern science" that threatened Christian duty to increase and multiply.[11] Clerics also adopted legal and scientific reasoning to undermine the credibility of eugenics. For Hervé Blais, eugenics posed "a moral and legal problem, concerning the conformity of its programmes with moral law or the rights of individuals or of society."[12] Doctrine, religious or political, was not the only basis for criticism. One French-Canadian pediatrician challenged eugenicists to support their claims scientifically, asking: "What does it mean to be feebleminded? Can it be measured with I.Q. tests? Or disabilities?"[13]

Recent research casts doubt on the notion that French Catholics rejected eugenics outright, however. Religious authorities certainly criticized eugenicists (including several high-profile members of the Eugenics Society of Canada, formed in 1930) who supported sterilization and birth control, measures that interfered with reproduction. But when it came to the goal of encouraging the fit to breed and discouraging dysgenic practices, objections melted away. Dominican M. C. Forest, for one, approved of the isolation and incarceration of the "unfit": "Segregation will do everything sterilization would do, and it will do it without violating the inalienable rights of the individual and upsetting the moral sense of the community." Statements such as these have urged historians to shift their focus from official church policy toward community sentiment and to individual decision-making on reproductive matters.[14] Clerics spoke for the people and for the French "race," but they did not necessarily shape private behavior. Children judged to be unfit could be placed in church-operated orphanages, and private sub rosa arrangements with doctors to prevent family members with mental or physical impairments from reproducing could be made. Just as recent studies have documented the compromises Catholic clergy made with married couples over their desire to limit family size,[15] so further research is required to determine whether eugenic decision-making may have entered into segregation and sterilization decisions.[16]

West of Quebec, the climate for eugenics was less hostile, allowing eugenicists to court and win popular as well as governmental support. Toronto, the country's second-largest city, was home to the nation's largest concentration of medical doctors, psychologists, and public health officials, many of whom translated eugenics from scientific discourse into social cause. More significantly, Ontario's Anglo-Protestant culture and its advanced penal-welfare apparatus proved receptive to expert claims-making. Helen MacMurchy (1862–1953), the first woman to receive a medical degree from the University of Toronto, became the country's pioneering propagandist for eugenics. In 1913 the Ontario government appointed her Canada's first "inspector of the feeble-minded," and she used this position to announce the bad news: venereal disease, alcoholism, crime, tuberculosis, epilepsy, and illegitimacy had spread to alarming levels. The root cause of these mass ills? Mental deficiency. Christian charity and philanthropy, along with the country's open door to immigrants, had tragically allowed feeblemindedness to flourish, she claimed. MacMurchy's 1920 tract, *The Almosts: A Study of the Feeble-minded* (1920), reached a lay audience reeling from wartime losses and receptive to her message: Canada's only hope to prevent the spread of feeblemindedness was the isolation and sterilization of the unfit.[17] Although it was little more than a messy mix of statistics and alarmist predictions, *The Almosts* won a popular audience and helped to make feeblemindedness a pressing national issue by the 1920s.

Managing the Menace

Although eugenicists garnered growing public support they complained that legislators were slow to respond. Dr. C. K. Clarke (1857–1924), dean of medicine and professor of psychiatry at the University of Toronto, was a perennial complainer who griped over inadequate state support for the segregation of mentally and physically defective people. Yet he managed to make effective use of provincial institutions to realize his eugenic goals. In 1909 he set up the Toronto Psychiatric Clinic, a psychometric and psycho-social sorting system that doubled as Toronto General Hospital's psychiatric outpatient clinic. As soon as the city established a juvenile court in 1912, its judge, a close associate of Clarke's, sent minors to the Clinic, where he also assessed the mentality of venereal disease patients from clinics and reformatories. Clarke subjected referrals to intelligence tests and took note of physical clues to mental subnormality—anything from cleft palate to uneven gait. Clarke's greatest concern was young, working-class women and their responses to his questions about their sexual behavior. In his expert opinion, these "thoughtless girls" with low "social and moral intelligence" were "high grade morons." This diagnostic category brought with it the potential for punitive consequences. Once labeled morally or mentally unfit, young women, and less frequently men, became candidates for incarceration at the Ontario Provincial Asylum for Idiots, Canada's largest institution of the sort. In 1919, when a mother dared to inquire about her child's progress, the superintendent replied with a dim prognosis: "Feeble-mindedness is something that no doctor or institution can cure."[18]

In other words, the incarceration of people identified as subnormal or inappropriately sexual accomplished eugenic objectives, even in provinces where eugenic policies were never codified in law. In 1924, lobbying by juvenile court judges across the country, including Regina's Ethel MacLachlan and Edmonton's Emily Murphy, produced an amendment to the federal Juvenile Delinquents Act, which empowered courts to intervene in cases involving "sexual immorality or any similar form of vice."[19] Although gender- and class-neutral in its wording, the statute, like those passed in many US states, placed young, working-class Anglo-Celtic and Aboriginal women more squarely in prosecutorial sight.[20] Studies based on institutional records and patient case files cast doubt on eugenicists' complaints over their incapacity to prevent "subnormal" people from procreating. Unlike prisons, whose inmates' sentences were statutorily limited, psychiatric hospitals, industrial schools, and training schools exercised their much wider latitude to segregate "unfit" individuals for indeterminate periods—even life sentences.[21]

CONSTITUTING CANADIAN CITIZENSHIP

Like the United States (and in contrast to other British Dominions), Canada adopted an aggressive pro-immigration policy in the 1890s, in a rush to populate the less-settled area of the vast country. The program successfully boosted and broadened Canada's population: three million immigrants arrived between 1896 and 1914, many to farm in the Prairies (particularly Manitoba, Saskatchewan, and Alberta). After suppressing the Northwest Rebellion in 1885 (the last major armed campaign by Aboriginal people to resist colonization and to retain their land), the federal government opened the resource-rich frontier to non-native immigrants, largely from eastern and southern Europe, Scandinavia, and the Russian empire. Coercive marital regulations were already pressing Aboriginals into the fold of moral citizenry,[22] but without similar mechanisms to "civilize" immigrants, arriving by hundreds of thousands each year, eugenicists worried that Canada's national character and fitness were under threat from unfit foreigners.[23]

Over the late nineteenth and early twentieth century, the proportion of foreign-born persons in its population exceeded even that of the United States.[24] This radical change helps to explain why so few Canadian eugenicists supported birth control: the best stock was dwindling, while alien "defectives" were procreating at alarming rates, producing the Canadian version of "race suicide." There was no need for experts to define the racial identity of Canada's "best": race in this iteration was an amalgam of biological, cultural, and geographical qualities that added up to whiteness. Eugenicists did not invent racism, but their hereditarian claims, articulated by medical and scientific experts, authorized it, and paved the way toward tighter immigration restrictions.[25]

Dealing with large intakes of immigrants inspired a variety of approaches, including efforts to develop immigrants' skills and resources and to improve health and housing conditions. Others were inclined to see immigrants' problems as inherited, on account of fixed racial characteristics and, in all cases, on account of bad breeding. Peter Bryce, the chief medical officer of the federal immigration department and an advocate of sterilization of the unfit, presented shocking evidence that feeblemindedness among

British immigrant children was twice that of Canadian-born children.[26] Inspections of schools, jails, and asylums confirmed that rates of physical, mental, and moral defects were highest among immigrants of all ethnicities. Helen MacMurchy confidently stated that "the number of recent immigrants that drift into institutions for the neuropathic, the feeble-minded and the insane is very great."[27] Thus, eugenicists believed some immigrants to be inferior on the basis (as with indigenous people) of fixed racial characteristics. But experts had to examine every immigrant to determine her or his suitability for Canada. "It is all very well to talk about pumping in the population," C. S. Clarke complained, "but surely the streams tapped should not be those reeking with degeneracy, crime and insanity."[28]

By the early 1900s, amendments to the Immigration Act began to attach eugenic objectives to immigration restrictions. An amendment in 1906 prohibited the landing of "feeble-minded" immigrants, as well as those convicted of "a crime involving moral turpitude." Significantly the 1906 amendment granted the Department of Immigration the legal power to deport immigrants whose undesirable qualities became evident after arriving in Canada. This new proactive role gave the federal government, in cooperation with provincial and municipal authorities, the power to expel undesirables. A 1910 amendment introduced racial characteristics among a list of vaguely defined criteria for rejection: "immigrants belonging to any race deemed unsuited to the climate or requirements of Canada, or of immigrants of any specified class, occupation or character" could be prevented from landing.[29] Explicitly race-based restrictions worked from 1885 to reduce Chinese immigration, and in 1923 a federal statute (named, ironically, the Chinese Immigration Act) prohibited immigrants of "Chinese origin or descent."[30]

Deportation orders also followed eugenic objectives, even if they were never implemented in strict accordance with expert assessments, as Clarke, MacMurchy, Bryce, and other eugenicists had urged. The Immigration Department's retrospective review of deportation, conducted in 1950, revealed that approximately 10 percent of the more than 80,000 persons deported between 1903 and 1939 were removed for medical reasons; of these deportees, half were expelled on the grounds of insanity or feeblemindedness.[31] Studies based on close readings of case files reveal how character assessments could be turned into grounds for deportation on the word of a physician. Men and women diagnosed with mental illness or judged morally defective were equally vulnerable. For example, when a Manitoba doctor treated a young English man with an "addiction" to masturbation, the physician's prognosis that the vice would "end in insanity" was sufficient reason for deportation. Generally, however, women were more likely than men to be deported on moral or medical grounds. Even those not found to be suffering from venereal disease were singled out: "she is presumably healthy enough, except that, being a prostitute, she is likely to spread sexual disorder," one doctor advised.[32] Judgments of this nature were acceptable and appropriate, according to William Scott (1861–1925), superintendent of immigration from 1908 to 1924: "It is intended that only the criminally inclined, mentally or physically incapable, and moral degenerates should be deported."[33]

The pace of deportations escalated by the 1930s, when public support for the indigent, as well as funding for hospitals, asylums, and prisons was stretched to the breaking point. But the logic of cost saving, institutional efficiency, and racial betterment found its way into more radical proposals as well. Over the 1920s and 1930s, disparate calls for the sterilization of the unfit united into a Canada-wide campaign, championed by two national organizations and endorsed by the country's leading business and political figures. Although British Columbia and Alberta were the sole provinces to pass institutional sterilization laws (with Alberta providing for non-consensual sterilization), negative eugenics was more than a western-Canadian phenomenon: extreme eugenic measures would never have been implemented so harshly in the west had medical and psychiatric experts from central and eastern Canada not promoted them so vigorously.

NATIONAL CAUSE, PROVINCIAL PATTERNS

Eugenicists faced their greatest challenge in dealing with native-born people whom they considered to be defective. These were white Canada's "Almosts"—people who could not be confined to reservations, sent to residential schools, or deported. After World War I, two organizations rallied public and political support for eugenic reforms across the nation. The first was the Canadian National Committee for Mental Hygiene (CNCMH), which psychologist Clarence Hincks (1885–1964) established in 1918[34] as hearings for Ontario's "Royal Commission on the Care and Control of the Mentally Defective and Feeble-Minded" were still underway.[35] The second was the Eugenics Society of Canada, established by Dr. William Hutton (1888–1958), a Toronto-area medical officer of health, and supported financially by businessman A. R. Kaufman (1889–1979), a controversial proponent of voluntary sterilization and birth control. While the former was instrumental in encouraging the governments of Alberta and British Columbia to introduce sterilization statutes, the latter organization formed out of a sense that the western provinces' innovations could pave the way for the nation-wide adoption of a full-blown eugenic program.

Although the country's leading mental hygienists came together in the CNCMH, its members had a range of views on eugenics. Some psychologists and psychiatrists were drawn to eugenics to the extent that it helped explain their incapacity to cure all of their patients. Yet many placed greater faith in therapy and rejected eugenics as gloomy hereditarianism. Dr. William Blatz (1895–1964), one of the country's first child psychologists, believed that improved scientific child study and parental training offered the best recipe for fit children.[36] Nevertheless, he and others who disavowed negative eugenics joined the CNCMH, as did many of the academics and medical experts who had participated in the Ontario Royal Commission, in addition to an extraordinary roster of the nation's business leaders and blue-blooded philanthropists.[37] Mental hygiene was a cause that embraced a range of perspectives on eugenics, and its president was a respected professional, a humanitarian campaigner, and an advocate of negative eugenics—all perfectly possible in postwar Canada.[38]

When government bodies and social welfare organizations, such as local councils of women, sought expert advice for solutions to such problems as juvenile delinquency, prostitution, and overcrowded asylums, the CNCMH was poised to respond with expert advice. The first major commission came from the governments of Manitoba, British Columbia, and Alberta in 1918 and 1919. Over the next three years, Hincks and his team provided mental hygiene reports for seven of the nine provinces. The conclusions the CNCMH reached, after investigating Canada's asylums, industrial schools, and prisons, as well as many of its public schools, were grim but predictable: the population of mental defectives was booming. The radical downturn in Canada's immigrant intake and the use of deportations were the first steps toward remedying the problem; the final was sterilization.

Because Alberta and British Columbia were the only provinces to enact sterilization laws (involuntary, in the case of Alberta), historians struggle to explain why that was the case. In most Canadian provinces, aside from Quebec, sterilization bills or commissions of inquiry brought negative eugenics to the brink of implementation, so which factors tipped these western governments over the edge? The answer lies in the unique range of demographic, political, and cultural factors at play. Alberta, along with Saskatchewan, became a self-governing province only in 1905. Compared to the longer-settled eastern provinces, Alberta's health and social service network was rudimentary and ill-equipped to service its disproportionate share of Canada's immigrants. Similarly British Columbia's major cities, Victoria and Vancouver, were prime entry points for Chinese and Indian immigrants. Although British Columbia's array of institutions for mentally and physically unfit people was larger than Alberta's, its public health system had also failed to keep pace with spikes in immigration early in the twentieth century.

Both provinces had local champions of eugenics who linked Canada-wide concerns about rising populations of suspect deficients to local conditions. In Edmonton, Police Magistrate Emily Murphy (1868–1933) headed an investigation into the province's asylums and jails as a national board member of the CNCMH. Vancouver had a larger cohort of feminists, including Mary Ellen Smith (1861–1933), who became a legislator and cabinet member in the provincial Liberal government, where she used her position to promote sterilization legislation. Western eugenicists supplemented local expertise with advice from central Canadian medical and psychiatric experts and they also looked southward, especially after California and Washington passed involuntary sterilization statutes in 1909. Alexandra Stern's analysis of the distinctive western cast to eugenics in the United States[39] might be extended transnationally, to incorporate Canada's western-most provinces into a wider frame that helps to analyze the regional preoccupation with the breeding of "human thoroughbreds."[40]

Eugenicists' efforts to secure the social good over individual rights came fully to fruition only in Alberta, where populism and western agrarianism swept aside doubts about the ethics and legalities of "asexualization." The United Farmers of Alberta (UFA) and its ally, the United Farm Women of Alberta Association, combined forces over the 1920s, using talk of animal husbandry and better breeding to appeal to the province's farmers.[41] In 1928, with the UFA forming a government, Alberta charged ahead with Canada's first Sexual Sterilization Act. A board comprised of two medical and two lay members was established to review the fitness of patients eligible for discharge from mental asylums. Where the board agreed that an individual's release presented "the danger of procreation with its attendant risk of multiplication of the evil by transmission of the disability to progeny," it could direct surgical sterilization to eliminate the danger.[42]

Initially the Act required mentally competent patients' consent, or permission from their guardians in the case of minors and individuals judged incompetent. An amendment in 1937 enhanced the board's powers and enlarged the scope of dangerous procreators to include "psychotics." The consent clause was struck, replaced by the board's unfettered power to order sterilizations, in cases in which any "mentally defective person" presented the "risk of mental injury either to such person or to his progeny."[43] Without governmental or public oversight, physicians and eugenics board members exercised their authority to prevent "defectives" from breeding, in a province whose political culture resembled that of the U.S. Deep South. There as well eugenicists on the periphery of scientific research held power and prestige, even as geneticists' doubts about the inheritability of defects mounted over the 1930s.[44] In this milieu a single individual, Alberta's first Eugenics Board head, who held his post from 1928 to 1965, endorsed over 3,200 sterilization orders, 60 percent of which were carried out, until the statute was eventually repealed in 1972.[45]

British Columbia's sterilization bill faced a rougher road to passage. BC's larger community of social welfare and medical experts included individuals who questioned the rush to sterilization. Some, like Vancouver's school inspector, favored education and integration: "the majority of morons....can be trained so that they can live in the outside world."[46] Environmental arguments of this nature pulled the province away from implementing involuntary sterilization. The report of the province's Royal Commission on Mental Hygiene in 1928 recommended sterilization legislation, but it demonstrated concern about the province's reputation and supported mental health care reforms over surgical solutions. A change of government delayed passage of a permissive sterilization bill until 1933, when the Liberals regained power amidst the Depression and committed the government to the use of sterilization. British Columbia's law also remained in effect until 1973, but its use declined after World War II, and it appears that far fewer institutionalized people (approximately 200) were sterilized. Still, it would be inappropriate to characterize British Columbia's sterilizations as "voluntary" and Alberta's as compulsory: when "asexualization" was presented as a condition of release and when guardians of minors or of those diagnosed as incompetent so wished, sterilizations occurred, with and without individuals' consent.

The Eugenics Society of Canada (ESC) hailed the western provinces' bold moves toward racial betterment, but it never managed to muster legislative support for eugenics elsewhere in the country. Its chief power base was Ontario and its principal support came from the medical profession in Ontario, although the province's Lieutenant Governor and Kaufman, a rubber manufacturer, became its most vocal spokesmen, who campaigned enthusiastically for sterilization. There was nothing new to their message, but the climate had shifted by the 1930s, as welfare relief rolls ballooned and the costs of incarcerating the unfit burdened taxpayers. Far from recoiling from an association with Nazi eugenic programs, Lieutenant Governor Bruce (1868–1963) urged Canada in 1938 to undertake a thorough "biological housecleaning" along the lines of Germany, which he praised for sterilizing "300,000 useless, harmful, and hopeless people."[47] Statements of this ilk had a darker ring after Canada joined the fight against Nazi Germany. Sterilizations continued to be performed in Alberta behind the walls of institutions (even exceeding California's and North Carolina's rates in the 1950s and 1960s) but the ESC, the public face of eugenics in Canada, declined by 1941.

EUGENICS' LONG HISTORY

The endurance of the CNCMH, renamed the Canadian Mental Health Association (CMHA) in 1950, signals that eugenic aspirations, not just policies, lingered on in postwar Canada. Prominent eugenicists remained active: Hincks in the CMHA until his death in 1964, and Kaufman in the contraception bureau he established in 1935 and headed until 1970. Many supporters of eugenics remained steady advocates, at least privately. Two-thirds of doctors polled in a 1970 medico-legal questionnaire supported the use of "forcible sterilization" for "mentally retarded" people, as well as the criminally insane. Others were moved to express their support publicly, as repeal campaigns gathered strength. In 1972 a superintendent of the Red Deer Training School for Mental Defectives, where compulsory sterilizations were still carried out, hoped that repeal agitation might prove nothing more than "a political storm in a tea cup."[48]

The minor storm that rose in the 1970s subsided quickly, only to gain far greater force in the 1990s, when individuals who had suffered from eugenic practices publicized their experiences. In a historical moment when claims for redress for past wrongs (such as institutional sexual abuse, wrongful convictions, and racist immigration and detention policies) were gaining political, legal, and cultural purchase, one woman—Leilani Muir (b. 1944)—became the public face of the harm inflicted in the name of eugenics[49] Sterilized without her knowledge or consent at 14 while she was an inmate of the Red Deer school, she sued the province of Alberta in 1996 for wrongful confinement and wrongful sterilization. The judgment in her favor was unequivocal: the "wrongful stigmatization of Ms. Muir as a moron…has humiliated Ms. Muir every day of her life…the community's, and the court's, sense of decency is offended."[50] Although the province resisted paying court-ordered compensation, over 700 people with experiences similar to Muir's, filed suits of their own.[51] A decade later, British Columbia's Public Guardian and Trustee represented individuals in that province who had been sterilized against their will, successfully claiming that the procedure constituted "battery."[52]

The history of eugenics in Canada (as in the United States and other jurisdictions with indigenous populations) is inseparable from racist assimilationist policies and practices. From the mid-nineteenth century, the national effort to reshape the character of Canada's indigenous population created a precedent for racially informed conceptions of fitness. Framed through colonial discourse and pathologized on account of Euro-Canadian readings of "instinct," Aboriginals were the nation's first "problem" population. Eugenics administrators who linked "Indian blood" to low intelligence were predisposed to diagnose indigenous people as "mentally defective" and incompetent: consequently they were judged unfit to make their own reproductive decisions. Detailed analysis of patient and inmate records in British Columbia and Alberta confirms that "Indian," "Métis," "half-breed," and "Eskimo" individuals, particularly young women already institutionalized for moral infractions, were assigned for sterilization at disproportionately high rates: three-quarters of Aboriginal people presented before Alberta's eugenics board were sterilized, compared to 47 percent of presentees of European descent.[53] Thus Canada's sterilization laws, while never explicitly race-specific in design or intent, were implemented to racist effect.

The people most affected by Canada's eugenic policies were those whose sexual morality and reproductive futures appeared suspect: young women. Gender disparities in institutional sterilizations were more marked than racial disparities, even though the girls and women who appeared before the eugenics boards of Alberta and British Columbia eugenics boards were less likely than men to be diagnosed as mentally defective. Similarly, the likelihood of sterilization was strongly associated with youth, largely because training schools for juveniles referred the bulk of inmates. Ultimately, the most consistent feature in the administration of negative and positive eugenics was its impact on the poor, who were most vulnerable to investigation by Canada's expanding welfare network of teachers, public health nurses, social workers, doctors, psychologists, and juvenile court judges. These were the professionals and experts whose reports could become the first links in the chain of eugenic inquiry, investigation, diagnosis, and segregation. For thousands, ultimately, the final link was non-consensual sterilization.

NOTES

1. Ian Robert Dowbiggin, *Keeping America Sane: Psychiatry and Eugenics in the United States and Canada, 1880–1940* (Ithaca, NY: Cornell University Press, 1997). In this article we stress the factors that made Canada distinct.

2. The only scholarly works published before McLaren's book are Terry L. Chapman, "The Early Eugenics Movement in Western Canada," *Alberta History* 25 (1977): 9–17; and Bernard M. Dickens, "Eugenic Recognition in Canadian Law," *Osgoode Hall Law Journal* 13 (1975): 547–577. Chapman and other more recent works rely on an unpublished research report by Timothy J. Christian, "The Mentally Ill and Human Rights in Alberta: A Study of

the Alberta Sexual Sterilization Act" (Faculty of Law, University of Alberta, 1974). Our account is heavily indebted to McLaren's interpretations and his citations in *Our Own Master Race: Eugenics in Canada, 1885–1945* (Toronto: McClelland and Stewart, 1990).

3. This argument has been used to discredit the Left. See Michael Coren, "Don't Blame Right-wing Thugs for Eugenics—Socialists Made it Fashionable," *National Post*, June 16, 2008, network.nationalpost.com/np/blogs/fullcomment/archive/2008/06/16/michael-coren-don-t-blame-right-wing-thugs-for-eugenics-socialists-made-it-fashionable.aspx (accessed August 5, 2008).

4. The Canadian Constitution Act 1867, Section 91(24), placed all matters regarding Canadian Aboriginal peoples and reserves set aside for them under federal jurisdiction, effectively defining Aboriginal people as wards of the state.

5. Mary Ellen Kelm, "Diagnosing the Discursive Indian: Medicine, Gender and the 'Dying Race,'" *Ethnohistory* 52, no. 2 (2005): 371–406.

6. Mariana Valverde, *The Age of Light, Soap and Water: Moral Reform in English Canada, 1885–1925* (Oxford and Toronto: Oxford University Press, 1991).

7. McGill pathologist, J. G. Adami (1862–1926), also published eugenic work. See "A Study in Eugenics: Into the Third and Fourth Generation," *Lancet* 2 (1912): 1199–1204.

8. Clarke to Mrs. Talbot Macbeth, 1896, quoted in Dowbiggin, *Keeping America Sane*, 140.

9. Derrick, December 21, 1915, quoted in Sebastien Normandin, "Eugenics, McGill and the Catholic Church in Montreal and Quebec, 1890–1942," *Canadian Bulletin of Medical History/Bulletin canadien d'histoire de la médecine* 15, no. 1 (1998): 68–69.

10. William Schneider makes this argument in *Quality and Quantity: The Quest for Biological Regeneration in Twentieth-Century France* (Cambridge: Cambridge University Press, 1990).

11. Normandin points out that this encyclical acknowledged eugenic ideals, but condemned any measures that interfered with reproduction. See his "Eugenics, McGill and the Catholic Church," 73.

12. Hervé Blais, *Les tendances eugénistes au Canada* (Montreal: L'Institut Familial, 1942), 133, quoted in Normandin, "Eugenics, McGill and the Catholic Church," 76.

13. Dr. Gaston Lapierre, "Les campagnes internationales actuelles d'eugenisme," *Revue trimestrielle canadienne* 21 (1935): 356–372, quoted in Normandin, "Eugenics, McGill and the Catholic Church," 79.

14. Denyse Baillargeon, *Un Québec en mal d'enfants. La médicalisation de la maternité, 1910–1970* (Montréal: Éditions du remue-ménage, 2004).

15. Dianne Gavreau, Peter Gossage, and Neil Sutherland, "Fécondité et contraception au Québec, 1920–60," *Revue d'histoire de L'Amerique francaise* 78, no. 3 (1997): 478–510.

16. Monique Benoit, "25 ans de pratique massive de la stérilisation tubaire au Québec: Les manifestations d'une crise de la fécondité," *Revue Sexologique* 5, no. 1 (1997): 48–49. Quebec established a provincial home for the feebleminded (École La Jemmerais) in 1928.

17. Dianne Dodd, "Advice to Parents: The Blue Books, Helen MacMurchy, MD, and the Federal Department of Health, 1920–34," *Canadian Bulletin of Medical History/Bulletin canadien d'histoire de la médecine* 8, no. 2 (1991): 203–230.

18. J. P. Downey to inmate mother (anonymized), quoted in Jessica Chupik and David Wright, "Treating the 'Idiot' Child in Early 20th-Century Ontario," *Disability and Society* 21, no. 1 (2006): 77.

19. Because juvenile court judges were not required to have law degrees, women were among the first appointees. Quebec, however, restricted judicial appointments to members of the bar.

20. Bruno Théoret, "Régulation juridique pénal des mineures et discrimination à l'égard des filles: La clause de 1924 amendant la *Loi sur les jeunes délinquents*," *Canadian Journal of Women and the Law* 4 (1990–1991): 539–555.

21. Deborah C. Park and John P. Radford, "From the Case Files: Reconstructing a History of Involuntary Sterilisation," *Disability and Society* 13, no. 3 (1998): 317–342.

22. This project was not exclusive to Canada. See Andrew Armitage, *Comparing the Policy of Aboriginal Assimilation: Australia, Canada and New Zealand* (Vancouver: University of British Columbia Press, 1995).

23. For an excellent collection of essays that takes a critical approach to Canadian population management, see Robert Adomoski, Dorothy E. Chunn, and Robert Menzies, eds., *Contesting Canadian Citizenship: Historical Readings* (Peterborough: Broadview Press, 2002).

24. Harold Palmer, ed., *Immigration and the Rise of Multiculturalism* (Toronto: University of Toronto Press, 1976), 4.

25. McLaren, *Our Own Master Race*, 49. See also Frank Dikötter, "Race Culture: Recent Perspectives on the History of Eugenics," *American Historical Review* 103, no. 2 (1998): 467–478.

26. Peter Bryce, "Medical Inspection in Schools," *Public Health Journal* 7 (1916): 59–62.

27. Helen MacMurchy, "Defective Children," *Social Service Congress: Ottawa 1914* (Toronto: Social Service Council, 1914), 101.

28. C. K. Clarke, "Defective and Insane Immigration," *Sessional Papers of Canada*, vol. 40, part 8 (Session 1908).

29. Canada, "An Act Respecting Immigration and Immigrants," *Revised Statutes of Canada*, Chapter 93, 1906, ss. 26, 29, 32; Canada, "An Act Respecting Immigration," *Statutes of Canada*, Chapter 27, 1910, s. 38 (b).

30. Canada, "Chinese Immigration Act," *Statutes of Canada*, Chapter 38, 1923.

31. Department of Citizenship and Immigration, "Immigration Studies with Special Reference to Mental Disease," National Archives of Canada, Ottawa, RG 29, vol. 3901, file 854–4–300, pt. 1-A, quoted in Robert Menzies, "Governing Mentalities: The Deportation of 'Insane' and 'Feeble-minded' Immigrants out of British Columbia from Confederation to World War II," *Canadian Journal of Law and Society* 13 (1998): 138.

32. Quoted in Fiona Alice Miller, "Making Citizens, Banishing Immigrants: The Discipline of Deportation Investigations, 1908–1913," *Left History* 7, no. 1 (2000): 79.

33. Barbara Roberts, *Whence They Came: Deportation from Canada, 1900–1935* (Ottawa: University of Ottawa Press, 1988), 55, 58, 60. Scott was responding to a mayor to underline that being a public charge was insufficient grounds for deportation.

34. At C. K. Clarke's suggestion, Hincks met the leader of the American National Committee for Mental Hygiene, Clifton Beers, in 1917. Ronald A. LaJeunesse, *Political Asylums* (Edmonton: Muttart Foundation, 2002), 63.

35. Frank E. Hodgins, *Report on the Care and Control of the Mentally Defective and Feeble-minded in Ontario* (Toronto: Queen's Printer, 1919).

36. Harley D. Dickinson, "Scientific Parenthood: The Mental Hygiene Movement and the Reform of Canadian Families, 1925–1950," *Journal of Comparative Family Studies* 24, no. 3 (1993): 387–402.

37. Charles G. Roland, *Clarence Meredith Hincks: Mental Health Crusader* (Toronto: Hannah Institute and Oxford University Press, 1990).

38. Hincks was sufficiently well respected to become the director of the US National Committee for Mental Hygiene in 1930.

39. Alexandra Minna Stern, *Eugenic Nation: Faults and Frontiers of Better Breeding in Modern America* (Berkeley, CA: University of California Press, 2005).

40. Emily Murphy famously used this phrase in 1932, in articles calling for steriliza-tion, which were published in the Vancouver *Sun* under the pseudonym "Janey Canuck." McLaren, *Our Own Master Race*, 101

41. The United Farmers of Alberta was established as a lobby group in 1909 and preferred not to operate as a party, even after it formed the government. Alvin Finkel, *The Social Credit Phenomenon in Alberta* (Toronto: University of Toronto Press, 1989).

42. Alberta, *Statutes of the Province of Alberta*, "The Sexual Sterilization Act," Chapter 37, 1928, s. 5.

43. Alberta, *Statutes of the Province of Alberta*, "An Act to Amend the Sexual Sterilization Act," Chapter 47, 1937, s. 5. The non-consent clause remained in effect until the Act was repealed, but it was amended in 1942 to apply to those diagnosed with neurosyphi-lis, epilepsy, and Huntington's chorea. Alberta, *Revised Statutes of Alberta*, "The Sexual Sterilization Act," Chapter 194, 1942.

44. Edward J. Larsen, *Sex, Race, and Science Eugenics in the Deep South* (Baltimore, MD: Johns Hopkins University Press, 1995).

45. Jana Marie Grekul, *Social Construction of the Feebleminded Threat— Implementation of the Sexual Sterilization Act in Alberta, 1929–1972*, (PhD diss., University of Alberta, 2002), 102–103; Jana Grekul, Harvey Krahn and Dave Odynak, "Sterilizing the 'Feeble-minded': Eugenics in Alberta, Canada, 1929–1972," *Journal of Historical Sociology* 17, no. 4 (2004): 359; K. J. McWhirter and J. Weijer, "The Alberta Sterilization Act: A Genetic Critique," *University of Toronto Law Journal*, 19 (1969): 424–431.

46. Quoted in Robert Menzies, "'Unfit Citizens and the B.C. Royal Commission on Mental Hygiene, 1925–28," in *Contesting Canadian Citizenship*, Adomoski et al., eds., 396, 392.

47. Bruce made this statement in a Canadian Broadcasting Company radio broadcast in 1938. Quoted in McLaren, *Our Own Master Race*, 124.

48. Quoted in Park and Radford, "From the Case Files," 340.

49. Gerald L. Gall, May M. Cheng, and Keiko Miki, "Redress for Past Government Wrongs," Advisory Committee to the Secretary of State (Multiculturalism) (Status of Women) on Canada's preparations for the UN World Conference Against Racism, January 2001, www.pch.gc.ca/progs/multi/wcar/advisory/redress_e.cfm (accessed August 5, 2008).

50. Muir v. The Queen in Right of Alberta, *Dominion Law Reports*, 132 (4th series, 1996), 696.

51. Grekul et al., "Sterilizing the 'Feeble-Minded,'" 380, n. 4.

52. In 2005 the British Columbia Court of Appeal ruled in favor of nine women, sterilized between 1940 and 1968, who received from $25,000 to $100,000 plus their legal costs in compensation. Grekul et al., "Sterilizing the 'Feeble-Minded,'" 382, n19.

53. Grekul et al., "Sterilizing the 'Feeble-Minded,'" 375.

FURTHER READING

Dickens, Bernard M. "Eugenic Recognition in Canadian Law," *Osgoode Hall Law Journal* 13 (1975): 547–577.

Dowbiggin, Ian Robert. *Keeping America Sane: Psychiatry and Eugenics in the United States and Canada, 1880–1940*, 2nd ed. (Ithaca, NY: Cornell University Press, 2003).

Grekul, Jana, Harvey Krahn, and Dave Odynak. "Sterilizing the 'Feeble-minded': Eugenics in Alberta, Canada, 1929–1972," *Journal of Historical Sociology* 17, no. 4 (2004): 358–384.

Kelley, Ninette, and Michael Treblicock. *The Making of the Mosaic: A History of Canadian Immigration Policy* (Toronto: University of Toronto Press, 1998).

Malacrida, Claudia. "Contested Memories: Efforts of the Powerful to Silence Former Inmates' Histories of Life in an Institution for 'Mental Defectives,'" *Disability and Society* 21, no. 5 (2006): 397–410.

McLaren, Angus. *Our Own Master Race: Eugenics in Canada, 1885–1945* (Toronto: McClelland and Stewart, 1990).

National Film Board of Canada, *The Sterilization of Leilani Muir* (Montreal, 1996).

Normandin, Sebastien. "Eugenics, McGill and the Catholic Church in Montreal and Quebec, 1890–1942," *Canadian Bulletin of Medical History/Bulletin canadien d'histoire de la médecine* 15, no. 1 (1998): 59–86.

Radford, John, and Deborah C. Park. "A Convenient Means of Riddance: Institutionalization of People Diagnosed as Mentally Defective in Ontario, 1876–1934," *Health and Canadian Society* 1 (1993): 369–392.

Stephen, Jennifer. "The 'Incorrigible,' the 'Bad,' and the 'Immoral': Toronto's 'Factory Girls' and the Work of the Toronto Psychiatric Clinic, 1918–1923," in *Law, State and Society: Essays in Modern Legal History*, eds. Louis Knafla and Susan Binnie (Toronto: University of Toronto Press, 1995), 405–439.

EPILOGUE:
WHERE DID EUGENICS GO?

ALISON BASHFORD

Historians always write about the beginning of eugenics, because they can: Galton coined the term "eugenics" in 1883. Identifying an end to eugenics is another story altogether. "Today, eugenics is back," claims one author.[1] Another argues that eugenics and genetics always had an "exquisitely close" relationship.[2] And a third refuses the connection, arguing for a marked division between population-level historical eugenics and contemporary choice-based medical genetics.[3]

There is often a gap between those who seek to write the history of eugenics, and those who seek answers to questions like "Is Gene Therapy a Form of Eugenics?"[4] One element of this gap is proper knowledge of the complexity of early eugenics, often sacrificed to political use of the term. As Lene Koch argues, "the witless reference to 'eugenics' with no further specification is empty and more often a function of our own projections and intentions than a reference to history."[5] And the history that is referred to is often flat and uniform. Not a few historians argue that selective understandings of the history of eugenics may seriously mislead contemporary efforts to regulate reproductive and genetic technologies, and be a questionable basis for policy decisions. Diane Paul puts it strongly: "It is time to be more sophisticated in our accounts of eugenics, not just for the sake of fidelity to the historical record but of a more adequate public policy."[6]

Another aspect of this gap between histories of eugenics and commentary on the "new eugenics" is the overall disinclination among historians to research eugenics after 1945. There is a popular and, in some instances, scholarly narrative that Nazi eugenics and its assessment (or presumed assessment) in the so-called doctors' trials, the genocide convention, and the United Nations human rights convention collectively marked the end of eugenics. Even though most historians are fully aware of the pre-, post-, and extra-Nazi history, periodizing the history of eugenics to 1945 remains reasonably common.[7] And yet, ongoing eugenic-genetic activity in the decades after 1945 was analyzed early by Daniel Kevles, and more recently by Alice Wexler and Ruth Schwartz Cowan, among others. As these historians show, in thinking about links between eugenics and developments in genetics and reproductive technologies (often conflated to "reprogenetics") the decades of continuous transition after World War II are especially revealing.[8]

In this chapter, I look at the history and historians of postwar eugenics, focusing on the Anglophone world. I survey several of the key substantive trajectories of eugenics: its connections with transhumanism; genetic counseling; sterility and infertility research; human and medical genetics. To suggest that any of these fields is historically connected to eugenics is quite different from arguing that it *is* "eugenics." There are benefits in pursuing a more strictly historical process of showing connections over time. And so, instead of asking "Is reprogenetics the new eugenics?," we might ask "Where did eugenics go?"

OLD EUGENICS, NEW EUGENICS, AND THE LONG TWENTIETH CENTURY

The term "new eugenics" (and the variants "eugenetics" and even "newgenics") is in increasingly common use, applied to various current reproductive and genetic procedures and possibilities.[9] It is often understood to be a wholly critical descriptor of current reprogenetics, an "almost universal agreement about the evils of eugenics."[10] This is overstated, however. Commentators use the idea and the term "new eugenics" from at least four different epistemological locations.

First, it needs to be recognized that eugenics is defended by some, an open and at times defiant claiming of the principles and objectives of eugenics from Galton onward. The term "new eugenics" was first used in this tradition. The molecular biologist Robert Sinsheimer labeled genetic engineering "new eugenics" favorably in 1969: "The old eugenics was limited to a numerical enhancement of the best of our existing gene pool. The horizons of the new eugenics are in principle boundless."[11] This position is often but not always presented in popular-level texts, John Glad's *Future Human Evolution: Eugenics in the Twenty-First Century,* for example.[12] A slightly more scholarly variation is *Dysgenics: Genetic Deterioration in Modern Population* by Richard Lynn, a 1996 book that draws a continuous history from Bénédict Morel (1809–1873) and Francis Galton through to the present. If eugenicists believed that modern populations were deteriorating, Lynn claims that "the evidence set out in this book shows they were correct," that this deterioration is ongoing, and that it should be addressed.[13]

Second, and more commonly, "new eugenics" signals a critique of current reprogenetics by disability scholars, some feminist scholars of reproductive politics, and some historians of eugenics. This is the tradition of Troy Duster's *Backdoor to Eugenics*,[14] and the work of Merryn Ekberg, who analyzes the arguments for discontinuity between eugenics and the new genetics and finds them wanting. "The old eugenics was genetics and the new genetics is eugenics," she concludes.[15] Philosophers and ethicists also utilize "new eugenics" in this way, in particular Jürgen Habermas, whose critical position on "the new liberal eugenics" has influentially focused a large amount of scholarship, extending the history of eugenics well outside the domains of history of science.[16]

Some, however, while recognizing a problematic "old eugenics," disagree that it is equivalent to current human application of molecular biology. Nikolas Rose takes this position in *The Politics of Life Itself*.[17] And from a very different tradition of scholarship, Ruth Schwartz Cowan has recently distinguished sharply between eugenics and later-twentieth-century genetic screening.[18]

A third group of commentators both critique and claim "eugenics" for the present. In *Eugenics: the Future of Human Life in the 21st Century*, molecular biologist David Galton argues for the continued use of the term "eugenics" because of its cautionary value: "Call it what you will," he writes, "but if your aim is to use scientific methods to make the best of the inherited component for the health and wellbeing of the children of the next generation, it is by definition eugenics. Sweeping the word under the carpet or sanitizing it with another name merely conceals the appalling abuses that have occurred in the past and may well lull people into a false sense of security."[19] "Reprogenetics" hides this history, while "eugenics" recognizes it, argues Galton, but this should not affect the ongoing development of genetic practices, in his view.[20]

The authors of *From Chance to Choice: Genetics and Justice* offer an "ethical autopsy" of eugenics in a thoughtful combination of good history and good bioethics. They question both the argument that "new genetics" is eugenics and therefore ethically unsound, and the argument that new genetics is unrelated to eugenics and therefore untainted by the problems of earlier eugenic practice. Early eugenics *was* unjust and problematic, they argue: "we can find, even given the most charitable understanding of its leaders' motives, a failure to deal adequately with the tension between social good and individual liberties, rights, and interests, which has long been the moral problem at the heart of the enterprise of public health."[21] Nonetheless, for these authors, this does not necessarily preclude just application of eugenic principles in the present or future. Their conclusion is that we need not abandon the central motivation of eugenics—"to endow future generations with genes that might enable their lives to go better"[22]—if this can be pursued and achieved justly. The rest of their book proceeds to test and, as they would have it, demonstrate the possibility of just and equitable application of the "new genetics."

In their effort to compare "old eugenics" and "new genetics," these authors point to two "eras" when there were "large-scale attempts to modify the pattern of human heredity for the better." The first era ("old eugenics") was from 1870 to 1950, and the second, the current era of molecular biology.[23] With some significant exceptions, this periodization is still a common feature in historiography and commentary on eugenics: authors often describe a discontinuous history in this fashion, interrupting at 1945 or 1950 what is really a continuous history of transformation in policy, science, technology, and politics. Many eugenic journals continued to publish after 1945, and some new titles were established, just one indicator of this postwar history. The journal *Eugenics Quarterly* was first published in 1954, changing its name in 1969 to *Social Biology,* becoming *Biodemography and Social Biology* in 2008. The *Bulletin* of the Eugenics Society (1969–1983) continued as *Biology and Society: The Journal of the Eugenics Society* (1984–1990), while *The Eugenics Review* (1909–1968) continued as the *Journal of Biosocial Science* (1969-). The Eugenics Society in England continued to meet in regular seminars and published volumes on all kinds of population-related questions.[24] Thus, while there is a common "old wine in new bottles" argument about eugenics, this reading disregards a rather more openly continuous history.[25]

INTERPRETING EUGENICS, RACE, AND GENOCIDE AFTER 1945

Even though it is widely known that eugenics emerged and flourished before and outside of the German Nazi regime, the connection between eugenics, genocide, and Nazism has been prominent in shaping interpretations of eugenics over the last 50 years: eugenics is often reduced to "racism" popularly, and in some scholarly circles. This is apparent, to take just one recent example, in the article, "Is China's Law Eugenic?" The defender of China's Law on Maternal and Infant Health argues that it is not eugenic specifically because "the law is not motivated by racism, but by a desire to reduce birth defects."[26] The reverse argument would be more historically correct. As many chapters in this volume show, eugenics was often, but not necessarily, driven by race questions in the first instance. Reduction in birth defects, on the other hand, was one consistent and central objective of eugenics in almost all national contexts. Eugenics and race, then, are often used interchangeably, in a way that flattens out this complicated history and that stems, in large part, from a still-common conflation of eugenics with Nazi racial hygiene.

While some Anglophone eugenic associations changed their names after 1945 to distance themselves from the Nazi medical experiments, others retained the name "eugenics" well into the 1980s. It proved easier to do so in Britain than in the United States. In general, those who argued most strongly to retain "eugenics" as a nomination for their work, or their organizations, were those who distanced themselves most from racial science. C. P. Blacker (1895–1975), for example, consistently argued that Nazi racial hygiene was an anomalous manifestation of eugenics, which should be dissociated from the thought and activity of his own society. He would not, and did not, cede the term "eugenics," and he expressed considerable discomfort with the shift toward race science under his successor at the Eugenics Society, Colin Bertram (1911–2001).[27] Julian Huxley (1887–1975), instrumental in the mid-twentieth century divorce between "biology" and "race," similarly promoted postwar eugenics, actively so in his 1947 UNESCO *Manifesto*. Even later, giving his Galton Lecture in 1962, Huxley never considered abandoning eugenics.

If those who defended eugenics were often anti-racists of various kinds, the reverse is also broadly correct. That is, those who *did* actively pursue race science in the postwar period, were likely to avoid the term "eugenics." Stefan Kühl has traced the connections between the U.S. Pioneer Fund's dreams of "race betterment" in the interwar years and ongoing race research in the United States from the 1950s to the 1980s. The latter was rarely labeled "eugenic," but nonetheless kept alive research questions about differential intelligence among races, the effects of interracial reproduction, and an overall thesis of genetic determinism entirely recognizable as one strand of eugenics in earlier generations.[28]

Defensive positions were certainly needed. When biologist Carl J. Bajema edited *Eugenics: Then and Now* in 1976, his introduction asked: "Does Eugenics Include the Racist Evolutionary Policies of Nazi Germany?" Yes, he thought, but only if one defined eugenics as "the social control of human genetic evolution." If, however, eugenics reached back to Galton's original statement that: (a) eugenics is the humane modification of natural selection, and (b) that it should lead to the genetic improvement of the human species, the Nazi program "fails both criteria," according to Bajema.[29] Bajema's efforts to distance eugenics from Nazi population policies tells us, among other things, that eugenics per se was by no means off-limits in the 1970s: at the same time as a strong anti-science, anti-psychiatry, and anti-racist critique of eugenics was taking shape, some scientists were defending eugenics as a legitimate research enterprise. And they were actively continuing the tradition of differentiating the Nazi version of racial hygiene from a "true" and beneficent eugenic path and purpose.

By the 1980s, the link between eugenics and Nazism was drawn afresh by a new generation of activists and scholars. This was a period when large volumes appeared refining understanding of German eugenics in the Nazi years.[30] The popular use of the connection between Nazism and eugenics became increasingly effective. It also became increasingly loose: ironic, given the new scholarship. As historian Stefan Kühl put it: "In the conflict about scientific racism, the word *Nazi* has degenerated into a term to be used in any situation to discredit the opponent."[31] This is the same broad comment that Lene Koch makes about the "witless" use of the term "eugenics" in discussion of contemporary reprogenetics[32]—and, one might add, the rhetorical use of the connection between eugenics and genocide in this period.

"Eugenics" and "genocide" came to be strongly linked over the 1970s and 1980s, often as a political response to then current health measures that were deeply problematic in terms of race and gender. Both "eugenics" and "genocide" were often deployed as an effective if imprecise code for "scientific racism" or "racist" health policy and/or research. The attempts at sickle-cell screening in the United States, strongly resisted by some African American groups, is an instance of the use of genocide charges in this period. This public health initiative targeted African Americans specifically, since a higher incidence was known, and aimed to limit reproduction of those screened positively. The combination of a race-based program with efforts to discourage reproduction is what gave rise to genocide charges.[33] In a different context, scholars were linking genocide to eugenics in the psychiatric domain: Lenny Lapon's 1986 book, *Mass Murderers in White Coats: Psychiatric Genocide in Nazi Germany and the United States,* is one example.[34] As Moses and Stone argue in this volume, however, eugenic "euthanasia" was largely performed on disabled Germans and therefore was not itself strictly genocidal. And the sterilization-race-genocide link is ongoing, as Johanna Schoen shows in her analysis of the recent apologies for sterilization by some U.S. states.[35] The eugenics-genocide connection also became a staple argument of eugenics scholarship, extending to historical sociology and political philosophy in the work of Zygmunt Bauman and Enzo Traverso, for example.[36]

In this popular and scholarly work, there is often a retrospective presumption that "eugenics" and "genocide" were actually linked in the postwar assessment of Nazism, specifically by the 1948 Genocide Convention. The intellectual history of the connection between eugenics, race, and the postwar Nazi trials needs further investigation and clarification, however. It was less the Genocide Convention of 1948 than the so-called Doctors' Trials of 1946–1947 that focused attention on eugenics: the X-ray, pharmaceutical, and surgical sterilization experiments and genetic-oriented twin experiments linked to the prior eugenic sterilization law.[37] Indeed, it is questionable whether "eugenics" per se actually arose in the Convention's debates at all. Analysis of 800 pages of transcript suggests not: neither the term "eugenics" nor "euthanasia" appear in these pages, and "sterilization" only twice.[38] In other words, it appears that the connection drawn by scholars and activists alike between eugenics and genocide was more strictly a phenomenon of the 1970s and 1980s, than of the 1940s and 1950s.

Transhumanism and Posthumanism

An insufficiently analyzed trajectory of eugenics is its place in the long history of human enhancement, imagined and realized, of which "transhumanism" and "post-humanism" are current versions. It was Julian Huxley who coined the term "transhumanism":

> The human species can, if it wishes, transcend itself—not just sporadically, an individual here in one way, an individual there in another way, but in its entirety, as humanity. We need a name for this new belief. Perhaps *transhumanism* will serve: man remaining man, but transcending himself, by realizing new possibilities of and for his human nature.[39]

Huxley is the direct link between eugenics and contemporary transhumanism: individuals and groups who embrace technological change that will enhance, as they see it, physical and mental capacity, extend human life and health, and render "posthuman" conditions possible. "Remaking ourselves," is possible, desirable, worthy, and can be socially just.[40] Transhumanist scholar Nick Bostrom argues that the "wisest approach" is to "embrace technological progress, while strongly defending human rights and individual choice." Though Bostrom draws from Aldous Huxley's *Brave New World* (1932), Aldous's brother Julian is a far closer antecedent. Current transhumanists own this connection with Julian Huxley in the etymological sense that he created the term. But the connection is also disowned in the sense that transhumanists typically distance themselves radically from eugenics. Transhumanists should defend "freedoms," Bostrom argues, and avoid "last century's government-sponsored coercive eugenics programs [which have been] thoroughly discredited."[41] Bostrom eschews any "necessary link with coercive eugenics, [n]or with the belief that some people are fundamentally inferior to others."[42] The irony is that eugenics advocate Julian Huxley himself would have entirely agreed with, indeed was partly responsible for, this discrediting of coercion.

Even distancing their project from eugenics, transhumanists are decried by their opponents as recapitulating Nazi visions: the Nazi meaning of eugenics remains almost impossible to circumvent, and transhumanists avoid eugenics for good strategic reasons. In any case, as Diane Paul points out, transhumanists have less in common with the radical Right, and more in common with the socialist utopian visions of scientists like J. B. S. Haldane (1892–1964). Origins of present-day transhumanism also lie in Nietzsche's ideas. His ideal race of *Übermenschen*, "over-human" or "beyond-man," inspired considerable eugenic interest. Statistician and evolutionary biologist R. A. Fisher (1890–1962), for example, strongly linked eugenics and Nietzsche, in attempts to think about developments of human capacity.[43] Pressing this trajectory further, Jennifer Robertson's work on *Robo sapiens Japanicus* is an important extension of eugenic history into the cyborg cultures of the late twentieth and twenty-first century.[44] Indeed, there is a long-twentieth-century history of enhancement, eugenics, and transhumanism waiting to be written, book-ended by Nietzsche's *Übermenschen* and Nicholas Agar's *Liberal Eugenics: In Defence of Human Enhancement* (2005).

REPRODUCTIVE POLITICS AND TECHNOLOGIES

Commentators on "new eugenics" are more likely to focus on the reproductive health domain than the broader field of transhumanism. But recent scholarly interest in high technology reprogenetics has tended to obscure far more normalized, even quotidian historical connections between interwar eugenics and postwar fertility control. There is a fairly straightforward history in which eugenics folded into family planning. In the 1950s and 1960s, eugenic advocates spoke of family planning and eugenics interchangeably, and some even saw birth control as eugenics' most important future. Occasionally, they would speak of the complementarity of the projects, foregrounding "planning." Blacker wrote in 1961, for example, that the objective of eugenics is "identical with the objective of the Family Planning Association. According to this objective, the particle *eu* in eugenics is reflected not in single attributes of parents such as intelligence, health, physique, etc, but in a performance test...begetting and rearing a happy and well-adjusted family, the children being wanted and conceived by design...eugenicists favour the planned as against the unplanned family."[45] The key to understanding this postwar history is in comprehending the extent to which eugenics was already part of birth control institutions, and fertility control was already part of eugenics.

Arguably the most overlooked trajectory of eugenics lies in its connection to the liberalization of abortion law. As Klausen and Bashford suggest in this volume, the Japanese Eugenic Law of 1948, which legalized abortion on eugenic grounds and on grounds of economic need, was an important early site where different kinds of reproductive politics shaded into one another. A common indication for abortion, as laws became liberalized from the 1960s, was the termination of a fetus likely to be born deformed, likely to carry a hereditary disease, or because of the mental state of the pregnant woman. As Johanna Schoen explains in the U.S. context: "In their fight for abortion reform, health and welfare officials across the country turned to the same financial and eugenic arguments that justified eugenic sterilization policies and that stood behind the 1960s push for family planning programs."[46]

The eugenic indication became especially significant once prenatal diagnosis technologies were refined. Ruth Schwartz Cowan details the history of fetal sex identification through amniocentesis (introduced in 1955–1956) and its application by Danish researchers to sex-linked hemophilia in 1959. This new knowledge could be "applied" because of the preexisting eugenic indication for legal abortion: the Danish 1938 eugenic law permitted abortion if there was a risk that the child would be born with "severe and non-curable abnormality of physical disease."[47] Where eugenic abortion laws were not available, the imperative to terminate a pregnancy, in light of the new diagnostic capacity, drove abortion's legalization, as much as did women's arguments for reproductive choice. This history links pre- and post–World War II eugenic-genetic history directly. And there are present-day manifestations of eugenics that embody this history, too. The 1995 Chinese Maternal and Infant Health Law, which was originally titled the "Eugenics Law," legislates for abortion after prenatal diagnosis of an abnormality in the fetus.[48]

STERILITY AND INFERTILITY

Various eugenic research institutions and societies took up the problems of sterility and infertility in the early twentieth century, connecting with later developments in "sperm banking" and in vitro procedures. The problem of sterility was comprehended by some as an element in positive eugenics. One contributor to *Eugenics*

Review put it in 1936 : "In meeting the problem of sterility, we may progress towards the central objectives of positive eugenics."[49] The study of "differential sterility" went along with the more common eugenic discussion of "differential fertility."[50] "Eutelegenesis," or donation of sperm, was regularly discussed in terms of men's infertility. Artificial insemination was researched first in the domain of animal husbandry, and the research link to animal breeding and agricultural science—always important for eugenics—is especially clear and pertinent in this field.[51]

Kevles and Stern have both written of the early commercial sperm bank, the Repository for Germinal Choice, established in San Diego in 1971.[52] "Germinal Choice" was derived from geneticist Hermann Muller's ideas, and the clear links to eugenics became known to some considerable controversy in 1980: the Repository collected sperm from Nobel Prize laureate donors and, according to the *Harvard Law Review,* dispensed it throughout the country "to recipients also selected for high intelligence." Physicist and engineer William Shockley identified himself as one of the donors.[53] Shockley was also deeply involved in questions of differential fertility among white and black Americans, arguing notoriously that those whose IQ was under 100 should be paid to undergo voluntary sterilization.[54]

Once in vitro fertilization (IVF) became possible in the early 1980s and increasingly widespread from the 1990s, the eugenic meaning of sperm banking shifted from the donor to the recipient. Intentional eugenic objectives of institutions like the Repository for Germinal Choice—seeking to disseminate "high quality" genes through high quality sperm—dropped away from the field, indeed were actively avoided by most clinics. Nonetheless, individual women, as well as homosexual and heterosexual couples, participating in sperm donor programs, made individual choices of donor gametes from a range of increasingly detailed information. Blacker foreshadowed the significance of this kind of individual decision in 1946: "It is usually desired that the donor should be a man resembling the legal father— i.e. that he should be of similar religious persuasion, physical type, race and social class. It has been argued that he should be of the same blood group. But the couple sometimes go further than this and ask that the donor should have special qualities such as outstanding intelligence, artistic gifts, physical excellences.... The practice has, in my view, useful potentialities as a demographic, eugenic and personal measure."[55] What pleased Blacker, however, has troubled more recent researchers and practitioners in the field of reproductive health. Many read the practices of selection of gametes by women, as well as selection of women for IVF, as problematically "eugenic."[56]

Stern argues that insemination with donor sperm, along with now routine procedures of prenatal screening and diagnosis, can easily be defined as eugenic "in outcome if not intent." But the more pressing issue, she continues, is less whether something "*is* or *is not* unequivocally eugenic, but whether reproductive and genetic practices or technologies are equitably distributed across the population."[57] The overall question of fitness and unfitness becomes less one of the biological überclass of William Shockley's dreams, and more one of the raced economies of a global "bio-underclass."[58]

HUMAN GENETICS AND SCREENING

One clear legacy of the eugenic voluntary sterilization and marriage screening/counseling projects of the 1920s and 1930s was genetic counseling, institutionalized from the late 1940s. Early- to mid-twentieth-century premarital clinics in the United Kingdom, Canada, Australia, and the United States undertook medical and psychiatric diagnoses of syphilis, tuberculosis, "perversions," alcoholism, speech defects, and "inherited diseases and tendencies."[59] This clinical diagnosis became probability and risk-based advice given to couples in the 1940s and 1950s, based on new genetic knowledge. From around the mid-1960s, clinics began to pursue prenatal diagnosis and carrier screening. It is here, in the field of medical genetics, more than any other field, that the label "the new eugenics" is used. But labeling itself reveals less than does scholarly documentation of the connections over time.

Pauline Mazumdar's work traces the emergence of human genetics in the 1920s and 1930s, analyzing both those geneticists deeply involved in organizational eugenics—R. A. Fisher, for example—and those deeply skeptical—such as J.B.S. Haldane. But despite left-wing geneticists' attacks, they "could not aim at expunging the entire eugenics problematic, since that was so intimately interwoven with all current research in human genetics."[60] Mazumdar argues that human geneticists were the successors of eugenicists: when the British Society finally wound up in 1989, it "changed its name and moved out of town, leaving the field to human genetics."[61] Everywhere, the postwar transition between eugenics and human genetics was taking place, sometimes smoothly, sometimes with considerable difficulty.[62] Perhaps most importantly, though, Mazumdar documents the continuity of the science that took place in this contested field. The Human Genome Project, for example, was the realization of the chromosome mapping and blood group linkage studies connecting the new human genetics of the 1930s through the 1960s and 1970s. This is a continuous, not a discontinuous history of science, both in institutional and in intellectual terms.[63]

In *Heredity and Hope*, Ruth Schwartz Cowan explores the specific history of genetic screening—prenatal, newborn, and carrier testing—presenting what she dubs an "ethical argument using historians' tools."[64] Her conclusion is that most current opponents of genetic screening are "misguided" on its ethics, and have got the history wrong. The historical connection with eugenics, she argues, needs to be closely investigated, not presumed. She finds the connection between medical genetics and eugenics elusive. Not only were the "founding fathers" of medical genetics—William Bateson and Archibald Garrod—unconnected to eugenics, but those at the real takeoff point of medical genetics in the 1960s "viewed their basic project as the relief of human suffering, not improvement of the race."[65] As classical genetics and medical genetics interwove over the century, they were "connected" with eugenics, she concedes, "but their fundamental beliefs are not the connection."[66] Her research adds up to this: "the history of genetics is indeed connected to the history of eugenics, but not in a way that affects the social, medical, or moral project of medical genetics."[67]

Cowan's insistence on distancing eugenicists from medical genetics certainly rescues the latter from opprobrium, but occasionally at the cost of simplifying the former. Many eugenicists would have considered their projects more consonant with the work of Cowan's "humanitarian" medical geneticists than she allows. Dr. Harry Haiselden understood his work to ease suffering, as he let deformed newborns die in Chicago during World War I, for example.[68] Even the strident racists of the Future Generations group can claim humanitarianism.[69]

The need to work as closely on the connections between eugenics and medical genetics as on the disconnections becomes evident when individual scientists' and clinicians' lives are analyzed. Medical geneticist Fraser Roberts (1900–1987), for example, established the earliest genetic counseling clinics in Britain, having worked before, during, and after World War II on blood groups and heritable disease, on mental deficiency, and on intelligence and fertility.[70] What he called "genetic hygiene" was simultaneously concerned with individual suffering and with population-level quality. "Look after the individuals and the families and offer them the best advice available and the population as a whole cannot fail to benefit." Genetic counseling through clinics was, he thought, the best guarantee by which "population quality is not forgotten."[71] But typically for British eugenicists, both before and after World War II, the voluntary ethic was critical for Roberts. "Any programme of genetic hygiene must be based on voluntariness. No such programme could be implemented before the public had been educated to understand the aims and purposes involved."[72]

Nonetheless, Cowan's book is especially valuable because it links as one twentieth-century narrative the emergence of eugenics and genetics, their transition in the middle of the century, and the place of the history of eugenics in shaping the politics of screening in the later twentieth century. Daniel Kevles's work also draws this long history, but allows for a slightly more derivative connection between eugenics and medical genetics: "In its efforts to encourage the use of genetics for medical purposes and to improve the biological quality of human populations, reform eugenics had helped lead to the opening of facilities devoted explicitly to genetic advisory services."[73] At the very least, we can map two trajectories of genetic counseling as Thom and Jennings have done, again in the case of Britain. They trace one direct lineage through Fraser Roberts and Cedric Carter (1917–1984), Eugenics Society mainstays and successive directors of the Clinical Genetics Research Unit in London. Another lineage is drawn through Lionel Penrose (1898–1972), who opposed eugenics, but whose very institutional position as Galton Chair at University College, London, always signaled the connection. "Human genetics owes its origins to eugenics," Thom and Jennings conclude, "but as the contrasting careers of Carter and Penrose show, origins do not determine outcomes."[74] Key insights into the past of human genetics are more likely to emerge from close analysis of the "transition" decades—what happened in the 1950s, 1960s, and 1970s—rather than in the "high eugenics" moment of the earlier twentieth century. Responding to Evelyn Fox Keller's *Century of the Gene,* Hilary Rose argues that the twentieth century was also "*the century of eugenics,* for genetics and eugenics, have, like conjoint twins, both individual and linked histories over the course of that one hundred years."[75]

REPROGENETICS

The 1980s saw considerable development in genomic research—the Human Genome Project, new possibilities not just of detection, but also correction of embryonic defect and, later, germ-line engineering.[76] Combined with great changes in the possibilities, successes, and uptake of in vitro and assisted reproduction technologies, "reprogenetics"—a term appearing around 1998—opened up another reassessment of eugenics and its legacies.[77] There was a marked trend to benchmark not just prenatal testing (when the woman is pregnant) against eugenics, but the new possibility of pre-implantation diagnosis and therapy (of the embryo outside the woman, in vitro).[78] Beginning in 1990, the Human Genome Project was also strongly debated in terms of eugenics,[79] and as we have seen, it coincided with a period of major new histories of eugenics. The Human Genome Project and Nazi history were quickly linked in public policy discussion. Several historians looked at the Commission of the European Communities' assessment of the human genome research program in the late 1980s. The report drew direct links with the Nazi past, insisting upon the "study of the history of and current trends in eugenics."[80] Some historians however—Daniel Kevles for example—minimized concerns about the recapitulation of the worst aspects of eugenics. "The eugenic past is prologue to the human genetic future in only a strictly temporal sense, that is, it came before."[81]

In all of this discussion of the eugenic past of reprogenetics, eugenics is presented as a historical phenomenon that threatens to return, or which already has. And yet it is again important to recognize (as Kevles, if anyone, knew well) that eugenics—even formal eugenics—never completely disappeared. In the 1980s when IVF, sex determination, and cloning were all on the table, feminist, disability rights groups, and anti-psychiatrists cautioned about the return of eugenics. But around the corner, as it were, all these matters were being considered at the annual Eugenics Symposium. The 1983 meeting, for example, discussed *Developments in Human Reproduction and Their Eugenic, Ethical Implications.* Cedric Carter considered the developments in his paper "Eugenic Implications of New Techniques," in which he listed (as negative and positive eugenics) new methods of contraception, genetic registers, carrier detection, prenatal diagnosis, artificial insemination by donor, in vitro fertilization, sex determination, and cloning.[82] This was the eugenics that never went away, in which all the new technological and genetic developments were folded into, and considered as part of, an ongoing eugenics.

Over the last few decades, two axes of analysis have governed much of the discussion about relations between eugenics and reprogenetics: the distinction between voluntarism and coercion, and the distinction between population-level and individual-level interventions and intentions. Coerced sterilization is often used to signal an older eugenic practice, but many historians have questioned how distinct the line between old and new really is. In the first place, commitment to "voluntarism" marked much early eugenics.[83] Second, the "freedoms" of contemporary reproductive choice are often overstated. Lene Koch argues that the common understanding that "old eugenics" represented coercive practices, while new genetics is marked by voluntary non-directive practice, is wrong on both counts. Eugenics "turns out to be a double helix with two strands of descendents: one is clinical genetics and genetic counseling where any coercion is now disavowed. But if the origin of the abnormality is considered social, compulsion is acceptable and widely practiced": removal of children, for example.[84] Rendering old/new equivalent to coercive/voluntary is neither useful nor accurate.

The second axis of analysis—contrasting population-level and individual decisions about reproductive and genetic futures—is on firmer ground. The clear population ambitions of the early eugenics' advocates must be distinguished from the current era, when population-level objectives are largely (though not wholly) absent, dominated instead by a discourse of individual choice and freedoms. Scholars of disability are sometimes unconvinced that this distinction is meaningful: "Today, unlike in the past, interventions that may result in a neoeugenics are usually masked by a rhetoric very different from that of the early twentieth century, one in which individual choice is dominant and in which the role of government is rendered invisible."[85] There is, nonetheless, a clear political difference between even a "masking" possibility of choice and the absence of choice. For example, the state promotion and implementation of reproductive and demographic plans in China from the late 1970s to date, which openly prioritize collective over individual needs, are significantly different from the choice-based ethic that governs the reproductive domain in many other national contexts.[86]

Some scholars distinguish between "private" and "public" eugenics.[87] Others have nominated a new "liberal eugenics" that is defiantly state-neutral.[88] But the implications and apparent freedoms of "liberal eugenics" are by no means clear. Diane Paul suggests that "[p]olicies are characterized as eugenic if their intent is to further a social or public purpose, such as reducing costs or sparing future generations unnecessary suffering. Expansion of genetic services motivated by concern for the quality of the *population* would be eugenic by this definition, while the same practices motivated by the desire to increase the choices available to individuals would not be."[89] Yet, as Paul continues, knowledge of motives around reproductive and genetic decisions is not always obvious and may likely be mixed. The individual-population distinction, apparently clear, is really a continuum. Indeed, early eugenics advocates themselves sometimes imagined certain practices on a personal-population continuum, as a "demographic, eugenic and personal measure."[90] And as Nils Roll-Hansen indicates in this volume, reproductive choices may have population-level "eugenic" effects, irrespective of policy intention, or even of an individual's critical attitude to eugenics.

CONCLUSION

While debates on new eugenics focus on freedom, choice, and coercion, the derivative question of selection is perhaps equally pertinent, and highlights a discursive continuity otherwise obscured. Active selection is everywhere in reprogenetics. It was there with early "artificial insemination" and IVF, when women and couples selected donor gametes. Selection intensified with the possibility of pre-implantation diagnosis, both of defect and disease, and of sex. The pursuit of selection, not manipulation, is the key to a beneficial future eugenics, write the authors of a 1995 article in *Human Reproduction:* selection through pre-implantation diagnosis is "an original tool for eugenics."[91] These authors write of the care needed to deal eugenically with embryos: "the viable embryos are transferred into the uterus, those not viable are eliminated from the human reproductive circuit, and the doubtful ones are in a stand-by unemployment population, in laboratory freezers."[92] This is a repetition— presumably witting, but perhaps not—of social categories of fitness, unfitness, and the "doubtful": the latter something like the passing feebleminded, or the "almosts."[93] Categorization and selection of fit and unfit biological elements—gametes, embryos, genes—represent a major discursive continuity with earlier selection of fit and unfit people. Whether or not this is called "eugenic" is less important than recognition that most men and women interested in eugenics in earlier periods would undoubtedly be delighted at contemporary possibilities for reproductive selections. Current capacity to select out, and select in, "viable" future lives is far more extensive and normalized than many early eugenicists would have ever imagined, and what's more, is largely voluntary. This was precisely the dream of most men and women who called themselves eugenicists in the past.

"New eugenics" and even "new genetics" implies that eugenics disappeared and returned. But if there was activity—however marginal—from the 1950s onward, eugenics more correctly waxed and waned than disappeared. As Nikolas Rose has put it: "There is and will be no single point of culmination or transformation. If mutations are occurring in the relation between life and politics, we are neither at the beginning nor at the end, but in the middle."[94] We should imagine—and research—a continuous modern discourse, a history of eugenics over the long twentieth century.

ACKNOWLEDGMENTS

My thanks to Roberta Bivins, Ann Curthoys, Philippa Levine, Dirk Moses, Dan Stone, Carolyn Strange, and Mathew Thomson for comments on drafts of this chapter. I am grateful to the Galton Institute for permission to access and quote from the Eugenics Society Papers.

NOTES

1. Christina Codgell, *Eugenic Design: Streamlining America in the 1930s,* (Philadelphia, PA: University of Pennsylvania Press, 2004), xiv.

2. Pauline M. H. Mazumdar, *Eugenics, Human Genetics and Human Failings: The Eugenics Society, Its Sources and Its Critics in Britain* (London and New York: Routledge, 1992), 267.

3. Ruth Schwartz Cowan, *Heredity and Hope: The Case for Genetic Screening* (Cambridge, MA: Harvard University Press, 2008).

4. John Harris, "Is Gene Therapy a Form of Eugenics?" *Bioethics* 7 (1993): 178–187. For an analysis of conversation between genetics and history, see Roberta Bivins, "Hybrid Vigour? Genes, Genomics, and History," *Genomics, Society, and Policy* 4, no. 1 (2008): 12–22.

5. Lene Koch, "The Meaning of Eugenics: Reflections on the Government of Genetic Knowledge in the Past and Present," *Science in Context* 17, no. 3 (2004): 329.

6. Diane B. Paul, "On Drawing Lessons from the History of Eugenics," in Lori P. Knowles and Gregory E. Kaebnick, *Reprogenetics: Law, Policy, and Ethical Issues,* (Baltimore, MD: Johns Hopkins University Press, 2007), 15. See also Alan Petersen, "Is the New Genetics Eugenic?: Interpreting the Past, Envisioning the Future," *New Formations* 60 (2006–2007): 80.

7. For example, Deborah Barrett and Charles Kerzman, "Globalizing Social Movement Theory: The Case of Eugenics," *Theory and Society* 33, no. 5 (2004): 487–527; Merryn Ekberg, "The Old Eugenics and the New Genetics Compared," *Social History of Medicine* 20, no. 3 (2007): 581.

8. Daniel Kevles, *In the Name of Eugenics: Genetics and the Uses of Human Heredity,* (Cambridge, MA: Harvard University Press, 1995) chaps. 14–18; Alice Wexler, *The Woman Who Walked into the Sea: Huntington's and the Making of a Genetic Disease* (New Haven, CT: Yale University Press: 2008), xxiii; Cowan, *Heredity and Hope.*

9. For "eugenetics," see Bill Armer, "Eugenetics: A Polemical View of Social Policy in the Genetic Age," *New Formations* 60 (2006–2007): 79–88.

10. Koch, "The Meaning of Eugenics in the Past and Present," 318.

11. Sinsheimer cited in Paul, "On Drawing Lessons from the History of Eugenics," 10.

12. John Glad', *Future Human Evolution: Eugenics in the Twenty-First Century,* (Schuylkill Haven, PA: Hermitage Publishers, 2006).

13. Richard Lynn, *Dysgenics: Genetic Deterioration in Modern Populations* (Westport, CT: Praeger, 1996), 210.

14. Troy Duster, *Backdoor to Eugenics* (London and New York: Routledge, 1990).

15. Ekberg, "The Old Eugenics and the New Genetics Compared" 581–593.

16. Jürgen Habermas, *The Future of Human Nature* (Cambridge: Polity Press, 2003); see also Catherine Mills, "Biopolitics, Liberal Eugenics and Nihilism," in *Giorgio Agamben: Sovereignty and Life,* ed. Matthew Calarco and Steven DeCaroli (Stanford, CA: Stanford University Press, 2007), 180–202; Lenny Moss, "Contra Habermas and Towards a Critical Theory of Human Nature and the Question of Genetic Enhancement," *New Formations* 60 (2006–2007): 139–149.

17. Nikolas Rose, *The Politics of Life Itself: Biomedicine, Power, and Subjectivity in the Twenty-First Century* (Princeton, NJ: Princeton University Press, 2008), 54–64.

18. Cowan, *Heredity and Hope.*

19. David Galton, *Eugenics: The Future of Human Life in the Twenty-First Century* (London: Abacus, 2002), xiii.

20. Ibid., 252.

21. Allen Buchanan, Dan W. Brock, Norman Daniels, and Daniel Wikler, *From Chance to Choice: Genetics and Justice* (Cambridge: Cambridge University Press, 2000), 30.

22. Ibid., 60.

23. Ibid., 27–28.

24. Bernard Benjamin, Peter R. Cox, John Peel, eds, *Population and the New Biology: Proceedings of the Tenth Annual Symposium of the Eugenics Society* (London: Eugenics Society, 1973); D. A. Coleman, ed., *Demography of Immigrants and Minority Groups in the United Kingdom: Proceedings of the Eighteenth Annual Symposium of the Eugenics Society* (London: Eugenics Society, 1981); Peter Diggory, Malcolm Potts, and Sue Teper, eds, *Natural Human Fertility: Social and Biological Determinants: Proceedings of the Twenty-Third Annual Symposium of the Eugenics Society* (London: Eugenics Society, 1986).

25. As Carolyn Burdett notes in the important special issue of *New Formations,* "In truth, and as many of the essays in this collection testify, eugenic thinking never really went away." Carolyn Burdett, "Introduction: Eugenics Old and New," *New Formations* 60 (2006–2007): 8.

26. Qiu Renzong, "Is China's Law Eugenic?" www.unesco.org/courier/1999_09/uk/dossier/txt07.htm. Accessed May 6, 2009. See also Frank Dikötter's response.

27. "Surely colour feeling is very largely prejudice and self-interest and has hardly any biological significance? Is there good scientific justification for making it biological?" Blacker to Bertram, "The Eugenic Aspects of West Indian Immigration: Some General Notes," n.d., Eugenics Society Papers, Wellcome Library, London, SA/EUG/D103.

28. Stefan Kühl, *The Nazi Connection: Eugenics, American Racism, and German National Socialism* (Oxford and New York: Oxford University Press, 1994), 5–6. See also Barry Mehler, "Foundation for Fascism: The New Eugenics Movement in the United States," *Patterns of Prejudice* 23, no. 4 (1989): 17–25; William H. Tucker, *The Funding of Scientific Racism: Wickliffe Draper and the Pioneer Fund* (Urbana, IL: University of Illinois Press, 2007); Gavin Schaffer, *Racial Science and British Society, 1930–62* (Basingstoke: Palgrave, 2008), 151–152. These generations are barely removed from our own. The current Galton Institute Web site (in 1989 the Eugenics Society changed its name) links to the current Pioneer Fund site, albeit with distancing commentary. And it links to the "Future Generations" site, which gathers together the small group of researchers who came to prominence in the 1980s—the scientific racists of whom Kühl wrote in 1994. "Future Generations" now announces itself thinly, as "humanitarian." The site promotes the ideas of a group of scientists and commentators known mostly for their insistence on race as a biological entity: John Glad, Marian Van Court, William Shockley, J. Philippe Rushton, and Harry Weyher (who negotiated with the Eugenics Society in the 1950s). "Future Generations" distances itself from Nazi eugenics, not by disclaiming Nazi sterilization and euthanasia—the more common strategy—but by denying that these practices stemmed from a eugenic/biological rationale at all, citing the notorious Holocaust-denier David Irving, among others. www.galtoninstitute.org.uk/index.html; www.eugenic.net/ Accessed March 20, 2009. Stephen B. Saetz, Marian Van Court, and Mark W. Henshaw, "Eugenics and the Third Reich," http://www.eugenics.net/papers/3rdreich.html Accessed March 20, 2009.

29. Carl J. Bajema, ed. *Eugenics: Then and Now* (Stroudsburg, PA: Dowden, Hutchinson & Ross, 1976), 5–6.

30. Benno Müller-Hill, *Murderous Science: Elimination by Scientific Selection of Jews, Gypsies, and Others, Germany 1922–1945* (Oxford and New York: Oxford University Press, 1987); Sheila Faith Weiss, *Race Hygiene and National Efficiency: The Eugenics of Wilhelm Schallmeyer* (Berkeley, CA: University of California Press, 1987); Peter Weingart, Jürgen Kroll, Kurt Bayertz, *Rasse, Blut und Gene: Geschichte der Eugenik und Rassenhygiene in Deutschland* (Frankfurt am Main: Surhrkamp, 1988); Robert Proctor, *Racial Hygiene: Medicine under the Nazis* (Cambridge, MA: Harvard University Press, 1989); Paul Weindling, *Health, Race and German Politics between National Unification and Nazism,*

1870–1945 (Cambridge: Cambridge University Press, 1989). There was also important work done in the 1970s through the Hastings Center.

31. Kühl, *The Nazi Connection,* 11.

32. Koch, "The Meaning of Eugenics," 329.

33. Cowan, *Heredity and Hope,* 227.

34. Lenny Lapon, *Mass Murderers in White Coats: Psychiatric Genocide in Nazi Germany and the United States* (Springfield, MA: Psychiatric Genocide Research Institute, 1986). See Kühl, *The Nazi Connection,* xv.

35. See Johanna Schoen, *Choice and Coercion: Birth Control, Sterilization and Abortion in Public Health and Welfare* (Chapel Hill, NC: University of North Carolina Press, 2005), 244–246.

36. Zygmunt Bauman, *Modernity and the Holocaust* (Cambridge: Polity Press, 1989); Enzo Traverso, *The Origins of Nazi Violence* (New York: The New Press, 2003). See Dirk Moses, "Genocide and Modernity," and Ann Curthoys and John Docker, "Defining Genocide," in *The Historiography of Genocide,* ed. Dan Stone (Basingstoke: Palgrave, 2008).

37. P. J. Weindling, *Nazi Medicine and the Nuremberg Trials: From Medical War Crimes to Informed Consent* (Basingstoke: Palgrave, 2005).

38. United Nations, *Official Records of the Third Session of the General Assembly,* Part 1, Legal Questions, Sixth Committee, Summary Records of Meetings 21 September—10 December 1948. This is ongoing research. My thanks to Dirk Moses and Dan Stone for discussion and documents on this point.

39. Julian Huxley, "Transhumanism," in *New Bottles for New Wine* (London: Chatto & Windus, 1957), 13–17.

40. Philip Kitcher, *The Lives to Come: The Genetic Revolution and Human Possibilities,* (New York: Simon and Schuster, 1996); see also Gregory Radick, "A Critique of Kitcher on Eugenic Reasoning," *Studies in the History and Philosophy of Biology and Biomedical Sciences* 32, no. 4 (2001), 741–751; Lee M. Silver, "Reprogenetics: How Reprogenetic and Genetic Technologies Will Be Combined to Provide New Opportunities for People to Reach Their Reproductive Goals," in *Engineering the Human Germline,* eds. Gregory Stock and John Campbell (New York: Oxford University Press, 2000), 57–71; see also Paul, "On Drawing Lessons from the History of Eugenics," 5–6.

41. Nick Bostrom, "In Defense of Posthuman Dignity," *Bioethics* 19, no. 3 (2005): 206.

42. Nick Bostrom and Rebecca Roache, "Ethical Issues in Human Enhancement," in *New Waves in Applied Ethics,* eds. Jesper Ryberg, Thomas S. Petersen, and Clark Wolf (Basingstoke: Palgrave, 2007). See also Nicholas Agar, *Liberal Eugenics: In Defence of Human Enhancement* (Malden: Blackwell, 2005).

43. For Nietzsche and eugenics, see Dan Stone, *Breeding Superman: Nietzsche, Race and Eugenics in Edwardian and Interwar Britain* (Liverpool: Liverpool University Press, 2002); Mazumdar, *Eugenics, Human Genetics, and Human Failings,* 103–106; Stefan Lorenz Sorgner, "Nietzsche, the Overhuman, and Transhumanism," *Journal of Evolution and Technology* 20, no. 1 (2009): 29–42.

44. Jennifer Robertson, "*Robo Sapiens Japanicus:* Humanoid Robots and the Posthuman Family," *Critical Asian Studies* 39, no. 3 (2007): 369–398.

45. C. P. Blacker typescript response to P. B. Medawar, "Principle and Paradox in Eugenics," *The Medical World* (1962) in Blacker Papers, Wellcome Library, PP/CPB/H1/47.

46. Schoen, *Choice and Coercion,* 143.

47. Cowan, *Heredity and Hope,* 90–93.

48. Frank Dikötter, *Imperfect Conceptions: Medical Knowledge, Birth Defects, and Eugenics* (New York: Columbia University Press, 1998), 174.

49. Herbert Brewer, "Eutelegenesis and Sterility," *Eugenics Review* 28 (1935–1936): 344. For histories of early artificial insemination, see Michael Finn, "Female Sterilization and Artificial Insemination at the French Fin de Siècle," *Journal of the History of Sexuality* 18, no. 1 (2009): 26–43; Christina Benninghaus, "Great Expectations: German Debates about Artificial Insemination in Humans around 1912," *Studies in the History and Philosophy of Biological and Biomedical Sciences* 38, no. 2 (2007): 374–392.

50. See, for example, Bernard Mallett, "The Population Union: Its Formation, Scheme, and Future Work," *Eugenics Review* 19 (1927–1928): 179.

51. Sarah Wilmot, "From "Public Service" to Artificial Insemination: Animal Breeding Science and Reproductive Research in Early Twentieth Century Britain," *Studies in History and Philosophy of Biological and Biomedical Sciences* 38, no. 2 (2007): 411–441.

52. Alexandra Minna Stern, *Eugenic Nation: Faults and Frontiers of Better Breeding in Modern America* (Berkeley, CA: University of California Press, 2005), 214; Kevles, *In the Name of Eugenics,* 262–263.

53. "Eugenic Artificial Insemination: A Cure for Mediocrity," *Harvard Law Review* 94, no. 8 (1981): 1850.

54. William Shockley, "Dysgenics, Geneticity, Raceology: A Challenge to the Intellectual Responsibility of Educators," *Phi Delta Kappan* 53, no. 5 (1972): 297–307.

55. "Artificial Insemination: Eugenic Aspects" October 3, 1946, Typescript, Blacker Papers, Wellcome Library, PP/CPB/H.1/6.

56. For example, Deborah Lynn Steinberg, "A Most Selective Practice: The Eugenic Logics of IVF," *Women's Studies International Forum* 20, no. 1 (1997): 33–48; Dorothy C. Wertz, "Eugenics Is Alive and Well: A Survey of Genetic Professionals around the World," *Science in Context* 11, no. 3–4 (1998): 493–510.

57. Stern, *Eugenic Nation,* 214–215. Original emphasis.

58. Laura Briggs, "Medicalizing Reproductive Economies: The 'Bio-Underclass,' Middle-Class Anxiety, and Transnational Adoption," Paper delivered to the Department of History of Medicine and Science, Yale University, January 23, 2006.

59. Racial Hygiene Association of New South Wales (1938–1939) in Alison Bashford, *Imperial Hygiene: A Critical History of Colonialism, Nationalism and Public Health* (Basingstoke: Palgrave, 2004), 175–176. See also Ruth Chadwick, "Can Genetic Counseling Avoid the Charge of Eugenics?" *Science in Context* 11, no. 3–4 (1998): 471–480; Robert G. Resta, "Eugenic Considerations in the Theory and Practice of Genetic Counseling," *Science in Context* 11, no. 3–4 (1998): 431–438

60. Mazumdar, *Eugenics, Human Genetics and Human Failings,* 196.

61. Ibid., 1, 257.

62. Kevles discusses Lionel Penrose's anxious attempts to dissociate himself from the eugenics that was in his very title. Kevles, *In the Name of Eugenics,* 252.

63. Mazumdar, *Eugenics, Human Genetics and Human Failings,* 257–268.

64. Cowan, *Heredity and Hope,* 9.

65. Ibid., 47–48, 236.

66. Ibid., 67.

67. Ibid., 68.

68. Martin S. Pernick, *The Black Stork: Eugenics and the Death of "Defective" Babies in American Medicine and Motion Pictures since 1915* (Oxford and New York: Oxford University Press, 1996).

69. www.eugenic.net/ Accessed March 20, 2009.

70. Marcus E. Pembrey, "Dr. John Alexander Fraser Roberts," *Journal of Medical Genetics* 24, no. 7 (1987): 442–444.

71. Fraser Roberts to Ruggles Gates, October 5, 1954, Eugenics Society Papers, Wellcome Library, SA/EUG/D104.

72. Fraser Roberts speaking at Working Party on the Relation between Fertility of Different Groups and the Development of Intelligence in New Generations, 1954. UNESCO Archives, Paris, UNESCO/SS/POP.M./Conf.1/1/S.R.1.

73. Kevles, *In the Name of Eugenics,* 253.

74. Deborah Thom and Mary Jennings, "Human Pedigree and the "Best Stock": From Eugenics to Genetics?" in *The Troubled Helix: Social and Psychological Implications of the New Human Genetics,* eds. Theresa Marteau and Martin Richards (Cambridge: Cambridge University Press, 1996), 232.

75. Hilary Rose, "Eugenics and Genetics: The Conjoint Twins?" *New Formations,* no. 60 (2006–2007): 14 (italics in original); Evelyn Fox Keller, *The Century of the Gene* (Cambridge MA: Harvard University Press, 2000).

76. For the latter, see Catherine Waldby and Robert Mitchell *Tissue Economies: Blood, Organs and Cell Lines in Late Capitalism* (Durham, NC: Duke University Press, 2006).

77. For example, Dorothy Nelkin and Laurence Tancredi, *Dangerous Diagnostics: The Social Power of Biological Information* (New York: Basic Books, 1989); Joel Howell, "The History of Eugenics and the Future of Gene Therapy," *Journal of Clinical Ethics* 2, no. 4 (1991): 274–278.

78. David S. King, "Preimplantation Genetic Diagnosis and the 'New' Eugenics," *Journal of Medical Ethics* 25 (1999): 176–182; J. Milliez and C. Sureau, "Pre-implantation Diagnosis and the Eugenics Debate: Our Responsibility to Future Generations," in *Ethical Dilemmas in Assisted Reproduction,* eds. F. Shenfield and C. Sureau (New York: Parthenon, 1997), 57–66.

79. For example, L. Gannett "Racism and Human Genome Diversity Research: The Ethical Limits of 'Population Thinking,'" *Philosophy of Science* 68 (2001): 479–489; Anne Kerr and Tom Shakespeare, *Genetic Politics: From Eugenics to Genome* (Cheltenham: New Clarion Press, 2002); Barbara Katz Rothman, *The Book of Life: A Personal and Ethical Guide to Race, Normality, and the Implications of the Human Genome Project* (Boston, MA: Beacon Press, 2001).

80. Mazumdar, *Eugenics, Human Genetics and Human Failings,* 266.

81. Daniel Kevles, "Is the Past Prologue? Eugenics and the Human Genome Project," *Contention Debates in Society, Culture and Science* 2 no. 3 (1993): 24.

82. C. O. Carter, "Eugenic Implications of New Techniques," in *Developments in Human Reproduction and Their Eugenic, Ethical Implications,* ed. C. O. Carter (London and New York: Academic Press, 1983), 205–211.

83. Paul, "On Drawing Lessons from the History of Eugenics," 4, 7–9; see also discussion by Petersen, "Is the New Genetics Eugenic?"

84. Koch, "The Meaning of Eugenics," 321–322.

85. Margaret Lock, "Genomics, Laissez-Faire Eugenics, and Disability," in *Disability in Local and Global Worlds,* eds. Benedicte Ingstad and Susan Reynolds Whyte (Berkeley, CA: University of California Press, 2007), 190.

86. Dikötter, *Imperfect Conceptions,* 123.

87. Jyotsna Agnihotri Gupta, "Private and Public Eugenics: Genetic Testing and Screening in India," *Bioethical Inquiry* 4 (2007): 217–228.

88. Agar, *Liberal Eugenics.*

89. Diane B. Paul, "Is Human Genetics Disguised Eugenics?" in *Genes and Human Self Knowledge,* eds Robert F. Weir et al. (Iowa City, IA: University of Iowa Press, 1994), 69.

90. "Artificial Insemination: Eugenic Aspects," October 3, 1946, Typescript, Blacker Papers, Wellcome Library, PP/CPB/H.1/6.

91. Jacques Testart and Bernard Sèle, "Towards an Efficient Medical Eugenics: Is the Desirable Always the Feasible," *Human Reproduction* 10, no. 12 (1995): 3086–3087. See also John Marks, "The New Eugenics: Jacques Testart and French Bioethics," *New Formations* 60 (2006–2007): 124–138.

92. Testart and Sèle, "Towards an Efficient Medical Eugenics," 3090.

93. Helen MacMurchy, *The Almosts: A Study of the Feeble-minded* (New York: Houghton Mifflin, 1920). My thanks to Carolyn Strange for this reference.

94. Rose, *The Politics of Life Itself,* 252.

FURTHER READING

Cowan, Ruth Schwartz. *Heredity and Hope: The Case for Genetic Screening* (Cambridge, MA: Harvard University Press, 2008).

Duster, Troy. *Backdoor to Eugenics* (London and New York: Routledge, 2000).

Ekberg, Merryn. "The Old Eugenics and the New Genetics Compared," *Social History of Medicine,* 20, no. 3 (2007): 581–593.

Falk, Raphael, Diane Paul, Garland Allen, and Snait Gissis, eds. *Eugenic Thought and Practice: A Reappraisal,* Special Issue of *Science in Context* 11, no. 3–4 (1998).

Fortun, Michael and Everett Mendelsohn, eds, *The Practices of Human Genetics* (Dordrecht: Kluwer, 1999).

Koch, Lene. "The Meaning of Eugenics: Reflections on the Government of Genetic Knowledge in the Past and Present," *Science in Context* 17, no. 3 (2004): 315–331.

Lock, Margaret. "Genomics, Laissez-Faire Eugenics, and Disability," in *Disability in Local and Global Worlds,* eds. Benedicte Ingstad and Susan Reynolds-Whyte (Berkeley, CA: University of California Press, 2007).

Marteau, Theresa, and Martin Richards, eds. *The Troubled Helix: Social and Psychological Implications of the New Human Genetics* (Cambridge and New York: Cambridge University Press, 1996).

Paul, Diane B. "Genetic Services, Economics and Eugenics," *Science in Context,* 11, no. 3–4 (1998): 481–491.

Paul, Diane B. "On Drawing Lessons from the History of Eugenics," in *Reprogenetics: Law, Policy, and Ethical Issues,* eds. Lori P. Knowles and Gregory E. Kaebnick (Baltimore, MD: Johns Hopkins University Press, 2007).

Petersen, Alan. "Is the New Genetics Eugenic? Interpreting the Past, Envisioning the Future," *New Formations* no. 60 (2006–2007): 79–88.

Robertson, Jennifer. "Dehistoricizing History: The Ethical Dilemma of 'East Asian Bioethics,'" *Critical Asian Studies* 37, no. 2 (2005): 233–250.

Rose, Nikolas. *The Politics of Life Itself: Biomedicine, Power, and Subjectivity in the Twenty-First Century* (Princeton, NJ: Princeton University Press, 2007).

CHRONOLOGY

....

Year	Publication, organization, or statute
1859	Charles Darwin, *On the Origin of Species by Means of Natural Selection*
1869	Francis Galton, *Hereditary Genius: An Inquiry into Its Laws and Consequences*
1871	Charles Darwin, *The Descent of Man, and Selection in Relation to Sex*
1877	Malthusian League, Britain
1882	Hindu Neo-Malthusian League, Madras, India
1883	First *eisei tenrankai* (hygiene exhibitions), Japan
1883	Francis Galton, *Inquiries into Human Faculty and Its Development.* It is in this work that Galton coined the term "eugenics."
1894	William Bateson, *Materials for the Study of Variation*
1895	An Act Concerning Crimes and Punishments (prohibiting marriage for epileptics, imbeciles, and the feebleminded), Connecticut, United States
1895	Alfred Ploetz, *Grundlinien einer Rassen-Hygiene* (The Foundations of Racial Hygiene)
1896	*Ligue de la régénération humaine* (League for Human Regeneration), France
1903	*Towarzystwo ku Zwalczaniu Zakaźnych Chorób Płciowych* (Society for Combating Sexually Transmitted Diseases), Poland
1903	American Breeders Association, United States
1904	Eugenics Record Office, London, Britain
1904	Friedrich Hertz, *Moderne Rassentheorien* (Modern Racial Theories)
1904	Carnegie Institution Station for Experimental Evolution, Cold Spring Harbor, New York, United States
1904	*Den Antropologiske Komité* (Anthropological Committee), Denmark
1905	*Gesellschaft für Rassenhygiene* (Society for Racial Hygiene), Germany
1906	Race Betterment Foundation, United States

(continued)

Year	Publication, organization, or statute
1906	Eugenics Committee created within the American Breeders Association
1907	Eugenics Record Office (1904) renamed Francis Galton Laboratory for the Study of National Eugenics, University College, London, Britain
1907	Compulsory Sterilization Law, Indiana, United States
1907	Civil Code (prohibiting marriage for mental defectives), Switzerland
1907	Permanent Commission for the Study of Métis, France
1907	Society for Racial Hygiene (1905) renamed *Internationale Gesellschaft für Rassenhygiene* (International Society for Racial Hygiene), Germany
1907	Eugenics Education Society, Britain
1904–1908	Royal Commission on the Care and Control of the Feeble-Minded, Britain
1909	*Svenska sällskapet för rashygien* (Swedish Society for Racial Hygiene)
1909	Eugenics Committee (1906) upgraded to Eugenics Section, American Breeders Association
1909	Sterilization laws passed, Washington and California, United States
1909	Francis Galton, *Essays in Eugenics*
1910	*Mendelska sällskapet* (Mendelian Society), Sweden
1910	Eugenics Record Office, Cold Spring Harbor, New York, United States
1910	*Deutsche Gesellschaft für Rassenhygiene* (German Society for Racial Hygiene) created as a national subdivision of the *Internationale Gesellschaft für Rassenhygiene*
1911	Mental Defectives Act, New Zealand
1911	Eugenics subcommittee, South Australian branch, British Science Guild, Australia
1911	Charles Davenport, *Heredity in Relation to Eugenics*
1911	Karl Pearson appointed first Galton Professor of Eugenics, University College, London, Britain
1912	Eugenics Education Society of New South Wales, Australia
1912	First International Eugenics Congress, London, Britain
1912	International Eugenics Committee, London, Britain
1912	*Société française d'eugénique* (French Eugenics Society)
1913	*Comitato per lo Studio della Eugenics* (Committee for the Study of Eugenics) created within the *Società Romana di Antropologia* (Roman Anthropological Society), Italy
1913	Eugenics Research Association, Cold Spring Harbor, New York, United States
1913	Mental Deficiency Act, Britain

Year	Publication, organization, or statute
1914	Eugenics Education Society of Melbourne, Australia
1914	*Egyesületközi Fajegészségügyi Bizottság* (Committee of the Eugenics Society), Hungary
1914	*Sektion für Sozialbiologie und Eugenik* (Section for Social Biology and Eugenics) created within the *Soziologische Gesellschaft* (Sociological Society), Austria
1915	Thomas Hunt Morgan, et al., *The Mechanism of Mendelian Heredity*
1915	Friedrich Hertz, *Rasse und Kultur* (Race and Civilization)
1915	Marriage Law (prohibiting marriage for the mentally retarded and mentally ill), Sweden
1916	*Institut Eksperimental'noi Biologii* (Institute of Experimental Biology), Moscow, Russia
1916	International Society for Racial Hygiene (1907) officially replaced by its national subdivision, the *Deutsche Gesellschaft für Rassenhygiene* (German Society for Racial Hygiene)
1916	*Institut for arvelighetsforskning* (Institute for Genetic Research), Oslo, Norway
1916	Mental Disorders Act, South Africa
1917	Law of Family Relations, Mexico
1917	*Magyar Fajegészségtani és Népesedéspolitikai Társaság* (Hungarian Society for Racial Hygiene and Population Policy), Budapest, Hungary
1917–1919	Royal Commission on the Care and Control of the Mentally Defective and Feeble-Minded in Ontario, Canada
1918	*Liga Pro-Saneamento do Brasil* (Pro-Sanitation League of Brazil)
1918	*Sociedade Eugênica de São Paulo* (Eugenics Society of São Paulo), Brazil
1918	Canadian National Committee for Mental Hygiene
1918	Galton Society, United States
1918	*Zjazd w Sprawie Wyludnienia Kraju* (Congress on the Depopulation of the Country), Poland
1919	*Société belge d'eugénique* (Belgian Eugenics Society)
1919	*Gosudarstvennyi Muzei Sotsial'noi Gigieny* (State Museum of Social Hygiene), Moscow, Russia
1919	*Società Italiana di Genetica ed Eugenica* (Italian Society of Genetics and Eugenics)
1919	*Norsk forening for arvelighetsforskning* (Norwegian Genetics Society)
1920	*Russkoe Evgenicheskoe Obshchestvo* (Russian Eugenics Society)
1920	*Evgenicheskii otdel* (Eugenics section) created within the Institute of Experimental Biology, Russia

(continued)

Year	Publication, organization, or statute
1920	*Pervoe Vserossiiskoe soveshchanie po okhrane materinstva i mladenchestva* (First all-Russian Conference on the Protection of Maternity and Infancy), Moscow, Russia
1921	Station for Experimental Evolution (1904) renamed Carnegie Institution Department of Genetics, Cold Spring Harbor, New York, United States
1921	*Biuro po Evgenike* (Bureau of Eugenics), Petrograd, Russia
1921	American Birth Control League, United States
1921	Standing Committee on Eugenics and Genetics created within the South African Association of Science
1921	Second International Eugenics Congress, New York, United States
1921	International Eugenics Committee (1912) renamed Permanent International Commission on Eugenics
1921	*Erste internationalen Tagung für Sexualreform auf sexualwissen-schaftlicher Grundlag* (First International Conference for Sexual Reform on a Scientific Basis), Berlin, Germany
1921	Indian Eugenics Society
1921	*Reale Società Italiana D'Igiene* (Royal Italian Society of Hygiene), Italy
1922	*Istituto Italiano di Igiene, di Assicurazione e di Assistenza Sociale* (Italian Institute of Hygiene, Insurance, and Social Assistance), Rome
1922	National Office of Eugenics, Solvay Institute, Brussels, Belgium
1922	*Biuro po izucheniiu normal'noi i patologicheskoi nasledstvennosti cheloveka* (Bureau for Studies in Normal and Pathological Human Heredity), Kiev, USSR
1922	*Julius Klaus Stiftung für Vererbungsforschung, Sozialanthropologie und Rassenhygiene* (Julius Klaus Foundation for Heredity Research, Social Anthropology and Racial Hygiene), Zürich, Switzerland
1922	Society for Combating Sexually Transmitted Diseases (1903) became *Polskie Towarzystwo Eugeniczne* (Polish Eugenics Society)
1922	*Statens institut för rasbiologi* (State Institute for Race Biology), Uppsala, Sweden
1922	Marriage Act (prohibiting marriage for the mentally retarded), Denmark
1922	American Eugenics Society
1922	Indian Birth Control Society
1922	Hans F. K. Günther, *Rassenkunde des deutschen Volkes* (Racial Study of the German People)
1923	*Oberösterreichische Gesellschaft für Rassenhygiene* (Upper Austrian Society for Racial Hygiene)

Year	Publication, organization, or statute
1923	*Liga Brasileira de Higiene Mental* (Brazilian Mental Hygiene League)
1924	*Centraal Comité van Samenwerkende Organisaties voor Erfelijkheidsonderzoek bij de Mens* (Central Committee of Collaborating Societies Promoting Research in Human Heredity), The Netherlands
1924	*Office national de l'hygiène sociale* (National Social Hygiene Office), Paris, France
1924	*Wiener Gesellschaft für Rassenpflege* (Viennese Society for Racial Hygiene), Austria
1924	*Nederlandsche Vereeniging ter Bevordering van Geestelijke Volksgezondheid* (Dutch Society for Mental Hygiene), The Netherlands
1924	*Mediko-Biologicheskii Institut* (Medico-biological Institute), Moscow, USSR
1925	Bureau of Eugenics (1921) renamed the *Biuro po Genetike i Evgenike* (Bureau of Genetics and Eugenics), USSR
1925	Permanent International Commission on Eugenics (1921) renamed the International Federation of Eugenic Organizations (IFEO)
1925–1928	Royal Commission on Mental Hygiene, British Columbia, Canada
1926	*Deutscher Bund für Volksaufartung und Erbkunde* (German Alliance for National Regeneration and the Study of Heredity)
1926	Race Improvement Society, Australia
1926	*Deutsche Gesellschaft für Blutgruppenforschung* (German Society for Blood Group Research), Austria
1926	Human Betterment Foundation, United States
1926	*Nippon yūsei undō kyōkai* (Eugenic Exercise/Movement Assocation), Japan
1926	*Kinder der Landstrasse* (Children of the Open Road) child-removal program, Switzerland
1926	Eugenics Education Society (1907) renamed Eugenics Society, Britain
1926	*Kaiser Wilhelm Institut für Anthropologie, menschliche Erblehre und Eugenik* (Kaiser Wilhelm Institute of Anthropology, Human Heredity, and Eugenics), Berlin, Germany
1926	Soviet Civil Code (prohibiting marriage between close relatives and between the mentally ill)
1927	*Deutsch-sowjetisches Institut für Rassenforschung* (German-Russian Racial Research Insitute), Moscow, USSR

(*continued*)

Year	Publication, organization, or statute
1927	*Oficina Central Panamericana de Eugenesia y Homicultura* (Pan American Central Office of Eugenics and Homiculture), Havana, Cuba
1927	US Supreme Court decision *Buck v. Bell* upheld Virginia's eugenic sterilization law
1927	*Secția Eugenică și Biopolitică a "Astrei"* (Eugenics and Biopolitical Section of the *Astra* Association), Romania
1927	*Eugenetische Vereeniging in Nederlansch-Indië* (Eugenics Society of the Dutch East Indies)
1927	*Primera Conferencia Panamericana de Eugenesia y Homicultura* (First Pan American Conference on Eugenics and Homiculture), Havana, Cuba
1927	International Federation of Eugenics Societies conference, Amsterdam, The Netherlands
1927	First *yūsei kekkon sōdansho* (eugenic marriage counseling centers), Japan
1928	Bureau of Genetics and Eugenics (1925) renamed the *Biuro po Genetike* (Bureau of Genetics), USSR
1928	Law on Coercive Sterilizations, canton of Vaud, Switzerland
1928	Sexual Sterilization Act, Alberta, Canada
1928	Madras Neo-Malthusian League, India
1928	*Bălgarsko družestvo za rasova higiena* (Bulgarian Society for Racial Hygiene)
1928	Eugenics Board, New Zealand
1928	Race Improvement Society (1926) renamed Racial Hygiene Association of New South Wales, Australia
1928	*Kabinet Nasledstvennosti i Konstitutsii* (Office of Human Heredity and Constitution) created at the *Mediko-Biologicheskogii Institut* (Medical-Biological Institute), Moscow, USSR
1928	*Weltliga für Sexualreform* (World League for Sexual Reform), Denmark
1928	*Segunda Conferencia Internacional de Emigración e Inmigración* (Second International Conference of Emigration and Immigration), Havana, Cuba
1929	*Sociedad Mexicana de Puericultura* (Mexican Puériculture Society)
1929	Sterilization Act, Denmark
1929	Sholapur Eugenics Education Society, India
1929	*Primeiro Congresso Brasiliero de Eugenia* (First Brazilian Congress of Eugenics), Rio de Janeiro, Brazil
1929	Marriage Act (prohibiting marriage on grounds of mental illness, idiocy, and epilepsy), Finland

Year	Publication, organization, or statute
1930	Eugenic Society, India
1930	Central Committee of Collaborating Societies Promoting Research in Human Heredity (1924) renamed *Nederlandsche Eugenetische Federatie* (Dutch Eugenics Federation)
1930	Encyclical *Casti Connubii* (On Christian Marriage) issued by Pope Pius XI
1930	*Nippon minzoku eisei gakkai* (Japanese Race Hygiene Society), Japan
1930	Race Welfare Society, South Africa
1930	Eugenics Society of Canada
1930	*Nederlandsche Vereeniging ter Bevordering van Geestelijke Volksgezondheid* (Dutch Society for Mental Hygiene) relaunched due to lack of activity since 1924, The Netherlands
1931	*Comissão Central Brasileira de Eugenía* (Brazilian Central Commission of Eugenics)
1931	Eugenics Clinic opened, Bombay, India
1931	*Sociedad Eugénica Mexicana para el Mejoramiento de la Raza* (Mexican Eugenics Society for the Betterment of Race)
1931	German Society for Racial Hygiene (1916) merged with the German Alliance for National Regeneration (1926) and the Study of Heredity to become *Deutsche Gesellschaft für Rassenhygiene (Eugenik)* (German Society for Racial Hygiene (Eugenics))
1932	Sterilization Law, Veracruz, Mexico
1932	Third International Eugenics Congress, New York, United States
1932	First birth control clinic opened, South Africa
1933	*Comité Pro-Raza de la Ciudad de México* (Pro-Race Committee for Mexico City)
1933	University of Western Australia Eugenics Society, Australia
1933	Kenya Society for the Study of Race Improvement
1933	*Gesetz zur Verhütung erbkranken Nachwuchses* (Law for the Prevention of Genetically Diseased Offspring, or "Sterilization Law"), Germany
1933	Sterilization Law, British Columbia, Canada
1933	German Society for Racial Hygiene (Eugenics) (1931) reverted to *Deutsche Gesellschaft für Rassenhygiene* (German Society for Racial Hygiene)
1934	Sterilization Act, Norway
1934	Sterilization Act, Sweden
1934	*Segunda Conferencia Panamerica de Eugenesia e Homicultura* (Second Pan American Conference of Eugenics and Homiculture), Buenos Aires, Argentina

(*continued*)

Year	Publication, organization, or statute
1934	*Verein für menschliche Vererbungslehre und Endokrinologie* (Association for Human Genetics and Endocrinology), Austria
1934	*Konferentsiia po Meditsinskoi Genetike* (Conference on Medical Genetics), Moscow, USSR
1935	*Fédération international latine des sociétes d'eugénique* (International Latin Federation of Eugenics Societies), Mexico
1935	Society for the Study and Promotion of Family Hygiene, India
1935	Sterilization Act, Finland
1935	*Reichsbürgergesetz* (Reich Citizenship Law) and *Gesetz zum Schutz des deutschen Blutes und der deutschen Ehre* (Blood Protection Law), together known as the *Nürnberger Gesetze* (Nuremberg Laws), Germany
1935	Medico-Biological Institute (1924) renamed *Institute Meditsinskoi Genetiki* (Institute of Medical Genetics), USSR
1935	*Societatea Regală Română de Eugenie şi Studiul Eredităţii* (Royal Romanian Society of Eugenics and Heredity)
1935	Marital Health Law (making premarital hereditary health examinations compulsory), Germany
1936	Eugenics League, Hong Kong
1936	Eugenics Society of Victoria, Australia
1936	International Federation of Eugenics Organizations conference, Scheveningen, The Netherlands
1936	*Zentralstelle zur Bekämpfung des Zigeunerunwesens* (Central Office to Combat the Gypsy Nuisance), Munich, Germany
1937	First family planning clinic, Colombo, Sri Lanka
1937	*Instituto Nacional de Puericultura* (National Institute of Puériculture), Rio de Janeiro, Brazil
1937	*Premier congrès latin d'eugénique* (First Latin Eugenics Congress), Paris, France
1938	Marriage Law (mandating premarital health certificates), Iran
1938	First All-India Conference on Family Hygiene, in conjunction with the All-India Conference on Population, Bombay, India
1939	Hermann J. Muller et al., *The Geneticists' Manifesto*
1939	Nazi practice of "euthanasia" of mentally ill, mentally defective, and disabled introduced, Germany
1940	Family Planning Society, India
1940	*Kokumin Yūsei Hō* (National Eugenic Law), Japan
1940	*Öröklési, Fajbiológiai és Eugenikai Osztály, A Magyar Nemzetbiológiai Intézet* (Heredity, Racial Biology, and Eugenics Section of the Hungarian Institute of National Biology), Budapest

Year	Publication, organization, or statute
1940	*Congresso Nacional sobre a Ciência da População* (National Congress on the Science of Population), Oporto, Portugal
1941	*Commissariat général aux questions juives* (Commissariat General for Jewish Affairs), France
1941	*Fondation française pour l'étude des problèmes humaines* (French Foundation for the Study of Human Problems), Paris, France
1942	Law of December 16, 1942, Relative to the Protection of Maternity and Newborns (including premarital medical examination), France
1946–1947	The "Doctors' Trial" (*United States of America v. Karl Brandt et al.*), first of the Nüremberg Trials
1948	United Nations Convention on the Prevention and Punishment of the Crime of Genocide
1949	Family Planning Society (1940) became the Family Planning Association of India
1949	Family Planning Association of Singapore
1949	*Nederlandse Anthropogenetische Vereniging* (Dutch Anthropogenetic Society)
1950	Canadian National Committee for Mental Hygiene (1918) renamed Canadian Mental Health Association
1950	Eugenics League (1936) renamed Family Planning Association of Hong Kong
1950	Immorality Amendment Act and Population Registration Act, South Africa
1952	Family Planning Assocation of Bangladesh
1953	Family Planning Association of Pakistan
1953	Family Planning Association of Sri Lanka
1953	*Elliniki Etaireia Evgonikis* (Hellenic Eugenics Society), Greece
1959	The Swedish Institute for Race Biology (1922) renamed Institutionen för medicinsk genetik (Department of medical genetics) and becomes a part of Uppsala University, Sweden
1960	Racial Hygiene Association of New South Wales renamed Family Planning Association of Australia
1963	Francis Galton Laboratory for the Study of National Eugenics (1907) renamed Galton Laboratory of the Department of Human Genetics and Biometry, University College, London, Britain
1973	American Eugenics Society (1922) renamed Society for the Study of Social Biology
1989	Eugenics Society renamed Galton Institute, London, Britain

INDEX

....

CPSIA information can be obtained
at www.ICGtesting.com
Printed in the USA
BVHW090509191222
654444BV00003B/5